Traditional Chinese Medicine

Traditional Chinese Medicine

Edited by **Penelope Williams**

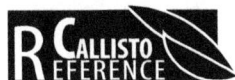

R CALLISTO REFERENCE

New York

Published by Callisto Reference,
106 Park Avenue, Suite 200,
New York, NY 10016, USA
www.callistoreference.com

Traditional Chinese Medicine
Edited by Penelope Williams

International Standard Book Number: 978-1-63239-735-5 (Hardback)

The publisher's policy is to use permanent paper from mills that operate a sustainable forestry policy. Furthermore, the publisher ensures that the text paper and cover boards used have met acceptable environmental accreditation standards.

Trademark Notice: Registered trademark of products or corporate names are used only for explanation and identification without intent to infringe.

Printed in the United States of America.

Contents

Preface

This book aims to highlight the current researches and provides a platform to further the scope of innovations in this area. This book is a product of the combined efforts of many researchers and scientists from different parts of the world. The objective of this book is to provide the readers with the latest information in the field.

Traditional Chinese medicine is based on the belief that body's vital energy circulates through channels called meridians that have branches running through the body. This branch of medicine tries to cure diseases with the help of acupuncture, herbal medicine, exercise and massage. It tries to diagnose problems by tracing symptoms to patterns of an underlying discord. This book provides significant information of this discipline to help develop a good understanding of chinese medicine and related fields. The readers would gain knowledge that would broaden their perspective about this area of study. The various advancements in chinese medicine are glanced at and their applications as well as ramifications are discussed in detail. This book will serve as a resource guide for students and experts alike.

I would like to express my sincere thanks to the authors for their dedicated efforts in the completion of this book. I acknowledge the efforts of the publisher for providing constant support. Lastly, I would like to thank my family for their support in all academic endeavors.

Editor

Ethno-Botanic Treatments for Paralysis (Falij) in the Middle East

Aref Abu-Rabia
Ben-Gurion University of the Negev, Beer-Sheva, Israel
Email: arefabu@gmail.com

ABSTRACT

The goal of this paper is to describe beliefs and treatments for specific forms of Paralysis (falij) and other nervous disorders in the Middle East. Themes to be investigated include, the traditional medicinal practices used to treat Paralysis, as well as their curative methods using traditional herbal medicine. This paper is based on first and secondary sources; interviews with traditional healers, as well as patients who suffered from these disorders. The author found 152 plants species belonging to 58 families (see Appendix) that treat paralysis and other nervous disorders. The most significant plants species are found in the six families of herbs: Labiatae, Compositae, Umbelliferae, Papilionaceae, Liliaceae, and Solanaceae.

Keywords: Paralysis; Ethno Botanic Medicine; Middle East

1. Introduction

The use of plant medicines in the Middle East has historical roots in Ancient Arabic medicine, which itself was influenced by the ancient medicinal practices of Mesopotamia, Greece, Rome, Persia, and India. During the Umayyad rule (661-750 A.D.), translations of ancient medical works began. The Abbasids dominated the sociopolitical life of the greater part of the Muslim world from 750 to 1258 A.D. Within a century, Muslim physicians and scientists were making original contributions to medical and botanical knowledge. In Baghdad, and in other parts of the Muslim world, centers of medical learning had already been founded. The next 3 centuries saw the synthesis and creation of new drugs and therapies [1].

One of the greatest and most famous Islamic doctors was Ibn Sina (Avicenna, 980-1037 A.D.), who combined the Canon of Medicine, which includes many descriptions of uses for medicinal plants. Another Arabic philosopher-physician was al-Razi (Rhazes, 865-923 A.D.), who composed a Comprehensive Book on Medicine. This material composed was arranged under the headings of different diseases, with separate sections on pharmacologic topics. Ibn al-Baytar's (1197-1248 A.D.) work, the Compendium of Simple Drugs and Food described more than 1400 medicinal drugs, including 300 previously undocumented drugs. This scholarly medical tradition which was molded in the tenth century matured through the eleventh and twelfth centuries, reached a peak in the thirteenth through sixteenth centuries, and later declined during the seventeenth through the nineteenth centuries. Medical information grounded in Arab classical medical scholarship of the Middle Ages was gradually transferred to local traditional healers and to the general public. Arabs relied primarily on their traditional medicine [2]. In this way, Arab classical medicine became the exclusive domain of traditional medicine and folk healers in the nineteenth and twentieth centuries [3]. Most of the herbs were used both as food and as medicine [4].

Many of the plants used by the Arab have direct effects on the body as purgatives, emetics, astringents, or tonics, or cause/prevent vomiting or diarrhea. This traditional medicine is based on a practical knowledge of plants and disease treatments over centuries. It should be noted that some plants are used similarly throughout the Middle East, while some plants have different uses in different countries in the region.

Based on their patterns of life, the Arab in the Middle East belongs to three distinct ethnic groups: the urbanized (hadar); the peasants (fallahin); and the nomads and seminomad Bedouin tribes (badu) [1].

2. Methodology

The data for this paper are derived from a broader study of ethno-botany and folk medicine of the Middle East over three decades. The paper is based on interviews with healers and patients. Unstructured interviews and the observation of participants were carried out in the informants' homes (men and women), as well as in the homes of traditional healers (men and women). Most of the healers were in the age range of forty to eighty years old. All the informants were married and over thirty years old. All the material was recorded in field logs, and some was tape-recorded. Plant samples were collected and identified by healers, tribal elders, and university botanists. The samples were identified and classified according to the plant seeds, leaves, fruit, taste, color and shape.

3. Results

This paper describes beliefs and treatments for specific forms of Paralysis and other nervous disorders in the Middle East by traditional herbalists among the Arabs in the Middle East. In this study, we found that Arab use various parts of the plants, including leaves, flowers, barks, stems, stalks, roots, rhizomes, bulbs, tubers, fruit, corns, shells, seeds, stones/pits (in fruits), soft seed pods, grain buds, shoots, twigs, stolons, oils, resins and gums. These parts are used fresh and soft, or cooked or dried. Toxic plants/bulbs are dried, boiled several times in water, or placed in hot ashes and then used for medicines or foods. The dosages for patients with the same diseases or disorders may vary, according to the ages and the structures of the patients' bodies.

The rich variety of approaches employed by different healers to treat specific forms of paralysis and other nervous disorders is indicative of the depth and breadth of indigenous medicine practiced among the Arab in the twentieth century. It should be noted that wild desert plants also contain a host of other biologically active compounds besides nutrients. The physiological effects of these other compounds in relation to plant nutrients are not well known, but could affect nutrient and medical utilization or other functions. These topics are of relevance for future research in terms of improving our understanding of human nutritional and medical requirements of the people in the Middle East.

Analysis of the findings shows that the Middle East is the geographic origin of both wild and cultivated medicinal plants. In this research the author found 152 plants species belonging to 58 families that treat parlaysis and other nervous disorders. The most significant plants species are found in the six families of herbs: Labiatae with 21 plants, Compositae with 15 plants, Umbelliferae with 15 plants, and Papilionaceae with 10 plants, Liliaceae with 7 plants, Solanaceae with 6 plants. The appendix shows the whole families with their plants species.

This paper deals with the six representative families; the Latin name of the species is given first followed by the Arabic and English names as described below:

4. Labiatae: (21 Plants)

4.1. *Ballota nigra* L.

Arabic: Ferasyoun aswad.
   English: Black hemp-nettle.
   Plant parts: The whole herb.
   Active constituents: Essential oil, tannin, gallic acid [5].
   Ethno-botanical use: Antispasmodic, to make one less nervous [5,6] and sedative (is a drug which quiets nervous activity). Flowering branches are an antispasmodic [7] and tranquilizer (a drug used in calming persons suffering from nervous tension and anxiety). Leaves and flowers are boiled in water: used as anti-spasmodic [8] and sedative.

4.2. *Coridothymus capitatus* (L.) Reichb

Arabic: Zahayfy, Za'tar Farisy.
   English: Wild thyme.
   Plant parts: Leaves and flowers.
   Active constituents: The essential oil contains phenols: carvacrol and thymol [9].
   Ethno-botanical use: Boil leaves and flowers in water, stay in the bathtub for one hour, once a day for one month to treat paralysis [10].
   To treat paralysis: Prepare a steam bath from the leaves and use it daily for a month.

4.3. *Lavandula officinalis*

Arabic: Khuzama, Khuzama ma'rufa.
   English: Common lavender.
   Plant parts: Leaves and flowers.
   Active constituents: Pinene, limonene, geraniol, borneol, essential oil, tannin [5,11]; lavender oil and coumarins [8].
   Ethno-botanical use: Infusion of flowering summits or lavender oil are antispasmodic [5,7,8].

4.4. *Melissa officinalis* L.

Arabic: 'Ishbit el-Nahel, Turunjan.
   English: Lemon-balm.
   Plant parts: Leaves, and flowers.
   Active constituents: Essential oil obtained from leaves contain citral and citronal [9].
   Ethno-botanical use: Leaves and flowers used to relieve convulsions [12]. A water infusion is used as a tranquilizer; extracts of the leaves relax muscle spasms [9]. Infusion of leaves is an antispasmodic [7].

4.5. *Mentha longifolia* L./*Mentha piperita* L./ *Mentha pulegium* L./*Mentha spicata* L.

Arabic: Na'na' barri, Na'na, Habaq.

English: Mint, Horse mint.

Plant parts: Leaves.

Active constituents: Menthol, tannin, essential oil, bitter principle [5]; Magnesium and potassium [13]; commercial menthe oil (menthylacetate, menthol and menthone) [14].

Ethno-botanical use: Preparation: boil in water and drink; boil the leaves in water and drink two to four cups a day as a sedative and relieves spasms [5]. Treat muscle spasms and convulsions, and pain of facial paralysis [12]; an antispasmodic [7]; to prevent muscle spasms [9].

4.6. *Micromeria fruticosa* (L.) Druce

Arabic: Qurnya, 'Ishbit esh-shai, Duqat 'Adas.

English: Thyme-leaved savory.

Plant parts: Leaves, flowers.

Active constituents: Essential oil: novel, natural monoterpene ketone [9].

Ethno-botanical use: Drink an infusion from the leaves and flowers in order to strengthen and calm the nerves [9].

4.7. *Nepeta cataria*

Arabic: Qatram, hashishat al-her.

English: Catmint, catnip.

Plant parts: Leaves, the whole plant.

Preparation: Boil leaves in water and drink.

Active constituents: Vitamin C [13]; thymol, carvacrol and lactones [8].

Ethno-botanical use: Antispasmodic [8].

4.8. *Ocimum basilicum* L.

Arabic: Rayhan.

English: Sweet basil, basilica.

Plant parts: Leaves and seeds.

Preparation: Boil in water and drink.

Active constituents: Essential oil, tannin [5]; oil is the active ingredient which consists: thymol, linalol, cineol, eugenol, terpenes, sesquiterpenes, and methylchavicol [11,14,15].

Ethno-botanical use: Used as a calming medicine [16]; used as a calming sedative and antispasmodic [8].

4.9. *Origanum vulgare* L.

Arabic: Mardagush.

English: Oregano, Organy, wild majorana.

Plant parts: Leaves, the whole herb.

Active constituents: Essential oil, tannin, thymol, carvacrol; and vitamin C [13].

Ethno-botanical use: Antispsmodic [5]. Treats pains of facial paralysis [11,12].

4.10. *Rosmarinus officinalis*

Arabic: Iklil al-Jabal, Hasalban.

English: Rosemary.

Plant parts: Leaves, flowers.

Preparation: Boil the leaves in water and drink.

Active constituents: Essential oil, cineol, borneol, tannin, acids, resin [5,11].

Ethno-botanical use: Antiepileptic [5] and antispasmodic [7].

4.11. *Salvia fruticosa* Mill/*Salvia officinalis* L.

Arabic: Marmarya, miramia, Na'ema.

English: Three-lobed sage, Sage.

Plant parts: Leaves, seeds and flowers.

Active constituents: Vitamin B complex [13]; leaves contain essential oil: phenols; and thujones which depress the central nervous system; to prevent convulsions [8,9], tannin, camphor, cineol, borneol, pinene, resin [5,11], sulfur and steroid substances [13].

Ethno-botanical use: Antispasmodic [5].

4.12. *Stachys lavandulaefolia*/*Stachys arabica* Hornem

Arabic: Sarmag.

English: Woundwort.

Plant parts: The whole herb.

Active constituents: Essential oil, tannins, alkaloids [5].

Ethno-botanical use: Antispasmodic [5].

4.13. *Thymbra spicata* L.

Arabic: Za'tar hmar, za'tar shibli.

English: Spiked thymbra.

Plant parts: Leaves and stalks.

Active constituents: Essential oil: Thujene, myrecene, alpha-terpinene, paracymene, gama-terpinene, linalool, carvacrol and betacaryophyllene [17].

Ethno-botanical use: boil green leaves and stalks in water, put in bath tub and soak your body for one hour, to treat paralyzed limbs [10].

4.14. *Thymus algeriensis* Boiss. & Reut./ *Thymus serpyllum* L./*Thymus vulgaris*

Arabic: Khieta, zahhayfy, za'tar.

English: Thyme.

Plant parts: The whole herb.

Active constituents: Essential oil, cymol, thymol, tannin [5].

Volatile oil: Phenols such as thymol, carvacrol, glycoside, and flavonoids [11,14,15].

Ethno-botanical use: Leaves and flowering branches are an antispasmodic [7] and sedative [5,14].

5. Compositae: (15 Plants)

5.1. *Achillea fragrantissima* (Forssk)/*Achillea millefolium*

Arabic: Qaysum, qisum, umm alf waraqa.
  English: Lavender cotton, yarrow.
  Plant parts: Leaves, flowers.
  Preparation: Boil in water and drink.

Active constituents: Flavonoids, sesquiterpene lactones, which relieve convulsions and inflammations [9]; terpenoids, sterols, lactones, and chamazulenes [14]; and Potassium [13].

Ethno-botanical uses: Used as an antispasmodic [12]. Make a vapor bath by boiling leaves and flowers, or prepare an infusion to drink, in order to treat convulsions and muscle spasms.

5.2. *Ambrosia maritima* L.

Arabic: Damsisa.
  English: Sea Ambrosia.
  Plant parts: Leaves, the whole plant.
  Preparation: Boil in water and drink.
  Active constituents: Chlorosesquiterpene lactones [14].

Ethno-botanical uses: The whole plant is used as an antispasmodic [14].

5.3. *Anacyclus pyrethrum* L. Link

Arabic: Oud el-'attas, Agargarha.
  English: Spanish pellitory.
  Parts used: Roots.
  Active constituents: The roots contain anacyclin [18].

Ethno-botanical use: A gargle of its infusion is prescribed for partial paralysis of the tongue and lips, relief of neuralgia and palsy [7].

5.4. *Artemisia absinthium* L./*Artemesia herba-alba* Asso

Arabic: Shih Rumi, Afsantin, Shih, sheeh.
  English: Wormwood, absinthium.
  Plant parts: Leaves, flowers.
  Preparation: Boil in water and drink, or eat.
Active constituents: Vitamin C [13]. Its active substances include silica, two bitter substances (absinthin and anabsinthine), thujone, tannic and resinous substances, malic acid, and succinic acid. Essential oil, resin, pinene, cadinen, tannin [5,11]; Santonin, sterols and thujones [11,19]; it also contains essential oils, sesquiterpene lactones and thymol; leaves and stems contain three nonglycosidic flavonoids [14].

Ethno-botanical uses: To treat nervousness: prepare a sweetened extract, from the leaves, in glass of water and drink it [9]; to treat paralysis [20]. It is also used as an

antispasmodic and calmative (having relaxing/quieting effect or pacifying properties).

5.5. *Atractylis gummifera* L.

Arabic: Heddad, Shawk el-'elk.
  English: White chameleon, Spindle wort.
  Plant parts: Leaves and flowers.
  Active constituents: Verapamil, or dithiothreitol [21].
  Ethno-botanical use: Root fumigant for paralysis; infusion of flowers for epilepsy and convulsions, paralysis of lips [7].

5.6. *Calendula officinalis* L.

Arabic: Uqhuwan.
  English: Marigold.
  Plant parts: Leaves, flowers and fruit.
  Preparation: Boil in water and drink.

Active constituents: Calendulin, essential oil, acids mucilage and carotenoides [5]; Vitamin A and phosphorrus [13].

Ethno-botanical uses: Flowers are used as an antispasmodic [7,11].

5.7. *Carthamus tinctorius* L.

Arabic: Qurtum, zafaran, 'usfur.
  English: Safflower.
  Plant parts: Flowers and seeds.

Active constituents: Carthamin, fixed oil, yellow and red coloring matters [5]. Safflower seeds are the source of oil [13]; flowers contain palmitic acid, myristic acid and lauric acid; flavonoids and sterols; seeds contain aphenolic amide [14].

Ethno-botanical use: Boil flowers in water for 15 minutes, filter, and drink five table spoons a day, to treat paralyzed body organs [10].

5.8. *Chrysanthemum coronarium* L.

Arabic: Bisbass, Sufirah, balsamiya.
  English: Chrysanthemum.
  Plant parts: Leaves and flowers.
  Active constituents: Sesquiterpene lactones [9].

Ethno-botanical use: Use the leaves in a steam bath to relieve muscle aches, nervousness and contractions of the uterus [9]; sedative and antispasmodic [8].

5.9. *Echinops ritro* L.

Arabic: Qunfudhiya.
  English: Globe thistle.
  Plant parts: Flowers and seeds.
  Active constituents: Echinospine, oil and minerals [5].
  Ethno-botanical use: Antispasmodic and neurotonic

[5].

5.10. *Inula viscose* (L.) Ait

Arabic: 'Irq al-Tayun, Tayun.

English: Inula, Elecampane, clammy inula.

Plant parts: Leaves, roots and the whole herb.

Preparation: Boil in water and drink.

Active constituents: Inulin, levulin, mucilage, essential oil [5]; flavonoids: Quercetin and inulin [9].

Ethno-botanical use: To cure muscle cramps—prepare a steam bath with the leaves or the whole herb; treat local paralysis: Extract oil from the leaves and massage the affected area. For nervousness, prepare a decoction from the roots and spread it on the body [9]. Or soak the leaves in water and drink a table spoon a day for one week as a tranquilizer.

5.11. *Lactuca serriola* L.

Arabic: Khass Barri.

English: Oil lettuce, Prickly lettuce.

Plant parts: Leaves, stems and stalks.

Preparation: Eat as raw salad.

Active constituents: Alkaloids, flavonoids and saponin [22].

Ethno-botanical use: Calmative and antispasmodic [7].

5.12. *Matricaria recutita* L.

Arabic: Uqhuwan, kahwan, babounaj.

English: Wild chamomile, German Chamomile.

Plant parts: Flowers, the whole herb.

Active constituents: Essential oil, vitamin C, coumarin, apigenin [5]; potassium [13]; volatile oil; proazulene, flavoles and coumarines; apigenin glycosides [14].

Ethno-botanical use: Flowers are an antispasmodic [7] and sedative [8].

5.13. *Silybum marianum* L.

Arabic: Khurfeish al-jamal, shouk al-jamal.

English: Milk thistle, St. Mary's Thistle.

Plant parts: Shoots, the whole herb, seeds.

Preparation: To be eaten as raw salad; or boiled in water and drank.

Active constituents: Tyramine, tannin, resin, fixed oil [5]; seeds contain a mixture of glycosides known as silymarine. Silymarine contain active ingredients: Silybin, silychristin, and silydianin [9].

Ethno-botanical use: Antispasmodic [5].

6. Umbelliferae: (15 Plants)

6.1. *Ammi visnage* L.

Arabic: Khella, Saq al-'Arus.

English: Bishop's weed.

Part used: Seeds.

Active constituents: In modern medicine-substances produced from this plant are: Khellin, visnagin, visnadin and khellol-they are spasmolytic agents, and relax various smooth muscles [9,11].

Ethno-botanical use: To prepare a water infusion of the crushed seeds, and drink one cup a day, as an antispasmodic [5,7], and to prevent muscle spasms [11,12].

6.2. *Anethum graveolens* L.

Arabic: Shebet, 'ayn Jaradeh.

English: Dill.

Plant parts: Seeds and flowers, fruit.

Active constituents: Essential oil, terpenes, carvone, fixed oil, tannin [5]; sulfur [13]; essential oil: carvone [9]; seeds contain volatile oil: Anethofuran, carvone and limonene [14].

Ethno-botanical use: Fruit is used as an antispasmodic and sedative [7]; and as tranquilizer.

6.3. *Apium graveolens* L.

Arabic: Karafs.

English: Celery.

Part used: Leaves, roots and seeds.

Active constituents: The seeds contain essential oils of which the main components are limonene and apiol [9,11]; Essential oil, apiin, asparagin, limonene [5].

Ethno-botanical uses: Roots are used in the form of infusion for relaxing nervous tension, and is antispasmodic [5,11].

6.4. *Carum carvi* L.

Arabic: Krawya, Karawiya.

English: Caraway, common caraway.

Plant parts: Flowers and seeds.

Active constituents: Essential oil, fixed oil, carvone, resin, tannin, coumarins [5]; and phosphorus [13].

Ethno-botanical use: Analgesic, ripe fruits are a nerve calmative; ripe seeds antispasmodic [7,11].

6.5. *Conium maculatum*

Arabic: Shiqran, Shawkaran.

English: Poison-hemlock, Hemlock.

Plant parts: Dried leaves, seeds and roots.

Preparation: The dried leaves are soaked in water and drunk, a table spoon a day for two weeks.

Active constituents: Essential oil, coniine, conhydrine, conicein [5]; alkaloids: Coniine, being the toxic constituent, found in all parts of the plant [9]; Coniilne and conhydrine [11].

Ethno-botanical use: Treat nervous excitability, acting

on the paralysis tremors. Young branches and ripe fruits is effective as a tranquilizer, analagesic, prophylactic muscle relaxant; neuroleptic, antidepressant, and anti-convulsant [5,9]. The tincture is prescribed as a neuro-muscular sedative and antispasmodic for a paralyzed respiratory system [7,11].

6.6. *Coriandrum sativum* L.

Arabic: kuzbarah, kusbara.
  English: Coriander.
  Plant parts: seeds and leaves.
  Preparation: boil in water and drink.
  Active constituents: Essential oil, corinadrol [5]; and Vitamin C [13]; essential oil from the fruit has high content of linalol, a material which is used in the production of vitamin A; leaves are a source of vitamin A, and C; and coriander oil [9]; fruit and leaves contain: fats, protein, volatile oil [14].
  Ethno-botanical use: The distilled essential oil from the fruits relieves muscle pains, and acts as a tranquillizer [9], antispasmodic [5], sedative and treat nervous disorders [7].

6.7. *Cuminum cyminum* L.

Arabic: Kamun, sannut.
  English: Cumin.
  Plant parts: Seeds.
  Active constituents: Cuminol, carvone, essential oil, cymol, cuminic aldehyde [5]; seeds contain volatile oil [14].
  Ethno-botanical use: infusion of fruits antispasmodic [7] and sedative [14].

6.8. *Daucus carota* L. Subsp

Arabic: Jazar barri, jiziyr.
  English: Wild carrot.
  Plant parts: fruit, roots and seeds.
  Preparation: eaten as raw food.
  Active constituents: Vitamin A and B, pytosterine, carotin, asparagine, minerals [5]; Vitamins A, B6, B complex, and C; Chloride compounds, magnesium, potassium, sodium and iron; it is a source of carbohydrates [13]; roots contain glucose, sucrose, protein, salts, pectin, carotene, vitamins and asparagine; seeds contain: pinene, limonene, carotol, daucol, isobutyric acid and asarone [14].
  Ethno-botanical use: fruits are an antispasmodic [7], and sedative [14].

6.9. *Eryngium creticum* Lam

Arabic: Kursannih.
  English: Eryngo, Snake root.

Plant parts: roots.
  Preparation: boil in water and drink.
  Active constituents: Sugar, saponins, essential oil [5].
  Ethno-botanical use: to strengthen the nerves, to treat paralysis and nervous diseases [14].

6.10. *Pimpinella anisum/Pimpinella cretica* Poirt

Arabic: Yansun.
  English: Anise, Sweet cumin, Aniseed plant.
  Plant parts: seeds and flowers.
  Active constituents: essential oil, anethol, fixed oil, choline, mucilage [5]; anisic acid, fats, protein and sugar [14].
  Ethno-botanical uses: To treat convulsion, facial paralysis boil seeds in water, and allow the body to obserb the steam. The steams contain essential oil which affect on the face convulsions and heal them [10]. Seeds treat spasms [6,11].

6.11. *Ferula asafetida/Ferula communis/Ferula narthex*

Arabic: haltit, Simgh al-Unjadhan, Jiddeh.
  English: Asafoetida.
  Plant parts: resin: oleo-gum-resin.
  Preparation: boiled in water and drunk, chewed, or burn on coals for inhaling the smoke.
  Active constituents: Sulfur [13]. The oleo-gum-resin, asafetida, is obtained from the plant's rhizome; it consist volatile oil which contain sulphur compounds; the resinous portion include asaresinol ferulate and free ferulic acid [11,23].
  Ethno-botanical use: the oleo-gum-resin is used as an antispasmodic [7,14].

6.12. *Foeniculum vulgare* Mill

Arabic: Shawmar.
  English: Fennel.
  Plant parts: Stems, leaves and seeds.
  Preparation: Boil leaves in water and drink two cups a day for three weeks.
  Active constituents: Essential oil, anethole, anisic acid, acids, fixed oil [5]; Potassium and sulfur [13]; from the fruit we get fennel oil: anethole and enol; liquorice and senna [9]; seeds contain volatile oil; phenolic anethole and a ketone fenchone [14].
  Ethno-botanical use: the fruit is an antispasmodic and calmative [7,11,12].

7. Papilionaceae: (10 Plants)

7.1. *Glycyrrhiza glabra* L.

Arabic: 'Irq al-sus, 'ud al-sus.

English: Liquorices, licorice.

Plant parts: leaves, rhizome.

Preparation: boil in water and drink.

Active constituents: Glycyrrhizin asparagine, liquirtin, coumarin, sugar, tannin [5], and phosphorus; and steroid substances [13]; glycyrrhizin and glycyrrhetic acid [9]; the plant is a source of licorice, the sweet taste due to glycyrrhizin (the calcium and potassium salts of glycyrrhizinic acid); flavonoids, starch, protein and bitter principles [11,14].

Ethno-botanical use: to relax uterine muscles, antispasmodic [7,8], and tranquilizer, sedative, rhizome is used for treating muscle pain [14].

7.2. *Lotus corniculatus*

Arabic: qarn al-ghazal, beseli.

English: Bird's foot.

Plant parts: flowers.

Active constituents: cyanogenetiques, flavonoides [8].

Ethno-botanical use: sedative and antispasmodic [8].

7.3. *Medicago sativa* L.

Arabic: khubz al-Ra'ay, barsim hijazy.

English: Medick, locerne, alfalfa.

Plant parts: leaves, seeds, and the whole herb.

Active constituents: Saponin, alkaloids [5]; Vitamins A, C, K and B complex; and enzymes [13]; saponin, glucose and medicagenic acid; lucernic acid, oil, flavonoids, alkaloids and phenols [14].

Ethno-botanical use: sedative which quiets nervous activity [14].

7.4. *Melilotus alba/Melilotus indicus* (L.) All

Arabic: nafal.

English: Scented trefoil.

Plant parts: leaves, and flowers.

Active constituents: coumarins and flavonoids, terpenoid glycosides, herniarin, choline and aromatic compound [14].

Ethno-botanical use: infusion of flowering branches is an antispasmodic [7].

7.5. *Retama raetam* (Forssk.) Webb

Arabic: ratam, ratama.

English: white broom, ratame.

Plant parts: The whole herb, flowers.

Active constituents: Essential oil [5]; alkaloids: retamine and sparteine [9].

Ethno-botanical use: to treat limb paralysis: use the upper branches to prepare a vapor bath; to treat local paralysis: use the roots-boil in water and spread the extract on the affected area [9].

7.6. *Trifolium arvense/Trifolium pratense/Trifolium purpureum*

Arabic: barsim ahmar, abu d'alabish, naflih.

English: red clover.

Plant parts: leaves and roots.

Active constituents: Tannin, trifoline, isotrifoline [5].

Ethno-botanical uses: used as sedative and an antispasmodic; treat emotional tension and strain [10,24].

7.7. *Vicia faba* L.

Arabic: Foul, fool.

English: broad bean.

Plant parts: broad bean/brown bean.

Preparation: eat as coked food, eat broad bean once a day for two to three weeks.

Active constituents: Vitamin B1, B complex; Phosphorus, potassium, copper and iron [13].

Ethno-botanical uses: flowers are an antispasmodic [7].

8. Liliaceae: (7 Plants)

8.1. *Asphodelus aestivus/Asphodelus fistulosus/Asphodelus ramosus/ Asphodelus microcarpus* Salzm. & Viv

Arabic: Swai.

English: Asphodel.

Plant parts: roots, leaves, flowers, seeds and bulbs.

Preparation: boil in water and drink.

Active constituents: Asphodeline, inuline, mucilage [5], Alkaloids, glycosides and anthraquinones [9].

Ethno-botanical use: antispasmodic [5]. Rubbing the body with roasted tubers and drinking decoction from leaves treats paralysis [7].

8.2. *Lilium candidum* L.

Arabic: Zanbaq, Sawsan abyad.

English: White lily.

Plant parts: flowers and bulbs, leaves or dried seeds.

Preparation: soak in water and drink.

Active constituents: Scillin, minerals, mucilage, pectinds [5].

Ethno-botanical use: antispasmodic [5].

8.3. *Ruscus aculeatus* L.

Arabic: Ass Barri, Khizana.

English: Butcher's broom, Kee holly.

Plant parts: roots, leaves.

Preparation: boil in water and drink.

Active constituents: mixture of sterols and fatty acids [9].

Ethno-botanical use: An infusion of the flowers tranquilizes the nerves and calms hysterical seizures and convulsions; a decoction of the branches mitigates convulsions [9].

8.4. *Urginea maritima* L. Bak

Arabic: halluf, 'Unsol, bussayl.
  English: Squil white.
  Plant parts: leaves, bulbs.
  Active constituents: Urginin, cardiotonic glycosides, scillaren, mucilage [5,11]; bulbs contain glycoside: proscillaridin A.
  Ethno-botanical uses: treatment of cathartic and upset nerves [7,11].

9. Solanaceae: (6 Plants)

9.1. *Atropa belladonna* L.

Arabic: Set al-Husn.
  English: Deadly nightshade, Belladona.
  Plant parts: leaves and roots.
  Active constituents: atrosin [5]; atropine, hyoscyamine and hyoscine cocaein [11].
  Ethno-botanical use: antispasmodic and sedative [5, 11].

9.2. *Datura stramonium* L.

Arabic: Daturah, Semm al-far.
  English: Jimsonweed, thorn-apple.
  Plant parts: leaves, seeds and roots.
  Active constituents: active ingredients like alkaloids of the tropane group, such as atropine, scopolamine and hyoscamine [9]; daturine, hyoscyamine, atropine, scopolamine, hyocine [5,11].
  Ethno-botanical use: sedative, analgesic, antispasmodic, for asthma and neuralgic pain; acts as a tranquillizer. Tincture of leaves prescribed for spasmodic coughs and asthma; leaves used in fumigations and in cigarettes to ease asthma attacks [5]. Atropine is one of the active ingredients in this plant. Its physiological activity is mainly on the central nervous system. It is used to prevent convulsions of the smooth muscles, especially in the lower part of the body [9]. Leaves acts as an antispasmodic and sedative [7,11].

9.3. *Hyoscyamus albus* L./*Hyoscyamus aureus*

Arabic: Sikiran, banj.
  English: White henbane.
  Part used: Leaves and seeds.
  Active constituents: Alkaloids, hyoscyamine, hyoscypicrin, essential oil [5]; atropine and hyoscine [11].
  Ethno-botanical use: plant alleviates nervous irritation such as various forms of hysteria [7]; calmative, tranquilizer for hysteria and nervousness [9,11].

9.4. *Nicotiana tabacum* L.

Arabic: teten, tebgh, dukhan
  English: Tobacco
  Plant parts: Leaves.
  Active constituents: Nicotine compounds [5]; nicotine and anabacine [11].
  Ethno-botanical use: CNS stimulant followed by depression, hypertensive [5]; smoking dried leaves as tranquilizer and antispasmodic.

9.5. *Solanum nigrum* L.

Arabic: Enab eddib, 'Enb al-Tha'lab.
  English: Black nightshade.
  Part used: The whole herb, fruit (berries) and seeds. Unripe berries are poisonous, ripe berries are edible.
  Active constituents: Saponin, solanine [5,9]; Vitamin C and carotenes [14]; solasodine [11].
  Ethno-botanical use: sedative, antispasmodic [5]. Leaves to relieve nervous pains: use the leaves, prepare a decoction and massage with it; the fruit have a narcotic and tranquilizing effect; extracts of this plant suppress the activity of the central nervous system and prevent muscle spasms [9].

REFERENCES

[1] A. Abu-Rabia, "Palestinian Plant Medicines for Treating Renal Disorders: An Inventory and Brief History," *Alternative & Complementary Therapies*, Vol. 11, No. 6, 2005, pp. 295-300. doi:10.1089/act.2005.11.295

[2] A. Abu-Rabia, "The Bedouin's Traditional Medicine," Mod Publishing, Tel-Aviv, 1999.

[3] E. Lev, "Reconstructed Material Medica of the Medieval and Ottoman al-Sham," *Journal of Ethnopharmacology*, Vol. 80, No. 2-3, 2002, pp. 167-179. doi:10.1016/S0378-8741(02)00029-6

[4] M. Ali-Shtayeh, Z. Yaniv and J. Mahajna, "Ethnobotanical Survey in the Palestinian Area: A Classification of the Healing Potential of Medicinal Plants," *Journal of Ethnopharmacology*, Vol. 73, No. 1-2, 2000, pp. 221-232. doi:10.1016/S0378-8741(00)00316-0

[5] F. Karim and S. Qura'an, "Medicinal Plants of Jordan," Yarmouk University, Irbid, 1986.

[6] J. Philips, "Lebanese folk cures," University Microfilms, Ann Arbor, 1958.

[7] L. Boulos, "Medicinal Plants of North Africa," Reference Publications, Algonac, 1983.

[8] H. Qubaysi, "Mu'jam al-a'Shab wal-Nabatat al-Tibbiya," Dar al-Kotob al-Ilmiyah-Publishing Haouse, Bayrut, 1998.

[9] D. Palevitch and Z. Yaniv, "Medicinal Plants of the Holy Land," Modan Publishing House, Tel-Aviv, 2000.

[10] N. Krispil, "Medicinal Plants in Israel and throughout the World: The Complete Guide," Hed Arzi Publishing House, Yehuda, 2000.

[11] A. Atyat, "Production and Processing of Medicinal and Aromatic Plants in the Arab World," Arab Institute for Research and Publications (in Arabic), Bayrut, 1995.

[12] A. Khalifa, "al-Nabatat: Saydaliyat al-Taby'ah," al-Markaz al-Thaqafi al-'Arabi (in Arabic), Bayrut, 1998.

[13] J. Lust, "The Herb Book," Bantam Books, Turonto and New York, 1980.

[14] S. Ghazanfar, "Handbook of Arabian Medicinal Plants," CRC Press, London, 1994.

[15] S. Ghazanfar and A. Al-Sabahi, "Medicinal Plants of Northern and Central Oman (Arabia)," *Economic Botany*, Vol. 47, No. 1, 1993, pp. 89-98. doi:10.1007/BF02862209

[16] M. Akhmisse, "Medicine, Magie et Sorcellerie au Maroc ou L'Art traditionnel de guerir," d'Impression Eddar el-Beida, Casablanca, 1985.

[17] M. Inan, M. Kirpik, K. Alpaslan and S. Kirici, "Effect of Harvest Time on Essential Oil Composition of Thymbra Spicata L. Growing in Flora of Adıyaman," *Advances in Environmental Biology*, Vol. 5, No. 2, 2011, pp. 356-358.

[18] O. Gautam, S. Verma and S. Jain, "Anticonvulsant and Myorelaxation Activity of *Anacyclus pyrethrum* DC. (Akarkara) Root Extract," *Pharmacologyonline*, Vol. 1, No. 1, 2011, pp. 121-125.

[19] P. Tal, "Medicinal Plants," Rshafim, Tel-Aviv, 1981.

[20] A. Ibn al-Baytar, "al-Jami' li-Mufradat al-Adwiya wa'l-Aghdhiya (Compendium of Simple Drugs and Food)," Dar al-Kutub al-'Ilmiya, Bayrut, 1992.

[21] C. Danielea, S. Dahamnab, O. Firuzia, N. Sekfalib, L. Sasoa and G. Mazzantia, "Atractylis Gummifera L. Poisoning: An Ethnopharmacological Review," *Journal of Ethnopharmacology*, Vol. 97, No. 2, 2005, pp. 175-181. doi:10.1016/j.jep.2004.11.025

[22] F. Mojab, K. Mohammad, N. Ghaderi and H. R. Vahidipour, "Phytochemical Screening of Some Species of Iranian Plants," *Iranian Journal of Pharmaceutical Research*, Vol. 2. No. 2, 2003, pp. 77-82.

[23] G. Appendino, S. Tagliapietra, G. M. Mano and J. Jakupovic, "Sesquiterpene Coumarin Ethers from Asafetida," *Phytochemistry*, Vol. 30, No. 1, 1994, pp. 183-186.

[24] C. Townsend and G. Evan, "Flora of Iraq," Ministry of Agriculture and Agrarian Reform of Iraq, Baghdad, 1974.

Appendix of Families and Their Plants Species

Amaryllidaceae: *Narcissus pseudo-narcissus.*
Anacardiaceae: *Pistacia lentiscus.*
Apocynaceae: *Adenium obesum.*
Araliaceae: *Hedera helix.*
Asclepiadaceae: *Calotropis procera.*
Asteraceae: *Santolina chamaecyparissus.*
Cannabaceae: *Cannabis sativa, Humulus lupulus.*
Capparaceae: *Capparis cartilaginea, Capparis spinosa.*
Caryophyllaceae: *Stellaria media.*
Celastraceae: *Catha edulis.*
Cesalpiniaceae: *Cassia italic.*
Chenopodiaceae: *Chenopodium ambrosioides, Chenopodium vulvaria.*
Compositae: *Achillea fragrantissima, Achillea millefolium, Ambrosia maritime, Anacyclus pyrethrum, Artemisia absinthium, Artemesia herba-alba, Atractylis gummifera, Calendula officinalis, Carthamus tinctorius, Chrysanthemum coronarium, Echinops ritro, Inula viscose, Lactuca serriola, Matricaria recutita, Silybum marianum.*
Cruciferae: *Anastatica hierochuntica.*
Cucurbitaceae: *Citrulus colocynthis Schirad, Ecballium elaterium.*
Cupressaceae: *Juniperus excelsa.*
Cyperaceae: *Cyperus rotundus.*
Euphorbiaceae: *Ricinus communis.*
Fabaceae: *Lablab purpureus.*
Fumariaceae: *Fumaria officinalis.*
Gramineae: *Avena sativa, Cymbopogon proximus, Lolium temulentum, Zea mays.*
Hypericaceae: *Hypericum perforatum.*
Juglandaceae: *Juglans regia.*
Iridaceae: *Crocus sativus.*
Labiatae: *Ballota nigra, Coridothymus capitatus, Lavandula officinalis, Melissa officinalis, Mentha longifolia, Mentha piperita, Mentha pulegium, Mentha spicata, Micromeria fruticosa, Nepeta cataria, Ocimum basilicum, Origanum vulgare, Rosmarinus officinalis, Salvia fruticosa, Salvia officinalis, Stachys lavandulaefolia, Stachys arabica Hornem, Thymbra spicata, Thymus algeriensis, Thymus serpyllum, Thymus vulgaris.*
Lauraceae: *Laurus nobilis.*
Leguminosaae: *Robinia pseudo-acacia.*
Liliaceae: *Asphodelus aestivus, Asphodelus fistulosus, Asphodelus ramosus, Asphodelus microcarpus, Lilium candidum, Ruscus aculeatus, Urginea maritime.*
Loranthaceae: *Viscum album, Viscum cruciatum.*
Lythraceae: *Lawsonia inermis.*
Malphigiaceae: *Acridocarpus orientalis.*
Mimosaceae: *Acacia nilotica, Acacia Arabica, Acacia ehrenbergiana, Prosopis farcta.*
Moraceae: *Ficus carica, Morus alba.*
Myristicaceae: *Myristica fragrans.*
Myrtaceae: *Eucalyptus globules.*
Nymphaeaceae: *Nymphaea alba.*
Paeoniaceae: *Paeonia coriacea, Paeonia officinalis.*
Papaveraceae: *Papaver somniferum.*
Papilionaceae: *Glycyrrhiza glabra, Lotus corniculatus, Medicago sativa, Melilotus alba/Melilotus indicus, Retama raetam, Trifolium arvense, Trifolium pretense, Trifolium purpureum, Vicia faba.*
Passifloraceae: *Passiflora incarnate.*
Pedaliaceae: *Sesamum orientale.*
Piperaceae: *Piper nigrum*
Primulaceae: *Cyclamen persicum.*
Punicaceae: *Punica granatum.*
Ranunculaceae: *Adonis aestivalis, Anemone coronaria, Delphinium staphisagria, Nigella sativa.*
Rhamnaceae: *Ziziphus lotus, Zizyphus spina-christi.*
Rosaceae: *Crataegus aronia/Crataegus monogyna, Rosa canina.*
Rubiaceae: *Rubia tinctorum, Rubia tenuifolia.*
Rutaceae: *Citrus aurantium, Haplophyllum tuberculatum, Ruta chalepensis,*
Salicaceae: *Salix alba.*
Solanaceae: *Atropa belladonna, Datura stramonium, Hyoscyamus albus, Hyoscyamus aureus, Nicotiana tabacum, Solanum nigrum.*
Scrophulariaceae: *Verbascum eremobium.*
Tiliaceae: *Tilia cordata.*
Umbelliferae: *Ammi visnage, Anethum graveolens, Apium graveolens, Carum carvi, Conium maculatum, Coriandrum sativum, Cuminum cyminum, Daucus carota, Eryngium creticum, Ferula asafetida, Ferula communis, Ferula narthex, Foeniculum vulgare, Pimpinella anisum, Pimpinella cretica Poirt.*
Urticaceae: *Urtica pilulifera.*
Verbenaceae: *Aloysia triphylla, Verbena officinalis, Vitex agnus-castus.*
Zingiberaceae: *Zingiber officinalis.*
Zygophyllaceae: *Balanites aegyptiaca, Peganum harmala, Tribulus terrestris.*

Holistic Psychopharmacology of *Fumaria indica* (Fumitory)

Anshul Shakya[1], Shyam Sunder Chatterjee[2*], Vikas Kumar[1]

[1]Neuropharmacology Research Laboratory, Department of Pharmaceutical Engineering, Indian Institute of Technology (Banaras Hindu University), Varanasi, India
[2]Stettiner Straße 1, Karlsruhe, Germany
Email: vikas.phe@iitbhu.ac.in

ABSTRACT

Fumaria indica is a medicinal plant of the fumitory family wildly growing throughout India. Classical texts of Ayurveda, *i.e.* the oldest traditionally known health care and medical system originating in Indian subcontinent, mentions diverse medicinal uses of the plant. During more recent decades broad spectrums of therapeutically interesting pharmacological properties of its extracts and secondary metabolites have also been reported. Recent observations made during efforts to define its pharmacological activity profile according to the Ayurvedic concepts of mind body medicine have revealed exceptionally broad spectrums of psychopharmacological activity profiles of diverse types of hydro alcoholic extracts of the plant. These effects of the extracts become apparent after their repeated daily doses only. Taken together with prior preclinical knowledge on the plant, these observations strongly suggest that *Fumaria indica* could be an easily available source for discovering and developing phyto-pharmaceuticals or drugs potentially useful for treatments of mental health problems commonly associated with numerous physical disorders and chronic diseases. Since several psychoactive and other phytochemical of *Fumaria indica* are also encountered in other plants commonly used in Chinese and other traditionally known medical systems, observations made and the holistic strategy used for defining its psychopharmacological activity profile could be of interest of others involved in efforts necessary for proper understanding of therapeutic potentials of many plants containing Fumaria alkaloids and other bioactive phytochemicals present in *Fumaria indica*.

Keywords: *Fumaria indica*; Fumitory Alkaloids; Ayurveda; Holistic Psychopharmacology; Comorbid Psychopathologies; Therapeutic Potential

1. Introduction

Medicinal uses of herbs and their combinations are common characteristics of Chinese as well as Indian systems of medicines. Ayurveda, *i.e.* the oldest and still the most popular health care system of India, and traditional Chinese medicine (TCM) have always been widely practiced in many Asiatic countries, and during more recent they have also been well accepted and adapted in many other parts of the economically more developed world. Such global popularity of these traditionally known medical systems, especially those of TCM [1], has increased the global demand of traditionally known herbal remedies, and has also triggered interests of numerous modern medical researchers and practitioners in properly understanding their therapeutic potentials in terms of modern medical sciences. However, despite extensive efforts and considerable progress made during past few decades, many therapy relevant questions concerning medicinal phytochemistry and pharmacology of numerous Chinese and Ayurvedic medicinal plants cannot yet be properly answered in terms of postmodern concepts of evidence based medicine. Consequently, novel strategies and paradigms are now being conceived and tried in many laboratories for clarifying them. Hereupon, more attention is paid to the molecular mechanisms and pharmacological targets based concepts of modern medicine than to the holistic principles of traditionally known medical systems like TCM or Ayurveda. However, in numerous laboratories, especially in India, China and other Asiatic countries, the conventionally known more holistic strategies and *in vivo* animal models for evaluating therapy relevant pharmacological properties of herbs are still widely practiced.

Phytochemical and pharmacological information now available on numerous traditionally known medicinal plants strongly suggest that most, if not all, of them could have modulating effects on the essential functions of the central

*Former Head of the Pharmacological Research Laboratories, Dr. Willmar Schwabe GmbH & Co. KG, Karlsruhe, Germany.

nervous system (CNS). Although several such plants have been more thoroughly explored and commercialized in the western world for combating mental health problems [2], as yet little concentrated efforts have been made verify mental health benefits of numerous others well known as accumulators of diverse CNS-active alkaloids and other phytochemicals. Recent efforts in our laboratories to define neuro-psychopharmacological activity profiles of some Indian medicinal plants [3] led us identify diverse psychotherapeutic potentials of several traditionally known medicinal plants, including those of *Fumaria indica* and some other currently popular Ayurvedic medicinal plants.

Fumaria indica is one such medicinal plant of the Fumitory species widely used in many other traditionally known medical systems commonly practiced in India and elsewhere. Several so called Fumitory alkaloids and other phytochemical encountered in *Fumaria indica* are structurally identical or similar to those of many other plants of the species, and several pharmacological properties of its extracts are also analogous or identical to those reported for extracts from other members of the family. However, potential roles of the psychoactive principles of *Fumaria indica* in therapeutically interesting pharmacological activity profiles of its diverse types of medicinally used extracts still remain speculative only. Efforts to clarify the situation is not only necessary for pharmacologically more rational standardization of its commercialized extracts, but also for identifying novel therapeutic leads potentially useful for combating co-morbid mental health problems commonly encountered in chronically ill patients. In this communication our current understanding on medicinal phytochemistry of *Fumaria indica* will be summarized, and usefulness of more holistic psychopharmacological strategies for more precisely defining its therapeutically interesting pharmacological activity profile will be pointed out.

2. Historical Background

Ayurveda is one of the three major traditionally known codified systems of medicine well integrated in the modern Indian health care system. Medicinal uses of many Ayurvedic plants, including those of *Fumaria indica*, are also known to practitioners of other traditionally known medical systems in India and elsewhere. Initially, Ayurvedic codes were in Sanskrit language. However, during more recent decades extensive efforts have been made to translate, de-codify, and understand its texts in English and other modern languages. It was only through such efforts that eventually *Fumaria indica* was identified as an Ayurvedic medicinal plant. Its medicinal values are often mentioned in classical texts like Charak Samhita [4], Dhanvantari Nighantu [5] and Bhava Prakash [6]. Botanically it belongs to the *Fumaria* species,

also commonly called "fumitory", "earth smoke", "beggary", "fumus", "fumittery" or "wax dolls" in English. These are annual weeds, growing wildly in plains and lower hills of India, Pakistan, Afghanistan, Turkey, Iran, Central Asia, North Dakota and Colorado [7,8]. The genus *Fumaria* (Fumariaceae/Papavaraceae) consists of many species [9], and the *Fumaria* species defined as *Fumaria indica* (Haussk) Pugsley (synonyms: *F. parviflora*, *F. vaillantii*), is now one of the most commonly used herbs in Ayurvedic, Unani and other folk medicine system of India. In Pakistan, it is traditionally used for treatment of dermatological diseases, topical diseases, cardio vascular complaints, circulatory disease, fever and headache [10]. The plant is now commonly known as "Pitpapda" in India, and as "Shahtra papra" in Pakistan [11,12]. Its diverse currently known medicinal uses are often in agreement with, or justified by, its broad spectrum of therapeutically interesting pharmacological activity profile unraveled mainly during the 20th century [11,13]. However, many questions concerning the details of its botanical identity, chemical constituents, bioactivities, and more appropriate medicinal values still remain to be more properly answered in terms of modern sciences.

3. Pharmacognostic Features

It has recently been ascertained [12] that the genus *Fumaria* L. (Papaveraceae) consists of 60 species and that *F. parviflora*, *F. indica*, and *F. vaillantii* are closely associated species. Various vernacular names of the plant used in Indian system of medicine are given in **Table 1** [14]. The macroscopic, microscopic, and chemotaxonomic characteristics of the plant are useful tools for pharmaceutical industries for identification and authentication of its commercial samples. The HPTLC profile using rutin and protopine as marker have recently been proposed to be useful means for quality control and affirming batch to batch consistency of the plant material used by the herbal industries for manufacturing pharmaceutical products [15]. It must be noted though, that both rutin and protopine are encountered also in numerous other plants, and that they are not the only extractable bioactive constituents of the plant.

3.1. Macroscopic and Microscopic Characteristics

F. indica is a pale green colored and highly branched annual herb. Roots of the plant are cream to buff in color and comprise of tap root system with numerous rootlets and root hairs. Transverse section of root has crushed epidermis followed by thin walled, irregular shaped, parenchymatous cortex merged with endodermis and well developed vascular bundles. Its stem is smooth and

Table 1. The vernacular names of *Fumaria indica*.

Vernacular names of *Fumaria indica* [14]			
Language	**Vernacular name**	**Language**	**Vernacular name**
Sanskrit	Parpata/Suksmapatra	Hindi	Pitpapra
English	Fumitory	Assamese	Shahtraj
Nepalese	Kairuwa	Kashmi	Shahterah
Sinhalese	Patha padagam	Bengali	Shotara/pipapapra/bandhania
German	Erdrauch	Gujrati	Pittapapdo
Chinese	Tuysha tu chian	Marathi	Pittapapra
Unani	Shahotarah	Kannada	Parpataka/Kallu sabbasige
Arabian	Shahtraj	Tamil	Thara/Tura/Thusha
Turkish	Sahtere	Telugu	Parpatakamu

light green in color. Transverse sections of stem is quadrangular to pentagonal in shape, and consist of single layered epidermis covered with cuticle followed by two distinct layer of cortex containing closed and bicollateral vascular bundles at the ridges, without endodermis. Leaves of the *Fumaria* are compound, 5 to 7 cm long, divided into narrow segments. The lamina of leaf is made up of single layer, thin walled, rectangular to oval shaped, parenchymatous epidermis on either side; mesophyll composed of oval to polygonal thin walled parenchymatous cells; vascular bundle are scattered throughout the mesophyll; anomocytic stomata present on both the surfaces. Inflorescence has 10 to 15 flowered racemes. Flowers are 6 to 7 mm long, composed of two whitish sepals, four purplish green petals, corolla in 2 whorls, stamens 3 + 3 and 3 to 4 mm long bi-lipped stigma. Fruits are capsules, sub round to ovate, and are single seeded. The seed is spherical to ellipsoid and has an apical pore and rib [12,15-18].

3.2. Phytochemicals

Extensive efforts made during the latter half to the 20th century in several Indian and other laboratories have led to the identification and characterization of numerous phytochemicals from the leaves, stem, root and seed of the *Fumaria indica*. The very first report on isolation, structure elucidation, and pharmacology of protopine and a few other alkaloids isolated from *Fumaria indica* appeared during 1971 [19]. Since then presence of numerous others alkaloids (often referred to as Fumitory alkaloids), flavonoids, glycosides, tannins, saponins, anthraquinones, steroids and triterpenoids in diverse parts of the plant have been reported [11,13,20]. Structures of the phytochemical isolated from different parts of *Fumaria indica* are given in **Table 2** [21-33]. Amongst them, a group of benzylisoquinoline alkaloids commonly known

as "protopine alkaloids" are encountered in all parts of the plant. It must be noted though that depending on the acidic environments protopine alkaloids can exist in two isomeric forms [34], which theoretically must not possess the same biological activities. Such characteristics of these and other alkaloids are often neglected by modern medicinal chemists and pharmacologists. Moreover, quantitatively as well as qualitatively the alkaloid contents of *Fumaria indica* extracts depend not only on the extraction procedure used, but also on the harvesting period of the plant itself [35], possible influences of such variations, and of drying and extraction procedures, on the pharmaceutical quality of *Fumaria indica* extracts have not yet been carefully examined. In view of the recent report [12] that drying induced morphological changes do occur in *Fumaria* species, such characteristics of a plant can not necessarily be used for acquiring its authentic samples for medicinal purposes. More detailed phytochemical analysis might be a better alternative for medicinal purposes. For such purposes, a simple, fast and efficient method based on the use of GC-MS technique for proper chemotaxonomic identification of plants of *Fumaria* species [9] has recently been published.

4. Medicinal Uses

Like for other traditionally known medical systems, the theories, principles, and practices of Ayurveda have little in common with those of the so called "western" medical systems. Details of Ayurvedic principles and medicinal recommendations for *Fumaria indica* are now available in authoritative publications in English [14,36]. Traditionally, the plant has been used as anthelmintic, antidyspeptic, blood purifier, anti periodic, cholagogue, diaphoretic, diuretic, laxative, stomachic, sedative, tonic [37], and has also been considered to be useful for treatment

Table 2. Structures of some bioactive phytochemicals of *Fumaria indica*.

S. No.	Chemical constituent	Plant part	Structure	Reference
		Alkaloids		
1.	Fuyuziphine	Whole plant		[21,22]
2.	(±)-α-Hydrastine	Whole plant		[22]
3.	Bicuculine	Whole plant		[22]
4.	Protopine	Whole plant, stem, leaves and seed		[19,23]
5.	Narlumicine	Stem		[23]
6.	Stylopine/ DL-Tetrahydrocoptisine	Whole plant, stem and seeds		[23]
7.	Narlumidine	Whole plant and stem		[23]

Continued

8.	Fumariline	Whole plant and seed		[24]
9.	(-)-8-methoxydihydrosanguinarine	Seed		[24]
10.	Oxysanguinarine	Seed		[24]
11.	Coptisine chloride	Whole plant		[25]
12.	Dehydrocheilanthifoline	Whole plant		[25]
13.	Narceimicine	Seed		[26,27]
14.	Papracinine	Aerial parts		[28]

Continued

15.	Paprazine	Aerial parts		[28]
16.	Fumaritine N-oxide	Whole plant and aerial parts		[28]
17.	Parfumine	Aerial parts		[28]
18.	Lastourvilline	Aerial parts		[28]
19.	Feruloyl tyramine	Aerial parts		[28]
20.	Fumariflorine	Aerial parts		[28]
21.	N-methyl corydaldine	Aerial parts		[28]
22.	Papraine	Aerial parts		[29]

Continued

23.	Fumarizine	Whole plant and aerial parts		[30]
24.	Paprafumine	Aerial parts		[31]
25.	Paprarine	Aerial parts		[31]
26.	Papraline	Aerial parts		[31]
27.	Cryptopine	Aerial parts		[31]
28.	Raddeanine	Aerial parts		[31]
29.	8-oxocoptisine	Aerial parts		[31]

Continued

| 30. | Berberine | Stem and leaves | | [32] |

Steroids

| 1. | *β*-sitosterol | Whole plant, stem, leaves and aerial parts | | [11,13] |

| 2. | Stigmasterol | Whole plant and aerial parts | | [11,13] |

| 3. | Campesterol | Whole plant and aerial parts | | [11,13] |

Organic acid and their esters

| 1. | Caffeic acid | Whole plant and aerial parts | | [11,13] |

| 2. | Fumaric acid | Whole plant and aerial parts | | [11,13] |

| 3. | Monomethyl fumarate | Whole plant and aerial parts | | [33] |

of abdominal cramps [38], diarrhea, fever [39], jaundice, leprosy and syphilis [18], blood disorders and tuberculosis [40]. The leaf paste has been used to treat headache and fever [41], and decoction and infusion of the herb are indicated for treatments of goiter, leprosy, constipation, jaundiance, chronic fevers and dyspepsia [42]. Fresh juice of the plant are administered orally for common fever, removing worms from the abdomen, blood purification and as liver tonic for hepatic ailment, and also used for the treatment of simple goitre, diabetes and bladder infection by taking its extraction early morning [43,44]. Whole plant of *F. indica* is an important ingredient of many common household, Ayurvedic, Unani medicinal preparations like *Ayurveda capsule, Parpatadi-kwath, parpatadya arista, Parpatadi-arka, trifala shahtara, Sharabat-pittapapada* [15,33], and other marketed polyherbal formulations such as *Livokriti syrup, Esno capsule* [45]. Examples of some such marketed formulations are given in **Table 3**. Furthermore, in Unani system of medicine, paste of fine powder of whole plant of *Fumaria indica* along with *Azadirachta indica* leaves, *Swertia chirata, Sphaeranthus indicus* flowers and *Rosa damascene* leaves in sufficient quantity of curd, has been used against pimples as routine home remedy [46].

5. Biological Activities and Safety

The very first reports on pharmacology of *Fumaria indica* concentrated mainly on the bioactivities of the alkaloids of the plant. Many of these alkaloids and other bioactive constituents of the plant are also encountered in other plants, and during more recent years the list of

therapeutically interesting bioactivities constituents of *Fumaria indica* has enlarged considerably. Diverse reported pharmacological properties of such secondary metabolites of *Fumaria indica* are summarized in **Table 4** [47-64]. The doses and routes of administrations used in these studies are also mentioned in this table. Other reports on therapeutically interesting pharmacological properties of different types of extracts obtained from the whole plant or from its areal parts and seeds have appeared also. **Table 5** [65-81] gives an overview of these reports which also includes the type of extracts and their doses used in the study. More detailed or critical analysis of available information on bioactivities and safety of *Fumaria indica* extracts and their bioactive constituents is beyond the scope of this communication. For such purposes a recent review [13] and several monographs now available on the plant can be consulted.

6. Psychopharmacological Aspects

Initial reports on psychopharmacology of *Fumaria indica* dealt mainly with the CNS function modulating effects of its alkaloids. Amongst them the so called benzylisoquinoline alkaloid protopine is one of the more well studied one, and it is also one of the quantitatively major alkaloid of *Fumaria indica*. Protopine was first

Table 3. Marketed formulations containing *Fumaria indica* extracts.

S. No.	Name of formulation	Indication(s)	Manufacturer
1.	Phytoliv tablets	Liver disorders	Tomer Laboratories 350 Campus Drive Somerset, New Jersey 08873 http://www.tomerlabs.com/
2.	Esno capsule	Chronic eosinophilla, cough and cold	Vita Health Private Limited Plot No. 753, At Rakanpur, Ta. Kalol, Gandhinagar-382721, Gujarat, India http://vitahealth.in/
3.	Livokriti syrup	Liver disorders	Elson Llc Wz-49h, 01st Floor, Budella, Vikas Puri, New Delhi-110018, India http://elsonusa.com/
4.	Valiliv forte tablets	Liver disorders	Unijules Life Sciences Limited Universal Square, 1505-1 Shantinagar Nagpur-440001, Maharashtra India http://www.unijules.com/
5.	Raktashodhak syrup	Blood purification	D.G. Ayurvedic Sangrah #14, J. P. Road, Opp. Ram Hanuman Mandir, Andheri West, Mumbai-400058, Maharashtra, India http://www.healthbyayurveda.in/
6.	Redliv DS caps	Liver disorders	Altis Life Sciences A-1/40, IIIrd floor, Sector-7, Rohini, Near M2K. Delhi-110085, India http://www.altislifesciences.com/

Table 4. Reported pharmacological activities of secondary plant metabolites isolated from *Fumaria indica*.

S. No.	Chemical Constituents	Pharmacological activities	Dose, duration and route of administration	References
1.	Fumariline	CNS depressant Anticonvulsant Analgesic Antifungal	10 - 50 mg/kg, single dose, i.p.	[47,48]
2.	Protopine	CNS stimulant Antidepressant Hepatoprotective Smooth muscle relaxation Choleretic Anti-thrombotic Anti-platelet aggregation Anti-inflammatory Anti-inflammatory Analgesic Anti-acetylcholinesterase Antifungal Antibacterial Antiviral	10 mg/kg, single dose, i.p. 5 - 20 mg/kg, single dose, p.o. 25 - 50 mg/kg, 7 days, p.o. 0.5 - 5 µg/ml *in vitro* 5 mg/kg, single dose, i.v. 50 - 100 mg/kg, single dose, i.p. 50 - 100 mg/kg, single dose, i.p. 50 - 100 mg/kg, single dose, i.p. 5 mg/kg, single dose, i.v. 10 - 40 mg/kg, single dose, s.c. 1.8 µM *in vitro* 8 - 64 µg/ml *in vitro*	[19,48-56]
3.	Narceimine, adlumidine and narlumidine	Anti-inflammatory Antifungal	10 mg/kg, single dose, i.p.	[48,49]
4.	*L*-tetrahydrocoptisine	Neuroleptic Antifungal	50, 100 mg/kg, 7 days, p.o.	[48,57]
5.	Monomethyl fumararte	Hepatoprotective Anti-inflammatory Anti-psoriatic Neuroprotective activity	50 mg/kg, 3 days, p.o. and 10 - 100 µg/ml *in vitro* 200 µM *in vitro*	[33,58-60]
6.	Fumaric acid	Neuroprotective Anti-psoriatic Immunomodulatory Anti-inflammatory	200 µM *in vitro* 95 mg, three times a day, p.o.	[58,59,61, 62]
7.	Fuyuziphine	Antifungal	1250 ppm *in vitro*	[21]
8.	Berberine iodide	Antifungal Antibacterial Antiviral	1.5 g/L *in vitro* 8 - 64 µg/ml *in vitro*	[32,56]
9.	N-octacosanol	Hepatoprotective	100 µg/ml *in vitro*	[63]
10.	Fatty acids	Antioxidant		[64]
11.	Caffeic acid	Anti-inflammatory Antinociceptive		[11]
12.	*β*-sitosterol	Anti-inflammatory Antinociceptive Antipyretic agent		[11]

isolated from opium during 1875, and since then it has been detected in numerous other medicinal plants, including several of them commonly used in TCM (**Table 6** [82-120]). During more recent decades diverse therapeutically interesting pharmacological properties of protopine have been identified, and many analogous activities have also been reported for extracts of diverse other protopine producing plants. One such report dealing with antidepressant like properties of the alkaloid revealed that it is a potent inhibitor of neuronal serotonin and noradrenaline transporter, and does not have any effects on dopamine or GABA transporters [50]. Despite exten-

sive efforts though, no antidepressant like activity of a hydro alcoholic *Fumaria indica* extract could be detected in rodent behavioural models commonly used for detecting such activities of synaptic serotonin and noradrenaline reuptake inhibitors [74]. Since protopine content of the tested extract is not known, no definitive statements on the role of protopine in psychotherapeutic potentially of *Fumaria indica* extracts can yet be made.

However, more recent efforts in our laboratories have revealed diverse therapeutically interesting psychopharmacological activities of hydro alcoholic extracts of *Fumaria indica*. They include their mental stress alleviating

Table 5. Reported pharmacological activities of *Fumaria indica* extracts.

S. No.	Type of extract	Plant part used	Pharmacological activity	Dose, duration and route of administration	References
1.	Aqueous-ethanolic	Whole plant	Anthelmintic	183 mg/kg, 13 days, p.o. 50 - 200 mg/kg, 14 days, p.o. 3.12 - 50 mg/ml *in vitro*	[65,66]
2.	Hydro-alcoholic	Whole plant	Spasmogenic Spasmolytic	1.0 - 5.0 mg/ml *in vitro* 0.1 - 1.0 mg/ml *in vitro*	[67]
3.	Aqueous-ethanolic	Whole plant	Anti-inflammatory and anti-nociceptive	100, 200 and 400 mg/kg, single dose, p.o.	[11]
4.	Aqueous, methanolic, petroleum ether	Whole plant	Hepatoprotective		[68]
5.	Hydro-ethanolic	Whole plant	Hepatoprotective	100 and 400 mg/kg, 7 days, p.o.	[51]
6.	Aqueous-methanolic	Whole plant	Hepatoprotective	500 mg/kg, twice daily for 2 days, p.o.	[69]
7.	Aqueous-methanolic	Whole plant	Potentiation of pentobarbital sleeping	500 mg/kg, single dose, p.o.	[69]
8.	Hydro-ethanolic	Seed	Antibacterial	100 µl *in vitro*	[70]
9.	Aqueous	Whole plant	Anti-hypochlorhydric	20 mg/kg, 14 days, p.o.	[8]
10.	Chloroform-methanolic	Whole plant	Anti-acetylcholinesterase Anti-butyrylcholinesterase	1 mg/ml *in vitro*	[71]
11.	Hydro-alcoholic	Whole plant	Antipyretic		[72]
12.	Aqueous-ethanolic	Whole plant	Hepatoprotective Antioxidant Anti-apoptotic	200 mg/kg, 5 days, p.o.	[73]
13.	Hydro-alcoholic	Whole plant	CNS depressant	100, 200 and 400 mg/kg, 7 days, p.o.	[74]
14.	Hydro-alcoholic	Whole plant	Safety profile: Acute toxicity Sub-chronic toxicity Chronic toxicity Cytotoxicity	1 - 5 g/kg, p.o. 100 - 400 mg/kg, 30 days, p.o. 100 - 400 mg/kg, 30 days, p.o. 50 - 100 µg/ml *in vitro*	[45,75]
15.	Hydro-alcoholic	Whole plant	Anti-stress	100, 200 and 400 mg/kg, 7 days, p.o.	[76]
16.	Hydro-alcoholic	Whole plant	Anti-aggressive	100, 200 and 400 mg/kg, 7 days, p.o.	[77]
17.	Hydro-alcoholic	Whole plant	Anti-anxiety	100, 200 and 400 mg/kg, 7 days, p.o.	[78]
18.	Aqueous-methanolic	Aerial parts	Prokinetic and laxative	30 - 100 mg/kg, single dose, p.o. 0.1 - 5 mg/ml *in vitro*	[20]
19.	Aqueous	Aerial parts	Gastroprotective Cytoprotective Anti-secretory Anti-ulcer Anti-*H. pylori*	100, 200 and 300 mg/kg, single dose, i.g. 100, 200 and 300 mg/kg, single dose, i.p. 0.25 - 1.0 mg/disc *in vitro*	[79]
20.	Aqueous	Whole plant	Dysentery		[80]
21.	Aqueous-ethanolic	Whole plant	Spermatogenesis	250 mg/kg, 5 days, p.o. 750 and 1050 mg/kg, 3 days, p.o.	[81]

[76], anti-aggressive [77], and anxiolytic [74,78] activities. During the course of these studies it became apparent also that the psychopharmacological activity profile

of a given *Fumaria indica* extract depends largely on the functional state of the central nervous system. Thus for example, although no antidepressant like effects of a

Table 6. Some plants known to contain protopine and other *Fumaria* alkaloids.

S. No.	Botenical name	Medicinal uses in Chinese medicine	Reference
1.	*Arctomecon alifornica*	-	[82]
2.	*Argemone Mexicana*	-	[83]
3.	*Aristotelia chilensis*	-	[84]
4.	*Aristolochia constricta*	-	[85]
5.	*Chelidonium majus*	Yes	[86,87]
6.	*Corydalis adunca*	Yes	[88]
7.	*Corydalis bungeana*	Yes	[89]
8.	*Corydalis calliantha*	-	[90]
9.	*Corydalis cava (C. tuberose)*	-	[91]
10.	*Corydalis crispa*	-	[92]
11.	*Corydalis decumbens*	Yes	[93]
12.	*Corydalis intermedia*	-	[94]
13.	*Corydalis marschalliana*	-	[95]
14.	*Corydalis meifolia*	-	[96]
15.	*Corydalis pumilis*	-	[94]
16.	*Corydalis racemose*	Yes	[97]
17.	*Corydalis solida*	-	[94]
18.	*Corydalis speciosa*	-	[98]
19.	*Corydalis tashiroi*	-	[99]
20.	*Corydalis ternate*	-	[100]
21.	*Corydalis thyrsiflora*	-	[101]
22.	*Corydalis yanhusuo*	Yes	[102]
23.	*Dactylicapnos scandens*	Yes	[103]
24.	*Eomecon chionantha*	Yes	[104]
25.	*Eschscholtzia californica*	-	[105]
26.	*Fumaria agrarian*	-	[9]
27.	*Fumaria bastardii*	-	[9]
28.	*Fumaria capreolata*	-	[9]
29.	*Fumaria densiflora*	-	[9]
30.	*Fumaria faurei*	-	[9]
31.	*Fumaria indica*	-	[19]
32.	*Fumaria macrosepala*	-	[9]
33.	*Fumaria officinalis*	-	[106]
34.	*Fumaria parviflora*	-	[107]
35.	*Fumaria petteri*	-	[9]
36.	*Fumaria schrammii*	-	[106]

Continued

37.	*Glaucium flavum*	-	[108]
38.	*Glaucium grandiflorum*	-	[109]
39.	*Glaucium oxylobum*	-	[110]
40.	*Glaucium pulchrum*	-	[111]
41.	*Glaucium vitellinum*	-	[111]
42.	*Hypecoum erectum*	Yes	[112]
43.	*Hypecoum lactiflorum*	Yes	[113]
44.	*Hypecoum leptocarpum*	Yes	[114]
45.	*Macleaya cordata*	Yes	[115]
46.	*Macleaya microcarpa*	Yes	[116]
47.	*Papaver bracteatum*	Yes	[117]
48.	*Papaver coreanum*	-	[118]
49.	*Papaver somniferum*	-	[117]
50.	*Sanguinaria canadensis*	-	[119]
51.	*Thalictrum rugosum*	-	[120]

hydro alcoholic *Fumaria indica* extract were detectable in non-stressed animals [74], such effects of the same extract was apparent in the same tests using mentally stressed animals [76]. It must be mentioned also that anxiolytics like and diverse other psychopharmacological activities of *Fumaria indica* extracts can be observed after their repeated daily doses only, and that their efficacies increase with the number of their daily oral doses administered. These and many other observations made to date with diverse types of *Fumaria indica* extracts and their bioactive constituents clearly reveal that their pharmacological targets and modes of actions are not like those of any known psychoactive drugs and other bioactive agents studied to date. It was only by the use of appropriate holistic psychopharmacological strategy, and proper choices of plant materials and extraction procedures, that these conclusions could be reached with certainty.

7. Concluding Remarks

It cannot be overemphasized that like many other medicinal plants *Fumaria indica* also produces structurally and functionally diverse bioactive secondary plant metabolites, not all of which can be extracted by a single solvent or extraction procedure. Moreover, therapeutically interesting bio-activity profile of a given plant extract is not only a resultant of the combined effects of all bioactive ingredients present in it, but also depends on its treatment regimen used to define its activity profile. Complexities arising from these facts clearly indicate that

translation of traditional knowledge on medicinal uses of *Fumaria indica*, or of any other medicinal plant, in terms of modern medical sciences is possible only when the plant is considered as a whole, and its diverse types of extracts are tested in a battery of therapy relevant animal models. Hereupon, due attention has to be paid to the psychopharmacological activity profiles of the extracts.

It is now well established that all chronic diseases, or illnesses, always causes mental health problems, and that bi-directional interactions between mental health problems and physical health is a common feature of almost all socioeconomically important health problems. Unfortunately, even today, modern medicinal phyto-chemists and pharmacologists pay little attention to these facts and continue to explore traditionally known medicinal plants as sources for structurally and functionally novel therapeutic lead molecules only. Lessons learned and experiences gained from extensive efforts made since decades in our laboratories and elsewhere strongly suggest that *Fumaria indica* could be a valuable tool for identifying novel pharmacological targets and mechanisms potentially useful for achieving better and reproducible successes with phyto-pharmaceuticals containing its extracts as active ingredients. Since *Fumaria indica* is a weed, and holistic pharmacological strategies can easily be practiced in many developing and underdeveloped countries, efforts to better understand and more precisely define its therapeutic potentials can be strongly recommended. Moreover, since the lists of plants producing the same or structurally analogous bioactive secondary metabolites of *Fumaria indica* are long (for example see **Table 6**), know how gained from the efforts to properly decode its pharmacology will certainly be useful for decoding medicinal values of many other as yet underexplored ones. In any case, experiences gained with *Fumaria indica* strongly suggest that repeated oral dose studies with psychoactive alkaloid containing plants could be the more appropriate ones for properly evaluating their psychotherapeutic potentials.

REFERENCES

[1] B. Patwardhan, D. Warude, P. Pushpagandan and N. Bhatt, "Ayurveda and Chinese Medicine: A Comparative Overview," *Evidence-Based Complementary and Alternative Medicine*, Vol. 2, No. 4, 2005, pp. 465-473. doi:10.1093/ecam/neh140

[2] W. C. McClatchey, G. B. Mahady, B. C. Bennett, L. Shiels and V. Savo, "Ethnobotany as a Pharmacological Eesearch Tool and Recent Developments in CNS-Active Natural Products from Ethnobotanical Sources," *Pharmacology and Therapeutics*, Vol. 123, No. 2, 2009, pp. 239-254.

[3] S. S. Chatterjee and V. Kumar, "Holistic Psychopharmacology and Promiscuous Plants and Principles of Ayurveda," *American Journal of Plant Sciences*, Vol. 3, No. 7, 2012, pp. 1015-1021. doi:10.4236/ajps.2012.327120

[4] P. V. Sharma, "Charak Samhita," Chaukhambha Orientalia, Varanasi, 1983.

[5] P. V. Sharma and G. P. Sharma, "Dhanvantari Nighantu," Chaukhambha Orientalia, Varanasi, 2008.

[6] B. Mishra and R. Vaishya, "Bhava Prakasha," Chaukhamba Sanskrit Bhawan, Varanasi, 2003.

[7] S. R. Baquar, "Medicinal and Poisonous Plants of Pakistan," Printas, Karachi, 1989.

[8] U. Mandal, D. K. Nandi, K. Chatterjee, K. M. Ali, A. Biswas and D. Ghosh, "Effect of Different Solvent Extracts of *Fumaria vaillantii* L. on Experimental Hypochlorhydria in Rat," *Asian Journal of Pharmaceutical and Clinical Research*, Vol. 4, No. 1, 2011, pp. 136-141.

[9] R. Suau, B. Cabezudo, R. Rico, F. Najera and J. M. Loppez-Romero, "Direct Determination of Alkaloid Contents in *Fumaria* Species by GC-MS," *Phytochemical Analysis*, Vol. 13, No. 6, 2011, pp. 363-367.

[10] W. Murad, A. Ahmad, S. A. Gilani and M. A. Khan, "Indigenous Knowledge and Folk Use of Medicinal Plants by the Tribal Communities of Hazar Nao Forest, Malakand District, North Pakistan," *Journal of Medicinal Plants Research*, Vol. 5, No. 7, 2011, pp. 1072-1086.

[11] C. V. Rao, A. R. Verma, P. K. Gupta and M. V. Kumar, "Anti-Inflammatory and Anti-Nociceptive Activities of *Fumaria indica* Whole Plant Extract in Experimental Animals," *Acta Pharmaceutica*, Vol. 57, No. 4, 2007, pp. 491-498.

[12] F. E. Araii, M. Keshavarzi, M. Sheidaii and P. Ghadam, "Fruit and Seed Morphology of the *Fumaria* L. Species (Papaveraceae) of Iran," *Turkish Journal of Botany*, Vol. 35, No. 2, 2011, pp. 167-173.

[13] P. C. Gupta, N. Sharma and C. V. Rao, "A Review on Ethnobotany, Phytochemistry and Pharmacology of *Fumaria indica* (Fumitory)," *Asian Pacific Journal of Tropical Biomedicine*, Vol. 2, No. 8, 2012, pp. 665-669.

[14] Anonymous, "The Ayurvedic Pharmacopoeia of India," Government of India Ministry of Health and Family Welfare Department of Ayush, Controller of Publications, New Delhi, 1999.

[15] A. A. Rajopadhya and A. S. Upadhye, "Botanical and Phytochemical Standardization of *Fumaria vaillantii*," *Indian Journal of Natural Products and Resources*, Vol. 2, No. 3, 2011, pp. 369-374.

[16] R. N. Chopra, S. L. Nayar and S. N. Chopra, "Glossary of Indian Medicinal Plants," National Institute of Science Communication and Information Resources (CSIR), New Delhi 1985.

[17] K. R. Kirtikar and B. D. Basu, "Indian Medicinal Plants," Lait Mohan Basu Publishers, Allahabad, 1985.

[18] K. M. Nadkarni, "Indina Materica Medica," Popular Prakashan, Bombay, 1976.

[19] V. B. Pandey, B. Dasgupta, S. K. Bhattacharya, R. Lal and P. K. Das, "Chemistry and Pharmacology of the Major Alkaloid of *Fumaria indica*," *Current Science*, Vol. 40, No. 17, 1971, pp. 455-457.

[20] N. U. Rehman, M. H. Mehmood, A. J. A. Rehaily, R. A. A. Mothana and A. H. Gilani, "Species and Tissue-Specificity of Prokinetic, Laxative and Spasmodic Effects of *Fumaria parviflora*," *BMC Complementary and Alternative Medicine*, Vol. 12, No. 16, 2012. doi:10.1186/1472-6882-12-16

[21] M. B. Pandey, A. K. Singh and U. P. Singh, "Inhibitive Effect of Fuyuziphine Isolated from Plant (Pittapapra) (*Fumaria indica*) on Spore Germination of Some Fungi," *Mycobiology*, Vol. 35, No. 3, 2007, pp. 157-158. doi:10.4489/MYCO.2007.35.3.157

[22] M. B. Pandey, A. K. Singh, J. P. Singh, V. P. Singh and V. B. Pandey, "Fuyuziphine, a New Alkaloid from *Fumaria indica*," *Natural Product Research*, Vol. 22, No. 6, 2008, pp. 533-536. doi:10.1080/14786410701592596

[23] V. K. Tripathi and V. B. Pandey, "Stem Alkaloids of *Fumaria indica*," *Phytochemistry*, Vol. 31, No. 6, 1992, pp. 2188-2189. doi:10.1016/0031-9422(92)80401-Y

[24] V. B. Pandey, A. B. Ray and B. Dasgupta, "Minor Alkaloids of *Fumaria indica* Seeds," *Phytochemistry*, Vol. 18, No. 4, 1979, pp. 695-696. doi:10.1016/S0031-9422(00)84306-X

[25] V. B. Pandey, A. B. Ray and B. Dasgupta, "Quaternary Alkaloids of *Fumaria indica*," *Phytochemistry*, Vol. 15, No. 4, 1976, pp. 545-546. doi:10.1016/S0031-9422(00)88969-4

[26] Y. C. Tripathi, V. B. Pandey, N. K. R. Pathak and M. Biswas, "A Seco-Pthalideisoquinoline Alkaloid from *Fumaria indica* Seeds," *Phytochemistry*, Vol. 27, No. 6, 1988, pp. 1918-1919. doi:10.1016/0031-9422(88)80485-0

[27] B. Dasgupta, K. K. Seth, V. B. Pandey and A. B. Ray, "Alkaloids of *Fumaria indica*: Further Studies on Narceimine and Narlumidine," *Planta Medica*, Vol. 50, No. 6, 1984, pp. 481-485. doi:10.1055/s-2007-969778

[28] A. U. Rahman, M. K. Bhatti and M. I. Choudhary, "Che-

mical Constituent of *Fumaria indica*," *Fitoterapia*, Vol. 63, No. 2, 1992, pp. 129-135.

[29] A. U. Rahman, M. K. Bhatti, H. Ahmed, H. U. Rehman and D. S. Rycroft, "A New Isoquinoline Alkaloid Papraine from *Fumaria indica*," *Heterocycles*, Vol. 29, No. 6, 1989, pp. 1091-1095. doi:10.3987/COM-89-4856

[30] A. U. Rahman, S. S. Ali, M. M. Qureshi, S. Hasan and M. K. Bhatti, "Fumarizine—A New Benzylisoquinoline Alkaloid from *Fumaria indica*," *Fitoterapia*, Vol. 60, No. 6, 1989, pp. 552-553.

[31] A. U. Rahman, M. K. Bhatti, M. I. Choudhary and S. K. Ahmad, "Alkaloidal Constituent of *Fumaria indica*," *Phytochemistry*, Vol. 40, No. 2, 1995, pp. 593-596. doi:10.1016/0031-9422(95)00038-9

[32] B. K. Sarma, V. B. Pandey, G. D. Mishra and U. P. Singh, "Antifungal Activity of Berberine Iodide, a Constituent of *Fumaria indica*," *Folia Microbiologica*, Vol. 44, No. 2, 1999, pp. 164-166. doi:10.1007/BF02816235

[33] K. S. Rao and S. H. Mishra, "Antihepatotoxic Activity of Monomethyl Fumarate Isolated from *Fumaria indica*," *Journal of Ethnopharmacology*, Vol. 60, No. 3, 1998, pp. 207-213. doi:10.1016/S0378-8741(97)00149-9

[34] J. Dostal, "Two Faces of Alkaloids," *Journal of Chemical Education*, Vol. 77, No. 8, 2000, pp. 993-998. doi:10.1021/ed077p993

[35] Y. C. Tripathi, M. Rathore and H. Kumar, "On the Variation of Alkaloidal Contents of *Fumaria indica* at Different Stages of Life Span," *Ancient Science of Life*, Vol. 13, No. 3-4, 1993, pp. 271-273.

[36] L. D. Kapoor, "Handbook of Ayurvedic Medicinal Plants," CRC Press, Boca Raton, 1990.

[37] K. Usmanghani, A. Saeed and M. T. Alam, "Indusyunic Medicine," University of Karachi Press, Karachi, 1997.

[38] J. A. Duke, M. J. Bogenschutz-Godwin, J. Ducelliar and P. K. Duke, "Handbook of Medicinal Herbs," 2nd Edition, CRC Press, Boca Raton, 2002. doi:10.1201/9781420040463

[39] I. U. Haq and M. Hussain, "Medicinal Plants of Mansehra," *Hamdard Medicus*, Vol. 36, No. 3, 1993, pp. 78-79.

[40] P. K. Singh, V. Kumar, R. K. Tiwari, A. Sharma, C. V. Rao and R. H. Singh, "Medico-Ethnobotany of 'Chatara' Block of District Sonebhadra, Uttar Pradesh, India," *Advances in Biological Research*, Vol. 4, No. 1, 2010, pp. 65-80.

[41] B. Uniyal and V. Shiva, "Traditional Knowledge on Medicinal Plants among Rural Women of the Garhwal Himalaya, Uttaranchal," *Indian Journal of Taridtional Knowledge*, Vol. 4, No. 3, 2005, pp. 259-266. doi:10.1055/s-2007-969166

[42] S. Z. Husain, R. N. Malik, M. Javaid and S. Bibi, "Ethonobotanical Properties and Uses of Medicinal Plants of Morgah Biodiversity Park, Rawalpindi," *Pakistan Journal of Botany*, Vol. 40, No. 5, 2008, pp. 1897-1911.

[43] R. Qureshi, A. Waheed, M. Arshad and T. Umbreen, "Medico-Ethnobotanical Inventory of Tehsil Chakwal, Pakistan," *Pakistan Journal of Botany*, Vol. 41, No. 2, 2009, pp. 529-538.

[44] M. Ahmad, R. Qureshi, M. Arshad, M. A. Khan and M.

Zafar, "Traditional Herbal Remedies Used for the Treatment of Diabetes from District Attock (Pakistan)," *Pakistan Journal of Botany*, Vol. 41, No. 6, 2009, pp. 2777-2782.

[45] G. K. Singh and V. Kumar, "Acute and Sub-Chronic Toxicity Study of Standardized Extract of *Fumaria indica* in Rodents," *Journal of Ethnopharmacology*, Vol. 134, No. 3, 2011, pp. 992-995.

[46] A. Jamal, A. Siddiqi and S. M. Ali, "Home Remedies for Skin Care in Unani System of Medicine," *Natural Product Radiance*, Vol. 4, No. 4, 2005, pp. 339-340.

[47] A. Kumar, V. B. Pandey, K. K. Seth, B. Dasgupta and S. K. Bhattacharya, "Pharmacological Actions of Fumariline Isolated from *Fumaria indica* Seeds," *Planta Medica*, Vol. 52, No. 4, 1986, pp. 324-325.

[48] R. A. Singh, U. P. Singh, V. K. Tripathi, R. Roy and V. B. Pandey, "Effect of *Fumaria indica* Alkaloids on Conidial Germination of Some Fungi," *Oriental Journal of Chemistry*, Vol. 13, No. 2, 1997, pp. 177-180.

[49] Y. C. Tripathi and R. K. Dwivedi, "Central Nervous System and Anti-Infammatory Activities of Alkaloid of *Fumaria indica*," *Natural Academy Science Letters*, Vol. 13, No. 6, 1990, pp. 231-233.

[50] L. F. Xu, W. J. Chu, X. Y. Qing, S. Li, X. S. Wang, G. W. Qing, J. Fei and L. H. Guo, "Protopine Inhibits Serotonin Transporter and Noradrenaline Transporter and Has the Antidepressant-Like Effect in Mice Models," *Neuropharmacology*, Vol. 50, No. 8, 2006, pp. 934-940.

[51] A. Rathi, A. K. Srivastava, A. Shirwaikar, A. K. S. Rawat and S. Mehrotra, "Hepatoprotective Potential of *Fumaria indica* Pugsley Whole Plant Extracts, Fractions and an Isolated Alkaloid Protopine," *Phytomedicine*, Vol. 15, No. 6-7, 2008, pp. 470-477.

[52] Y. H. Huang, Z. Z. Zhang and J. X. Jiang, "Relaxant Effects of Protopine on Smooth Muscles," *Zhongguo Yao Li Xue Bao*, Vol. 12, No. 1, 1991, pp. 16-19.

[53] S. A. Saeed, A. H. Gilani, R. U. Majoo and B. H. Shah, "Anti-Thrombotic and Anti-Inflammatory Activities of Protopine," *Pharmacological Research*, Vol. 36, No. 1, 1997, pp. 1-7. doi:10.1006/phrs.1997.0195

[54] Q. Xu, R. L. Jin and Y. Y. Wu, "Opioid, Calcium, and Adrenergic Receptor Involvement in Protopine Analgesia," *Acta Pharmaceutica Sinica*, Vol. 14, No. 6, 1993, pp. 495-500.

[55] B. Sener and I. Orphan, "Molecular Diversity in the Bioactive Compounds from Turkish Plants—Evaluation of Acetylcholinesterase Inhibitory Activity of *Fumaria* Species," *Journal of the Chemical Society of Pakistan*, Vol. 26, No. 3, 2004, pp. 313-315.

[56] I. Orhan, B. Ozçelik, T. Karaoglu and B. Sener, "Antiviral and Antimicrobial Profiles of Selected Isoquinoline Alkaloids from *Fumaria* and *Corydalis* Species," *Zeitschrift für Naturforschung C*, Vol. 62, No. 1-2, 2007, pp. 19-26.

[57] V. K. Tripathi and V. B. Pandey, "Stem Alkaloids of *Fumaria indica* and Their Biological Activity," *Planta Medica*, Vol. 58, No. S7, 1992, pp. 651-652.

[58] R. De Jong, A. C. Bezemer, T. P. Zomerdijk, P. K. T.

Vande, T. H. Ottenhoff and P. H. Nibbering, "Selective Stimulation of T Helper 2 Cytokine Responses by the Anti-Psoriasis Agent Monomethyl Fumarate," *European Journal of Immunology*, Vol. 26, No. 9, 1996, pp. 2067-2074.

[59] D. H. Lee, R. A. Linker, M. Stangel and R. Gold, "Fumarate for the Treatment of Multiple Sclerosis: Potential Mechanism of Action and Clinical Studies," *Expert Review of Neurotherapeutics*, Vol. 8, No. 11, 2008, pp. 1683-1690. doi:10.1586/14737175.8.11.1683

[60] M. Lukashev, W. Zeng, S. Goelz, R. Linker and R. Gold, "Activation of Nrf2 and Modulation of Disease Progression in EAE Models by BG00012 (Dimethyl fumarate) Suggests a Novel Mechanism of Action Combining Anti-inflammatory and Neuroprotective M. S. Modalities," *Multiple Sclerosis*, Vol. 13, No. S2, 2007, p. S149.

[61] U. Mrowietz and K. Asadullah, "Dimethyl fumarate for Psoriasis: More than a Dietary Curiosity," *Trends in Molecular Biology*, Vol. 11, No. 1, 2007, pp. 43-48.

[62] S. Schilling, S. Goelz, R. Linker, F. Luehder and R. Gold, "Fumaric Acid Esters Are Effective in Chronic Experimental Autoimmune Encephalomyelitis and Suppress Macrophage Infiltration," *Clinical and Experimental Immunology*, Vol. 145, No. 1, 2006, pp. 101-107.

[63] I. E. Orhan, B. Sener and S. G. Musharraf, "Antioxidant and Hepatoprotective Activity Appraisal of Four Selected *Fumaria* Species and Their Total Phenol and Flavonoids Quantities," *Experimental and Toxicologic Pathology*, Vol. 64, No. 3, 2012, pp. 205-209. doi:10.1016/j.etp.2010.08.007

[64] F. H. Tirtash, M. Keshavarzi and F. Fazeli, "Antioxidant Components of *Fumaria* Species (Papaveraceae)," *World Academy of Science, Engineering and Technology*, Vol. 50, No. 2, 2011, pp. 233-236.

[65] P. Hordegen, H. Hertzberg, J. Heilmann, W. Langhans and V. Maurer, "The Anthelmintic Efficacy of Five Plant Products against Gastrointestinaltrichostrongylids in Artificially Infected Lambs," *Veterin Parasitology*, Vol. 117, No. 1-2, 2003, pp. 51-60.

[66] I. R. M. Al-Shaibani, M. S. Phulan and M. Shiekh, "Anthelmintic Activity of *Fumaria parviflora* (Fumariaceae) against Gastrointestinal Nematodes of Sheep," *International Journal of Agriculture and Biology*, Vol. 11, No. 4, 2009, pp. 431-436.

[67] A. H. Gilani, S. Bashir, K. H. Janbaz and A. Khan, "Pharmacological Basis for the Use of *Fumaria indica* in Constipation and Diarrhoea," *Journal of Ethnopharmacology*, Vol. 96, No. 3, 2005, pp. 585-589. doi:10.1016/j.jep.2004.10.010

[68] S. R. Kurma and S. H. Mishra, "Hepatoprotective Activity of the Whole Plant of *Fumaria indica*," *Indian Journal of Pharmaceutical Sciences*, Vol. 59, No. 4, 1997, pp. 165-170.

[69] A. H. Gilani, K. H. Janbaz and M. S. Akhtar, "Selective Protective Effect of an Extract from *Fumaria parviflora* on Paracetamol-Induced Hepatotoxicity," *General Pharmacology*, Vol. 27, No. 6, 1996, pp. 979-983. doi:10.1016/0306-3623(95)02140-X

[70] J. Parekh and S. Chanda, "*In Vitro* Screening of Antibac-terial Activity of Aqueous and Alcoholic Extracts of Various Indian Plant Species against Selected Pathogens from Enterobacteriaceae," *African Journal of Microbiology Research*, Vol. 1, No. 6, 2007, pp. 92-99.

[71] I. Orhan, B. Sener, M. I. Choudhary and A. Khalid, "Acetylcholinesterase and Butyrylcholinesterase Inhibitory Activity of Some Turkish Medicinal Plants," *Journal of Ethnopharmacology*, Vol. 91, No. 1, 2004, pp. 57-60. doi:10.1016/j.jep.2003.11.016

[72] S. G. Khattak, S. N. Gilani and M. Ikram, "Antipyretic Studies on Some Indigenous Pakistani Medicinal Plants," *Journal of Ethnopharmacology*, Vol. 14, No. 1, 1985, pp. 45-51. doi:10.1016/0378-8741(85)90027-3

[73] M. Tripathi, B. K. Singh, S. Raisuddin and P. Kakkar, "Abrogation of Nimesulide Induced Oxidative Stress and Mitochondria Mediated Apoptosis by *Fumaria parviflora* Lam Extract," *Journal of Ethnopharmacology*, Vol. 136, No. 1, 2011, pp. 94-102. doi:10.1016/j.jep.2011.04.014

[74] G. K. Singh and V. Kumar, "Neuropharmacological Screening and Lack of Antidepressant Activity of Standardized Extract of *Fumaria indica*: A Preclinical Study," *Electronic Journal of Pharmacology and Therapy*, Vol. 3, No. 5, 2010, pp. 19-28.

[75] G. K. Singh, S. K. Chauhan, G. Rai and V. Kumar, "*Fumaria indica* Is Safe during Chronic Toxicity and Cytotoxicity: A Preclinical Study," *Journal of Pharmacology and Pharmacotherapeutics*, Vol. 2, No. 3, 2011, pp. 191-192. doi:10.4103/0976-500X.83287

[76] G. K. Singh, G. Rai, S. S. Chatterjee and V. Kumar, "Beneficial Effects of *Fumaria indica* on Chronic Stress-Induced Neurobehavioral and Biochemical Perturbations in Rats," *Chinese Medicine*, Vol. 3, No. 1, 2012, pp. 49-60.

[77] G. K. Singh, G. Rai, S. S. Chatterjee and V. Kumar, "Anti-Aggressive, Brain Neurotransmitters and Receptor Binding Study of *Fumaria indica* in Rodents," *Current Psychopharmacology*, Vol. 1, No. 3, 2012, pp. 195-202. doi:10.2174/2211556011201030195

[78] G. K. Singh, G. Rai, S. S. Chatterjee and V. Kumar, "Potential Antianxiety Activity of Fumaria *indica*: A Preclinical Study," *Pharmacognosy Magazine*, 2012.

[79] Rifat-uz-Zaman and Attiq-ur-Rehman, "Anti-*Helicobacter pylori* and Protective Effects of Aqueous *Fumaria vaillantii* L. Extract in Pylorus-Ligated, Indomethacin- and Toxic-Induced Ulcers in Rats," *African Journal of Pharmacy and Pharmacology*, Vol. 4, No. 5, 2010, pp. 256-262.

[80] S. Mitra and S. K. Mukherjee, "Ethnomedicinal Usages of Some Wild Plants of North Bengal Plain for Gastro-Intestinal Problems," *Indian Journal of Traditional Knowledge*, Vol. 9, No. 4, 2010, pp. 705-712.

[81] M. H. Nasrabadi, H. Aboutalebi and M. Naseri, "Effect of *Fumaria parviflora* Alcoholic Extract on Male Rat's Reproductive System," *Journal of Medicinal Plants Research*, Vol. 6, No. 10, 2012, pp. 2004-2010.

[82] F. R. Stermitz and V. P. Muralidharan, "Alkaloids of the Papaveraceae. VI. Protopine and Allocryptopine from *Arctomecon alifornica*," *Journal of Pharmaceutical Sciences*, Vol. 56, No. 6, 1967, p. 762. doi:10.1002/jps.2600560625

[83] A. Capasso, S. Piacente, C. Pizza, N. De Tommasi, C. Jativa and L. Sorrentino, "Isoquinoline Alkaloids from *Argemone mexicana* Reduce Morphine Withdrawal in Guinea Pig Isolated Ileum," *Planta Medica*, Vol. 63, No. 4, 1997, pp. 326-328. doi:10.1055/s-2006-957693

[84] O. Munoz, P. Christen, S. Cretton, N. Backhouse, V. Torres, O. Correa, E. Costa, H. Miranda and C. Delporte, "Chemical Study and Anti-Inflammatory, Analgesic and Antioxidant Activities of the Leaves of *Aristotelia chilensis* (Mol.) Stuntz, Elaeocarpaceae," *Journal of Pharmacy and Pharmacology*, Vol. 63, No. 6, 2011, pp. 849-859. doi:10.1111/j.2042-7158.2011.01280.x

[85] L. Rastrelli, A. Capasso, C. Pizza, N. De Tommasi and L. Sorrentino, "New Protopine and Benzyltetrahydroprotoberberine Alkaloids from *Aristolochia constricta* and their Activity on Isolated Guinea-Pig Ileum," *Journal of Natural Products*, Vol. 60, No. 11, 1997, pp. 1065-1069. doi:10.1021/np960710b

[86] J. E. Park, T. D. Cuong, T. M. Hung, I. Lee, M. Na, J. C. Kim, S. Ryoo, J. H. Lee, J. S. Choi, M. H. Woo and B. S. Min, "Alkaloids from *Chelidonium majus* and Their Inhibitory Effects on LPS-Induced NO Production in RAW264.7 Cells," *Bioorganic and Medicinal Chemistry Letters*, Vol. 21, No. 23, 2011, pp. 6960-6963. doi:10.1016/j.bmcl.2011.09.128

[87] M. Gilca, L. Gaman, E. Panait, I. Stoian and V. Atanasiu, "*Chelidonium majus*—An Integrative Review: Traditional Knowledge versus Modern Findings," *Forsch Complemented*, Vol. 17, No. 5, 2010, pp. 241-248. doi:10.1159/000321397

[88] Y. L. Tang, A. M. Yang, Y. S. Zhang and H. Q. Wang, "Studies on the Alkaloids from the Herb of *Corydalis adunca*," *Zhongguo Zhong Yao Za Zhi*, Vol. 30, No. 3, 2005, pp. 195-197.

[89] L. Y. He and Y. B. Zhang, "TLC Separation and Densitometric Determination of Six Isoquinoline Alkaloids in *Corydalis bungeana*," *Yao Xue Xue Bao*, Vol. 20, No. 5, 1985, pp. 377-382.

[90] P. Wangchuk, J. B. Bremner, S. R. Rattanajak and S. Kamchonwongpaisan, "Antiplasmodial Agents from the Bhutanese Medicinal Plant *Corydalis calliantha*," *Phytotherapy Research*, Vol. 24, No. 4, 2010, pp. 481-485. doi:10.1002/ptr.2893

[91] V. Preininger, R. S. Thakur and F. Santavy, "Isolation and Chemistry of Alkaloids from Plants of the Family Papaveraceae LXVII: *Corydalis cava* (L.) Sch. et K. (*C. tuberosa* DC)," *Journal of Pharmaceutical Sciences*, Vol. 65, No. 2, 1976, pp. 294-296. doi:10.1002/jps.2600650230

[92] P. Wangchuk, P. A. Keller, S. G. Pyne, M. Taweechotipatr, R. Rattanajak, A. Tonsomboon and S. Kamchonwongpaisan, "Phytochemical and Biological Activity Studies of the Bhutanese Medicinal Plant *Corydalis crispa*," *Natural Product Communication*, Vol. 7, No. 5, 2012, pp. 575-580.

[93] Y. Shen, C. Han, B. Xia, Y. Zhou, C. Liu and A. Liu, "Determination of Four Alkaloids in *Corydalis decumbens* by HPLC," *Zhongguo Zhong Yao Za Zhi*, Vol. 36, No. 15, 2011, pp. 2110-2112.

[94] S. Sturm, C. Seger, M. Godejohann, M. Spraul and H. Stuppner, "Conventional Sample Enrichment Strategies Combined with High-Performance Liquid Chromatography-Solid Phase Extraction-Nuclear Magnetic Resonance Analysis Allows Analyte Identification from a Single Minuscule *Corydalis solida* Plant Tuber," *Journal of Chromatography*, Vol. 1163, No. 1-2, 2007, pp. 138-144. doi:10.1016/j.chroma.2007.06.029

[95] H. G. Kiryakov, E. Iskrenova, B. Kuzmanov and L. Evstatieva, "Alkaloids from *Corydalis marschalliana*," *Planta Medica*, Vol. 41, No. 3, 1981, pp. 298-302. doi:10.1055/s-2007-971718

[96] D. S. Bhakuni and R. Chaturvedi, "The Alkaloids of *Corydalis meifolia*," *Journal of Natural Products*, Vol. 46, No. 3, 1983, pp. 320-324. doi:10.1021/np50027a004

[97] X. Jiang, J. Ye, J. Zeng, X. Zou and J. Wu, "Determination of Protopine in *Corydalis racemose* by HPLC," *Zhongguo Zhong Yao Za Zhi*, Vol. 35, No. 17, 2010, pp. 2315-2317.

[98] D. K. Kim, K. T. Lee, N. I. Baek, S. H. Kim, H. W. Park, J. P. Lim, T. Y. Shin, D. O. Eom, J. H. Yang and J. S. Eun, "Acetylcholinesterase Inhibitors from the Aerial Parts of *Corydalis speciosa*," *Archives of Pharmacal Research*, Vol. 27, No. 11, 2004, pp. 1127-1131. doi:10.1007/BF02975117

[99] J. J. Chen, Y. L. Chang, C. M. Teng, W. Y. Lin, Y. C. Chen and I. S. Chen, "A New Tetrahydroprotoberberine N-Oxide Alkaloid and Anti-Platelet Aggregation Constituents of *Corydalis tashiroi*," *Planta Medica*, Vol. 67, No. 5, 2001, pp. 423-427. doi:10.1055/s-2001-15820

[100] S. R. Kim, S. Y. Hwang, Y. P. Jang, M. J. Park, G. J. Markelonis, T. H. Oh and Y. C. Kim, "Protopine from *Corydalis ternata* Has Anticholinesterase and Antiamnesic Activities," *Planta Medica*, Vol. 65, No. 3, 1999, pp. 218-221. doi:10.1055/s-1999-13983

[101] Y. W. Li and Q. C. Fang, "Isoquinoline Alkaloids from *Corydalis thyrsiflora* Prain," *Yao Xue Xue Bao*, Vol. 26, No. 4, 1991, pp. 303-306.

[102] Z. Lu, W. Sun, X. Duan, Z. Yang, Y. Liu and P. Tu, "Chemical Constituents from *Corydalis yanhusuo*," *Zhongguo Zhong Yao Za Zhi*, Vol. 37, No. 2, 2012, pp. 235-237.

[103] X. Wang, H. Dong, B. Yang, D. Liu, W. Duan and L. Huang, "Preparative Isolation of Alkaloids from *Dactylicapnos scandens* Using pH-Zone-Refining Counter-Current Chromatography by Changing the Length of the Separation Column," *Journal of Chromatography B, Analytical Technologies in the Biomedical and Life Sciences*, Vol. 879, No. 31, 2011, pp. 3767-3770. doi:10.1016/j.jchromb.2011.10.013

[104] F. Du, S. Wang and Z. Xie, "Concentration of Four Alkaloids in the Aerial Parts of *Eomecon chionantha* from Different Month in Year," *Zhong Yao Cai*, Vol. 23, No. 4, 2000, pp. 189-190.

[105] T. Tanahashi and M. H. Zenk, "New Hydroxylated Benzo[c] Phenanthridine Alkaloids from *Eschscholtzia californica* Cell Suspension Cultures," *Journal of Natural Products*, Vol. 53, No. 3, 1990, pp. 579-586. doi:10.1021/np50069a007

[106] J. Vrba, E. Vrublova, M. Modriansky and J. Ulrichova,

"Protopine and Allocryptopine Increase mRNA Levels of Cytochromes P450 1A in Human Hepatocytes and HepG2 Cells Independently of AhR," *Toxicology Letters*, Vol. 203, No. 2, 2011, pp. 135-141. doi:10.1016/j.toxlet.2011.03.015

[107] I. Valka, D. Walterova, M. E. Popova, V. Preininger and V. Simanek, "Separation and Quantification of Some Alkaloids from *Fumaria parviflora* by Capillary Isotachophoresis1," *Planta Medica*, Vol. 51, No. 4, 1985, pp. 319-322. doi:10.1055/s-2007-969501

[108] A. Shafiee, I. Lalezari, S. Lajevardi and F. Khalafi, "Alkaloids of *Glaucium flavum* Grantz, Populations Isfahan and Kazerun," *Journal of Pharmaceutical Sciences*, Vol. 66, No. 6, 1977, pp. 873-874. doi:10.1002/jps.2600660636

[109] T. Gozler, "Alkaloids of Turkish *Glaucium* Species," *Planta Medica*, Vol. 46, No. 3, 1982, pp. 179-180. doi:10.1055/s-2007-971209

[110] A. Shafiee, I. Lalezari and M. Mahjour, "Alkaloids of *Glaucium oxylobum* Boiss and Buhse, Population Ab-Ali," *Journal of Pharmaceutical Sciences*, Vol. 66, No. 4, 1977, pp. 593-594. doi:10.1002/jps.2600660437

[111] A. Shafiee, I. Lalezari and O. Rahimi, "Alkaloids of Papaver Genus IX. Alkaloids of *Glaucium vitellinum* Boiss and Buhse, Population Seerjan and *Glaucium pulchrum* Stapf, Population Elika," *Lloydia*, Vol. 40, No. 4, 1977, pp. 352-355.

[112] D. S. Bae, Y. H. Kim, C. H. Pan, C. W. Nho, J. Samdan, J. Yansan and J. K. Lee, "Protopine Reduces the Inflammatory Activity of Lipopolysaccharide-Stimulated Murine Macrophages," *Journal of Biochemistry and Molecular Biology*, Vol. 45, No. 2, 2012, pp. 108-113.

[113] S. Philipov, R. Istatkova, P. Denkova, S. Dangaa, J. Samdan, M. Krosnova and C. Munkh-Amgalan, "Alkaloids from Mongolian Species *Hypecoum lactiflorum* Kar. et Kir. Pazij," *Natural Product Research*, Vol. 23, No. 11, 2009, pp. 982-987. doi:10.1080/14786410802133878

[114] B. Z. Chen and Q. C. Fang, "Chemical Study on a Traditional Tibetan Drug *Hypecoum leptocarpum*," *Yao Xue Xue Bao*, Vol. 20, No. 9, 1985, pp. 658-661.

[115] P. Kosina, J. Gregorova, J. Gruz, J. Vacek, M. Kolar, M. Vogel, W. Roos, K. Naumann, V. Simanek and J. Ulrichova, "Phytochemical and Antimicrobial Characterization of *Macleaya cordata* Herb," *Fitoterapia*, Vol. 81, No. 8, 2010, pp. 1006-1012. doi:10.1016/j.fitote.2010.06.020

[116] K. Pencikova, J. Urbanova, P. Musil, E. Taborska and J. Gregorova, "Seasonal Variation of Bioactive Alkaloid Contents in *Macleaya microcarpa* (Maxim.) Fedde," *Molecules*, Vol. 16, No. 4, 2011, pp. 3391-3401. doi:10.3390/molecules16043391

[117] P. G. Vincent and B. F. Engelke, "High Pressure Liquid Chromatographic Determination of the Five Major Alkaloids in *Papaver somniferum* L. and Thebaine in *Papaver bracteatum* Lindl. Capsular Tissue," *Journal-Association of Official Analytical Chemists*, Vol. 62, No. 2, 1979, pp. 310-314.

[118] D. U. Lee, J. H. Park, L. Wessjohann and J. Schmidt, "Alkaloids from *Papaver coreanum*," *Natural Product Communication*, Vol. 6, No. 11, 2011, pp. 1593-1594.

[119] M. Bambagiotti-Alberti, S. Pinzauti, G. Moneti, P. Gratteri, S. A. Coran and F. F. Vincieri, "Characterization of *Sanguinaria canadensis* L. Fluid Extract by FAB Mass Spectrometry," *Journal of Pharmaceutical and Biomedical Analysis*, Vol. 9, No. 10-12, 1991, pp. 1083-1087. doi:10.1016/0731-7085(91)80048-E

[120] W. N. Wu, J. L. Beal, G. W. Clark and L. A. Mitscher, "Antimicrobial Agents from Higher Plants. Additional Alkaloids and Antimicrobial Agents from *Thalictrum rugosum*," *Lloydia*, Vol. 39, No. 1, 1976, pp. 65-75.

3

Health Problem and Occupational Stress among Chinese Doctors

Xiaojun Chen[1,2], Xuerui Tan[1], Liping Li[2*]

[1]Department of Cardiovascular Diseases, The First Affiliated Hospital of Shantou University
Medical College, Shantou, China
[2]Injury Prevention Research Center, Shantou University Medical College, Shantou, China
Email: *lpli@stu.edu.cn

ABSTRACT

This paper provides an overview of research into mental health problem and occupational stress among Chinese doctors in recent 10 years. It indicates that doctors in general hospitals have worse mental status. Occupational stress comes from over workload, high demanding from patients, occupational risk, effort-reward imbalance and fierce competition for job promotion. For medical staffs battling against severe acute respiratory syndrome (SARS), or working in catastrophic Wenchuan earthquake-affected areas, they have elevated stress and worrying levels of psychological distress. Post-traumatic stress disorder (PTSD) is a common mental health problem among them. The most common diseases the Chinese doctors usually suffered were cervical spondylosis, hyperlipidemia, hypertension, fatty liver and hyperglycemia. It could be important for health administrators to note that mental health appears to be an increasing problem in Chinese doctors and corresponding helping measure should be made.

Keywords: Mental Health; Stress; Doctors; Physical Health; China

1. Introduction

China is a country with the largest population in the world. The rapid economic growth in this developing country gives rise to many social problems. Mental health is one of them but the research on individual behavior and psychology start late and behind. A study in China had found that there were serious mental health problems in the occupational population in China [1]. Doctor is an occupation coping with the cure of patients and directly confronts severe illness and death. The huge population base in China results in an increasing number of patients. These facts seem to aggravate the occupational stress of Chinese doctors. The ratio of doctors to general population in China is 1:735, considerably lower than that in western countries (1:280 - 1:640) [2]. Large population basis, increasing health consciousness and overload working have made doctors exhausted with dealing with patients. Consequently, they find it very difficult to give enough care and time in explanation to patients, then it may easily leads to a tensional doctor-patient relationship, which aggravates the pressure and mental health among doctors [3]. However, few studies have been concentrated on the assessment of mental health and its related factors among Chinese doctors.

Only several related research on nurses in English version can be found. Therefore, an updated English review of studies in Chinese doctor is expected to put it in the research of international literatures on mental health. This article summarized the published studies on mental health in Chinese doctor. It presents studies of doctors' health problems, in particular mental health problems and occupational stress studies. In conclusion information is given about the intervention suggestion.

2. Methods

This literature review using PubMed database and Chinese journal database searched with key words "doctor" "physician" and "medical staff". From retrieved article the relevant keywords "mental health", "mental disorder", "psychological problem" were identified and researched. Publications from the past 20 years were included with priority given to studies in recent 10 years. Literatures must be representative, concerning doctor's well-being, mental status, health-related behavior, working pressure and ways of relaxation. Studies on medical students or nurses were not included. **Table 1** gives an overview of the selected studies between 2001 and 2011 published in Chinese medical journals. We lack an updated review in English of the contribution from this research programme.

---

*Corresponding author.

3. Results

There were 73 references located including investigation and review, of which 32 belong to epidemiological survey of mental health problems in medical staff. The rest of them excluded were viewpoints, ideas, proposal of helping measures. **Table 1** lists the studies on mental health in doctor in Chinese medical institutions from year 2001 to 2011. There were several investigation sample exceed 1000 with the majority were between 100 - 300 interviewers. Most of them were investigating with

Table 1. Studies on mental health among chinese doctors 2001-2011.

Year	Sample (N)	Measures	Major finding and conclusions
2011	Case = 257 Control = 300	SAS, SDS, SCL-90	Mental health of case group was worse than the control group
2011	1208	SCL-90	Scores of all items for doctors in rural area were higher than Chinese norm
2011	114	SCL-90	Harmonious doctor-patient's relationship was good for mental health of medical staff
2011	368	SCL-90	Continuing physiological education for doctors was imminent as their mental health was decreasing.
2010	225	SCL-90	Score of major items for doctor in rural area were higher than Chinese norm. Doctor's mental health should receive enough attention
2010	239	SCL-90	Mental health of doctor in general dept. were obviously lower than ordinary people
2010	213	SCL-90	Mental health of community doctors were relatively better
2010	102	SCL-90, SCSQ	Mental health of psychiatrist were poorer than national level
2010	109	SCL-90	Mental health of doctor was similar to ordinary population
2010	200	SCL-90	Major factors influencing doctor's mental health were high working pressure, low salary and job dissatisfaction
2009	267	SCL-90	Overall mental health of doctor was good
2009	1763	SCL-90	More than one third of the medical staffs are in a constant mental string state of depression, compulsion and anxiety.
2009	500	PCL-C, SAS, SDS	Provenance of PTSD, anxiety and depression for medical personnel involved in rescue working were still high one year after earthquake
2009	130	HAMA	1 year after disaster rescuing work, depression and anxiety of doctors were higher than before. Social support was limited.
2009	262	SCL-90	Different level of mental disorder existed in medical staff
2009	481	PTSD, SDS, SAS	The prevalence of PTSD, SAS, and SDS within medical staffs who took part in rescue in the disaster area after Wenchuan Earthquake was higher than in the non-disaster area.
2008	543	MBI-GS	The main significant predictors of exhaustion were role overload, responsibility, physical environment and self care.
2008	1418	SCL-90	Score of medical practitioner in general hospital were better than national norm. Health of male staff was better than females.
2008	405	SCL-90	Appearances of psychological problems of different nationality were different.
2008	159	SCL-90, SAS	Scores of mental health for psychiatrist were higher than Chinese norm
2007	176	SCL-90	Overall mental health of medical staffs in township hospitals were good
2007	116	SCL-90	Occupational risk factors have long-term negative effect on mental health of medical staff in dept. of infectious disease. Intervention was necessary.
2006	126	SCL-90	Mental health of clinical practitioners was worse than Chinese norm.
2006	328	SCL-90	there are significant mental health problems especially emergency department and the surgeons in general hospital doctors
2006	282	SCL-90, SCSQ	Psychological health status of doctors was similar to Chinese norm. Gender, professional titles were related.
2005	198	SCL-90, SCSQ	Active and passive measure coping with depression were helping factors in mental health
2005	133	GHQ-12, EPQ-RSC	Personality character was an influencing factor in doctor's mental health
2004	106	SCL-90	Physiological health surveillance should be done in medical staff after outbreak of SARS
2004	201	SCL-90	Mental health scores of doctors dealing with SARS were significantly higher than Chinese norm
2003	316	SCL-90	Mental health was good in community medical workers
2002	486	SCL-90	Education of psychological promotion combined with ideological and political education could strengthen mental health of young doctors

Symptom Checklist-90 (SCL-90) Chinese version and not all of the conclusions were inconsistence.

3.1. General Mental Health among Doctors

Doctor in general hospitals have worse mental status as most of their scores were higher than the Chinese norm, especially those worked in the departments of surgery, emergency and infectious disease [4,5]. The scores of somatization, interpersonal sensitivity, depression, anxiety, hostility, and paranoid ideation were significantly higher in male than female doctors [6]. Total scores of clinical doctors were significantly higher than those non-clinical medical staffs [7]. Doctors in community or township hospitals, or military hospital had better mental health. The latest cross-sectional study conducted in 7 teaching hospitals found the average standard scores of Self-Rating Anxiety Scale (SAS) for the male and female doctors were 46.8 and 46.7 [8], higher than the China norm in general population, and even higher than the level (45.36) among inhabitants in Wenchuan County after the 5.12 Sichuan earthquake [9].

The consensus suggestions were the same that attention from authorities should be paid to these medical practitioners as they were facing mounting pressure and thus the corresponding social and health services were in urgent demand. Positive relief-helping measures should be taken individually or by the institution to dealing with professional pressure.

3.2. Occupational Stress in Medical Professional

Occupational stress is a result of combined exposure to several factors in work environment and employment conditions [10]. The huge population in China has resulted in increasing number of patients and the health care system reform has enhanced patients' demand from doctors. The increasing numbers of patients and health consciousness in recent year have imposed heavy burdens on doctors. The burdens deteriorating their physical and mental health were multiple occupational pressures coming from over workload, high demanding from patients, occupational risk, effort-reward imbalance and fierce competition for title promotion [11]. The studies concentrated on the assessment of occupational stress and its related factors among Chinese doctors were limited. Hui Wu *et al.* using the Chinese version Personal Strain Questionnaire in 1587 doctors found that major factors associated with occupational stress differed between male and female doctors. Role boundary and role insufficient were the most crucial factors in male and female doctors respectively [12]. Siying Wu *et al.* explored the job burnout and associated variables among 543 Chinese doctors and found that the main significant predictors of exhaustion were role overload, responsibil-

ity, physical environment and self care [13].

Several studies indicate a high prevalence of stress and psychological problems among doctors. It was revealed that Traditional Chinese Medicine doctors (TCM), in terms of job satisfaction, general psychological health, stress and coping were much more favorable than non TCM doctors. Additionally, the general health questionnaire (GHQ) of TCM doctors is higher than that of western medicine doctors [14]. In another research showed that doctors who experienced medium and high degree of stress accounted for 19.5% and 2.3% respectively. The highest stressors were caused by working treatment and load, professional level and medical treatment risk, which of these seriously influences their mental health [15]. In terms of working hours, a connection has been shown between sleep and mental health problems among doctors [16]. Emotional pressure and demanding patients were also related to mental health problems.

3.3. Mental Health of Medical Staffs in Special Events

Among the investigation researches collected, there were reports exploring the psychological status of medical practitioners involving in large-scale disaster rescuing work. One was the 2002-2003 severe acute respiratory syndrome (SARS) outbreak infected 8422 individuals leading to 916 deaths around the world [17]. China became the focus of worldwide attention when the coronavirus that causes SARS emerged. Sudden onset of SARS has the features of easy contagion, fast spread and high mortality, posing a great threat to human health. It was a major public health disaster. Post-traumatic stress disorder (PTSD) was one of the most prevalent long-term psychiatric diagnoses among medical staffs participating in war of SARS [18]. One year after the outbreak, SARS battling doctors still had elevated stress levels and worrying levels of psychological distress. The total mean score and factor scores except somatization were significantly lower in the hospital employees than the national norm [19]. The coping style for medical staff was very defective and their negative response equalization was significantly higher than the norm. Its main psychological symptoms lied in somatization, anxiety, terror and obsessive compulsion [20-21].

The other research focus was the catastrophic Wenchuan earthquake measuring 8.0 on the Richter scale occurred in Sichuan province of southwest China. During the earthquake, 69,227 people were killed, 374,643 injured, 17,923 listed as missing, and about 4.8 million were left homeless [22]. The symptoms of posttraumatic stress disorder and associated risk factors were investigated among health care workers in earthquake-affected areas in southwest China. These findings suggest that

PTSD is a common mental health problem among health care workers in earthquake-affected areas. The prevalence of PTSD for overall was 23.3%, anxiety was 21.6%, depression was 49.9%, and the anxiety plus depression was 19.54% [23]. The basic medical personnel in 6 severe disaster-stricken areas still show obvious mental distress at 14 months after the earthquake, some even have suicide attempt and symptoms of depression and PTSD [24]. The average standard score of SDS and the average crude score o f SAS of 142 healthcare workers were significant higher than the national norm [25]. Abnormal of the mental health status in the medical staff was outstanding after Wenchuan earthquake. The situation should be given the enough attention.

3.4. General Physical Health Status

Doctor is a health care provider who practices the profession of medicine, which is concerned with promoting, maintaining or restoring human health through the study, diagnosis, and treatment of disease or injury. Doctors should have the less health problems than the rest of the population as they have the professional knowledge. However, doctor's physical health appears not as good as it thought it would be or even worse than that of the general population in China. Studies on health status of doctors in medical institution are abundant and repeated. The prevalence of chronic disease among doctors was 32.17% [26], prevalence of chronic illness increased with age growth. The analysis result was worrying and the consistence common diseases were cervical spondylosis, hyperlipidemia, hypertension, fatty liver and hyperglycemia [27-29]. Besides, female doctors also suffered from uterine fibroids. Yang Jie *et al.* analyzed 1723 medical staffs aged at 35 - 88 and found that the top five prevalences were hyperlipidemia (53.1%), overweight and obesity (50.1%), hypertension (31.2%), fatty liver (25.4%) and hyperglycemia (17.8%) [30]. Another routine health check-up in 2877 medical staffs found that hyperlipidemia (45%), fatty liver (37.5%), hyperglycemia (11.7%), hypertension (10.7%) [31]. While among doctors with associate and senior professional titles, cervical spondylosis listed the top [27]. In a survey of 2423 health workers in a certain Beijing hospital found that cervical spondylosis was the most annoying disease [32]. While in hospitals in southern China, the perseverance of these chronic diseases was relatively lower. A research demonstrated that hyperlipidemia (34.6%), Fatty liver (16.07%), hypertension (5%), diabetes (4.5%) in a hospital in Hainan province [33]. Prevalence of sub-health in doctors was 66.5% and even higher with significant difference between male and female. The most common symptom was mental stress [34]. All these chronic diseases were closely related to fast-pace of work, high concentration of energy, long time overloaded and high pressure.

4. Discussion

In China, medical college requires 5 years for graduate course, 3 years for postgraduate course and 3 years for doctorate course. As for education, doctors started to take medical education course directly after they graduate from high school and, then, go to practice. While practicing as a doctor, some will prefer to take further education course. It is not easy to become a doctor, and it is even tougher to serve as a qualified doctor in the country with huge population. Moreover, China is undertaking health care system reform in which the focus is transforming from disease to health and from sustaining life to quality of life. The traditional disease-centered care model had been gradually replaced by the patient-centered care model.

In health care practice, patients have limited medical knowledge but impose high expectation in treatment effect. It could possibly lead to tensional doctor-patient relationship, driving doctor more frustrated. As a result, medical disputes would occur more frequently than before. Insufficient doctors increase their nightshifts and extending working hours. Working on Saturday, Sunday and even national legal holidays are often seen in doctors. Their rest time is considerably less than other occupational population. In addition to stress in hospital, doctors have their individual professional pressure. To keep up with the constantly updated medical knowledge and technology, doctor has to spent time on leaning after work. Besides, the professional promotion is fiercely competitive that young doctor need to pursuit higher educational degree and writing papers to be qualified. Senior doctors are undertaking scientific research project and teaching task for medical students. Excessive working hours and heavy workload do not exchange with high financial reward is one of the major complains for job dissatisfaction among Chinese doctors. Experiencing heavier occupational stress and lower job satisfaction may directly attribute to poor mental health in doctor.

The reform in present medical system is expected to inevitably deteriorate the mental health problems of doctors. It has been reported that, at present, most Chinese doctors suffer from depressive symptom [35]. Studies have revealed that the increased prevalence of mental health problems among doctors is most likely caused by occupational stress and individual factors. Pressure of overload working, demanding patients, life-long learning for medical knowledge and risk of medical treatment is related to their mental problems.

For doctors participating in life-threatening rescuing medial work, their mental health status is even worse.

During the SARS epidemic, the working and living environment of the ward is isolated. Communication with the outside world is also subject to restrictions. The original pace of life and work had been disrupted, it not easy for them to adapt quickly; and also the fear of being infected by SARS virus all contribute to psychological stress factors [36]. Therefore, in the future disaster prevention, preparedness and disaster relief measures, unexpected major public health emergency response and rescue strategies and plans, psychological intervention measure should be carried out, so as to reduce the psychological damage caused by the disaster reduction and subsequent psychosocial problem [37].

In our review studies, chronic diseases of cervical spondylosis, hyperlipidemia, hypertension, fatty liver and hyperglycemia were common among Chinese doctors. It is different from that in Finnish study which chronic eczema, stomach and intestinal disorder, back complaints as the common physical disease in doctors. It could be different in another country as the work load and working condition are very different. However, either in developing countries or developed countries, doctors had to absorb the latest knowledge to improve their ability besides the routine works. Poor physical condition was able to aggravate work burden in comparison to good health.

5. Conclusion

Overall, this literature review shows that studies reveal a high prevalence of stress-related and mental disorders among doctors, and their physical health is not as good as people regarded. Doctors participating in the life-threatening major public health events should therefore be ensured psychiatric treatment afterward.

REFERENCES

[1] S. F. Yu, S. Q. Yao, H. Ding, L. Q. Ma, Y. Yang and Z. H. Wang, "Relationship between Depression Symptoms and Stress in Occupational Populations," *Chinese Journal of Industrial Hygiene and Occupational Diseases*, Vol. 24, 2006, pp. 129-133.

[2] J. Li, W. Yang and S. I. Cho, "Gender Differences in Job Strain, Effort Reward Imbalance, and Health Functioning among Chinese Physicians," *Social Science & Medicine*, Vol. 62, No. 5, 2007, pp. 1066-1077. doi:10.1016/j.socscimed.2005.07.011

[3] X. J. Feng, "Causes and Respond of Mental Health Problems in the Medical Staff," *Chinese Medicine Modern Distance Education of China*, Vol. 8, No. 15, 2010, pp. 152-153.

[4] H. Z. Jia, J. Shan and Y. Zhao, "A Survey on Psychological Status of Medical Staff in Infectious Department in Hengshui," *Chinese Nursing Management*, Vol. 11, 2007, pp. 28-29.

[5] L. Tu, X. Q. Zhang, N. Ren and H. Peng, "Current Situation and Analysis of the Medical Staff'S Psychological Health in China," *Medicine & Philosophy*, Vol. 30, No. 7, 2009, pp. 44-46.

[6] X. H. Xue, T. L. Zhao and J. G. Hu, "Mental Health of Doctors in General Hospital," *Chinese Journal of Clinical Psychology*, Vol. 14, No. 3, 2006, pp. 324-325.

[7] Y. B. Li, W. Zhong and P. Wang, "Study on Mental Health and Correlating Factors of Clinical Doctor vs Non-Clinical Doctor," *Chinese Journal of Health Psychology*, Vol. 13, No. 2, 2005, pp. 94-95.

[8] W. Sun, J. L. Fu, Y. Chang and L. Wang, "Epidemiological Study on Risk Factors for Anxiety Disorder among Chinese Doctors," *Occupational Health*, Vol. 54, No. 1, 2012, pp. 1-8. doi:10.1539/joh.11-0169-OA

[9] M. Guo, Y. Gao, X. Wang and X. Jiang, "Survey of Anxiety and Depression of People during Wenchuan Earthquake," *China Tropical Medicine*, Vol. 19, 2009, pp. 383-384.

[10] S. Y. Wu, H. Y. Li, X. R. Wang, S. J. Yang and H. Qiu, "A Comparison of the Effect of Work Stress on Burnout and Quality of Life between Female Nurses and Female Doctors," *Archives of Environmental and Occupational Health*, Vol. 66, No. 4, 2011, pp. 193-200. doi:10.1080/19338244.2010.539639

[11] Y. Tu, X. Y. Dou and R. Y. Yang, "On the Mental Health Survey of Doctors and Counter Measure," *Journal of Yunan University*, Vol. 31, No. S1, 2009, pp. 415-418.

[12] H. Wu, Y. Zhao, J. N. Wang and L. Wang, "Factors Associated with Occupational Stress among Chinese Doctors: A Cross-Sectional Survey," *International Archives of Occupational and Environmental Health*, Vol. 83, No. 2, 2010, pp. 155-164. doi:10.1007/s00420-009-0456-z

[13] B. L. Lin, S. R. Gao, L. H. Cheng, Y. H. Sun and H. Luo, "Occupational Stress and Psychological Health between Traditional Chinese Medicine and Western Medicine Doctors in China," *Chinese Mental Health Journal*, Vol. 21, No. 11, 2007, pp. 779-782.

[14] S. Y. Wu, W. Zhu, H. Y. Li, Z. M. Wang and M. Z. Wang, "Relationship between Job Burnout and Occupational Stress among Doctors in China," *Stress and Health*, Vol. 24, No. 2, 2008, pp. 143-149. doi:10.1002/smi.1169

[15] Y. J. Shi and L. F. Wang, "Doctors Professional Stress and Its Relation with Their Mental Health," *Chinese Journal of Public Health*, Vol. 23, No. 5, 2007, pp. 529-531.

[16] R. Tyssen, "Health Problems and the Use of Health Services among Physicians: A Review Article with Particular Emphasis on Norwegian Studies," *Industrial Health*, Vol. 45, No. 5, 2007, pp. 599-610. doi:10.2486/indhealth.45.599

[17] "Summary of Probable SARS Cases with Onset of Illness from 1 November 2002 to 7 August 2003," http://www.who.int/csr/sars/country/country2003_08_15.pdf

[18] C. Y. Lin, Y. C. Peng, Y. H. Wu, J. Chang, C. H. Chan and D. Y. Yang, "The Psychological Effect of Severe Acute Respiratory Syndrome on Emergency Department Staff," *Emergency Medicine Journal*, Vol. 24, No. 1, 2007, pp. 12-17. doi:10.1136/emj.2006.035089

[19] M. Gu, Y. Gu, Y. M. Mei, J. H. Lu and R. B. Yu, "Survey on Mental Health Status of Medical Practitioners in Comprehensive Hospitals of Jiangsu," *Chinese Journal of Public Health*, Vol. 24, No. 8, 2008, pp. 921-922.

[20] Z. H. Zhou, X. M. Li, K. N. Chen, X. Q. Li, Y. Dong and J. B. Zhao, "Relation of Mental Health and Coping Style for First-Line Medical Staff in SARS Battle," *Chinese Journal of Behavioral Medical Science*, Vol. 13, No. 3, 2004, p. 305.

[21] L. Shao, S. H. Xiao, T. Y. Cao, J. Xia and X. D. Li, "Survey on Mental Health of Young Medical Staff during SARS Period," *Medical Journal of National Defending Forces in North China*, Vol. 16, No. 3, 2004, p. 209.

[22] L. Wang, Y. Zhang, W. Wang, Z. Shi, J. Shen, M. Li, *et al.*, "Symptoms of Posttraumatic Stress Disorder among Adult Survivors Three Months after the Sichuan Earthquake in China," *Journal of Traumatic Stress*, Vol. 22, No. 5, 2009, pp. 444-450. doi:10.1002/jts.20439

[23] Z. Li, J. Li, Y. Liu, H. Liao, Y. Feng and X. L. Sun, "A Mental Health Survey of Medical Staffs Who Took Part in Rescue in Disaster Area after Wenchuan Earthquake," *Chinese Journal of Evidence-Based Medicine*, Vol. 9, No. 11, 2009, pp. 1151-1154.

[24] W. J. Mao, T. Zhang, W. J. Min, *et al.*, "The Association Analysis of Rural Doctor'S Mental Heath Status and Social Supports after Earthquake in Dujiangyan," *Sichuan Medical Journal*, Vol. 30, No. 10, 2009, pp. 1649-1651.

[25] B. Zhou, Y. Hu, L. M. Yang, J. Xiao, L. Zheng and C. Yang, "Investigation the Mental Health Status of the Medical Staff after Wenchuan Earthquake," *Sichuan Medical Journal*, Vol. 30, No. 10, 2009, pp. 1652-1654.

[26] Z. L. Guo, C. R. Zhang and C. Y. Chen, "Survey on Health Status of Medical Staff in a District in Guangzhou City," *Chinese Journal of Coal Industry Medicine*, Vol. 14, No. 5, 2011, pp. 724-725.

[27] J. Tang, B. Lv, J. Sun and J. Song, "Analysis on the Health Status of Senior Medical Staff," *Chinese Journal of Health Education*, Vol. 23, No. 10, 2007, pp. 784-785.

[28] Z. Y. Sun and Y. F. Wu, "Healthy Situation of the Medical Staff in a Hospital from 2006 to 2008," *China Foreign Medical Treatment*, Vol. 9, 2010, p. 150.

[29] L. P. Wang, Z. Y. Zhu, Y. B. Lin and D. Nie, "The Follow-Up Analysis about Circumstances of Health Physical Examination of Medical Staff," *Chinese Journal of Clinical Healthcare*, Vol. 9, No. 5, 2006, pp. 436-437.

[30] J. Yang, H. Zhao, H. Xin and Y. Q Liu, "Investigation of Health Check Results of Medical Staff in a Beijing Hospital in 2010," *Chinese Journal of Misdiagnose*, Vol. 11, No. 3, 2011, pp. 749-750.

[31] H. Xing and X. F. Wang, "Analysis of the Health Situation of the Medical Staff in a Hospital," *Hebei Medicine*, Vol. 11, No. 4, 2005, pp. 337-338.

[32] L. N. Lai, L. N. Yang, W. W. Lu and Y. Dai, "Survey on Health and Working Conditions of Medical Staff Members in a Third: A Comprehensive Hospital in Beijing," *Modern Hospital Management*, Vol. 42, No. 3, 2011, pp. 58-60.

[33] D. L. Nie, "Results of Health Check-Up of Medical Workers," *China Tropical Medicine*, Vol. 9, No. 3, 2009, p. 589.

[34] X. L. Gan, Q. Y. Chen and X. Z. Liu, "Sub-Health Status of Doctors in 3A Grade Hospital of Guangzhou and Its Characteristic Analysis," *Chinese General Practice*, Vol. 11, No. 9A, 2009, pp. 1573-1574.

[35] J. N. Wang, W. Sun, T. S. Chi, H. Wu and L. Wang, "Prevalence and Associated Factors of Depressive Symptoms among Chinese Doctors: A Cross-Sectional Survey," *International Archives of Occupational and Environmental Health*, Vol. 83, No. 8, 2010, pp. 905-911. doi:10.1007/s00420-010-0508-4

[36] Y. Cao and Y. Qi, "Psychological Status and Effect of Psychological Intervention in SARS Patients," *Chinese Journal of Nursing*, Vol. 38, No. Suppl, 2003, pp. 233-234.

[37] J. Gan, X. Q. Li, W. H. Zhang, C. Y. Gao, D. D. Yang, Y. N. Zhao, *et al.*, "Relative Factors of Mental Health of Anti-SARS Medical Staff," *Practical Journal of Medicine & Pharmacy*, Vol. 21, No. 1, 2004, pp. 42-43.

4

Chronic Subdural Haematoma in a Case of Hyperthyroidism Presenting with Papilledema

Somya Dulani*, Rajesh Dulani, Seema Lele, Sachin Diagavane,
Sandeep Anjankar, Netra Jaiswal, Prem S. Subramaniam, Rakesh Juneja

Ophthalmology JNMC DattaMeghe, Institute of Medical Sciences, Wardha, India

Email: *somya1010@rediffmail.com, rajeshkdulani@gmail.com, drseemalele@gmail.com, drsachin391977@gmail.com,
drsdanjankar@yahoo.co.in, netra_jaiswal@yahoo.com, psubram1@jhmi.edu, dr_rakeshjuneja555@yahoo.com

ABSTRACT

Subdural hematomas are often life-threatening when acute but chronic subdural hematomas, however, have better prognosis if properly managed. Chronic subdural hematomas are common in the elderly due to shrinkage of brain tissue, but in young patient mostly associated with head injury. It is seen also in young having various coagulopathies associated with blood disorders or drug-induced, but it is very rare. Propylthiouracil (PTU) is an oral medication that is used in treatment of hyperthyroidism approved by FDA in July 1947. This medication may rarely cause very serious blood disorders (such as a low number of red cells, white cells, and platelets), especially during the first few months of treatment. We are reporting a rare case of PTU-induced thrombocytopenia leading to chronic subdural haematoma, which presented with established papilledema and signs of raised ICP in a hyperthyroid female and she responded well to surgical management.

Keywords: Propylthiouracil (PTU); Thrombocytopenia; Papilledema

1. Introduction

A subdural hematoma, a form of traumatic brain injury in which, blood gathers within the outermost meningeal layer, between the dura mater, which adheres to the skull, and the arachnoid mater, which envelops the brain. Usually resulting from tears in bridging veins which cross the subdural space, subdural hemorrhages may cause an increase in intracranial pressure (ICP), which can cause compression of and damage to delicate brain tissue. Chronic subdural bleeds develop over a period of days to weeks, often after minor head trauma, though such a cause is not identifiable in 50% of patients [1]. Head injury is the most common cause of this lesion, but several predisposing factors such as coagulopathy, alcoholism, cerebrospinal fluid shunt procedures, vascular malformations, seizure disorders, and metastatic tumours must also be considered [2]. Hyperthyroidism, a hypermetabolic clinical syndrome which occurs, when there are elevated serum levels of T3 and/or T4. As there is too much thyroid hormone, every function of the body tends to speed up with symptoms like nervousness, irritability, increased perspiration, heart racing, hand tremors, anxiety, difficulty sleeping, thinning of the skin, fine brittle hair, and muscular weakness.

Thyrostatics (antithyroid drugs) are drugs that inhibit the production of thyroid hormones, such as carbimazole (used in UK) and methimazole (used in US), and propylthiouracil. Propylthiouracil (PTU) also works outside the thyroid gland, preventing conversion of (mostly inactive) T4 to the active form T3. It decreases production of thyroid hormone and also interferes with the conversion of T4 to T3, and, since T3 is more potent than T4, this also reduces the activity of thyroid hormones. In most cases, adverse effects are minor and transient. The most dangerous effect is agranulocytosis, which occurs in 0.1 to 0.5% of patients. Other major adverse effects aplastic anaemia, thrombocytopenia, lupus erythematosus-like syndrome, vasculitis are exceedingly rare [3].

2. Case Report

A forty five year hyperthyroid female (**Figure 1**) presented in eye clinic with a complaint of severe headache in fronto-parietal region which was radiating in the neck. Along with throbbing headache she also had nausea and vomiting since one month. Previously one year back, she presented with similar complaints of raised intracranial pressure. At that time she was onantithyroids drugs for hyperthyroidism since three years and but inadequate treatment as her T3-517 ng/dl, T4 > 30 ng/dl and TSH-13 ul/mL. She was advised to take adequate treatment and

---

*Corresponding author.

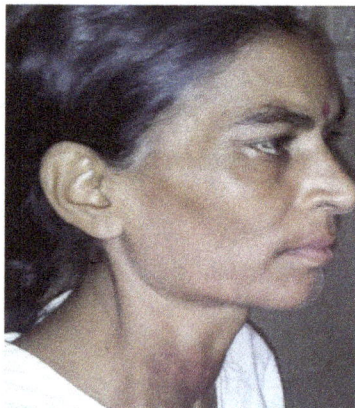

Figure 1. Clinical photograph of patient with mild swelling in neck.

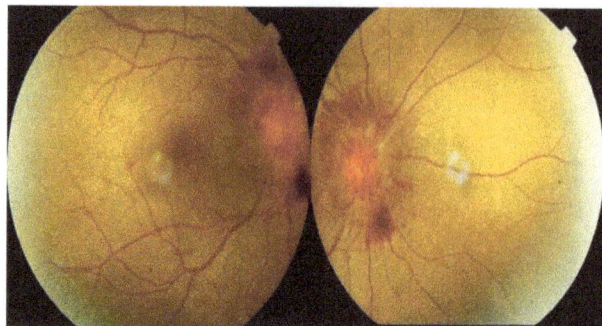

Figure 2. Fundus photograph showing established papilledema in both right and left eye before treatment.

her symptoms responded well to the treatment. But this time, patient was on regular antithyroid treatment and her thyroid profile was normal, so she was evaluated further. On ocular examination her visual acuity was 20/30 in both eyes with Marcus—Gunn pupillary reaction in both eyes. Fundus examination revealed well established papilledema in both eyes with disc swelling more than 5 disc diopters in both eyes (**Figure 2**).

She was advised MRI of brain, to rule out space occupying lesion which revealed, subacute extra-axial (subdural) hemorrage in right frontoparieto and occipital region in different stages causing midline shift to left side by 4 mm with cerebral oedema (**Figures 3** and **4**).

She had no history of head injury in past years. Her haemoglobin was 9.3 gm% and platelet count was very low that is 40,000/cu.mm. Systemic examination was done but other signs of thrombocytopenia were not present except excessive menstrual bleeding. Her drug history was taken, she was on PTU, a drug used as antithyroids since 3 months. She was advised to stop PTU drug and carbimazole was started. She was operated for subdural haematoma by a neurosurgeon after Fresh Frozen Plasma (FFP) transfusion to increase platelet count. Her post operative period was uneventful and within 2 days her papilledema reduced and on 5th day she had near to normal optic disc (**Figure 5**).

3. Discussion

One of the rare side effect of PTU is, decrease in blood platelets (thrombocytopenia). Since platelets are important for the clotting of blood, thrombocytopenia may lead to excessive bleeding [4]. A study of Subduralhaematoma among people who have hyperthyroidism, regardless of type of antithyroid drug taken was done [5]. On 2 July 2012, 1604 people who have hyperthyroidism are studied. Among them, 2 (0.12%) have Subdural Haematoma, and both were female, though the cause was not discussed. In our case probable cause is PTU-induced.

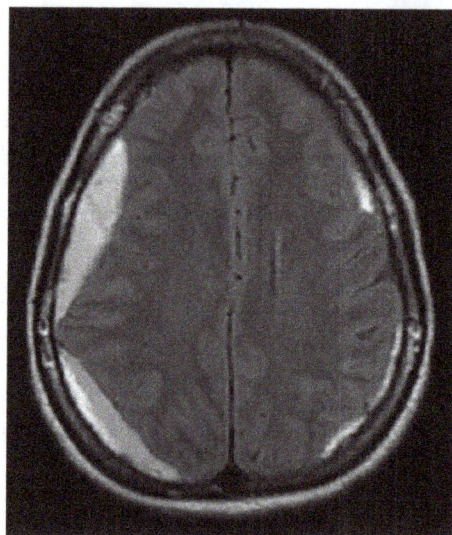

Figure 3. T-1 weighted Axial section MRI shows subacute extra-axial (subdural) hemorrhage in right frontoparieto and occipital region causing midline shift to left side by 4 mm with cerebral oedema.

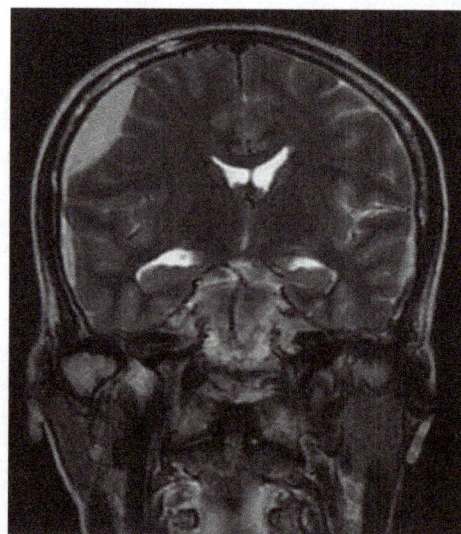

Figure 4. T-2 weighted Coronal section MRI shows subdural hemorrhage in parietal and occipital region causing midline shift to left side.

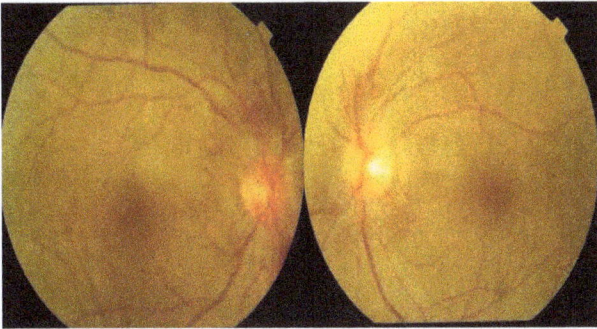

Figure 5. Fundus photograph showing resolving papilledema in both right and left eye after surgical management of subdural haematoma.

Yaka [6] and Herwig [7] presented a case of hyperthyroidism which was associated with symptoms of raised intracranial pressure which responded to antithyroids drugs because it was due to hyperactivity of thyroid hormone, similarly in our case first presentation that is one year before was due to deranged thyroid profile but second time it was due to chronic subdural haematoma.

Pseudotumorcerebri (PTC) is an entity characterized by elevated intracranial pressure with normal cerebrospinal fluid (CSF) and no structural abnormalities detected on brain MRI scans. The neurological symptoms and signs can be totally attributed to intracranial hypertension, and papilledema being the hallmark of PTC and its common cause is hyperthyroidism [8]. Thyroid testing may be useful for differential diagnosis of chronic headache, and indicates that headache could be caused by hyperthyroidism [9].

Chronic subdural hematoma is an important reversible cause of dementia and disability in the elderly. A sufficiently high level of clinical suspicion and prompt radiographic evaluation may allow for timely treatment to avoid poor outcomes. Thankfully, the routine use of computed tomographic scanning in most emergency facilities has made the diagnosis of these lesions common place [10]. Though there are cases of hyperthyroid females reported in literature associated with optic disc swelling, but drug-induce chronic subdural haematoma leading to papilledema in these patient is not reported till date.

REFERENCES

[1] A. Downie, "Tutorial: CT in Head Trauma," 2007.

[2] A. Prystupa, E. Kurys-Denis, T. Łopatyński, J. Baraniak and W. Krupski, "Case Report: Chronic Subdural Haematoma in a Patient with Arterial Hypertension and Alzheimer's Disease," *Journal of Pre-Clinical and Clinical Research*, Vol. 3, No. 2, 2009, pp. 127-129.

[3] L. Bartalena, F. Bogazzi and E. Martino, "Adverse Effects of Thyroid Hormone Preparations and Antithyroid Drugs," *Adverse Effects of Thyroid Hormone Preparations and Antithyr*, Vol. 15, No. 1, 1999, pp. 53-63. doi:10.2165/00002018-199615010-00004

[4] Medicine Net.com, "Newsletter Medicationspropylthiouracil Drug Monograph," 2012. http://www.medicinenet.com

[5] eHealth Me, "Real World Drug Outcomes. Could Hyperthyroidism Causes Subdural Haematoma," 2012. http://www.ehealthme.com

[6] E. Yaka and R. Çakmur, "Increased Intracranial Pressure Due to Hyperthyroidism," *Cephalalgia*, Vol. 30, No. 7, 2010, pp. 878-880.

[7] U. Herwig and M. Sturzenegger, "Hyperthyroidism Mimicking Increased Intracranial Pressure," *Headache: The Journal of Head and Face Pain*, Vol. 39, No. 3, 1999, pp. 228-230.

[8] E. Coutinho, A. M. Silva, C. Freitas1 and E. Santos, "Graves' Disease Presenting as Pseudotumorcerebri: A Case Report," *Journal of Medical Case Reports*, Vol. 5, 2011, p. 68. doi:10.1186/1752-1947-5-68

[9] U. Herwig and M. Sturzenegger, "Brief Communication: Thyroid Function in Patients with Chronic Headache," *International Journal of Neuroscience*, Vol. 57, No. 3-4, 1991, pp. 263-267.

[10] J. C. T. Chen and M. L. Levy, "Causes, Epidemiology and Risk Factors of Chronic Subdural Hematoma," *Neurosurgery Clinics of North America*, Vol. 11, No. 3, 2000, pp. 399-406.

5

The Eastern Cultural Signature of Traditional Chinese Medicine: Empirical Evidence and Theoretical Perspectives

Huanhua Lu[*], **Yi'nan Wang**[*], **Yiying Song, Jia Liu**[#]

State Key Laboratory of Cognitive Neuroscience and Learning, Beijing Normal University, Beijing, China

Email: [#]liujia@bnu.edu.cn

ABSTRACT

Background: Holistic thinking, which is rooted in Eastern culture, is assumed to be the core of traditional Chinese medicine (TCM). Recently, such holistic thinking has been proposed to be applicable to Western medicine practices for alleviating serious side effects; however, the obscure and often ill-defined terms of TCM, such as *qi*, *yin yang*, and *wuxing*, pose considerable obstacles for further understanding TCM. In the present study, we explored whether and how TCM is actually related to the scientific construct of holistic thinking, to elucidate the particular cultural signature of TCM. **Methods:** A random sample of 101 college students majoring in TCM and 93 non-medical college students was recruited for the study. Two psychological scales—the Chinese Holistic Thinking Scale and the TCM Competence Scale were used respectively to measure the holistic thinking and participants' ability to apply the TCM in practice. **Results:** We found that individuals who thought more holistically were better at applying TCM to modern medical problems. Interestingly, TCM was associated with holistic thinking in both TCM and non-medical students, suggesting that this association is intrinsic. Further exploration revealed that the association and variability facets of Eastern holistic thinking—which emphasize that the world is interconnected and ever-changing, respectively—significantly accounted for the individual differences in competence in utilizing TCM in practice. **Conclusion:** In short, our study provides the first empirical evidence linking TCM to the Eastern holistic thinking style, which not only deepens the understanding of TCM from a scientific perspective but also promotes dialogue between TCM and Western medicine for building safer and more effective health care systems.

Keywords: Association; Eastern Holistic Thinking; Individual Difference; Traditional Chinese Medicine (TCM); Variability; Western Medicine

1. Introduction

Traditional Chinese medicine (TCM) is a complete and independent medical system, which has been used to diagnose, treat, and prevent illnesses for thousands of years. Ever since the World Health Organization began exploring TCM in the 1950s, interest in it has been growing rapidly beyond China because of its particular therapeutic methods and effects. Currently, in many countries, TCM is practiced alongside Western medicine, providing patients with a wide array of therapeutic options. Thus, the integration of two medical traditions can take advantage of the strong points of both traditions to facilitate safer, faster, and more effective health care [1-4].

Because Western medicine and TCM arise in different cultural backgrounds, they show different characteristics, especially in the thinking styles for making diagnoses [1]. Western medicine primarily examines the material aspects of the body and treats illnesses by using drugs, radiation, and surgery, relying on a wide body of scientific evidence. In contrast, TCM emphasizes a more holistic approach and aims to cure and maintain balance in the body through more natural treatments [5-7]. In other words, TCM treats patients as an integrated whole, while Western medicine focuses on the specific symptoms associated with illness [3,8]. Therefore, although Western medicine is generally more effective in treating acute diseases than TCM, such treatment is usually accompanied by serious side effects, such as fatigue, nausea, or hair loss [9,10]. Therefore, Western medicine may bene-

---

[*]Huanhua Lu and Yi'nan Wang contributed equally to this study.
[#]Corresponding author.

fit from the acquisition of a more holistic approach, which can be obtained by using the techniques and thinking style of TCM to alleviate or even eliminate the unpleasant side effects of drugs and radiation therapy [2,3].

As a discipline rooted in Eastern traditional culture, TCM is not just a medical system, but also an important branch of Eastern philosophy and the Chinese healing arts. Therefore, TCM uses symbolic concepts to emphasize the integration of the body and mind. According to TCM terminology, health is thought to result from a delicate balance between *yin* (negativity) and *yang* (positivity) in the body. The body is thought to be constituted of *qi* (vital energy) and blood instead of tissues and organs. Furthermore, the body is divided into five functional sub-systems—*liver*, *heart*, *spleen*, *lungs*, and *kidneys*, corresponding to the Taoist concept of *wuxing* (five elements) [1]. However, these obscure concepts are often regarded as inaccurate descriptions of the human body in the eyes of Western medical practitioners [11]; this notion greatly interferes with appropriate understanding of TCM from a Western medicine perspective. Therefore, in the present study, we explore the particular cultural characteristics of TCM by using a well-established scale assessing Eastern holistic thinking style in an empirical study.

The core of holistic thinking is the belief that every element in the world is interconnected [12-16]. In the past two decades, numerous cross-cultural studies have demonstrated that East Asians, especially Chinese, prefer to think in a holistic way, whereas Westerners tend to engage more in analytic thinking [15,17-19]. For example, East Asians often pay more attention to context and the relationships between issues, while Westerners are more attentive to distinctive features [20-27]. Furthermore, East Asians are more likely to attribute behaviors to contextual factors than to personal dispositions, while Westerners do the opposite [28-35]. Finally, East Asians show more tolerance for contradiction and are more likely to expect changes in current trends, while Westerners prefer non-contradictory arguments and often predict that current trends will continue [36-41].

Despite theories assuming that TCM is rooted in holistic thinking, to our knowledge, no empirical study has directly examined the relationship between holistic thinking and TCM. To fill this gap, we investigated whether and how TCM relates to Eastern holistic thinking style by using two psychological scales—the Chinese Holistic Thinking Scale (CHTS) [42-45] and the Traditional Chinese Medicine Competence Scale (TCMCS), which was designed for this study. We investigated whether individuals who scored higher on the CHTS possessed greater competence in TCM practice, as measured by the TCMCS. In addition, we tested both students of TCM and non-medical students to examine whether the relationship between TCM and holistic thinking, if observed, is intrinsic, and therefore independent of TCM education.

2. Method

2.1. Participants

One hundred and one college students majoring in TCM at the Beijing University of Chinese Medicine (67 women; mean age = 20.86, SD = 0.61) and 93 non-medical college students at Beijing Normal University (64 females; mean age = 20.54, SD = 0.59) participated in the study. At the time of testing, the TCM students had already taken at least one year of core courses on TCM and had been trained in clinical practices such as acupuncture and moxibustion. The non-medical students had no history of any medical training. The study was approved by the institutional review board of Beijing Normal University. All subjects were informed that they were participating in a social and behavioral survey, and that their answers would be used only for the purposes of scientific research and would be kept strictly confidential. Before testing, written informed consent was obtained from all participants.

2.2. Measures

Eastern holistic thinking style was measured with the CHTS [44], a 26-item questionnaire using a 7-point Likert-type scale from "completely disagree" (1) to "completely agree" (7). The CHTS contains three facets: association, variability, and contradiction. The association facet consists of 13 questions such as "I always think about all of the aspects of others," which asserts that everything in the world is interconnected and nothing can be separated from the rest of the world. The contradiction facet consists of nine questions such as "I often do something which I do not really like," which holds that the world is a contradictory entity with old and new, good and bad, strong and weak opposites, coexisting in everything. Finally, the variability facet contains four items such as "I think that a person's habits are difficult to change," which emphasizes that everything in the world is changeable and flexible, and nothing can stand still or remain fixed. The CHTS has excellent reliability and validity [42-45]. Both the total score and the score of each facet were used in the following analyses.

To assess participants' ability to apply TCM theories in tackling medical problems, we created the TCMCS. To conceptualize TCM competence and generate items to assess it, we generated 60 items on the use of TCM to diagnose medical problems by reviewing the literature on TCM. An example item is "In my opinion, illness is related to one's living environment, daily diet, and mood states." Of these 60, 25 were selected by eleven TCM experts from the Beijing University of Chinese Medicine and the Chinese Academy of Traditional Chinese Medicine. A pilot study revealed sixteen items that had high internal consistency and test-retest reliability; these were selected as the items of the TCMCS (see Appendix for all items). All were rated on a 7-point Likert-type scale from "completely disagree" (1) to "completely agree" (7). Individuals who scored higher on the TCMCS were better at applying the TCM in practice.

Nine participants were excluded because of missing items in the questionnaire. Three additional participants (1.5% of the sample) with outlier responses—that is, scoring over three SDs from the group mean—were excluded from further analyses. Therefore, the final sample comprised 182 participants (92 TCM students; 90 non-medical students).

3. Results

The CHTS, which was used to measure Eastern holistic thinking style, had high internal consistency reliability (Cronbach's $\alpha = 0.73$). The reliability of its three subscales was also adequate (association: $\alpha = 0.79$; variability: $\alpha = 0.83$; contradiction: $\alpha = 0.65$). Similarly, the TCMCS, which was used to measure participants' competence in TCM practice, also had high internal consistency reliability (Cronbach's $\alpha = 0.75$). Participants with TCM training (i.e., TCM students) scored significantly higher on the TCMCS than did the non-medical students; TCM students: mean = 92.9, $SD = 9.64$; non-medical students: mean = 82.8, $SD = 9.19$; t(180) = 7.2, $p < 0.001$; these data indicate that the TCMCS had high construct validity. Next, we investigated whether participants who preferred to think holistically were better at TCM practice.

First, we examined the relationship between holistic thinking and TCM competence in TCM students. The significant positive correlation found between holistic thinking and TCM competence (r = 0.27, $p = 0.009$; Figure 1(a)) suggested that individuals who had an Eastern holistic thinking style exhibited greater TCM competence. To further examine whether this association was established through education on TCM, or whether it was an intrinsic property of Eastern culture, we examined the association in a group of non-medical students who had no experience with or knowledge of TCM. Interestingly, in this sample, we observed a similar association (r = 0.38, $p < 0.001$; Figure 1(b)); this was further confirmed by Fisher's Z-test analysis, in that there was no significant group difference in the correlation (Z < 1). Therefore, we conclude that the association between Eastern holistic thinking and TCM competence is intrinsic, and independent of TCM education. Taken together, our findings indicate that TCM competence is the realization of Eastern holistic thinking in practice.

To further examine which specific facets of Eastern

holistic thinking (as measured by the CHTS) affect TCM competence, we performed a stepwise multiple regression analysis. To increase the statistical power, both the TCM and non-medical students were included in the analysis because they showed the same pattern in the association between holistic thinking and TCM competence. In this analysis, we used TCM competence as the dependent variable, and the three facets of Eastern holistic thinking (i.e., association, variability, and contradiction) as covariates of interest, controlling for gender and age. The regression analysis revealed that both the association and variability facets, not the contradiction facet, significantly predicted TCM competence (Table 1), together accounting for 11.8% of the variance in TCM competence. The finding was further confirmed by correlation analyses between the three facets of Eastern holistic thinking and TCM competence (association: r = 0.17, $p = 0.02$; variability: r = 0.27, $p < 0.001$; contradiction: r = −0.01, $p = 0.86$; Figure 2).

4. Discussion

Holistic thinking and TCM are arguably the most representative markers of Eastern culture. Many theorists believe that TCM naturally embeds holistic thinking in medical practice [5,7,19]. Our study used the individual differences approach to provide the first empirical evidence supporting this speculation. That is, individuals who preferred to think holistically were more competent in putting TCM into practice. Importantly, this link was observed even in individuals who had no knowledge of TCM, suggesting that the link is intrinsic, and independent of education on TCM.

Our study not only adds to the findings of previous cross-culture studies on thinking style but also deepens the understanding of TCM. In previous studies on the differences in thinking style between people from Eastern and Western cultures, researchers focused on cultural influences on cognitions as tested in laboratories, such as attention, categorization, and attribution, and rarely on

Table1. Multiple regression analysis testing the relationship between TCM competence and the three facets of holistic thinking.

	beta	t-value	p-value
Dependent variable: TCM competence (N = 182)			
variability	0.303	4.262	<0.001
association	0.209	2.940	0.004
contradiction	0.016	0.223	0.824
gender	−0.024	−0.332	0.740
age	0.042	0.582	0.561
	R^2	F	p
	0.118	11.934	<0.001

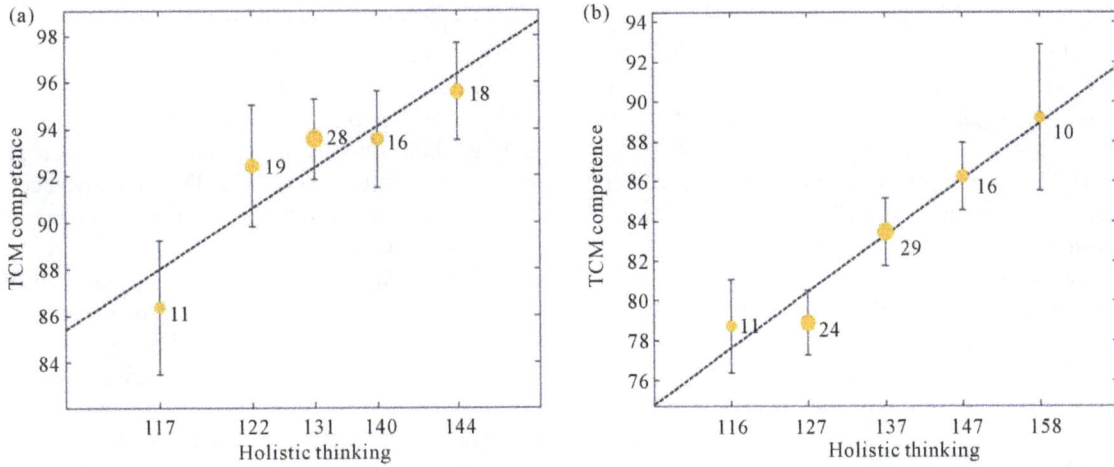

Figure 1. Binned scatter plots between TCM competence and Eastern holistic thinking in (a) TCM students, (b) non-medical students. The x-axis denotes participants' scores on the Chinese Holistic Thinking Scale (CHTS), with higher scores indicating preference for holistic thinking. The y-axis denotes participants' scores on the Traditional Chinese Medicine Competence Scale (TCMCS), with higher scores indicating higher competence in TCM practice. To avoid overlap between participants with similar scores, participants were binned into groups according to holistic thinking scores. Dot size is proportional to the number of observations, which are listed next to each dot. Error bars indicate standard errors of the mean.

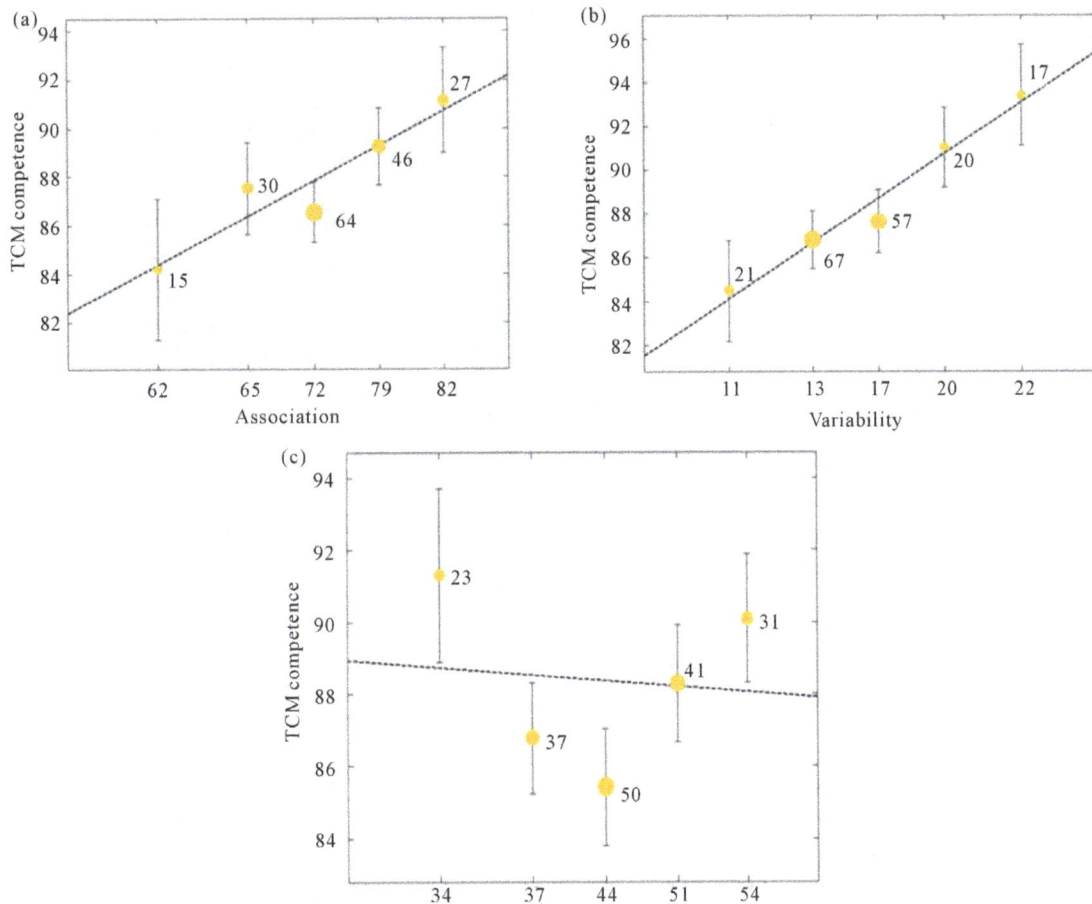

Figure 2. Binned scatter plots between TCM competence and the three facets of Eastern holistic thinking: (a) association, (b) variability, and (c) contradiction. To avoid overlap between participants with similar scores, participants were binned into groups according to scores for association, variability, and contradiction facets. Dot size is proportional to the number of observations, which are listed next to each dot. Error bars indicate standard errors of the mean.

daily activities or common practices [20,21,28,46-50]. The link between holistic thinking and TCM observed in this study thus provides a new platform for further investigation of how Eastern culture affects daily behaviors through thinking in general, and of the culture difference between TCM and Western medicine in particular. Furthermore, our study aids in understanding the obscure concepts in TCM such as *yin yang*, *wuxing*, and *qi* by making the thinking style through which they were formed more accessible to scientific study. In TCM, *yin* and *yang* are complementary opposites that are interdependent; *wuxing* emphasizes dynamic interactions and the balance of organs; and *qi* is regarded as the ultimate constituent of the world, the nature of the cosmic movement, and the medium that connects everything in the universe [7,51,52]. Our finding that the association and variability facets of CHTS were correlated with TCM competence confirmed the hypothesis that the *yin yang*, *wuxing*, and *qi* concepts in TCM derive from the associative and flexible nature of Eastern holistic thinking [7,51].

Why is there an association between holistic thinking and TCM? One possible reason is that both originate from the agrarian culture of Eastern societies and philosophy [5,7,15,19]. In Eastern societies, irrigated agriculture and changeable climatic conditions require cooperation and coordination with a substantial number of individuals for effective economic activities. Therefore, individuals living in such an interdependent social environment may have needed to attend more to interpersonal relationships and to emphasize the harmony between human and nature, which are core tenets of Eastern holistic thinking [15,19]. In parallel, TCM, which stems from practices in agricultural production, uses metaphors to understand the body (e.g., *liver*, *heart*, *spleen*, *lungs*, and *kidneys*) in terms of natural phenomena (e.g., metal, wood, water, fire, and earth), and thus integrates the body and nature into a unified whole. From the perspective of Eastern philosophy, the *Yi Jing* (the Book of Changes), the first Chinese philosophy book written during the *Zhou* Dynasty (1111-721 BC), offers a comprehensive view on the interconnected and everchanging nature of the universe and human societies. Therefore, the holistic thinking style suggested by Chinese philosophy likely serves as a cognitive schema in TCM practice, where TCM doctors are more likely to search for integrated patterns among seemingly fragmented elements. Taken together, because of the shared source of the agrarian culture and the common root of Chinese philosophy, it is not surprising that the link between holistic thinking and TCM competence was also found in individuals who were naïve to TCM. This observation has considerable implications in practice. In medical schools that teach TCM, education on traditional

Chinese philosophy and culture could improve students' TCM competence. Conversely, studying TCM may help people master Eastern holistic thinking styles [8,53].

Our study further demonstrated that the association and variability facets, and not the contradiction facet, of the CHTS were correlated with TCM competence, which may help enrich the thinking style of Western medicine. In terms of the association facet, diseases are not only caused by particular types of viruses, but also by lifestyles or emotion states. That is to suggest, therapy should focus more on the person with the disease, instead of the disease itself. Similarly, the variability facet suggests the benefits of individualized therapy based on a combination of treating symptoms and monitoring patients' physical conditions, and even their psychological traits. With future studies on the relation between Western analytical thinking and Western medicine, we can deepen our understanding of the cultural signatures of both TCM and Western medicine, which may help in building a safer and more effective system to promote physical health and well-being.

5. Conclusion

Our study used the individual differences approach to provide the first empirical evidence linking TCM to the Eastern holistic thinking style. That is, individuals who preferred to think holistically were more competent in applying TCM in practice. Importantly, this link was observed even in individuals who had no knowledge of TCM, suggesting that the link is intrinsic, and independent of education on TCM, which not only deepens the understanding of TCM from a scientific perspective but also promotes dialogue between TCM and Western medicine for building safer and more effective health care systems.

6. Acknowledgements

This study was funded by the National Social Science Foundation of China (11&ZD187) and the National Basic Research Program of China (2011CB505402).

REFERENCES

[1]   K. Chen and H. Xu, "The integration of Traditional Chinese Medicine and Western Medicine," *European Review*, Vol. 11, No. 2, 2003, pp. 225-235.

[2]   I. Holliday, "Traditional Medicines in Modern Societies: An Exploration of Integrationist Options through East Asian Experience," *Journal of Medicine and Philosophy*, Vol. 28, No. 3, 2003, pp. 373-389. doi:10.1076/jmep.28.3.373.14587

[3]   J. Lake, "The Integration of Chinese Medicine and Western Medicine: Focus on Mental Illness," *Integrative Medicine*, Vol. 3, No. 4, 2004, pp. CB-CJ.

[4]   G. J. Andrews, J. Evans and S. McAlister, "Creating the Right Therapy Vibe: Relational Performances in Holistic Medicine," *Social Science & Medicine*, Vol. 83, April 2013, pp. 99-109. doi:10.1016/j.socscimed.2013.01.008

[5]   T. J. Kaptchuk, "The Web That Has No Weaver: Understanding Chinese Medicine," McGraw-Hill, New York, 2000.

[6]   E. Yu, "Essential Traditional Chinese Medicine: Western Scientific Medicine Perspective," *Hong Kong Practitioner*, Vol. 23, No. 1, 2001, pp. 20-27.

[7]   D. E. Kendall, "Dao of Chinese Medicine: Understanding an Ancient Healing Art," Oxford University Press, Oxford, 2002.

[8]   M. Koo and I. Choi, "Becoming a Holistic Thinker: Training Effect of Oriental Medicine on Reasoning," *Personality and Social Psychology Bulletin*, Vol. 31, No. 9, 2005, pp. 1264-1272. doi:10.1177/0146167205274692

[9]   T. P. Lam, "Strengths and Weaknesses of Traditional Chinese Medicine and Western Medicine in the Eyes of Some Hong Kong Chinese," *Journal of Epidemiology and Community Health*, Vol. 55, No. 10, 2001, pp. 762-765. doi:10.1136/jech.55.10.762

[10] D. Normile, "The New Face of Traditional Chinese Medicine," *Science*, Vol. 299, No. 5604, 2003, pp. 188-190. doi:10.1126/science.299.5604.188

[11] J. Qiu, "Traditional Medicine: A Culture in the Balance," *Nature*, Vol. 448, No. 7150, 2007, pp. 126-128. doi:10.1038/448126a

[12] D. J. Munro, "Individualism and Holism: Studies in Confucian and Taoist Values," Center for Chinese Studies, University of Michigan, Ann Arbor, 1985.

[13] H. Nakamura, "Ways of Thinking of Eastern Peoples," University of Hawaii Press, Honolulu, 1964.

[14] J. Needham, "Science and Civilisation in China. Vol. 4: Physics and Physical Technology," Cambridge University Press, Cambridge, 1962.

[15] R. E. Nisbett, K. Peng, I. Choi and A. Norenzayan, "Culture and Systems of Thought: Holistic Versus Analytic Cognition," *Psychological Review*, Vol. 108, No. 2, 2001, p. 291. doi:10.1037/0033-295X.108.2.291

[16] D. Oyserman and S. W. Lee, "Does Culture Influence What and How We Think? Effects of Priming Individualism and Collectivism," *Psychological Bulletin*, Vol. 134, No. 2, 2008, pp. 311-342. doi:10.1037/0033-2909.134.2.311

[17] R. E. Nisbett and T. Masuda, "Culture and Point of View," *Proceedings of the National Academy of Sciences*, Vol. 100, No. 19, 2003, pp. 11163-11170. doi:10.1073/pnas.1934527100

[18] R. E. Nisbett and Y. Miyamoto, "The Influence of Culture: Holistic versus Analytic Perception," *Trends in Cognitive Sciences*, Vol. 9, No. 10, 2005, pp. 467-473. doi:10.1016/j.tics.2005.08.004

[19] R. E. Nisbett, "The Geography of Thought: How Asians and Westerners Think Differently and Why," Free Press, New York, 2003.

[20] H. F. Chua, J. E. Boland and R. E. Nisbett, "Cultural Variation in Eye Movements during Scene Perception," *Proceedings of the National Academy of Sciences*, Vol. 102, No. 35, 2005, pp. 12629-12633. doi:10.1073/pnas.0506162102

[21] L.-J. Ji, K. Peng and R. E. Nisbett, "Culture, Control, and Perception of Relationships in the Environment," *Journal of Personality and Social Psychology*, Vol. 78, No. 5, 2000, pp. 943-955.

[22] A. Boduroglu, P. Shah and R. E. Nisbett, "Cultural Differences in Allocation of Attention in Visual Information Processing," *Journal of Cross-Cultural Psychology*, Vol. 40, No. 3, 2009, pp. 349-360. doi:10.1177/0022022108331005

[23] S. Duffy and S. Kitayama, "Mnemonic Context Effect in Two Cultures: Attention to Memory Representations?" *Cognitive Science*, Vol. 31, No. 6, 2007, pp. 1009-1020. doi:10.1080/03640210701703808

[24] M. Doherty, H. Tsuji and W. A. Phillips, "The Context-Sensitivity of Visual Size Perception Varies across Cultures," *Perception*, Vol. 37, No. 9, 2008, pp. 1426-1433. doi:10.1068/p5946

[25] T. Masuda, R. Gonzalez, L. Kwan and R. E. Nisbett, "Culture and Aesthetic Preference: Comparing the Attention to Context of East Asians and Americans," *Personality and Social Psychology Bulletin*, Vol. 34, No. 9, 2008, pp. 1260-1275. doi:10.1177/0146167208320555

[26] K. Rayner, X. Li, C. C. Williams, K. R. Cave and A. D. Well, "Eye Movements during Information Processing Tasks: Individual Differences and Cultural Effects," *Vision Research*, Vol. 47, No. 21, 2007, pp. 2714-2726. doi:10.1016/j.visres.2007.05.007

[27] X. Li, J. Zhang, Y. Huang, M. Xu and J. Liu, "Nurtured to Follow the Crowd: A Twin Study on Conformity," *Chinese Science Bulletin*, Vol. 58, No. 10, 2013, pp. 1175-1180. doi:10.1007/s11434-013-5701-x

[28] I. Choi and R. E. Nisbett, "Situational Salience and Cultural Differences in the Correspondence Bias and Actor-Observer Bias," *Personality and Social Psychology Bulletin*, Vol. 24, No. 9, 1998, pp. 949-960. doi:10.1177/0146167298249003

[29] I. Choi, R. E. Nisbett and A. Norenzayan, "Causal Attribution across Cultures: Variation and Universality," *Psychological Bulletin*, Vol. 125, No. 1, 1999, pp. 47-63. doi:10.1037/0033-2909.125.1.47

[30] Lee F, Hallahan M, Herzog T: Explaining real-life events: How culture and domain shape attributions. *Personality and Social Psychology Bulletin*, Vol. 22, No. 7, 1996, pp. 732-741. doi:10.1177/0146167296227007

[31] M. W. Morris and K. Peng, "Culture and Cause: American and Chinese Attributions for Social and Physical Events," *Journal of Personality and Social Psychology*, Vol. 67, No. 6, 1994, pp. 949-949. doi:10.1037/0022-3514.67.6.949

[32] T. Masuda and S. Kitayama, "Perceiver-Induced Constraint and Attitude Attribution in Japan and the US: A Case for the Cultural Dependence of the Correspondence Bias," *Journal of Experimental Social Psychology*, Vol. 40, No. 3, 2004, pp. 409-416.

doi:10.1016/j.jesp.2003.08.004

[33] Y. Miyamoto and S. Kitayama, "Cultural Variation in Correspondence Bias: The Critical Role of Attitude Diagnosticity of Socially Constrained Behavior," *Journal of Personality and Social Psychology*, Vol. 83, No. 5, 2002, pp. 1239-1248. doi:10.1037/0022-3514.83.5.1239

[34] A. Norenzayan, I. Choi and R. E. Nisbett, "Cultural Similarities and Differences in Social Inference: Evidence from Behavioral Predictions and Lay Theories of Behavior," *Personality and Social Psychology Bulletin*, Vol. 28, No. 1, 2002, pp. 109-120. doi:10.1177/0146167202281010

[35] M. D. Lieberman, J. M. Jarcho and J. Obayashi, "Attributional Inference across Cultures: Similar Automatic Attributions and Different Controlled Corrections," *Personality and Social Psychology Bulletin*, Vol. 31, No. 7, 2005, pp. 889-901. doi:10.1177/0146167204274094

[36] K. Peng, "Naive Dialecticism and Its Effects on Reasoning and Judgment about Contradiction," University of Michigan, Ann Arbor, 1997.

[37] K. Peng and R. E. Nisbett, "Culture, Dialectics, and Reasoning about Contradiction," *American Psychologist*, Vol. 54, No. 9, 1999, pp. 741-754. doi:10.1037/0003-066X.54.9.741

[38] I. Choi and R. E. Nisbett, "Cultural Psychology of Surprise: Holistic Theories and Recognition of Contradiction," *Journal of Personality and Social Psychology*, Vol. 79, No. 6, 2000, pp. 890-905. doi:10.1037/0022-3514.79.6.890

[39] L.-J. Ji, R. E. Nisbett and Y. Su, "Culture, Change, and Prediction," *Psychological Science*, Vol. 12, No. 6, 2001, pp. 450-456. doi:10.1111/1467-9280.00384

[40] L.-J. Ji, Z. Zhang and T. Guo, "To Buy or to Sell: Cultural Differences in Stock Market Decisions Based on Price Trends," *Journal of Behavioral Decision Making*, Vol. 21, No. 4, 2008, pp. 399-413. doi:10.1002/bdm.595

[41] J. Spencer-Rodgers, M. J. Williams and K. Peng, "Cultural Differences in Expectations of Change and Tolerance for Contradiction: A Decade of Empirical Research," *Personality and Social Psychology Review*, Vol. 14, No. 3, 2010, pp. 296-312. doi:10.1177/1088868310362982

[42] Y. Hou, "Research Progress in Thinking Styles from the Perspective of Cultural Psychology," *Advances in Psychological Science*, Vol. 15, No. 2, 2007, pp. 211-216.

[43] Y. Hou, M. Zhang and X. Wang, "The Relationship between Adolescents' Thinking Style and their Coping Style," *Chinese Mental Health Journal*, Vol. 21, No. 3, 2007, pp. 158-161.

[44] Y. B. Hou and Y. Zhu, "The Chinese Holistic Thinking Styles: Their Structure and Effect," *APA Annual Symposium*, Chicago, 22-25 August 2002, pp. 22-25.

[45] Y. Hou, Y. Zhu and K. Peng, "How the Thinking Style Affect Managers' Attribution," In: D. Wang and Y. Hou, Eds., *Personality and Social Psychology*, Peking University Press, Beijing, 2004, pp. 115-130.

[46] L.-J. Ji, Z. Zhang and R. E. Nisbett, "Is It Culture or Is It Language? Examination of Language Effects in Cross-Cultural Research on Categorization," *Journal of Personality and Social Psychology*, Vol. 87, No. 1, 2004, pp. 57-65.

[47] A. Norenzayan, E. E. Smith, B. J. Kim and R. E. Nisbett, "Cultural Preferences for Formal versus Intuitive Reasoning," *Cognitive Science*, Vol. 26, No. 5, 2002, pp. 653-684. doi:10.1207/s15516709cog2605_4

[48] E. E. Buchtel and A. Norenzayan, "Which Should You Use, Intuition or Logic? Cultural Differences in Injunctive Norms about Reasoning," *Asian Journal of Social Psychology*, Vol. 11, No. 4, 2008, pp. 264-273. doi:10.1111/j.1467-839X.2008.00266.x

[49] L.-J. Ji, T. Guo, Z. Zhang and D. Messervey, "Looking into the Past: Cultural Differences in Perception and Representation of Past Information," *Journal of Personality and Social Psychology*, Vol. 96, No. 4, 2009, pp. 761-769. doi:10.1037/a0014498

[50] W. W. Maddux and M. Yuki, "The 'Ripple Effect': Cultural Differences in Perceptions of the Consequences of Events," *Personality and Social Psychology Bulletin*, Vol. 32, No. 5, 2006, pp. 669-683. doi:10.1177/0146167205283840

[51] Y. H. Zhang and K. Rose, "A Brief History of Qi," Paradigm Publications, Brookline, 2001.

[52] L. Lao, L. Xu and S. Xu, "Traditional Chinese Medicine," In: A. Längler, P. J. Mansky and G. Seifert, Eds., *Integrative Pediatric Oncology*, Springer, Berlin, 2012, pp. 125-135. doi:10.1007/978-3-642-04201-0_9

[53] C.-Y. Kim and B. Lim, "Modernized Education of Traditional Medicine in Korea: Is It Contributing to the Same Type of Professionalization Seen in Western Medicine?" *Social Science & Medicine*, Vol. 58, No. 10, 2004, pp. 1999-2008. doi:10.1016/S0277-9536(03)00405-2

Appendix:

Traditional Chinese Medicine Competence Scale (TCMCS)

1)* The brain is the organ of thinking; therefore, mental disorders damage the brain, not the five viscera.

2)* Health and disease are always contradictory.

3) There are multiple ways to reach the truth of a complicated issue.

4)* Using metaphors to understand the functionality of organs in terms of natural phenomena cannot lead to correct answers.

5) In my opinion, illness is related to one's living environment, daily diet, and mood states.

6) The dysfunction of an organ can result in the change of its structure.

7)* Scientific studies show that gypsum contains no antiviral ingredient, so it is useless for patients with viral influenza.

8)* On the issue of health, I prefer to trust reports from medical instruments, rather than subjective feelings.

9) How an illness manifests itself in the body is constantly changing.

10)* The human body is similar to a delicate machine, which will operate perfectly so long as the exact problem is identified and fixed.

11)* Meridians and collaterals do not really exist in the body; they are imaginary.

12)* There is no connection between abnormal feces and dysfunctions in the lungs, liver, spleen, or kidneys.

13)* To treat coughing or shortness of breath, we must focus on the lungs, and not on the liver or kidneys.

14)* Since the body is a natural phenomenon, it must be measured with scientific standards that are the same as those used in physics and chemistry.

15) In order to understand the laws of life, we must study health and diseases from multiple angles, such as their physiological structures, psychological factors, environmental factors, and nature.

16)* I believe that killing cancer cells is the only way to cure cancer.

*: reversed-scored items.

6

The Effects of *Ganoderma lucidum* on Initial Events Related to the *Bacillus Calmette-Guérin* Efficacy and Toxicity on High-Risk Uroepithelial Cells: An *in Vitro* Preliminary Study

John Wai-Man Yuen[1*], Mayur-Danny I. Gohel[2], Chi-Fai Ng[3]

[1]School of Nursing, The Hong Kong Polytechnic University, Hong Kong, China
[2]Department of Medical Science, Tung Wah College, Hong Kong, China
[3]Department of Surgery, The Chinese University of Hong Kong, Hong Kong, China
Email: *john.yuen@polyu.edu.hk, dannygohel@twc.edu.hk, ngcf@surgery.cuhk.edu.hk

ABSTRACT

A novel prophylactic regimen is demanded for preventing bladder cancer recurrence, because of the high side-effect tolls of conventional adjuvant *Bacillus Calmette-Guérin* (BCG) immunotherapy, in addition to its only moderate efficacy. *In vitro* and animal studies have demonstrated the anti-cancer properties of a medicinal mushroom called *Ganoderma lucidum* (GL). In this study, a pre-malignant human uroepithelial cells (HUC-PC) model was utilized to compare the effectiveness between ethanol extract of GL (GLe) and BCG on interleukin-6 (IL-6) secretion and lactate dehydrogenase (LDH) cytotoxicity. Additionally, parameters relevant to the BCG efficacy and safety, including free soluble fibronectin (FN) and cell-surface glycosaminoglycans (GAGs) levels were tested, following the exposure of GLe to the cells. GLe at 100 µg/ml and BCG at 4.8×10^7 CFU were shown to induce equivalent levels of IL-6, suggesting the potential synergism, while the tested concentrations of GLe were non-cytotoxic. During the initial four hours of GLe exposure, the free FN concentrations in harvested media were significantly reduced that might facilitate the binding of BCG for uroepithelial internalization to enhance BCG efficacy. Furthermore, the cell membrane-bound GAGs levels of HUC-PC cells were significant increased in response to GLe to suggest cellular protection from BCG infection. In summary, current findings suggest the potential additive synergism of GLe with the BCG efficacy, as well as its protective effects, and thus reducing the BCG toxicity.

Keywords: *Ganoderma lucidum*; *Bacillus Calmette-Guérin*; Bladder Cancer; Uroepithelial Cells; Synergism

1. Introduction

Ganoderma lucidum (GL), a popular ancient medicinal mushroom ranked as a superior tonic in traditional Chinese medicine, is commonly used for health promotion and longevity. Nowadays, the mushroom is being used by many cancer patients because of its perceived health benefits including immunomodulating properties and antitumorigenicity. In the recent years, our research team and collaborators have focused on bladder cancer, and reported a range of *in vitro* chemopreventive activities for GL. It was demonstrated that remarkable growth inhibitory effects via G2/M phase cell cycle arrest [1] and apoptosis [2] were exhibited by a defined ethanol extract

of GL (GLe) on the pre-malignant human uroepithelial cell line (HUC-PC). The GLe-treated HUC-PC cells were also characterized to have significant oxidative DNA damage [3] and secretion of several cytokines including IL-2, IL-6 and IL-8, [4] altogether suggesting the proinflammatory mechanism for adverse cell eradication. Furthermore, GLe was found to suppress the migration and telomerase activity that induced by a bladder cancer-relevant carcinogen 4-aminobiphenyl [1,2].

The recurrence rate of superficial transitional cell carcinoma (TCC) of bladder remains exceptionally high even with the effective transurethral resection (TUR) technique [5]. Refers to the "field cancerization hypothesis" and "seeding theory", residual cells at treated and adjacent sites are highly susceptible for mutagenic attacks

---

*Corresponding author.

and can potentially develop into tumors again, and hence powerful chemopreventive agents are demanded for prophylaxis [6]. *Bacillus Calmette-Guérin* (BCG), is currently the most effective prophylactic agent available and, when introduced intravesically, it triggers a local inflammatory response inside the urinary bladder [7,8]. In response to BCG, host leukocytes infiltrate into the urothelial wall and are responsible for most of the urinary cytokine secretion [9,10]. Evidence has also indicated that in situ lymphocytes are able to eradicate BCG-internalizing tumor cells through specific cell lysis against mycobacterial antigens [11]. However, only certain cytokines, including IL-2, IL-6 and TNF-α, are detectable in a patient's urine within the first 24 hours upon BCG instillation [12]. Particularly, the two pro-inflammatory cytokines, IL-6 and TNF-α, could also be secreted from various human bladder cancer cell lines [13-15]. Interestingly, well-differentiated bladder tumor cells that are incapable of internalizing BCG were also unable to up-regulate IL-6 expression [16]. In contrast, normal urothelial cells and poorly differentiated TCC cells were able to internalize BCG and produce IL-6 [11,16]. Therefore, IL-6 cytokine was considered as an indicative marker for BCG internalization [17]. Given that binding of BCG to the urothelial surface is a pre-requisite for successful internalization [17], the urothelium and mycobacterium are linked through fibronectin (FN) opsonization [18-20]. Formation of FN bridges might facilitate the process of BCG internalization [17-19]. Such linkage induces the expression of the IL-6 gene through NF-κB and AP-1 signal transducers in bladder tumor cells [21]. However, excess free FN was reported to be competitive with each other for the limited binding sites on urothelium and BCG surface, and thus impairing the internalization of BCG and its subsequent responses [22]. Besides its efficacy, BCG instillation also has high side-effect tolls of up to 90% of the patients develop cystitis and haematuria [8]. Patients receiving BCG treatment are taking the risk of systemic mycobacterial infection that could be lethal, although it is rare [23]. In fact, direct adhesion is not required for the process of BCG internalization, where a close-docking distance (70 - 100A) is set by the repellent force between BCG and urothelium [24,25]. The luminal wall of the bladder is protected by the mucosal lining that is covered with negatively charged glycosaminoglycans (GAGs), which keeping away the bacteria and toxins from certain distance of the anionic urothelial mucosa.[17] Thus, free FN concentration and cell surface-bound GAGs are two relevant biomarkers for BCG binding efficiency as well as potential toxicity.

In the present study, the HUC-PC cell model is continuously being utilized, firstly to compare between the effectiveness of GLe and BCG on the cytotoxicity and IL-6 secretion. IL-6 has been suggested to be responsible for the cytotoxicity of BCG on several TCC cell lines [26,27].

Whether BCG and GLe would both be cytotoxic to HUC-PC was determined using the LDH cytotoxicity assay, if they are capable of inducing IL-6 secretion. Secondly, the effects of GLe on extracellular FN and cell surface GAGs are explored. These findings will aid in elucidating whether GLe is a possible candidate to supplement or even replace the BCG immunotherapy.

2. Materials and Methods

2.1. Preparation of GLe and BCG

The active ingredients of RishiMax GLP^{TM} G. lucidum (Pharmanex, Hong Kong) were commercially standardized to 13.5% polysaccharides and 6% triterpenes. Powdered G. lucidum from capsules was re-extracted as previously described [3,4]. GLe was dissolved freshly in absolute ethanol (0.1% v/v) and diluted with culture medium to make a 1000 μg/ml stock solution. The whole vial (dry weight 81 mg) of live attenuated BCG (IMMUCYST®, Aventi, Toronto, Ontario, Canada) was reconstituted with 3 ml of the accompanying diluents to make a suspension containing a minimal dosage of 6.6×10^8 colony forming units (CFU). A 4.8×10^7 CFU BCG stock solution was prepared with culture medium. For assays, working assay media were prepared by further diluting the stock solutions of GLe and BCG into the concentrations of test ranges. Solvent media containing the maximal amount of corresponding solvent, *i.e.* 0.1% v/v ethanol for GLe and 33% v/v diluents for BCG, were used as controls. Furthermore, GLe and BCG were checked using Limulus Amebocyte Lysate (LAL) endpoint chromogenic kit assay (CAPE CO, E. Falmouth, MA, USA) for lipopolysaccharides (LPS) contamination. Glucashield^{TM} buffer (CAPE COD) was used to reconstitute pyrochrome to inhibit possible (1,3)-β-D-glucan presented in samples, and thus avoiding potential interference in the assay. Aseptic techniques were strictly applied throughout the procedures.

2.2. Cell Culture for Assays

The HUC-PC cell line was derived in the Department of Human Oncology, University of Wisconsin Medical School, and gifted by Dr. Rao from the University of California, Los Angeles. The cell line was cultured in F12 Ham enriched Dulbecco's Modified Eagle's Meium (F12/DMEM purchased from Sigma, St. Louis, MO) with 1% penicillin (10,000 μg/ml) and streptomycin (10,000 mg/ml) and 10% Fetal Bovine Serum (GIBCO BRL Isaland, New York, USA). Logarithmically growing HUC-PC cells were harvested and seeded in 96-well flat-bottle tissue culture plate (Greiner bio-one, Germany) at a concentration of 5×10^4 cells per microtitre well for cytotoxicity, FN and GAGs measurement. In parallel experiments, 1×10^6 cells were also seeded in 100-mm tissue culture dishes (Greiner bio-one, Germany) for IL-6 assay.

2.3. Lactate Dehydrogenase (LDH) Cytotoxicity Assay

Cytotoxicity of GLe and BCG was assayed by measuring LDH released from cells with LDH Cytotoxicity Detection kit (TaKaRa Bio Inc., Shiga, Japan). Following the manufacturer's instructions, the cells were incubated with assay media containing GLe or BCG for 24 hours in microtitre plate wells (Thermo Labsystems, Franklin, MA). No significant cytotoxicity was observed with the solvent controls. The release of LDH from cells was measured at 490 nm with reference wavelength at 690 nm, using TECAN SPECTRA Fluor Plus microplate reader (TECAN Austria GmbH, Grodig, Austria). Untreated cells were used as low controls to measure the spontaneous LDH release, and Triton X-100 treated cells were used as high controls to measure the maximum releasable LDH activity. No interference was observed from any test substances used in the assay. Cytotoxicity was calculated as a percentage of LDH release with the following formula:

$$\text{Cytotoxicity} = \frac{\left(A_{490}\left[\text{Experiment}\right] - A_{490}\left[\text{Low control}\right]\right)}{\left(A_{490}\left[\text{High control}\right] - A_{490}\left[\text{Low control}\right]\right)} \times 100$$

2.4. Enzyme-Linked Immunosorbent Assay (ELISA) for IL-6 Cytokine

Cultured supernatants were collected to measure the IL-6 secretion with the Endogen® Human IL-6 ELISA kit (Pierce Biotechnology Inc, Rockford, USA). The manufacturer's instructions were followed. Culture medium was used to prepare the standard curve by serial dilutions (ranging from 0 pg/ml to 400 pg/ml). Absorbance of the reaction microplate wells was measured at 450 nm on microplate reader (TECAN, Austria).

2.5. Enzyme Immunoassay (EIA) for Fibronectin Quantitation

Conditioned media were harvested from cell-seeded microtitre plate after four hours (for avoiding cytotoxic effects based on previous findings of apoptosis) of treatment with GLe. The TaKaRa Fibronectin EIA kit (TAKARA Bio Inc., Japan) was used for assay. Following the kit instructions, a 100 µl of sample/standard was added into an ELISA well coated with human anti-fibronectin and incubated for one hour at 37°C. The microtitre wells were washed four times and then 100 µl of substrate solution was added and incubated for 15

minutes at room temperature. 1 N Sulphuric acid (H_2SO_4) was added to stop the reaction. Finally, absorbance was read against diluent blank at 450 nm, using TECAN SPECTRA Fluor Plus microplate reader (TECAN, Austria).

2.6. Dimethylmethylene Blue (DMMB) Method for GAGs Quantitation

After four hours of incubation, same as for FN assay, membrane-bound GAGs from HUC-PC cells were extracted by a 0.1 M sodium acetate buffer at pH 5.8 in a microtitre plate overnight, in accordance with previous publication [28] with minor modifications. The supernatant was collected and digested overnight with 20 µl of papain (Merck, UK) at 65°C. The isolated GAGs were assayed by the DMMB method [29]. A 50 µl of sample/standard was added into each well of a new microtitre plate, which was followed by an addition of 200 µl of working DMMB (Aldrich, USA) reagent. Absorbance of the microtitre wells was read immediately against milliQ blank at 620 nm. GAGs solution (mixture of hyaluronate, chondroitin, sulphate, Keratan sulphate and heparan sulphate) at 0, 4, 8, 16, and 32 µg/ml concentrations was used as standards.

2.7. Statistical Analysis

Each study group was run in triplicate and duplicated samples from each group were measured for each variable. Differences between means were determined using Student's t-test (GraphPad Prism version 3.0 for Windows, San Diego California, USA). Statistical significance was sought at two tailed P-value of 0.05.

3. Results

3.1. Cytotoxicity and IL-6 Secretion Induced by GLe and BCG

Results indicated that both BCG and GLe were clearly capable of inducing dose-dependent IL-6 secretion in the HUC-PC culture (**Figure 1**). GLe was shown to be cytotoxic to the HUC-PC cells. No LPS was detected in the β-D-glucan-inhibited fractions of GLe, while approximately 0.4 EU/ml of LPS was detected in BCG at 1.2×10^7 CFU. By serial dilution, 100% ± 12% (Mean ± SEM) of the cells was killed by 250 µg/ml of GLe, and the cytotoxic effects reached a plateau of 100% at concentrations ranged 250 - 1000 µg/ml (**Figure 2(a)**). LD_{50} for GLe is between 180 - 190 µg/ml for GLe, the dose-dependence was confirmed by repeating LDH cytotoxicity assay with GLe concentrations at 40, 80, 100 and 200 µg/ml. Results indicated that 100% ± 5% and 13.8% ± 2% (Mean ± SEM) of cells were killed, by 200 µg/ml and 100 µg/ml of GLe respectively, but no cytotoxicity was found at 80

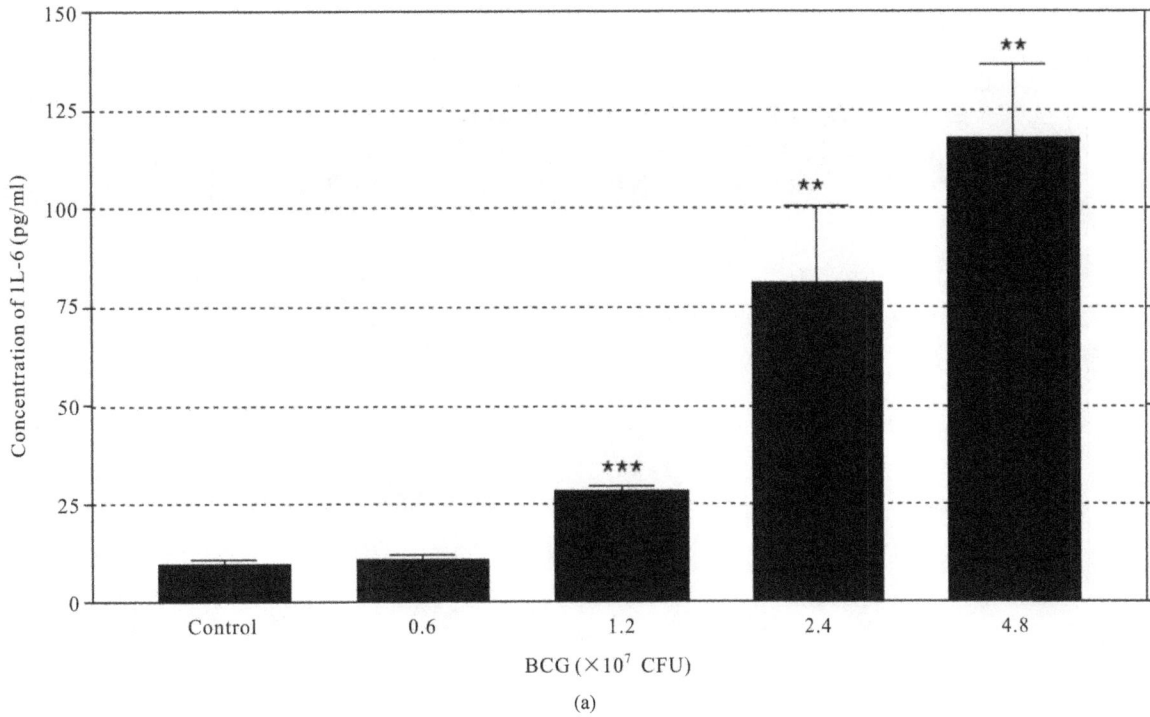

(a)

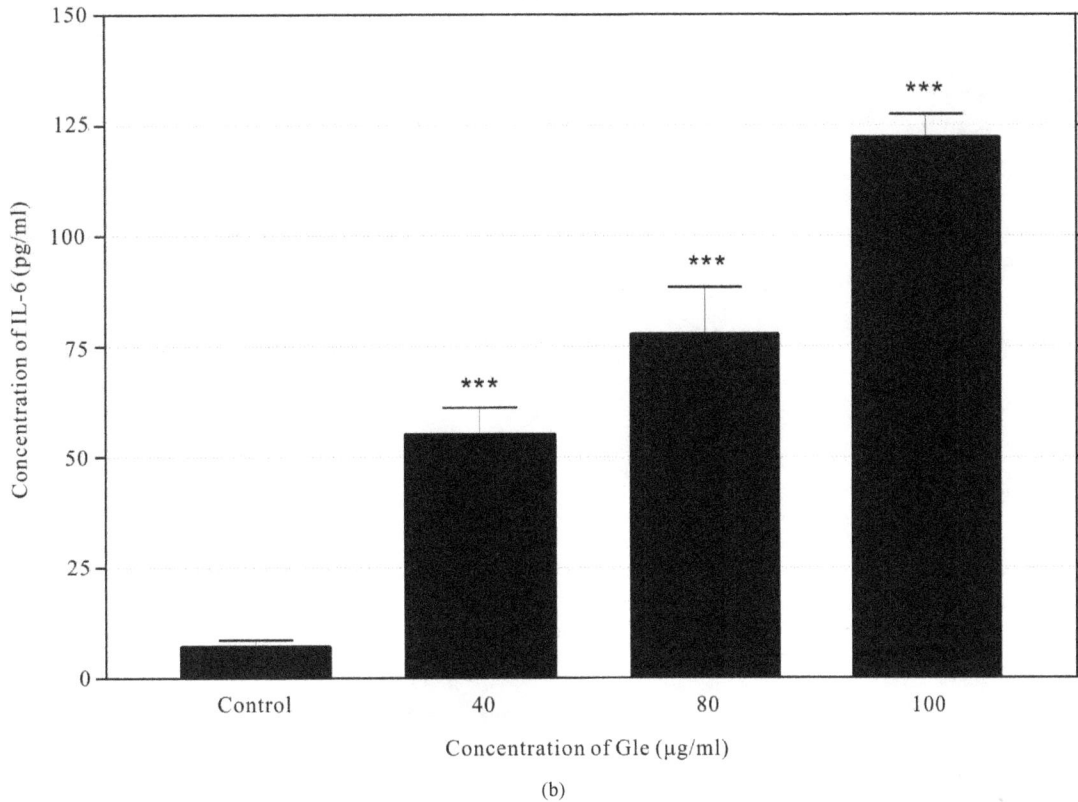

(b)

Figure 1. Dose-dependent IL-6 secretion was induced by BCG (a) and GLe (b). Culture media were harvested and measured at 24 hours after incubating with BCG at concentrations between $0.6 - 4.8 \times 10^7$ CFU while with GLe between 40 - 100 µg/ml (n = 3, error bar: SEM, $^{**}P < 0.01$; $^{***}P < 0.001$).

µg/ml or lower GLe concentration (**Figure 2(b)**). However, after the 24 hours exposure, no significant cytotox-icity was observed by BCG up to dosage at 4.8×10^7 CFU (**Figure 2(a)**).

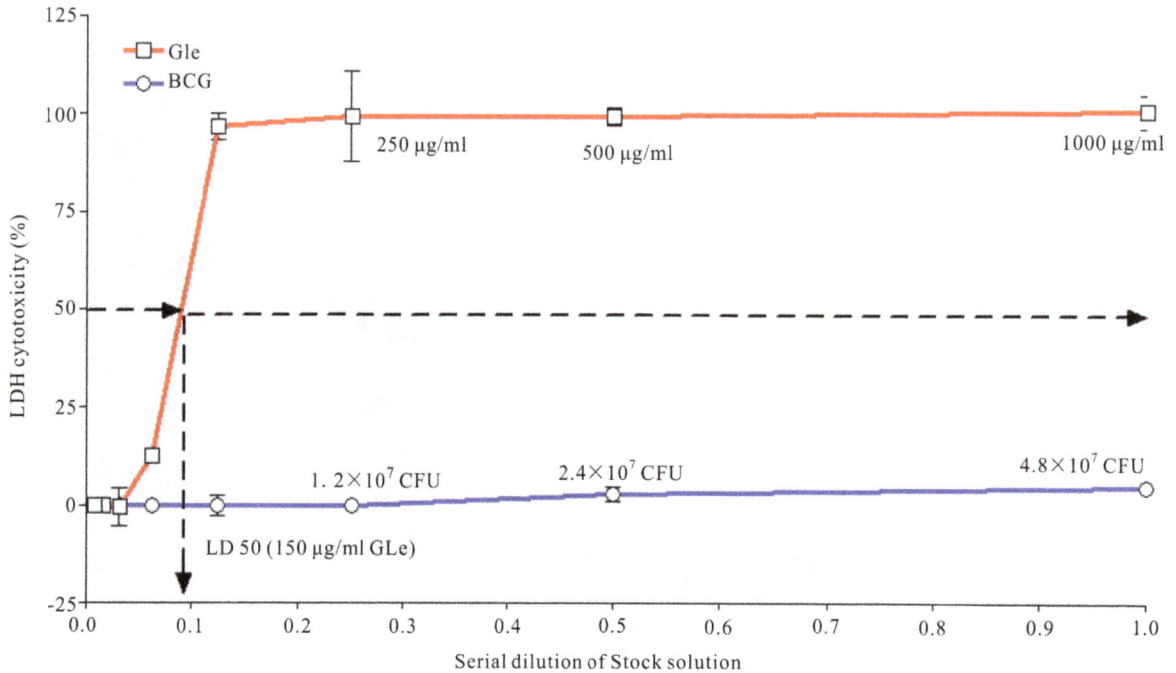

(a)

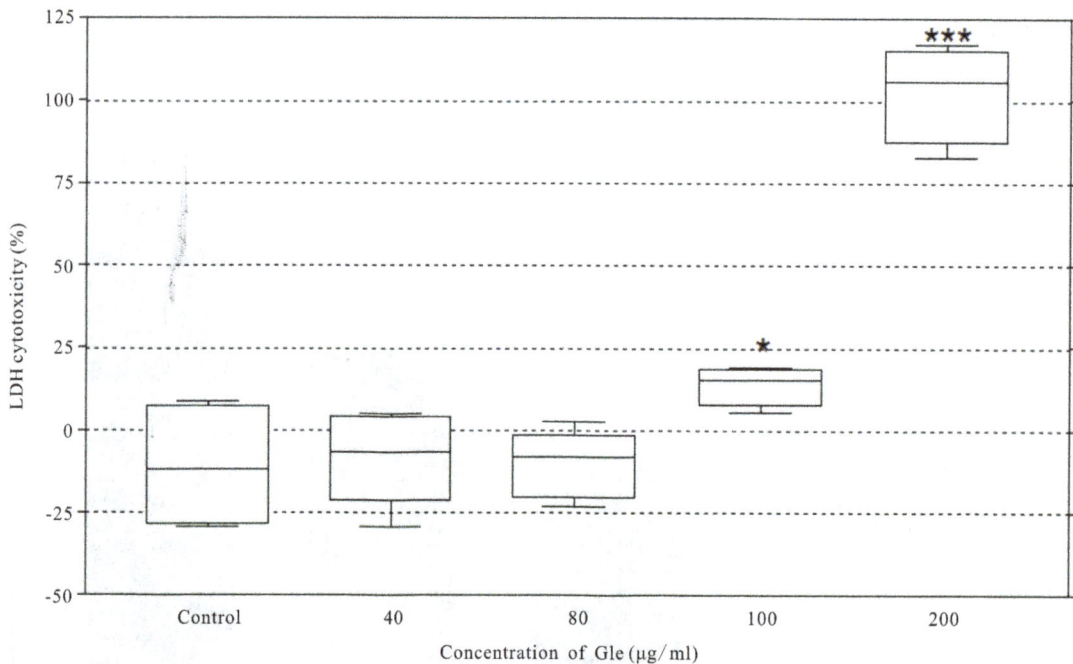

(b)

Figure 2. Cytotoxicties of BCG and *G. lucidum* on HUC-PC cells measured by LDH cytotoxicity assay after 24-hour incubation. (a) Serial dilution of GLe and BCG (starting concentrations of 1000 µg/ml and 4.8 × 10^7 CFU) were incubated with the cells. LD50 (→) was determined as 150 µg/ml for GLe (n = 3, error bar: SEM); (b) Dose-dependent cytotoxic effects of GLe at concentrations 40, 80, 100 and 200 µg/ml (n = 3, error bar: SEM). No cytotoxicity was detected at 40 and 80 µg/ml of GLe (*P < 0.05; ***P < 0.001).

3.2. The Modulation of Extracellular FN and Cell-Surface GAGs by GLe

About 15% of the free FN in the cultured media was sig-

nificantly (P < 0.01) reduced by GLe at concentrations of 40 - 100 µg/ml (**Figure 3(a)**). Such reduction may not be the maximum effects of GLe, as it was measured at 4 hours after incubation to avoid the cytotoxic artefact. On

(a)

(b)

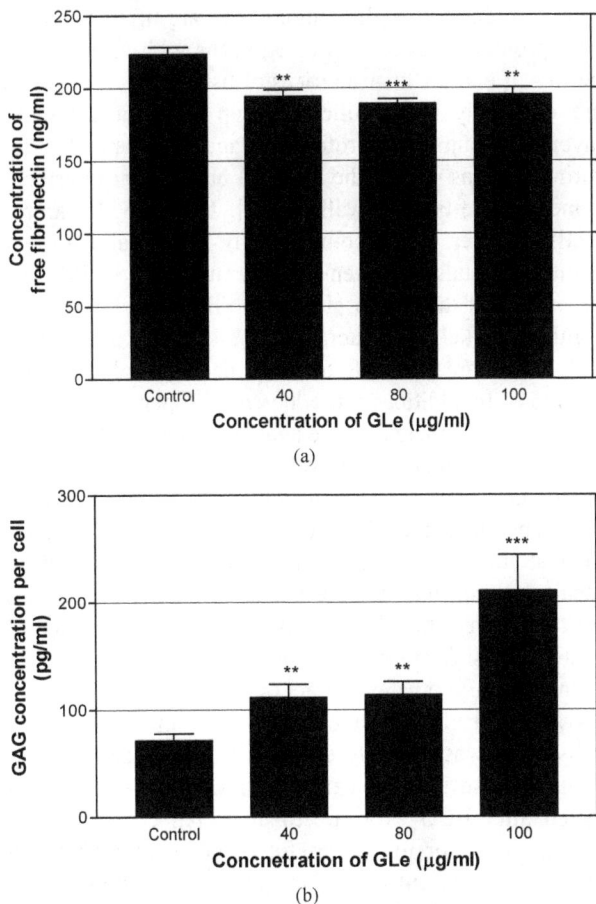

Figure 3. Culture media were harvested and measured at 4 hours after incubating with GLe (40, 80 and 100 μg/ml), which indicated the GLe-mediated reduction of extracellular FN (n = 3, error bar: SEM, ***P < 0.001; **P < 0.01). Whilst cultured cells were harvested at the same time and treated for measurement, which indicated the elevat of cell surface GAGs (n = 3, error bar: SEM, ***P < 0.001; **P < 0.01).

the other hand, the cell-membrane bound GAGs levels on HUC-PC cells were significantly (P < 0.01) increased (**Figure 3(b)**).

4. Discussion

In accordance with one of our recent publications [4], GLe has shown to be capable of stimulating IL-6 production in the HUC-PC cells. Current results indicated that the IL-6 secretions induced by GLe at 100 μg/ml and BCG at 4.8 × 107 CFU were almost quantitatively equivalent. This is consistent with reports on the HPV-immortalized Hu35E6E7 HUC cell line [21] and other bladder cancer cells [11,13-16] that IL-6 was commonly up-regulated by BCG. Lipopolysaccharide (LPS), a potent immune-stimulator is found in gram-negative bacteria but also easily being extracted from GL by ethanol [30,31]. However, results of LAL test indicated that

unlike the BCG, GLe used in current study was negative for LPS. Thus, the BCG-mediated IL-6 secretion was at least partly owned to its LPS activities while the IL-6 induced by GLe was not. At molecular level, the expression of IL-6 mRNA in the Hu35E6E7 HUC cells was found to be exclusively triggered by BCG through the toll-like receptor (TLR) signaling [21]. NF-κB and AP-1 are the main signaling pathways responsible for IL-6 expression immediately upon BCG stimulation [32]. Coherently, we have reported that GLe also enhanced the p50/p65 NF-κB activity during the immunological events in the HUC-PC cells [4]. In response to BCG, the NF-κB-mediated pathways and thus the IL-6 promoter constructs were triggered through the cross-linking of α5β1 integrin on the surface of human TCC cells and that able to induce cell cycle arrest [26,33]. The idea of "IL-6-activated tumor inhibition" has been proposed earlier [34]. IL-6 of autocrine and recombinant natures were demonstrated to be antiproliferative in TCC cell lines [26, 35-37]. The inhibition of leukaemia cells mediated by GL was also once suggested to be responsible by the increased IL-6 secretion [38,39]. However, the conceptual role of cytotoxic IL-6 is arguable with the fact that normal and low-grade bladder cancer cells which have high capacity of internalizing BCG to induce IL-6 are less efficient being killed by BCG [16]. Cytotoxicity of BCG was shown to be more potent on poorly-differentiated highgrade bladder cancer cells than the low-grade ones [27]. This is further confirmed by the present results where BCG was shown to be non-cytotoxic to the HUC-PC cells, at least after 24-hour incubation that IL-6 was significantly induced. In contrast, cytotoxic effects of GLe and IL-6 induction were explicitly demonstrated at 24 hours. Therefore, IL-6 is important to be an inductive marker for BCG internalization rather than its cytotoxicity in BCG-mediated prophylaxis in bladder cancer.

The α5β1 integrin is a classic cellular receptor presented on the malignant urothelium for fibronectin (FN) [26,33]. Expression of α5 and β1 mRNA could be promoted by exogenous and autocrine IL-6, while competitive inhibitors of FN inhibit BCG-induced NF-κB signaling pathways [33,40]. Furthermore, autocrine IL-6 enhanced BCG adherence to the 253J TCC cell line through the up-regulation of α5β1 integrin receptor for FN [40]. In the present study, the up-regulation of IL-6 secretion in response to BCG suggested the HUC-PC cells are capable of internalizing BCG, despite further elucidation is needed. FN is an essential adhesion glycoprotein for BCG binding to the surface of urothelium, internalization and production IL-6 [17,41,42]. There are two forms of FN: soluble and surface-bound [43]. Loss of cell surface FN on transformed cells is correlated with acquisition of tumorigenicity [44] and metastatic potential [45]. Such FN losses are mainly due to reduced synthesis, reduced binding and increased degradation rate, and increased FN release into the extracellular matrix [43]. These FN molecules facilitate cell-substrate adhesion, and thus enhance the interaction between the urothelium and extracellular matrix, and ultimately affect the cell morphology, cytoskeletal organization, migration and differentiation [46]. About 90% of urothelial tumor stroma was positive for FN immunohistochemical expression [47]. Expression of extracellular FN is correlated with tumor progression for invasiveness and aggressiveness [47,48]. Blocking of FN attachment sites on TCC cells inhibits the tumor outgrowth *in vivo* [49]. The diagnostic roles of soluble FN in urine have been proposed and its elevated levels are associated with tumor stage, degree of differentiation, tumor size, multifocal nature or macroscopic appearance [46,50]. Clinical data supported that persistent elevation of urinary FN causes BCG failure after complete TUR [51]. Excess soluble FN, whether from exogenous or autocrine origin, also saturates mycobacterial and cell surface FN receptors simultaneously, and precludes the bridging ability of a single FN molecule, impairing $\alpha5\beta1$ integrin/integrin mediated NF-κB signal transduction which is considered to be critical for BCG prophylaxis [22]. Thus, free FN in the culture media is regarded as a key factor for both carcinogenesis of urothelial cells and BCG binding. In contrast, cell surface expression of FN is comparatively less important regarding its roles in bladder chemoprevention. Current findings indicated that free FN was reduced in the culture media of treated HUC-PC cells by GLe.

Furthermore, the expression of GAGs on the HUC-PC cell surface was also increased by GLe. Formerly known as mucopolysaccharides, GAGs are long unbranched po-lysaccharides, are highly anionic and are often bound to core proteins to become proteoglycans with varying properties of extracellular matrices of tissues [52,53]. GAGs are extremely hydrophilic and trap water at the outer layer of the umbrella urothelium, and this trapped water forms a gel as part of the mucosal barrier that interfaces urine and the bladder wall [54,55]. This provides a protective barrier that becomes highly impermeable to any solutes, crystals and even bacteria in urine [54,56]. The disruption of this mucosal permeability is pathologically significant such that interstitial cystitis (IC) occurs [54, 57]. GAGs are also able to repair damaged bladder mucosa [54]. In addition, anti-adherence properties of GAGs have primary innate defence against bacterial attacks [52, 54,56]. Experimental removal of GAGs from the urothelial surface causes a ten-fold higher bacterial adherence [58]. Therefore, the effects of GLe on cell-surface GAGs may strengthen the mucosal barrier of the urothelium, repair the urothelial damage induced by BCG therapy, as well as prevent the side effects of BCG therapy, such as cystitis and infections.

In summary, ethanol extract of GL exerted as a similar activator for IL-6 production as BCG in the HUC-PC cells. IL-6 was the only cytokine selected for measurement because it is the earliest cytokine that can be detected after BCG exposure to urothelial cells and it is also an indicator for successful BCG internalization by these cells. Current results suggested that combinational use of GLe and BCG may exert synergistic effects in several ways (**Figure 4**): Firstly, the cytotoxic and cytokine secretion can be additive to BCG activities; Secondly, the reduction of free FN can facilitate BCG binding to the

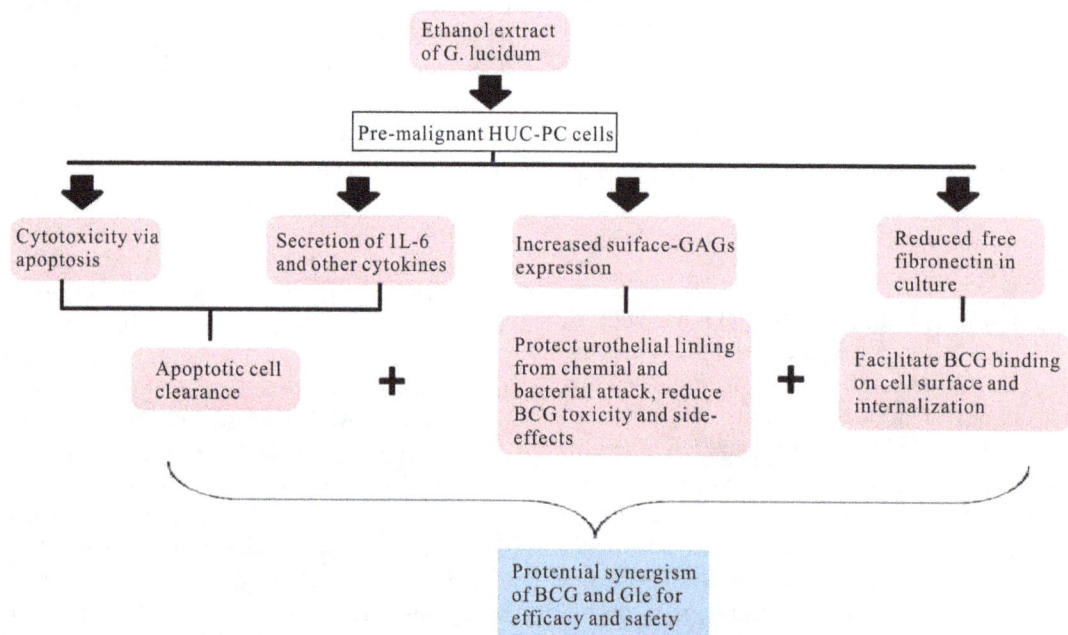

Figure 4. A summary of GLe effects on the HUC-PC cells to deduce the potential synergism between BCG and GLe.

urothelial surface for subsequent internalization and IL-6 secretion, particularly for cells at normal or low grades. Nonetheless, the reduction of free FN, by itself may also suggest being tumor suppressive to inhibit the growth and progression by reducing unnecessary cell-substrate interactions; and thirdly, the increased cell surface GAGs expression provide additional protection from chemical and bacterial attacks, and thus is potential in reducing side-effects caused by BCG. Further experiments are underway to define the synergism of GLe and BCG as well as to investigate the underlying mechanisms. No doubt, the anticancer activities of GLe were demonstrated in the HUC-PC cell model to suggest the associations between IL-6 induction, FN reduction, and BCG-GLe synergism were suggested. However, the cause-and-effect mechanism needs to be confirmed by further careful scientific investigation.

5. Acknowledgements

This project was supported by the Research Committee of the Hong Kong Polytechnic University for the postgraduate scholarship (RGH8) and Sir Edward Youde Memorial Fellowship awarded to Dr. John Yuen. The authors are grateful to Dr. J. Y. Rao (UCLA Medical Center, USA) for providing the HUC-PC cell line and professional advice.

REFERENCES

[1] Q. Y. Lu, Y. S. Jin, Q. Zhang, Z. Zhang, D. Heber, V. L. Go, et al., "Ganoderma lucidum Extracts Inhibit Growth and Induce Actin Polymerization in Bladder Cancer Cells in Vitro," Cancer Letters, Vol. 216, No. 1, 2004, pp. 9-20. doi:10.1016/j.canlet.2004.06.022

[2] J. W. Yuen, M. D. Gohel and D. W. Au, "Telomerase-Associated Apoptotic Events by Mushroom Ganoderma Lucidum on Premalignant Human Urothelial Cells," Nutrition and Cancer, Vol. 60, No. 1, 2008, pp. 109-119. doi:10.1080/01635580701525869

[3] J. W. Yuen and M. D. Gohel, "The Dual Roles of Ganoderma Antioxidants on Urothelial Cell DNA under Carcinogenic Attack," Journal of Ethnopharmacology, Vol. 118, No. 2, 2008, pp. 324-330. doi:10.1016/j.jep.2008.05.003

[4] J. W. Yuen, M. D. Gohel and C. F. Ng, "The Differential Immunological Activities of Ganoderma lucidum on Human Pre-Cancerous Uroepithelial Cells," Journal of Ethnopharmacology, Vol. 135, No. 1, 2011, pp. 711-718. doi:10.1016/j.jep.2011.04.005

[5] W. Oosterlinck, "The Management of Superficial Bladder Cancer," BJU International, Vol. 87, No. 2, 2001, pp. 135-140. doi:10.1046/j.1464-410x.2001.00948.x

[6] J. T. Leppert, O. Shvarts, K. Kawaoka, R. Lieberman, A. S. Belldegrun and A. J. Pantuck, "Prevention of Bladder Cancer: A Review," European Urology, Vol. 49, No. 2,

2006, pp. 226-234. doi:10.1016/j.eururo.2005.12.011

[7] P. Tyagi, P. C. Wu, M. Chancellor, N. Yoshimura and L. Huang, "Recent Advances in Intravesical Drug/Gene Delivery," Molecular Pharmaceutics, Vol. 3, No. 4, 2006, pp. 369-379. doi:10.1021/mp060001j

[8] D. L. Lamm, W. R. McGee and K. Hale, "Bladder Cancer: Current Optimal Intravesical Treatment," Urologic Nursing, Vol. 25, No. 5, 2005, pp. 323-326, 331-332.

[9] K. Taniguchi, S. Koga, M. Nishikido, S. Yamashita, T. Sakuragi, H. Kanetake, et al., "Systemic Immune Response after Intravesical Instillation of Bacille Calmette-Guerin (BCG) for Superficial Bladder Cancer," Clinical & Experimental Immunology, Vol. 115, No. 1, 1999, pp. 131-135. doi:10.1046/j.1365-2249.1999.00756.x

[10] M. Sanchez-Carbayo, M. Urrutia, R. Romani, M. Herrero, J. M. Gonzalez de Buitrago and J. A. Navajo, "Serial Urinary IL-2, IL-6, IL-8, TNF Alpha, UBC, CYFRA 21-1 and NMP22 during Follow-Up of Patients with Bladder Cancer Receiving Intravesical BCG," Anticancer Research, Vol. 21, No. 4B, 2001, pp. 3041-3047.

[11] J. J. Patard, F. Saint, F. Velotti, C. C. Abbou and D. K. Chopin, "Immune Response Following Intravesical Bacillus Calmette-Guerin Instillations in Superficial Bladder Cancer: A Review," Urological Research, Vol. 26, No. 3, 1998, pp. 155-159. doi:10.1007/s002400050039

[12] T. M. de Reijke, E. C. de Boer, K. H. Kurth and D. H. Schamhart, "Urinary Cytokines during Intravesical Bacillus Calmette-Guerin Therapy for Superficial Bladder Cancer: Processing, Stability and Prognostic Value," Journal of Urology, Vol. 155, No. 2, 1996, pp. 477-482. doi:10.1016/S0022-5347(01)66424-3

[13] T. M. de Reijke, P. C. Vos, E. C. de Boer, R. F. Bevers, W. H. de Muinck Keizer, K. H. Kurth, et al., "Cytokine Production by the Human Bladder Carcinoma Cell Line T24 in the Presence of Bacillus Calmette-Guerin (BCG)," Urological Research, Vol. 21, No. 5, 1993, pp. 349-352. doi:10.1007/BF00296835

[14] K. Esuvaranathan, A. B. Alexandroff, M. McIntyre, A. M. Jackson, S. Prescott, G. D. Chisholm, et al., "Interleukin-6 Production by Bladder Tumors Is Upregulated by BCG Immunotherapy," Journal of Urology, Vol. 154, No. 2, 1995, pp. 572-575. doi:10.1016/S0022-5347(01)67113-1

[15] Y. Zhang, R. Mahendran, L. L. Yap, K. Esuvaranathan and H. E. Khoo, "The Signalling Pathway for BCG-Induced Interleukin-6 Production in Human Bladder Cancer Cells," Biochemical Pharmacology, Vol. 63, No. 2, 2002, pp. 273-282. doi:10.1016/S0006-2952(01)00831-0

[16] R. F. Bevers, E. C. de Boer, K. H. Kurth and D. H. Schamhart, "BCG-Induced Interleukin-6 Upregulation and BCG Internalization in Well and Poorly Differentiated Human Bladder Cancer Cell Lines," European Cytokine Network, Vol. 9, No. 2, 1998, pp. 181-186.

[17] R. F. Bevers, K. H. Kurth and D. H. Schamhart, "Role of Urothelial Cells in BCG Immunotherapy for Superficial Bladder Cancer," British Journal of Cancer, Vol. 91, No. 4, 2004, pp. 607-612.

[18] L. R. Kavoussi, E. J. Brown, J. K. Ritchey and T. L. Ratliff, "Fibronectin-Mediated Calmette-Guerin Bacillus At-

tachment to Murine Bladder Mucosa. Requirement for the Expression of an Antitumor Response," *The Journal of Clinical Investigation*, Vol. 85, No. 1, 1990, pp. 62-67. doi:10.1172/JCI114434

[19] T. L. Ratliff, J. O. Palmer, J. A. McGarr and E. J. Brown, "Intravesical Bacillus Calmette-Guerin Therapy for Murine Bladder Tumors: Initiation of the Response by Fibronectin-Mediated Attachment of Bacillus Calmette-Guerin," *Cancer Research*, Vol. 47, 1987, pp. 1762-1766.

[20] J. Aslanzadeh, E. J. Brown, S. P. Quillin, J. K. Ritchey and T. L. Ratliff, "Characterization of Soluble Fibronectin Binding to Bacille Calmette-Guerin," *Journal of General Microbiology*, Vol. 135, No. 10, 1989, pp. 2735-2741.

[21] J. Miyazaki, K. Kawai, T. Oikawa, A. Johraku, K. Hattori, T. Shimazui, et al., "Uroepithelial Cells Can Directly Respond to Mycobacterium Bovis Bacillus Calmette-Guerin through Toll-Like Receptor Signaling," *BJU International*, Vol. 97, No. 4, 2006, pp. 860-864. doi:10.1111/j.1464-410X.2006.06026.x

[22] G. Zhang, F. Chen, Y. Xu, Y. Cao, S. Crist, A. McKerrow, et al., "Autocrine over Expression of Fibronectin by Human Transitional Carcinoma Cells Impairs Bacillus Calmette-Guerin Adherence and Signaling," *Journal of Urology*, Vol. 172, No. 4, 2004, pp. 1496-1500. doi:10.1097/01.ju.0000140193.95528.91

[23] Z. Akbulut, A. E. Canda, A. F. Atmaca, H. I. Cimen, C. Hasanoglu and M. D. Balbay, "BCG Sepsis Following Inadvertent Intravenous BCG Administration for the Treatment of Bladder Cancer Can Be Effectively Cured with Anti-Tuberculosis Medications," *The New Zealand Medical Journal*, Vol. 123, No. 1325, 2010, pp. 72-77.

[24] D. H. Schamhart, E. C. De Boer, R. Vleeming and K. H. Kurth, "Theoretical and Experimental Evidence on the Use of Glycosaminoglycans in BCG-Mediated Immunotherapy of Superficial Bladder Cancer," *Seminars in Thrombosis and Hemostasis*, Vol. 20, No. 3, 1994, pp. 301-309. doi:10.1055/s-2007-1001917

[25] D. H. Schamhart, E. C. de Boer and K. H. Kurth, "Interaction between Bacteria and the Lumenal Bladder Surface: Modulation by Pentosan Polysulfate, an Experimental and Theoretical Approach with Clinical Implication," *World Journal of Urology*, Vol. 12, No. 1, 1994, pp. 27-37. doi:10.1007/BF00182048

[26] F. Chen, G. Zhang, Y. Iwamoto and W. A. See, "BCG Directly Induces Cell Cycle Arrest in Human Transitional Carcinoma Cell Lines as a Consequence of Integrin Cross-Linking," *BMC Urology*, Vol. 5, 2005, p. 8. doi:10.1186/1471-2490-5-8

[27] Y. Zhang, H. E. Khoo and K. Esuvaranatha, "Effects of Bacillus Calmette-Guerin and Interferon-Alpha-2B on Human Bladder Cancer *in Vitro*," *International Journal of Cancer*, Vol. 71, No. 5, 1997, pp. 851-857. doi:10.1002/(SICI)1097-0215(19970529)71:5<851::AID-IJC25>3.0.CO;2-9

[28] R. W. Farndale, C. A. Sayers and A. J. Barrett, "A Direct Spectrophotometric Microassay for Sulfated Glycosaminoglycans in Cartilage Cultures," *Connective Tissue Research*, Vol. 9, No. 4, 1982, pp. 247-248. doi:10.3109/03008208209160269

[29] R. W. Farndale, D. J. Buttle and A. J. Barrett, "Improved Quantitation and Discrimination of Sulphated Glycosaminoglycans by Use of Dimethylmethylene Blue," *Biochimica et Biophysica Acta*, Vol. 883, No. 2, 1986, pp. 173-177. doi:10.1016/0304-4165(86)90306-5

[30] W. T. Chung, S. H. Lee, J. D. Kim, Y. S. Park, B. Hwang, S. Y. Lee, et al., "Effect of Mycelial Culture Broth of *Ganoderma lucidum* on the Growth Characteristics of Human Cell Lines," *Journal of Bioscience and Bioengineering*, Vol. 92, No. 6, 2001, pp. 550-555.

[31] H. S. Chen, Y. F. Tsai, S. Lin, C. C. Lin, K. H. Khoo, C. H. Lin, et al., "Studies on the Immuno-Modulating and Anti-Tumor Activities of *Ganoderma lucidum* (Reishi) Polysaccharides," *Bioorganic & Medicinal Chemistry*, Vol. 12, No. 21, 2004, pp. 5595-5601.

[32] F. Chen, P. Langenstroer, G. Zhang, Y. Iwamoto and W. A. See, "Androgen Dependent Regulation of Bacillus Calmette-Guerin Induced Interleukin-6 Expression in Human Transitional Carcinoma Cell Lines," *Journal of Urology*, Vol. 170, No. 5, 2003, pp. 2009-2013.

[33] F. Chen, G. Zhang, Y. Iwamoto and W. A. See, "Bacillus Calmette-Guerin Initiates Intracellular Signaling in a Transitional Carcinoma Cell Line by Cross-Linking Alpha 5 Beta 1 Integrin," *Journal of Urology*, Vol. 170, No. 2, 2003, pp. 605-610.

[34] P. Musiani, A. Modesti, M. Giovarelli, F. Cavallo, M. P. Colombo, P. L. Lollini, et al., "Cytokines, Tumour-Cell Death and Immunogenicity: A Question of Choice," *Immunology Today*, Vol. 18, No. 1, 1997, pp. 32-36.

[35] A. Sasaki, S. Kudoh, K. Mori, N. Takahashi and T. Suzuki, "Are BCG Effects against Urinary Bladder Carcinoma Cell Line T24 Correlated with Apoptosis *in Vitro*?" *Urology International*, Vol. 59, No. 3, 1997, pp. 142-148.

[36] E. C. Borden, D. S. Groveman, T. Nasu, C. Reznikoff and G. T. Bryan, "Antiproliferative Activities of Interferons against Human Bladder Carcinoma Cell Lines *in Vitro*," *The Journal of Urology*, Vol. 132, No. 4, 1984, pp. 800-803.

[37] A. M. Jackson, A. B. Alexandroff, D. Fleming, S. Prescott, G. D. Chisholm and K. James, "Bacillus Calmette-Guerin (BCG) Organisms Directly Alter the Growth of Bladder Tumour Cells," *International Journal of Oncology*, Vol. 5, No. 3, 1994, pp. 697-703.

[38] International Agency for Research on Cancer, "Monographs on the Evaluation of Carcinogenic Risk of Chemicals," World Health Organization, Geneva, 1972.

[39] S. Y. Wang, M. L. Hsu, H. C. Hsu, C. H. Tzeng, S. S. Lee, M. S. Shiao, et al., "The Anti-Tumor Effect of Ganoderma Lucidum Is Mediated by Cytokines Released from Activated Macrophages and T Lymphocytes," *International Journal of Cancer*, Vol. 70, No. 6, 1997, pp. 699-705. doi:10.1002/(SICI)1097-0215(19970317)70:6<699::AID-IJC12>3.0.CO;2-5

[40] G. J. Zhang, S. A. Crist, A. K. McKerrow, Y. Xu, D. C. Ladehoff and W. A. See, "Autocrine IL-6 Production by Human Transitional Carcinoma Cells Upregulates Expression of the alpha5beta1 Fibronectin Receptor," *The Journal of Urology*, Vol. 163, No. 5, 2000, pp. 1553-1559.

doi:10.1016/S0022-5347(05)67678-1

[41] W. Zhao, J. S. Schorey, M. Bong-Mastek, J. Ritchey, E. J. Brown and T. L. Ratliff, "Role of a Bacillus Calmette-Guerin Fibronectin Attachment Protein in BCG-Induced Antitumor Activity," *International Journal of Cancer*, Vol. 86, No. 1, 2000, pp. 83-88. doi:10.1002/(SICI)1097-0215(20000401)86:1<83::AID-IJC13>3.0.CO:2-R

[42] A. Bohle, E. van der Sloot, E. Richter, J. Gerdes, W. G. Wood and J. Gerdes, "Binding to Fibronectin (FN)—A Prerequisite Step? Investigations on the Role of FN in Intravesical BCG Immunotherapy," *Investigative Urology*, Vol. 5, 1994, pp. 100-104.

[43] R. O. Hynes and K. M. Yamada, "Fibronectins: Multi-functional Modular Glycoproteins," *The Journal of Cell Biology*, Vol. 95, No. 2, 1982, pp. 369-377. doi:10.1083/jcb.95.2.369

[44] R. O. Hynes, A. T. Destree, M. E. Perkins and D. D. Wagner, "Cell Surface Fibronectin and Oncogenic Transformation," *Journal of Supramolecular Structure*, Vol. 11, No. 1, 1979, pp. 95-104. doi:10.1002/jss.400110110

[45] H. S. Smith, J. L. Riggs and M. W. Mosesson, "Production of Fibronectin by Human Epithelial Cells in Culture," *Cancer Research*, Vol. 39, No. 10, 1979, pp. 4138-4144.

[46] N. Mutlu, L. Turkeri and K. Emerk, "Analytical and Clinical Evaluation of a New Urinary Tumor Marker: Bladder Tumor Fibronectin in Diagnosis and Follow-Up of Bladder Cancer," *Clinical Chemistry and Laboratory Medicine*, Vol. 41, No. 8, 2003, pp. 1069-1074. doi:10.1515/CCLM.2003.165

[47] E. Ioachim, M. Michael, N. E. Stavropoulos, E. Kitsiou, M. Salmas and V. Malamou-Mitsi, "A Clinicopathological Study of the Expression of Extracellular Matrix Components in Urothelial Carcinoma," *BJU International*, Vol. 95, No. 4, 2005, pp. 655-659. doi:10.1111/j.1464-410X.2005.05357.x

[48] T. Saito, Y. Tomita, T. Kawasaki, V. Bilim and K. Takahashi, "Subsequent Activation of Mitogen-Activated Protein Kinase after Adhesion of Transitional Cell Cancer Cells to Fibronectin," *Urologia Internationalis*, Vol. 69, 2002, pp. 125-128. doi:10.1159/000065561

[49] A. Bohle, A. Jurczok, P. Ardelt, T. Wulf, A. J. Ulmer, D. Jocham, *et al.*, "Inhibition of Bladder Carcinoma Cell Adhesion by Oligopeptide Combinations *in Vitro* and *in Vivo*," *The Journal of Urology*, Vol. 167, No. 1, 2002, pp. 357-363. doi:10.1016/S0022-5347(05)65468-7

[50] V. Menendez, A. Fernandez-Suarez, J. A. Galan, M. Perez and F. Garcia-Lopez, "Diagnosis of Bladder Cancer by Analysis of Urinary Fibronectin," *Urology*, Vol. 65, No. 2, 2005, pp. 284-289. doi:10.1016/j.urology.2004.09.028

[51] M. Laufer, I. Kaver, B. Sela and H. Matzkin, "Elevated Urinary Fibronectin Levels after Transurethral Resection of Bladder Tumour: A Possible Role in Patients Failing Therapy with Bacillus Calmette-Guerin," *BJU Internation*, Vol. 84, No. 4, 1999, pp. 428-432. doi:10.1046/j.1464-410x.1999.00208.x

[52] R. E. Hurst, "Structure, Function, and pathology of Proteoglycans and Glycosaminoglycans in the Urinary Tract," *World Journal of Urology*, Vol. 12, No. 1, 1994, pp. 3-10. doi:10.1007/BF00182044

[53] K. H. Kurth, "Glycosaminoglycans and Proteoglycans in the Urinary Tract," *World Journal of Urology*, Vol. 12, No. 1, 1994, p. 2.

[54] C. L. Parsons, "The Role of the Urinary Epithelium in the Pathogenesis of Interstitial Cystitis/Prostatitis/Urethritis," *Urology*, Vol. 69, No. 4, 2007, pp. 9-16. doi:10.1016/j.urology.2006.03.084

[55] J. N'Dow, N. Jordan, C. N. Robson, D. E. Neal and J. P. Pearson, "The Bladder Does Not Appear to Have a Dynamic Secreted Continuous Mucous Gel Layer," *The Journal of Urology*, Vol. 173, No. 6, 2005, pp. 2025-2031. doi:10.1097/01.ju.0000158454.47299.ae

[56] C. L. Parsons, "A Model for the Function of Glycosaminoglycans in the Urinary Tract," *World Journal of Urology*, Vol. 12, No. 1, 1994, pp. 38-42. doi:10.1007/BF00182049

[57] V. B. Lokeshwar, M. G. Selzer, W. H. Cerwinka, M. F. Gomez, R. R. Kester, D. E. Bejany, *et al.*, "Urinary Uronate and Sulfated Glycosaminoglycan Levels: Markers for Interstitial Cystitis Severity," *The Journal of Urology*, 2005, Vol. 174, No. 1, pp. 344-349. doi:10.1097/01.ju.0000161599.69942.2e

[58] C. L. Parsons, S. G. Mulholland and H. Anwar, "Antibacterial Activity of Bladder Surface Mucin Duplicated by Exogenous Glycosaminoglycan (Heparin)," *Infection and Immunity*, Vol. 24, No. 2, 1979, pp. 552-557.

7

Clinical Analysis of Influenza A (H1N1) Viral Pneumonia Complicated with Bacterial Infection

Xixin Yan, Haibo Xu, Fangfang Qu, Yue Liu, Xiumin Zhang

Department of Respiratory Medicine, The Second Affiliated Hospital, Hebei Medical University, Shijiazhuang, China

Email: superxuhaibo123@163.com

ABSTRACT

Purpose: We investigated the efficacy of potent or combined antibiotics in patients suffering bacterial infections secondary to H1N1 by retrospectively analyzing their bacterial pathogen spectrum and clinical characteristics. **Methods:** Multi-center retrospective analysis was performed using clinical data of H1N1 patients from 27 hospitals in Hebei Province, China, from November 1 to December 31, 2009. **Results:** Of 480 H1N1-infected patients enrolled from an inpatient clinic, 91 were positive for bacterial culture. Bacteria were detected in sputum culture at 7.00 ± 8.87 days post-admission. Compared with the negative group, the patients in the positive sputum culture group had a higher mean age and prevalence of basic diseases, higher APECHEII (Acute Physiology and Chronic Health Evaluation II) score within 24 hours of admission, longer hospital stays, and higher mortality. In total, 189 bacterial strains were isolated, with the majority of samples testing positive for *Acinetobacter baumanii* (47), *Streptococcus viridians* (26), or *Pseudomonas aeruginosa* (19). *S. viridians* was the major cause of infection within 3 days of admission, while *A. baumanii* infection was more prevalent from 4 days post-admission; there was a significant difference in the constituent ratio between the two pathogens ($p < 0.001$). Compared with patients administered common antibiotics, the potent antibiotics group showed no significant difference in hospitalization time, time until bacterial detection, mortality, or detection ratio of resistant strains ($p > 0.05$). **Conclusions:** Complicated bacterial infection in H1N1 patients increases hospitalization time and mortality. Gram-negative bacilli and multi-resistant strains are the main sources of infection. Early administration of potent or combined antibiotics, even during the period of rapid onset, may not be suitable in H1N1-infected patients, particularly previously healthy young patients.

Keywords: Influenza A H1N1; Bacteria; Antibiotics; Mortality

1. Introduction

The influenza A (H1N1) virus (2009) has universal susceptibility in population. Although there is no clear pattern of global incidence or data for patient mortality, there are three major causes of death in influenza A-infected patients: primary viral infection directly results in fatal respiratory failure; secondary bacterial infection affects the recovery of pulmonary function and ultimately results in death due to complications; and viral infection; or secondary bacterial infection induces deterioration of basic diseases. Previous investigations of the 1918-1919 influenza A pandemic found that most healthy young patients died from a single influenza viral infection, while mortality in older patients, particularly those with pre-existing conditions, was mainly due to complicated bacterial infection in the later stages of viral infection. From this standpoint, it is important to identify the number of cases of bacterial infection, and catalog the related clinical characteristics of influenza A (H1N1) patients, particularly where influenza A becomes a major infectious pathogen of the respiratory tract.

In this report, we described the bacterial pathogen spectrum and clinical characteristics of patients suffering bacterial infections secondary to H1N1, and analyzed the efficacy of potent or combined antibiotics.

2. Materials and Methods

2.1. Patients

The study included influenza A (H1N1) patients from 27 hospitals in Hebei Province, China, with samples collected from November-December 2009. The criteria for diagnosis of influenza A viral infection, severe and critical cases, met the Diagnosis and Therapy Strategy of Influenza A (H1N1) Virus (2009) requirements, as determined by the Ministry of Health of the People's Republic of China [1]. A confirmed case was a person whose influenza A (pH1N1) was verified by real-time reverse-transcriptase polymerase chain reaction (rRT-PCR) with or without the presentation of other clinical symptoms.

2.2. Collection of Patient Data

With the cooperation of the Department of Medical Policy, Provincial Health Bureau of Hebei, the data from original medical record were collected using a questionnaire that was designed according to the Clinical Research Project of Severe Influenza A (H1N1) Patients, established by the Division of Medical Policy, the Ministry of Health of the People's Republic of China.

2.3. Statistical Analysis

Means (standard deviations, SD) or medians (inter-quartiles, IQR) were calculated as summaries of continuous variables. For categorical variables, percentages of patients in each category were calculated. We compared clinical characteristics and clinical outcomes by using an ANOVA test, chi-square test, or Fisher's exact test or Wilcoxon rank-sum test as necessary. A p value of less than 0.05 was considered to indicate statistical significance. All analysis was carried out using SPSS for Windows (release 13.0).

3. Results

3.1. General Clinical Conditions

In total, 480 influenza A (H1N1) patients were enrolled in Hebei Province, including 192 males and 288 females, with an average age of 30.1 ± 18.7 years, and hospitalization duration of 1 - 85 days (mean 12.9 ± 10.4 days). Sixty-one patients died during the course of the study (12.7%), and the infection in 124 was further complicated by pre-existing conditions, including hypertension (47), diabetes (27), coronary artery disease (15), congestive heart failure (5), chronic obstructive pulmonary disease (10), stroke (5), hematological disease (10), and malignant tumors (5). Ninety-one patients showed positive bacterial culture (non-pre-existing), with an average

hospitalization period of 7.00 ± 8.87 days. The clinical characteristics are listed in **Table 1**.

3.2. Pathogen Data

A total of 189 bacterial isolates were identified from infected patients, including *Acinetobacter baumannii* (47), *Streptococcus viridans* (26), *Pseudomonas aeruginosa* (19), *Staphylococcus aureus* (16), *Neisseria* sp. (15), *Klebsiella pneumonia* (14), other *Staphylococcus* sp. (10), *Stenotrophomonas maltophilia* (8), and other species (34). There were 86 multi-drug resistant strains, including *S. aureus* (12), other strains (16), *P. aeruginosa* (5), and *Acinetobacter calcoaceticus* (4), as well as *A. baumannii* resistant to carbapenems (34), *K. pneumonia* producing extended-spectrum beta-lactamases (ESBL) (10), and *Staphylococcus* (5) resistant to methicillin.

The distribution of pathogens causing secondary bacterial infection and the clinical characteristics of patients within 3 days of hospitalization and at later time points are listed in **Tables 2** and **3**.

3.3. Antibiotic Treatment

There were 463 patients (96.5%) treated with antibiotics during hospitalization. Review of the initial antibiotic strategy showed that 211 patients were administrated potent antibiotics (including carbapenems, β-lactams/β-lactamase inhibitors against *P. aeruginosa* activity, fourth generation cephalosporins, vancomycin, teicoplanin, linezolid), while 200 patients were administrated a combination of two types of antibiotics. The prognoses of patients treated with the different antibiotic strategies for initial therapy post-admission are listed in **Table 4**.

4. Discussion

Previous influenza pandemics have shown that secondary bacterial infection and the aggression of underlying diseases are important factors contributing to mortality. Based on current data, influenza A (H1N1) patients with secondary bacterial infections are not uncommon. The

Table 1. Clinical characteristics of positive and negative bacterial culture groups.

	Positive group	Negative group	p value
Age (year)	35.77 ± 22.03	28.74 ± 17.59	0.001
APECHEII score	9.84 ± 6.15	6.77 ± 5.02	<0.001
Hospitalization (days)	20.23 ± 14.35	11.14 ± 8.37	<0.001
Percentage of patients with basic disease	29.0%	17.7%	0.04
Percentage of application of non-invasive ventilation	12.09%	13.88%	0.65
Percentage of application of invasive ventilation	54.94%	14.14%	<0.001
Mortality	20.88%	10.80%	0.009

Table 2. Distribution of bacterial strains at different periods of hospitalization.

	≤3 days	>3 days
Acinetobacter baumannii	1	46
Pseudomonas aeruginosa	2	17
Streptococcus viridans	13	13
Staphylococcus aureus	3	13
Klebsiella pneumoniae	2	12
Staphylococcus	0	10
Neisseria	6	9
Stenotrophomonas maltophilia	0	8
Other	4	30
Total	31	158

There was a statistical difference in the constituent ratio of pathogens between within 3 days of hospitalization and at later time points group (p < 0.001).

Table 3. Clinical characteristics of patients with bacterial infection at different periods of hospitalization.

	<3 days (30 cases)	>3 days (61 cases)	p value
Age (year)	33.47 ± 20.63	36.48 ± 22.60	0.53
WBC (×109)	7.05 ± 4.64	7.89 ± 6.16	0.50
N (×109)	5.30 ± 4.37	6.29 ± 5.43	0.37
T (°C)	37.31 ± 1.09	37.16 ± 0.90	0.49
APECHEII score	9.80 ± 7.11	9.80 ± 5.64	1
Hospitalization (days)	14.72 ± 7.71	24.93 ± 17.58	0.003
Ratio of multi-drug resistant bacteria	25.81%	49.37%	0.003
Mortality	12.12%	24.56%	0.15

Centers for Disease Control in the United States performed pathological analyses of 77 lethal cases of the most recent influenza A infection (2009) and found 22 cases with infection of the lower respiratory tract, including 10 cases with Streptococcus pneumoniae, 10 cases with other streptococcal infection, seven cases with *S. aureus* (five methicillin-resistant *S. aureus*), one case with Hemophilus influenzae, and 16 cases with underlying conditions such as asthma and cardio-cerebral vascular disease [2]. Researchers in Korea retrospectively analyzed reports from 115 deceased patients and found that 28 patients presented with positive bacterial sputum cultures, predominantly *S. aureus* and *K. pneumoniae* [3]. Louie *et al.* reported that in 1088 cases of influenza A (H1N1) infection, 46 cases were diagnosed with secondary bacterial pneumonia, mainly caused by common pathogens such as *S. pneumoniae*, *S. aureus*, group A Streptococcus, and various Gram-negative bacteria. Most patients with secondary infection caused by Gram-negative bacilli suffered basic pulmonary diseases such as cystic fibrosis [4]. These results are similar to our present findings. Single-species infections caused by *S. aureus*, *S. viridans*, *A. baumannii*, and *P. aeruginosa* accounted for a certain percentage of disease, which is more common in the middle-aged and elderly populations already complicated with underlying conditions, and results in prolonged hospitalization and increased mortality. Differences in infectious isolates are related to region, climate, inclusion criteria, pathogen prevalence, drug administration, and drug resistance.

The bacteria detected in sputum cultures taken 3 days post-hospitalization were predominantly Gram-negative bacilli and multi-drug resistant bacteria. Of these, 54.9% were detected in patients undergoing invasive ventilation, implicating these bacteria in ventilator-associated pneumonia. Interestingly, there was no obvious difference in the use of non-invasive ventilation between bacterial positive and negative groups, suggesting that there is no direct relationship between non-invasive ventilation and the detection of bacteria from the lower respiratory tract. This also indirectly implies that, in the therapy of influ-

Table 4. Comparison of prognoses between initial antibiotic strategies post-hospitalization.

	Potent antibiotics[a] (211 cases)	Impotent antibiotics[a] (252 cases)	Combined antibiotics[b] (200 cases)	Non-combined antibiotics[b] (263 cases)
Hospitalization time (days)	12.75 ± 9.74	14.15 ± 11.37	12.86 ± 9.28	13.91 ± 11.78
Initial detection of bacteria (days)	5.39 ± 6.01	8.05 ± 10.08	5.35 ± 5.13	8.78 ± 11.20
Mortality	13.22%	12.41%	11.00%	14.07%
Detection ratio of multi-drug resistant bacteria	35.48%	50.00%	46.51%	43.48%

[a]No statistical difference was observed between the potent antibiotic group and the Impotent antibiotic group in hospitalization time, initial detection of bacteria, mortality, or detection ratio of multi-drug resistant bacteria (p >0.05). [b]No statistical difference was observed between the combined antibiotic group and the non-combined antibiotic group in hospitalization time, initial detection of bacteria, mortality, or detection ratio of multi-drug resistant bacteria (p > 0.05).

enza A cases, non-invasive ventilation should be the first choice for respiratory support to correct hypoxemia, and should be performed as early as possible to avoid intubation [5,6]. These steps may reduce the risk of ventilator-associated pneumonia in the future.

Previous studies indicated that the incidence of secondary bacterial infection following influenza A (H1N1) infection tend to increase, which may be related to the facts that the virus can damage the mucosal epithelium of the airway, reduce the function of immune factors, and impair the bacterial defense of the organ [7,8]. Therefore, application of antibiotics is an important therapeutic strategy. However, antibiotics are not recommended for adult influenza patients who were previously healthy, are not complicated with pneumonia, or who have acute bronchitis without pneumonia. Previously healthy adult patients should only be given antibiotics if there are signs of deterioration, such as recurrent fever or obvious dyspnea. Generally, pneumonia in the middle and late stages (≥5 days) is characterized by pulmonary consolidation with lobe or segment base as determined by imaging. Continuous fever and cough with yellowish purulent sputum suggest bacterial pneumonia and requires administration of antibiotics, which should be chosen as described above. Pneumonia acquired during hospitalization (including during a period of mechanical ventilation) for severe influenza should be treated with antibiotics appropriate for hospital acquired pneumonia [9]. Our results indicated that there were 31 cases of positive bacteria culture within 3 days of admission, mainly caused by Gram-positive cocci such as *S. viridans*, and the incidence of multi-drug resistant bacteria was 25.8%. These etiological features suggest that antibiotics covering Gram-positive cocci should be the first choice for empiric treatment during the early stages of hospitalization. We found that administration of high-dose or combined antibiotics in the early stages could not shorten the hospitalization period, prevent bacterial infection, reduce the detection rate of multi-drug resistant bacteria, or decrease mortality, which may be related to the lower incidence of bacterial infection or multi-drug resistant bacterial infection of influenza A patients upon early hospitalization. Because the current influenza A virus represents a novel sub-type, the condition and prognosis of patients receives more social attention, and there is still no standard criteria for the detection of bacteria from the lower respiratory tract. Therefore, some of the detected bacteria may be commensal or even contaminating bacteria (non-quantitative culture), and excessive administration of high-dose antibiotics may have serious consequences. Therefore, high-dose or combined antibiotics should not be the first choice of treatment for influenza A patients within 3 days of admission.

In summary, secondary bacterial infection following influenza A (H1N1) pneumonia is more common in the older population with complicated underlying conditions, which will prolong the duration of hospitalization and increase mortality. Nosocomial infection accounts for the majority of secondary infections, and influenza A patients should be closely monitored to detect any changes in the bacteria recovered from the lower respiratory tract. Secondary bacterial infection can be diagnosed early, by comprehensive analysis combined with sputum sampling and imaging of the lung. The empirical use of antibiotics and whether administration of antibiotics in the early stages of admission can improve long-term prognosis remain to be investigated. However, we conclude that it is not necessary to use high-dose or combined antibiotics as a first choice in the early stages of treatment.

REFERENCES

[1] The Ministry of Health of People's Republic of China, "Diagnosis and Therapy Strategy of Influenza A (H1N1) of the Ministry of Healthy of People's Republic of China (Version 3)," 2009. http://www.moh.gov.cn

[2] R. J. Leggiadro, "Bacterial Coinfections in Lung Tissue Specimens from Fatal Cases of 2009 Pandemic Influenza A (H1N1)—United States, May-August 2009," *Morbidity and Mortality Weekly Report*, Vol. 58, No. 38, 2009, pp. 1071-1074.

[3] H. S. Kim, J. H. Kim, S. Y. Shin, Y. A. Kang, H. G. Lee, J. S. Kim, J. K. Lee and B. Cho, "Fatal Cases of 2009 Pandemic Influenza A (H1N1) in Korea," *Journal of Korean Medical Science*, Vol. 26, No. 1, 2011, pp. 22-27. doi:10.3346/jkms.2011.26.1.22

[4] J. K. Louie, M. Acosta, K. Winter, C. Jean, S. Gavali, R. Schechter, D. Vugia, K. Harriman, B. Matyas, C. A. Glaser, et al., "Factors Associated with Death or Hospitalization Due to Pandemic 2009 Influenza A (H1N1) Infection in California," *Journal of the American Medical Association*, Vol. 302, No. 17, 2009, pp. 1896-1902. doi:10.1001/jama.2009.1583

[5] B.-W. Dai, W. Tan, L.-F. Sun, et al., "Clinical Analysis of 75 Severe and Critical Patients with Novel Influenza A (H1N1)," *Chinese Journal of Practical Internal Medicine*, Vol. 30, No. 1, 2010, pp. 6-9.

[6] T. Teke, R. Coskun, M. Sungur, et al., "2009 H1N1 Influenza and Experience in Three Critical Care Units," *International Journal of Medical Sciences*, Vol. 8, No. 3, 2011, pp. 270-277. doi:10.7150/ijms.8.270

[7] J. A. McCullers and K. C. Bartmess, "Role of Neuraminidase in Lethal Synergism between Influenza Virus and *Streptococcus pneumoniae*," *The Journal of Infectious Diseases*, Vol. 187, No. 6, 2003, pp. 1000-1009. doi:10.1086/368163

[8] J. A. McCullers, "Insights into the Interaction between Influenza Virus and Pneumococcus," *Clinical Microbiology Reviews*, Vol. 19, No. 3, 2006, pp. 571-582. doi:10.1128/CMR.00058-05

[9] N.-S. Zhong, C. Wang, G.-F. Wang, et al., "Guidance of Diagnosis and Therapy of Influenza," *Journal of Community Medicine*, Vol. 9, No. 5, 2011, pp. 66-74.

8

The Essential Oil of *Eucalyptus grandis* W. Hill ex Maiden Inhibits Microbial Growth by Inducing Membrane Damage

Oluwagbemiga Sewanu Soyingbe[1], Adebola Oyedeji[2], Albert Kortze Basson[1], Andy Rowland Opoku[1*]

[1]Department of Biochemistry and Microbiology, University of Zululand, Empangeni, South Africa
[2]Department of Chemistry, Walter Sisulu University, Mthatha, South Africa
Email: *OpokuA@unizulu.ac.za

ABSTRACT

Eucalyptus grandis is a medicinal plant which has been indicated by Zulu traditional healer in the treatment of respiratory tract infections, bronchial infections, asthma and cough. The investigation of the essential oil of this plant could help to verify the rationale behind the use of the plant as a cure for these illnesses. Essential oil was hydro-distilled from the fresh leaves and characterised for the chemical constituents and bioactivity. The main constituents of the oil of the *E. grandis* are α-Pinene (29.69%), p-Cymene (19.89%), 1,8-cineole (12.80%), α-Terpineol (6.48%), Borneol (3.48%) and D-Limonene (3.14%). The essential oil of *E. grandis* showed high scavenging of DPPH and ABTS radicals, and was actively against 13 of the 16 organisms tested with the MIC ranging from 0.625 mg - 5.0 mg/ml; the MBC value ranged from 2.5 mg - 10 mg/ml. The essential oil also inhibited the growth of 7 of the 8 antibiotic resistant bacteria tested, with MIC ranging from 5 mg/ml - 10 mg/ml. The DNA extracted from the affected microorganisms did not show any damage. However, there was an increase of released cytosolic LDH activity. We conclude that the antibacterial activity of the essential oil was exhibited through cell membrane damage rather than the damage of the DNA. It is apparent that the bioactivity of the essential oil of *E. grandis* plays an important role in the plants' use in folk medicine for the treatment of respiratory tract illnesses.

Keywords: Essential Oil; Antioxidant; Antimicrobial Activity; LDH

1. Introduction

Medicinal plants form a sizeable component of traditional medicine and are mainstay for about 80% of the people in developing nations [1]. The use of medicinal plants is a basic part of African culture [2] and it is one of the oldest and most diverse all over the world [3]. In South Africa indigenous African medicine is used alongside Western allopathic medicine [4], which caters for different people of different cultures. Traditional healing which makes use of local herbs is widely practised in Zululand [5]. The medicinal effect of various plants traditionally used by the Zulus to cure different ailments has been well documented [1,6-9].

E. grandis (**Figure 1**) belongs to the Myrtaceae family previously native to Australia. Massive planting programs have been carried out in the Republic of South Africa, Zambia and Zimbabwe. The leaves are leathery in texture, hang oblique or vertically, and are studded with glands containing a fragrant volatile oil.

The flowers in bud are covered with a cup-like membrane (whence the name of the genus, derived from the Greek word "eucalyptus" meaning well covered), which is thrown off as lid when the flower expands. Eucalyptus trees are quick growers and many species reach great heights [10].

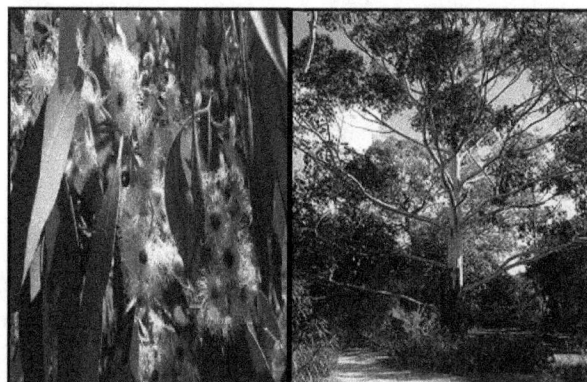

Figure 1. *Eucalyptus grandis* W. Hill ex Maiden (www.forestryimages.org).

---

*Corresponding author.

Traditional healer use *Eucalyptus* to treat many illnesses such as infections, colds, flu, sore throats, bronchitis, pneumonia, aching, stiffness, neuralgia [2], and as an antibiotic [11]. Vivik [12] reported its use as an antifungal agent for some skin infections.

Studies on other species from the *Eucalyptus* family (*Eucalyptus globules* and *Eucalyptus citriodora*) indicate 70% of their constituents to be 1,8 cineol (Eucalyptol) which has been reported to stimulate respiration, relieve coughing, helps to expel mucus, relax the respiratory muscles, and it is thus used for the management of bronchitis, asthma, catarrh, sinusitis and throat infections [13, 14]. To the best of our knowledge, little or no reports exist on the essential oil of *E. grandis*. Due to geographical and species differences, we investigated the chemical composition, the antioxidant and the antibacterial activity of the essential oil of the *E. grandis* of South Africa.

2. Methods

2.1. Plant Material and Extraction of Essential Oil

Eucaylptus grandis Hill ex Maiden was collected from the Mbakanathubana area of Eshowe, KwaZulu Natal, South Africa. The plant was taken to the Department of Botany, University of Zululand, KwaDlangezwa for identification and voucher specimens (OS.01UZ) were deposited at the University Herbarium. The leaves were picked and were subjected to more than three hours of hydrodistillation using a Clevenger-type apparatus. The essential oil so obtained was dried over anhydrous sodium sulfate, dissolved in methanol and then stored at −4°C until required.

2.2. GC-MS

Gas Chromatography/Mass Spectrometer (GC/MS) of the essential oils was carried out using an Agilent Gas Chromatography (7890A) equipped with a capillary column (Agilent 190915 30 m × 250 μm × 0.25 μm calibrated) attached with an Agilent mass spectrometer system (5975C VL MSD with Triple Axis Detector). The oven temperature was programmed from 45°C - 310°C. Helium was used as the carrier gas at a flow rate of 5 ml/min with a split ratio of 1:200. The essential oil (1 μl) was diluted in hexane and 0.5 μl of the solution was manually injected into the GC/MS. The chemical compositions of the essential oil of the fresh leave of *E. grandis* was determined according to their retention time, and spectrometric electronic libraries (WILEY NIST) Equations.

2.3. Microorganisms

Bacteria strains (**Table 1**) used in this study consisted of

Table 1. List of organisms.

No.	Bacteria strains	Reference number
1.	*Escherichia coli*	(ATCC 8739)
2.	*Pseudomonas aeruginosa*	(ATCC 19582)
3.	*Staphylococcus aureus*	(ATCC 6538)
4.	*Staphylococcus faecalis*	(ATCC 29212)
5.	*Bacillus cereus*	(ATCC 10702)
6.	*Bacillus pumilus*	(ATCC 14884)
7.	*Pseudomonas aeruginosa*	(ATCC 7700)
8.	*Enterobacter cloacae*	(ATCC 13047)
9.	*Klebsiella pneumoniae*	(ATCC 4352)
10.	*Serratia marcescens*	(ATCC 6830)

Environmental strains.

No.	Bacteria strains	Reference Strains
1.	*Acinetobacter calcoaceticus anitratus*	(CSIR)
2.	*Bacillus subtilis*	(KZN)
3.	*Shigella flexineri*	(KZN)
4.	*Salmonella spp*	(KZN)
5.	*Staphylococcus epidermidis*	(KZN)
6.	*Enterococcus faecalis*	(KZN)

Antibiotic resistant strains

No.	Antibiotic resistant strains	Reference number
1.	*Staphylococcus aureus*	(B10808)
2.	*Staphylococcus aureus*	(P12763)
3.	*Staphylococcus aureus*	(P12702)
4.	*Staphylococcus aureus*	(P12724)
5.	*Pseudomonas aeruginosa*	(T3374)
6.	*Streptococcus viridians*	(S17141)
7.	*Klebsiella pneumoniae*	(S17298)
8.	*Klebsiella pneumoniae*	(S17302)

reference strains identified and obtained from the Microbiology Department, University of Zululand; also included in this study were environmental strains and Antibiotic resistant strains of clinical isolates obtained from the Lancet pathology laboratory (Durban, South Africa).

The stock cultures were maintained at 4°C on Mueller-

Hinton agar (Merck catalogue number 1.05435.0500).

2.4. Antimicrobial Assay

The antibacterial properties of the essential oils were done using the agar disk diffusion method [15]. Bacteria were grown in 20 ml nutrient broth at 37°C overnight. The cultures were then diluted to the McFarland No.5 standard (1.0×10^8 CFU/ml). Standard Petri dishes containing nutrient agar were then inoculated with the bacteria suspension (1.0×10^8 CFU/ml). Sterile paper disks (6 mm) were placed on the inoculated plates and 10 μl of 10 mg/ml of the essential oils in 1% DMSO were added to the paper disk. The plates were then incubated at 37°C for 24 hrs and the zone of inhibition measured. Tests were performed in triplicate and the mean values reported; Ampicillin and Neomycin were used as positive controls.

The minimum inhibitory concentration (MIC) of the essential oils was determined by the method of Eloff [16]. Nutrients broth (50 μl) was added to all wells of the microtitre plate; 50 μl of the essential oils (10 mg/ml) in 1% DMSO was added to the well in row A and then serially diluted down the rows from row A. The remaining 50 μl was discarded. Bacteria culture (50 μl) of McFarland standard was then added to all the wells and then incubated at 37°C for 24 hrs. P-iodonitrotetrazolium violet (INT) solution (20 μl of 0.2 mg/ml) was then added to each well and incubated at 37°C for 30 mins. The MIC is the lowest concentration at which no visible microbial growth is observed. The minimum bactericidal concentration (MBC) is the lowest concentration of the sample at which inoculated bacterial strains are completely killed. This was confirmed by re-inoculating 10 μl of each culture medium from the microtiter plates on nutrient agar plates and incubating at 37°C for 24 hrs. Bacteria treated with Ampicillin and Neomycin, were used as positive controls.

2.5. Antioxidant Activity

The essential oil was screened for antioxidant activity: The (DPPH:1.1-diphenyl-2-picrylhydrazyl; ABTS: 2,2-azino-bis (3-ethylebenzthiazoline-6-sulfonic acid); NO: (nitric oxide radicals) scavenging activity, Fe^{2+} chelating oil was determined by the methods previously outlined [6, 17].

Unless otherwise stated, ascorbic acid, Trolox and BHT were used as standards. All assays were done in triplicate. The inhibitory effect of the extract on each parameter was calculated as:

$$\% \text{ Inhibition} = \left(1 - A_t / A_0\right) \times 100$$

where, A_0 is the absorbance value of the fully oxidized control and A_t is the absorbance of the extract. The inhibitory concentration providing 50% inhibition (IC_{50}) was determined using statistical package Origin 6.1.

2.6. DNA Damage (Cleavage)

The ZR Fungal/bacterial DNA MiniPrep™ kit (Zymo Research, USA) was used for this study. Fresh bacterial cultures were treated with the essential oils (MBC concentration). Treated as well as untreated cultures were centrifuged and the pellets obtained were re-suspended in the lysis solution for 5min and centrifuged (10,000 g for 10 min). Fungal/Bacterial DNA Binding Buffer was then added to the suspension and centrifuged (10,000 g for 10 min). The supernatant collected was added to a DNA Pre Wash Buffer and again centrifuged, after which Fungal/Bacterial Washing Buffer was added and then centrifuged. The precipitated DNA was then eluted with the elution buffer and centrifuged. Cleavage products were analysed by agarose gel electrophoresis (120 v for 1 hr) along with standard DNA maker. The DNA was then visualized using a vilberlourmate Gel documentation system [18,19].

2.7. Lactate Dehydrogenase (LDH) Release Assay (Membrane Damage)

The cytosolic LDH release assay was carried out according to the method previously described [20-22]. The susceptible organisms were grown and incubated with the MBC concentration of the essential oil overnight. The microbial cultures were then centrifuged (5000 g; 5 mins). The supernatant (100 μl) was then mixed with 100 μl of lactic acid dehydrogenase substrate mixture of 54 mM lactic acid, 0.28 mM of phenazinemethosulfate, 0.66 mM p-iodonitrotetrazolium violet, and 1.3 mM NAD^+. The pyruvate-mediated conversion of 2,4-dinitrophenylhydrazine into visible hydrazone precipitate was measured on an auto microplate reader (BiotekELx 808) at 492 nm. The total loss of membrane integrity resulting in complete loss of cell viability was determined by lysing the cells of untreated organisms with 3% Triton X-100 and using this sample as a positive control. The cytotoxicity in the LDH release test was calculated using the formula: (E-C)/(T-C) × 100, where E is the experimental absorbance of the cell cultures, C is the control absorbance of the cell medium, and T is the absorbance corresponding to the maximal (100%) LDH release of Triton X-100 lysed cells (positive control).

2.8. Statistical Analysis

The mean and standard error mean of three experiments were determined. Statistical analysis of the differences between mean values obtained were calculated using Microsoft excel program, 2007 and Origin 6.0 for IC_{50}.

3. Results and Discussion

3.1. Percentage Composition

The percentage yield of the essential oils from the leaves of *E. grandis* was 1.78%. The oil was light green in colour and with an aromatic smell. The percentage composition and the retention time of the essential oil are listed in **Table 2**. The major components of the oil were α-Pinene (29.69%), p-Cymene (19.89%), 1,8-cineole (12.80%), α-Terpineol (6.48%), Borneol (3.43%) and D-Limonene (3.14%). The result is similar to those reported for the other Eucalyptus species [23-26] however, while 1,8-cineole was observed to be the major component of the other species [27], we found 1,8-cineole to be only 12.8% of the components of the essential oil of fresh leaves of *E. grandis* in our study. Chemical variations within species have been attributed to factors like climatic and environmental conditions [28,29].

3.2. Antioxidant Activity

Table 3 shows the summary of the antioxidant activities of the essential oils of *E. grandis*. Free radicals (which are by-products of normal biochemical processes such as mitochondrial respiration and liver oxidases and xanthine oxidase activity, atmospheric pollutants, drugs and xenobiotics metabolism [30]) have been implicated to be the causative agents of some pathophysiological conditions such as neurodegenerative diseases, autoimmune diseases, arthritis, cardiovascular diseases and even aging [31, 32]. Major damages occur when free radicals attack cellular components such as DNA, or cell membranes. Antioxidants interact with free radicals and neutralize the chain reaction before tissues and other organs are damaged. There is an increasing interest in the search for natural antioxidants [6,9]. Antioxidant activities of essential oils have been studied widely and reported. Ramzi [33] working with the essential oils of *Nepetade flersiana* growing in Yemen showed that the oil was able to reduce DPPH and to demonstrate a moderate antioxidant activity; the observed low antioxidant activity was associated with low content of phenolic compounds such as thymol and carvacrol in the investigated oil. The essential oils from guava stem bark were seen to be weak proton donors in DPPH reaction [34]. Kadri *et al.* [35] while working on the essential oil from aerial parts of *Artemisia herba-alba* grown in Tunisian semi-arid region postulated that antioxidant activities of the essential oil studied may be a potential source of natural antioxidants in foods and the pharmaceutical industry for the prevention and the treatment of various human diseases. Antioxidant properties of essential oils may make them a very good candidate for use as natural antioxidants and also a model for new free radical scavenging drugs. With the observed high

Table 2. Volatile constituents of the essential oil of *E. grandis*.

Peak No.	Constituent	Retention time	% concentration	KI*
1.	α-Pinene	8.104	29.67	936
2.	Camphene	8.506	1.52	950
3.	p-Cymene	10.725	19.89	1025
4.	D-Limonene	10.840	3.14	1029
5.	1,8-cineole	10.926	12.80	1031
6.	γ-Terpinene	11.718	2.16	1060
7.	Terpinolene	12.602	0.35	1089
8.	Careen	12.906	0.26	1148
9.	β-Fenchol	13.352	1.21	1122
10.	*trans*-pinocarveol	13.730	0.60	1139
11.	Camphor	14.114	2.52	1146
12.	Sabinyl acetate	14.821	0.31	1166
13.	Borneol	14.906	3.43	1169
14.	Terpinen-4-ol	15.223	0.82	1177
15.	α-Terpineol	15.625	6.48	1189
16.	cis-Carveol	16.387	0.43	1231
17.	Thymol	18.197	0.26	1290
18.	Carvacrol	18.636	0.37	1299
19.	Terpinyl acetate	19.977	1.60	1349
20.	Caryophyllene	21.903	0.24	1419
21.	Alloaromadendrene	26.127	1.88	1441
22.	γ-Gurjunene	25.536	0.39	1447
23.	Viridiflorene	22.836	1.51	1497
24.	α-calacorene	24.878	0.45	1546
25.	Spathulenol	25.768	1.49	1578
26.	caryophyllene oxide	25.926	0.45	1583
27.	α-Eudesmol	26.355	0.78	1632
28.	cis-cadin-4-en-7-ol	26.652	1.77	1637
29.	epoxy-allo-alloaromadendrene	26.822	1.05	1641
30.	Cadine-1,4-diene	26.822	0.47	1646
31.	Amiteol	27.139	0.18	1660

*Kovats index on a DB-5 column in reference to n-alkanes (Adams 1995, 2001). MS, NIST and Wiley libraries spectra and the literature; KI, Kovats index.

Table 3. The antioxidant activity of the essential oils of *E. grandis*.

	Antioxidant activities IC$_{50}$ (mg/ml)			
	DPPH	ABTS	Nitric oxide	Fe^{2+} Chelating
Essential oil of *E. grandis*	1.36	7.94l	7.31l	> 10
Trolox	>10	>10		
Ascorbic acid	1.02	3.94	5.77l	
BHT		<5.00		
Citric acid				8.46
EDTA				15.63

scavenging activity of DPPH and NO radicals, it is apparent that the essential oil of *E. grandis* could be a candidate for plant-derived antioxidants.

3.3. Antimicrobial Activity

The results (MIC and MBC values) of the antibacterial activity of the essential oil are presented in **Table 4**. **Table 5** shows the essential oil's activity against antibiotic resistant organisms. The essential oil of *E. grandis* ex-

hibited activity comparable to the standards and was seen to be broad spectrum in nature as it affected both Gram positive and Gram negative bacteria. It is also worth noting that the oil effectively inhibited the growth of antibiotic-resistant organisms. The oils antimicrobial activity could be attributed to the presence of compounds like 1,8 cineole, α and β pinene, and limonene which have been reported [36] to have antimicrobial properties.

3.4. DNA Cleavage

The mechanisms of action of most plant extracts with antimicrobial activity have been poorly studied. The effect of the essential oil on the DNA and membrane of the affected microorganisms are presented in **Figure 2** and **Table 6**, respectively. It is apparent from the DNA cleavage studies that, unlike cajanol [19] and monoterpenoid-indole alkaloid [20] that was able to damage microbial DNA, the *E. grandis* essential oil did not affect the DNA of the organisms studied.

3.5. LDH Activity

The essential oil however, damaged the membrane integrity of the organism resulting in the release of the cytosolic enzyme, lactate dehyrogenase (LDH). This result

Table 4. Minimum inhibitory concentration (MIC) and minimum bactericidal concentration (MBC) of the essential oil of *E. grandis*.

Bacteria strains	MIC of essential oil of *E. grandis* (mg/ml)	MIC of Ampicillin (mg/ml)	MBC of essential oil of *E. grandis* (mg/ml)
Esherichia coli (ATCC 8739)	0.625	1.25	2.5
Psuedomonas aeruginosa (ATCC 19582)	10	5	10
Staphylococcus aureus (ATCC 6538)	1.25	2.5	3.25
Streptococcus faecalis (ATCC 29212)	2.5	5	5.5
Bacillus cereus (ATCC 10702)	0.625	5	3.25
Bacillus pumilus (ATCC 14884)	0.625	2.5	3.25
Psuedomonas aeruginosa (ATCC 7700)	0.625	5	4.5
Enterobacter cloacae (ATCC 13047)	1.25	1.25	10
Klebsiella pneumonia (ATCC 10031)	1.25	2.5	2.5
Serratia marcescens (ATCC 6830)	5	NA	10
Acinetobacter calcoaceticus anitratus (CSIR)	2.5	NA	2.5
Bacillus subtilis (KZN)	2.5	0.625	10
Shigella flexineri (KZN)	2.5	5	4.25
Salmonella spp. (KZN)	5	5	5.5
Staphylococcus epididirmis (KZN)	10	10	>10
Enterococcus faecalis (KZN)	2.5	5	5.25

MIC values given as mg/ml for essential oils, ND = not determined NA = not active, DMSO = dimethyl sulfoxide.

Table 5. Zone of inhibition, MIC and MBC of the essential oil of *E. grandis* (antibiotic resistant microorganism).

Antibiotic resistant bacteria strains	Antibiotic resistant to	Zone of inhibition (mm)	MIC (mg/ml)	MBC (mg/ml)
Staphylococcus aureus P12702	CIPRO: Levo Clindamycin	19 ± 0	2.5	2.5
Staphylococcus aureus P12763	CIPRO: Levo Clindamycin	14 ± 0.1	10	>10
Staphylococcus aureus P12724	CIPRO: Levo Clindamycin	14 ± 0.1	10	>10
Staphylococcus aureus B10808	Oxa:Clox, Oxa: meth, Gentamicin, Penicillin	14 ± 0.1	10	>10
Str. viridans S17141	Oxa: meth, OxaClox	18 ± 0.1	5	5.25
Psuedomonas aeruginosa T 3374	Cotrimoxazole	NA	NA	ND
Klebsiella Spp. S 17302	Ampicillin	20 ± 0	2.5	2.5
Klebsiella pneumonia S 17298	Ampicillin	21 ± 0.1	2.5	5.25

*Oxa: Oxacillin; Clox: Cloxacillin; Meth: Methicillin; Levo: Levofloxacin; CIPRO Ciprofloxacin. ND = Not determined NA = Not acti.

shown in **Table 6** is similar to previous studies of Mirzoeva *et al.* [37] and Sánchez-González *et al.* [38] which showed that extracts of medicinal plants damaged microbial cell membranes. Essential oils target negatively charged bacterial surfaces and disrupt microbial cytoplasmic membranes, causing increased permeability of cell membranes or lysis of cell walls and loss of cellular constituents. Since penicillin- and mutation-resistant strains of microbial pathogens are on the increase, there is a need to search for new compounds (that are not penicillin based) that inhibit microbial growth. The antibacterial activity of the *E. grandis*' essential oil coupled to its antioxidant properties presents the oil as a good candidate for the search of therapeutic agents.

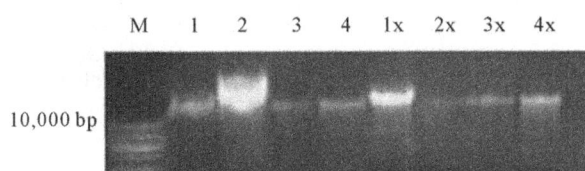

Figure 2. DNA cleavage activity of the essential oil of *E. grandis* against *Esherichia coli* (ATCC 8739), *Bacillus pumilus* (ATCC 14884), *Enterobacter cloacae* (ATCC 13047) and *Bacillus subtilis* (KZN). M = DNA maker, lane 1 - 4 are untreated DNA respectively and lane 1x - 4x are treated DNA respectively.

Table 6. LDH release (membrane damage) activity of the essential oil of *E. grandis*.

Bacteria	% LDH releases in relation to Triton X-100
Esherichia coli (ATCC 8739)	36.44%
Bacillus pumilus (ATCC 14884)	65.91%
Enterobacter cloacae (ATCC 13047)	69.40%
Bacillus subtilis (KZN).	58.76%

4. Conclusions

Despite the many and varying pharmaceutical properties of *E. grandis* that are exploited by traditional healers, there has been little or no scientific verification of their therapeutic activities. Various respiratory pathogens that affect the respiratory tracts lead to oxidative stress which in turn triggers asthmatic attack. Substances such as allergens, pollutants, chemicals, drugs, bacteria and viruses [39], lead to the recruitment and activation of inflammatory cells which have an exceptional capacity for producing oxidants in asthmatic airways [40]. It is apparent that the search for an effective drug to manage asthma and other related complications should be directed towards agents that are antioxidant, antimicrobial, anti-inflammatory, anti-allergic, and immune-boaster in nature.

The essential oil of *E. grandis* contained 1,8-cineole (Eucalyptol) which has been reported to stimulate respiration and relieve coughing, helps to expel mucus, relax the respiratory muscles, and it is thus used for the management of bronchitis, asthma, catarrh, sinusitis and throat infections [13,14]. The observed antimicrobial and antioxidant activities in this study suggest the rational for the traditional use of *E. grandis* for therapeutic purposes.

5. Acknowledgements

The authors are grateful to the University of Zululand research committee for financial support.

REFERENCES

[1] J. George, M. D. Laing and S. E. Drewes, "Phytochemical Research in South Africa," *Journal of Science South Africa*, Vol. 97, 2001, pp. 93-105.

[2] A. Hutchings, A. H. Scott, G. Lewis and A. Cunningham, "Zulu Medicinal Plants: An Inventory," University of Natal Press, Scottsville, 1996.

[3]   B. Van Wyk and M. Wink, "Medicinal Plants of the World," Briza Publications, Queenswood, 2004.

[4]   B. Van Wyk and N. Gericke, "Peoples Plants. A Guide to Useful of Southern Africa," Briza Publications, Queenswood, 2003.

[5]   M. V. Gumede, "In Traditional Healers: A Medical Doctors Perspective," Skotaville Press, Johannesburg, 1989.

[6]   A. R. Opoku, N. F. Maseko and S. E. Terblanche, "The in Vitro Antioxidative Activity of Some Traditional Zulu Medicinal Plants," Phytotherapy Research, Vol. 16, No. S1, 2002, pp. S51-S56. doi:10.1002/ptr.804

[7]   A. Jean-Paul, F. Lorna and S. Huw, "Plant Active Components: A Resource for Antiparasitic Agents?" Trends in Parasitology, Vol. 21, No. 10, 2005, pp. 442-468.

[8]   E. O. Iwalewa, L. J. Mc Gaw, V. Naidoo and J. N. Eloff, "Inflammation: The Foundation of Disease and Disorders. A Review of Phytomedicines of South African Origin Used to Treat Pain and Inflammatory Conditions," African Journal of Biotechnology, Vol. 6, No. 25, 2007, pp. 2868-2885.

[9]   H. Bibhabasu, B. Santanu and M. Nripendranath, "Antioxidant and Free Radical Scavenging Activity of Spondiaspinnata," BMC Complementary and Alternative Medicine, Vol. 8, 2008, pp. 63.

[10]   M. Jacobs, "Eucalypts for Planting," Food and Agriculture Organization of the United Nations, Rome, 1976, 398 p.

[11]   D. Hopkins-Broyles, Y. Rieger, A. Grim, D. Nihill, M. Jones, R. Damiano, D. K. Warren and V. J. Fraser, "Risk Factors for Staphylococcus aureus Colonization in a Cardiac Surgery Population," American Journal of Infection Control, Vol. 32, No. 3, 2004, p. 119 doi:10.1016/j.ajic.2004.04.176

[12]   K. Vivek, S. S. Bajpai and C. K. Sun, "Chemical Composition and Antifungal Activity of Essential Oil and Various Extract of Silenearmeria L.," Bioresource Technology, Vol. 99, No. 18, 2008, pp. 8903-8908. doi:10.1016/j.biortech.2008.04.060

[13]   F. Sisay, L. T. Gil, W. E. Tolosana and R. López, "Eucalyptus Species Management, History, Status and Trends in Ethiopia," Proceedings from the Congress, Addis Ababa, 15-17 September 2010, pp. 62-68.

[14]   F. A. Santos and V. S. Rao, "Anti Inflammatory and Antinociceptive Effects of 1,8-Cineole, a Terpenoid Oxide Present in Many Plant Essential Oils," Phytotherapy Research, Vol. 14, No. 4, 2000, pp. 240-244. doi:10.1002/1099-1573(200006)14:4<240::AID-PTR573>3.0.CO;2-X

[15]   S. F. Van Vuuren and A. M. Viljoen, "A Comparative Investigation of the Antimicrobial Properties of Indigenous South African Aromatic Plants with Popular Commercially Available Essential Oils," Journal of Essential Oil Research, Vol. 18, 2006, pp. 66-71.

[16]   J. N. Eloff, "A Sensitive and Quick Method to Determine the Minimal Inhibitory Concentration of Plant Extracts for Bacteria," Planta Medica, Vol. 64, No. 8, 1998, pp. 711-713. doi:10.1055/s-2006-957563

[17]   M. B. C. Simelane, O. A. Lawal, T. G. Djarova and A. R. Opoku, "In Vitro Antioxidant and Cytotoxic Activity of Gunnera perpensa L. (Gunneraceae) from South Africa," Journal of Medicinal Plants Research, Vol. 4, No. 21, 2010, pp. 2181-2188.

[18]   X. Liu, X.-J. Zhang, Y.-J. Fu, Y. G. Zu, N. Wu, L. Liang and T. Efferth, "Cajanol Inhibits the Growth of Escherichia coli and Staphylococcus aureus by Acting on Membrane and DNA Damage," Planta Medica, Vol. 77, No. 2, 2011, pp. 158-163. doi:10.1055/s-0030-1250146

[19]   M. Wu, P. Wu, H. H. Xie, G. J. Wu and X. Y. Wei, "Monoterpenoid Indole Alkaloids Mediating DNA Strand Scission from Turpinia arguta," Planta Medica, Vol. 77, No. 3, 2011, pp. 284-286. doi:10.1055/s-0030-1250239

[20]   C. Korzeniewski and D. M. Callewaert, "An Enzyme-Release Assay for Natural Cytotoxicity," Journal of Immunological Methods, Vol. 64, No. 3, 1983, pp. 313-320. doi:10.1016/0022-1759(83)90438-6

[21]   V. Badovinac, V. Trajkovic and M. Mostarica-Stojkovic, "Nitric Oxide Promotes Growth and Major Histocompatibility Complex-Unrestricted Cytotoxicity of Interleukin-2-Activated Rat Lymphocytes," Scandinavian Journal of Immunology, Vol. 52, No. 1, 2000, pp. 62-70. doi:10.1046/j.1365-3083.2000.00753.x

[22]   V. M. Tadić, I. Jeremic, S. Dobric, A. Isakovic, I. Markovic, V. Trajkovic, D. Bojovic and I. Arsic, "Anti-Inflammatory, Gastroprotective, and Cytotoxic Effect of Sideritis scardica Extracts," Planta Medica, Vol. 78, No. 5, 2012, pp. 415-427. doi:10.1055/s-0031-1298172

[23]   A. Lucia, P. Gonzalez Audino, E. Seccacini, S. Licastro, E. Zerbra and H. Masuh, "Larvicidal Effect of Eucalyptus grandis Essential Oil and Turpentine and Their Major Component on Aedesaegypti Larvae," Journal of the American Mosquito Control Association, Vol. 23, No. 3, 2007, pp. 299-303. doi:10.2987/8756-971X(2007)23[299:LEOEGE]2.0.CO;2

[24]   I. A. Ogunwande, O. O. Nureni, A. A. Kasali and A. K. Wilfried, "Chemical Composition of the Essential Oils from the Leaves of Three Eucalyptus Species Growing in Nigeria," Journal of Essential Oil Research, Vol. 15, No. 5, 2003, pp. 297-301. doi:10.1080/10412905.2003.9698595

[25]   K. Cimanga, S. Apers, T. Bruyne, S. Van Miert, N. Hermans, J. Totte, L. Pieters and A. J. Vlietinck, "Chemical Composition and Antifungal Activity of Essential Oils of Some Aromatic Medicinal Plants Growing in the Democratic Republic of Congo," Journal of Essential Oil Research, Vol. 14, No. 5, 2002, pp. 382-387. doi:10.1080/10412905.2002.9699894

[26]   E. Dagne, D. Bisrat, M. Alemayehu and T. Worku, "Essential Oils of Twelve Eucalyptus Species from Ethiopia," Journal of Essential Oil Research, Vol. 12, No. 4, 2000, pp. 467-470. doi:10.1080/10412905.2000.9699567

[27]   Y. C. Su, C.-L. Ho, E.-C. Wang and S.-T. Chang, "Antifungal Activities and Chemical Compositions of Essential Oils from Leaves of Four Eucalypts," Taiwan Journal of Forest Science, Vol. 21, No. 1, 2006, pp. 49-61.

[28]   S. M. A. Zobayed, F. Afreen and T. Kozai, "Temperature Stress Can Alter the Photosynthetic Efficiency and Secondary Metabolite Concentrations in St. John's Wort," Plant Physiology and Biochemistry, Vol. 43, No. 10-11,

2005, pp. 977-984. doi:10.1016/j.plaphy.2005.07.013

[29] A. Kirakosyan, E. Seymour, P. B. Kaufman, S. Warber, S. Bolling and S. C. Chang, "Antioxidant Capacity of Polyphenolic Extracts from Leaves of *Crataegus laevigata* and *Crataegus monogyna* (Hawthorn) Subjected to Drought and Cold Stress," *Journal of Agricultural and Food Chemistry*, Vol. 51, No. 14, 2003, pp. 3973-3976. doi:10.1021/jf030096r

[30] M. R. Saha, A. Alam, R. Akter and R. Jahangir, "*In Vitro* Free Radical Scavenging Activity of *Ixoracoccinea* L.," *Bangladesh Journal of Pharmacology*, Vol. 3, No. 1, 2008, pp. 90-96. doi:10.3329/bjp.v3i2.838

[31] C. Y. Hsu, Y. P. Chan and J. Chang, "Antioxidant Activity of Extract from *Polygonum cuspidatum*," *Biological Research*, Vol. 40, No. 1, 2007, pp. 13-21. doi:10.4067/S0716-97602007000100002

[32] G. Ambrosio, I. Tritto and P. Golino, "Reactive Oxygen Metabolites and Arterial Thrombosis (Review)," *Cardiovascular Research*, Vol. 34, No. 3, 1997, pp. 445-452. doi:10.1016/S0008-6363(97)00101-6

[33] A. M. Ramzi, "Chemical Composition, Antimicrobial and Antioxidant Activities of the Essential Oil of *Nepetade flersiana* Growing in Yemen," *Records of Natural Products*, Vol. 6, No. 2, 2011, pp. 189-193.

[34] R. T. Fasola, G. K. Oloyede and B. S. Aponjolosun, "Chemical Composition, Toxicity and Antioxidant Activities of Essential Oils of Stem Bark of Nigerian Species of Guava (*Psidium guajava* linn.)," *EXCLI Journal*, Vol. 10, No. 1, 2011, pp. 34-43.

[35] A. Kadri, B. C. Ines, Z. Zied, B. Ahmed, G. Néji, D. Mohamed and G. Radhouane, "Chemical Constituents and Antioxidant Activity of the Essential Oil from Aerial Parts of *Artemisia herbaalba* Grown in Tunisian Semi-Arid Region," *African Journal of Biotechnology*, Vol. 10, No. 15, 2011, pp. 2923-2929.

[36] G. Raju and M. Maridas, "Composition, Antifungal and Cytotoxic Activities of Essential Oils of *Piper barberi* Fruits," *International Journal of Biological Technology*, Vol. 2, No. 2, 2011, pp. 100-105.

[37] O. K. Mirzoeva, R. N. Grishanin and P. C. Calder, "Antimicrobial Action of Propolis and Some of Its Components: The Effects on Growth, Membrane Potential and Motility of Bacteria," *Microbiological Research*, Vol. 152, No. 3, 1997, pp. 239-246. doi:10.1016/S0944-5013(97)80034-1

[38] L. Sánchez-González, M. Vargas, C. González-Martínez, A. Chiralt and M. Cháfer, "Use of Essential Oils in Bioactive Edible Coatings: A Review," *Food Engineering Reviews*, Vol. 3, No. 1, 2011, pp. 1-16. doi:10.1007/s12393-010-9031-3

[39] S. J. Levine, "Bronchial Epithelial Cell-Cytokine Interactions in Airway Inflammation," *Investigative Medicine*, Vol. 43, 1995, pp. 241-249.

[40] S. Pinto, A. V. Rao and A. Rao, "Erythrocyte and Plasma Antioxidant in Bronchial Asthma before and after Homeopathic Treatment," *Journal of Homeopathy & Ayurvedic Medicine*, Vol. 1, No. 1, 2012, p. 13. doi:10.4172/2167-1206.1000103

9

Associations of Education with Blood Pressure in Hypertensive Patients: A Chinese Community Survey

Xiaojun Chen, Xuerui Tan[*]

Department of Cardiovascular Diseases, The First Affiliated Hospital of Shantou University Medical College, Shantou, China
Email: [*]tanxuerui@vip.sina.com

ABSTRACT

Objective: To examine the association between education and blood pressure in hypertensive Chinese. **Methods:** A cross-sectional study was conducted at the health care center of a university affiliated hospital in 2008 to enroll 502 mild to moderate essential hypertensive patients. All participants completed a questionnaire addressing their sociodemographic information before they were given a routine physical check-up. Results: The baseline blood pressure was 151.87/95.76 mmHg for 277 females and 149.80/97.74 mmHg for 225 males. Only few women reported smoke (4%, n = 11) or drink alcohol (6.9%, n = 19). Over half of men smoke and drink (63.2% and 52.9% respectively). Alcohol consumption was found different among educational attainment groups in males. Correlation analyses demonstrated that education was inversely related to systolic blood pressure in female hypertensives. **Conclusion:** Education is associated with blood pressure in females.

Keywords: Education; Blood Pressure; Hypertension; Survey

1. Introduction

Incidence of cardiovascular disease was consistently inversely associated with education and other measures of socioeconomic position, such as occupation and income [1]. As a major risk factor for cardiovascular disease, blood pressure was often analyzed to be related with improper daily habits [2]. As for relation to socio-economic status measure, elevated blood pressure has also been explored but only in white and black people and there was a slight inconsistence in the result [3,4]. The applicability of their findings was uncertain to other races/ethnicities. The objective of this study was to explore the association between educational attainment and blood pressure in Orientals.

2. Methods

2.1. Study Sample

A cross-sectional survey was conducted from year 2007 to 2008 in Shantou city, Eastern China. The study population was a random cluster sample from individuals for annual physical examination in the hospital health care center. Finally 502 eligible participants with mild to moderate essential hypertension out of 4020 individuals were recruited, as their 3 consecutive sitting diastolic blood pressure ≥ 90 and <110 mmHg and/or sitting systolic blood pressure ≥ 140 and <180 mmHg, coinciding with WHO/ISH Hypertension guidelines. The collection of clinical and sociodemographic data and answers of the questionnaires were carried out on an individual basis by the same researcher and took approximately twenty minutes.

2.2. Education

Education level was one item of the questionnaire mentioned above. The participants' education was recorded into 3 categories: ≤6 years (reflecting primary school or less), 7 - 12 years (indicative of high school or less including technical school) and ≥13 year's education (those with more than an undergraduate college degree).

2.3. Blood Pressure

Enroll participants were asked to stop anti-hypertensive medication for 24 h before investigation. Blood pressure was measured after a 5-minute rest in a seated position with a mercury sphygmomanometer on 3 separate visits in the morning. The average of these readings was used for analyses.

---

[*]Corresponding author.

2.4. Covariates

Covariates were collected by self-report at each questionnaire. Daily habits of alcohol consumption and cigarette smoking were classified as never, moderate or heavy. We defined moderate smoking as fewer than 5 cigarettes/day and heavy smoking as 20 or more cigarettes/day [5]. We categorized participants as moderate or heavy alcohol consumption if his or her intake of total alcohol of beer, wine was less than 20 g/day and more than 20 g/day respectively [6]. Occupational status was self-reported and categorized as unemployment, intellectuals work and physical labor work. Body mass index (BMI) was calculated as the weight in kilograms divided by the square of the height in meters (kg/m^2). Current antihypertensive medication use was self-reported and modeled as a binary variable (yes/no).

2.5. Statistical Analysis

The data collected were processed and analyzed by using routine statistical methods and a $P < 0.05$ level was taken to indicate the significant difference. Measures of association were analyzed by correlation analysis. All the statistics was performed by using the SPSS version 15.0.

3. Results

The baseline blood pressure of 277 hypertensive females was 151.87 ± 10.13 mmHg for SBP and 95.76 ± 8.04 mmHg for DBP. The baseline blood pressure of 225 hypertensive males was 149.80 ± 11.13 mmHg for SBP 97.74 ± 8.43 mmHg for DBP. Only few women reported smoke (4%, n = 11) or drink alcohol (6.9%, n = 19). Over half of men smoke and drink (63.2% and 52.9% respectively). Alcohol consumption was found different among educational attainment groups in males. There was no difference between 3 educational attainment groups in SBP, DBP, anti-hypertension medication, BMI index and smoking either for female or male groups (**Table 1**). In females, correlation analyses demonstrated that education was inversely associated with baseline values of SBP (**Table 2**); in males, education was inversely associated with age only. Education level was significantly associated with occupational position. The fewer educational years, the more low occupation status reported.

4. Discussion

Elevated blood pressure has been demonstrated in cross-sectional studies to be associated with low education and lower levels of other socio-economic status measures [7]. Several large scale epidemiological studies have been done in different races/ethnicities and there was a slight inconsistence in the result. The recent research, Framingham Offspring Study was one of the few studies in-

vestigating longitudinal blood pressure trajectories over a substantial proportion of life course, have showed fairly robust inverse association with SBP and DBP in female than in male white participants [3]. This association was weaker in black participants as Strand and his colleagues had demonstrated that education was inversely associated with increases over time in SBP in males and females [4].

However, little is known about sex-specific associations between education and blood pressure and the effects of using antihypertensive medications, BMI, alcohol consumption, smoking or other potential mechanisms in Asian people. Findings in this paper demonstrated that education was inversely associated with mean SBP in female hypertensives. It suggests that low education may have an impact on blood pressure in females. Associations of education with DBP were not yet detected for both females and males. Conventional risk factors including antihypertensive medication, smoking, BMI and alcohol consumption were not related with educational attainment, neither exerting an effect on association between blood pressure and education.

Previous research in Western countries have resort individuals of low education to high strain jobs, characterized by high demand and low control, which have been associated with elevated blood pressure [8]. Other related mechanisms involve stress induced sympathetic nervous system activation due to stressful conditions outside of work were also associated with low educational attainment. These may be particularly important for women. Women with low education may have higher possibility of poor health, single-parenting, depression, income below the poverty threshold, and unemployment, compared to men with low education [9]. It could be the same with Asian women. In this study, women who received only primary school education were basically in low level occupational status (92.8%) compared to those had college education (40%). Research has found that education reduces the probability of unhealthy behavior over the life course [10], while healthy lifestyle factors reduced the risk of hypertension remarkably. Low socioeconomic position may be a stronger determinant of hypertension risk in women compared with men. Further, SBP tends to increase steadily with age, while DBP tends to increase until age 50 years [11], therefore, the DBP was not yet detected to be related.

However, there remained plausible as childhood socioeconomic circumstances are associated with adulthood education and blood pressure [12], parental blood pressure may be associated with offspring education and blood pressure [13]. With regard to weaknesses, the research sample of our study was relatively small as the subjects were enrolled in a Chinese community, however, the trend of association could be found out though it was

Table 1. Characteristics of participants in cross-sectional study according to educational attainments.

	Participants	Educational Attainment (years)			
		≤6	7 - 12	≥13	P
Female					
N	277	139	123	15	
Age (years)	49.35 ± 6.69	49.81 ± 6.91	49.11 ± 6.32	47.07 ± 7.45	0.27
Systolic Blood Pressure, mmHg	151.87 ± 10.13	153.32 ± 11.59	150.70 ± 11.93	148.07 ± 7.06	0.10
Diastolic Blood Pressure, mmHg	95.76 ± 8.04	95.76 ± 8.04	95.99 ± 8.42	93.27 ± 5.78	0.46
Anti-Hypertensive Medication, %	86(31)	40(46.5)	42(48.8)	4(4.7)	0.60
Body Mass Index, kg/m^2	25.58 ± 3.16	25.58 ± 3.33	25.63 ± 2.98	25.18 ± 3.16	0.87
Smoker, %	11(4.0)	8(72.7)	3(27.3)	0	0.63
Alcohol Consumption, %	19(6.9)	7(36.9)	11(57.8)	1(5.3)	0.39
Low Occupational Position	218(78.7)	129(59.2)	83(38.1)	6(2.7)	0.00
Male					
N	225	34	149	42	
Age (years)	49.16 ± 7.55	51.97 ± 6.58	48.81 ±7.17	48.10 ± 7.07	0.05
Systolic Blood Pressure, mmHg	149.80 ± 11.13	152.26 ± 12.17	149.64 ± 11.35	148.38 ± 10.74	0.37
Diastolic Blood Pressure, mmHg	97.74 ± 8.43	97.59 ± 8.55	97.73 ± 8.39	97.90 ± 8.66	0.98
Anti-Hypertensive Medication,%	82(36.4)	8(9.7)	55(67.1)	19(23.2)	0.14
Body Mass Index, kg/m^2	25.34 ± 3.39	25.12 ± 3.36	25.29 ± 3.63	25.67 ± 2.48	0.75
Smoker, %	140(63.2)	22(15.7)	97(69.2)	21(15.0)	0.45
Alcohol Consumption, %	119(52.9)	12(36.3)	79(53.0)	28(66.7)	0.28
Low Occupational Position	78(34.6)	27(34.6)	45(57.7)	6(7.7)	0.00

To test the trend across education level, we used one-way ANOVA analysis for variables, Pearson chi-square tests comparing males and females for proportion taking anti-hypertensive medication, and proportion of current smokers and alcohol consumption (those reported moderate or heavy consumption). Low occupational position indicates unemployment or labor workers.

Table 2. Associations between educational attainment and blood pressure as well as conventional factors in linear analysis.

Sex (n)	Educational Attainment (years)					
	Age	SBP	DBP	Smoking	Alcohol consumption	Medication usage
Female (277)	−0.08	−0.13*	−0.04	−0.09	0.07	0.03
Male (225)	−0.14*	−0.09	0.01	−0.09	0.11	0.13

*Correlation is significant at the 0.05 level.

weak. Secondly, there is area bias as this result was obtained from a city community. It may not be generalized before multi-center research conducted for further testifies.

5. Conclusion

This study demonstrated that education is inversely associated with systolic blood pressure in female hypertensives, which adding evidence to the research of this kind in Chinese population.

6. Acknowledgements

This work was supported by the National Natural Science Foundation of China (No. 30771836) and Project for High-level Talents in Guangdong Higher Education (No. [2010]79).

REFERENCES

[1] M. A. Gonzalez, F. Rodriguez Artalejo, et al., "Relationship between Socioeconomic Status and Ischaemic Heart Disease in Cohort and Case Control Studies: 1960-1993," International Journal of Epidemiology, Vol. 27, No. 3, 1998, pp. 350-358. doi:10.1093/ije/27.3.350

[2] D. Gu, R. P. Wildman, X. Wu, et al., "Incidence and Predictors of Hypertension over 8 Years among Chinese Men and Women," Journal of Hypertension, Vol. 25, No. 3, 2007, pp. 517-523. doi:10.1097/HJH.0b013e328013e7f4

[3] E. B. Loucks, M. Abrahamowicz, Y. Xiao, et al., "Associations of Education with 30 Year Life Course Blood

Pressure Trajectories: Framingham Offspring Study," *BMC Public Health*, Vol. 28, No. 11, 2011, p. 139.

[4] B. H. Strand and A. Tverdal, "Trends in Educational Inequalities in Cardiovascular Risk Factors: A Longitudinal Study among 48,000 Middle-Aged Norwegian Men and Women," *European Journal of Epidemiology*, Vol. 21, No. 10, 2006, pp. 731-739. doi:10.1007/s10654-006-9046-5

[5] M. Hukkinen, J. Kaprio, U. Broms, *et al.*, "Characteristics and Consistency of Light Smoking: Long-Term Follow-Up among Finnish Adults," *Nicotine & Tobacco Research*, Vol. 11, 2009, pp. 797-805. doi:10.1093/ntr/ntp065

[6] M. T. Streppel, M. C. Ocké, H. C. Boshuizen, *et al.*, "Long-Term Wine Consumption Is Related to Cardiovascular Mortality and Life Expectancy Independently of Moderate Alcohol Intake: The Zutphen Study," *Journal of Epidemiology & Community Health*, Vol. 63, 2009, pp. 534-540. doi:10.1136/jech.2008.082198

[7] H. M. Colhoun, H. Hemingway and N. R. Poulter, "Socio-Economic Status and Blood Pressure: An Overview Analysis," *Journal of Human Hypertension*, Vol. 12, No. 2, 1998, pp. 91-110. doi:10.1038/sj.jhh.1000558

[8] A. Steptoe and G. Willemsen, "The Influence of Low Job Control on Ambulatory Blood Pressure and Perceived Stress over the Working Day in Men and Women from the Whitehall II Cohort," *Journal of Hypertension*, Vol. 22, No. 5, 2004, pp. 915-920. doi:10.1097/00004872-200405000-00012

[9] R. C. Thurston, L. D. Kubzansky, I. Kawachi, *et al.*, "Is the Association between Socioeconomic Position and Coronary Heart Disease Stronger in Women than in Men?" *American Journal of Epidemiology*, Vol. 162, No. 1, 2005, pp. 57-65. doi:10.1093/aje/kwi159

[10] A. Brännlund, A. Hammarström and M. Strandh, "Education and Health-Behaviour among Men and Women in Sweden: A 27-Year Prospective Cohort Study," *Scandinavian Journal of Public Health*, Vol. 41, No. 3, 2013, pp. 284-292. doi:10.1177/1403494813475531

[11] B. Williams, L. H. Lindholm and P. Sever, "Systolic Pressure Is All That Matters," *Lancet*, Vol. 371, No. 9631, 2008, pp. 2219-2221. doi:10.1016/S0140-6736(08)60804-1

[12] R. Hardy, D. Kuh, C. Langenberg and M. E. Wadsworth, "Birthweight, Childhood Social Class, and Change in Adult Blood Pressure in the 1946 British Birth Cohort," *Lancet*, Vol. 362, No. 9391, 2003, pp. 1178-1183. doi:10.1016/S0140-6736(03)14539-4

[13] A. P. van den Elzen, M. A. de Ridder, D. E. Grobbee, *et al.*, "Families and the Natural History of Blood Pressure. A 27-Year Follow-Up Study," *American Journal of Hypertension*, Vol. 17, No. 10, 2004, pp. 936-940. doi:10.1016/S0895-7061(04)00871-4

10

Hints at Quantum Characteristics of Light Signals Measured from a Human Subject

David Racine[1], Anshu Rastogi[2], Rajendra P. Bajpai[3*]
[1]School of Physics, Trinity College, Dublin, Ireland
[2]Department of Biophysics, Palack University, Olomouc, Czech Republic
[3]Division of Analytical BioSciences, Leiden University, The Netherlands
Email: racined@tcd.ie, anshusls@gmail.com, *rpbajpai@gmail.com

ABSTRACT

We measure ultra-weak photon signals emitted from the hand of a human subject, either spontaneously or gradually decaying after local stress has been induced with five concentrations of H_2O_2. We analyze the photon distributions of both spontaneous and stimulated number of photons per measuring interval (bin sizes) according to statistics measure Fano Factor which leads to quantum optics, $g^{(2)}(0)$. We also fit either semi-classical based exponential or quantum grounded hyperbolic curves to the decays. Both indicators point towards an adequate description of the photon signal in an interpretation that is quantum. We extend the interpretation towards the suggestion of a quantum coherent aspect of the subject which, once placed in a therapeutic perspective, links to the holistic views on health.

Keywords: Biophotons; Holistic Health; Quantum Coherence

1. Introduction

The phenomenon of spontaneous and incessant emission of, mainly visible range, photons by all living systems defies conventional interpretation. The phenomenon is called ultra-weak photon or biophoton emission and the emitted photon signals have been labeled biophoton signals [1]. A biophoton signal has many features which defy common interpretations in the living system. Two of these features are the visible range of photons (above the currency of biochemical energy) and non-decaying nature of signal. Both features make the incorporation of biophoton emission in the (semi)classical framework difficult.

The basic premises of the classical framework are composite structure of living system, contact interaction of constituents and preservation of the integrity (chemical and physical action) of constituents in biological processes. The constituents are the biomolecules. They cause and manifest all biological processes [2]. They emit photon signal in probabilistic transitions from higher to lower energy states. The probabilistic transitions of one type of biomolecules confer exponential decay shape to the emitted photon signal. Its wavelength, decay rate and strength are related to the properties of biomolecules emitting it [3]. The shape of signal emitted in the transitions of more than one type of biomolecules is the sum of exponential decay terms.

On the other hand, a non-decaying signal requires coordinated and continuous replenishing of the population of biomolecules in higher energy state through a mechanism, which in case of biophoton signals remains operative at all time. The absence of such a mechanism puts biophoton signals beyond the reach of classical framework. Visible range photons require a mechanism to supply more than 3 eV of energy to a biomolecule in one act for its transition from lower to higher energy state [4]. Cooperative occurrence of many chemical reactions can possibly upgrade their heat of reactions into an energy mode of more than 3 eV. The mechanism ensuring cooperative functioning of biomolecules is given the name coherence; the participating biomolecules cohere and the phenomena emanating from it are called coherent. The coherent phenomena need a different description using attributes that characterize synergetic/holistic functioning of biomolecules. The transfer of instructions/information between cohering biomolecules via interaction may or may not happen in coherent phenomena. If it happens or could happen, then it is classical coherence otherwise it is quantum coherence.

---

*Corresponding author.

Both coherence and its nature are inferred from the properties of a phenomenon. The main objectives of biophoton research, therefore, have been to establish the coherence of biophoton signal, determine its nature, discover holistic attributes and identify cohering biomolecules. Progress has been made in fulfilling all but the last objective. The measurement of the conditional probability of not detecting subsequent photon in a small interval after the detection of a photon provided information on coherence in biophoton signals [5]. This probability behaves differently in coherent and incoherent signals when signal strength goes to zero. It was measured for intervals (10 μs-1 ms) in biophoton signals and signals emitted by a light emitting diode [6]. The measurements pointed towards the coherence of biophoton signals without information transfer to cohering biomolecules by molecular and sound signals. Progress achieved in fulfilling the other two objectives is presented in the next two sections. We present analysis of biophoton signal emitted either spontaneously or after chemically-induced stress.

2. Quantum Coherence of Spontaneous Biophoton Signals

The quantum nature of coherence is easier to establish in a spontaneous biophoton signal because its statistical properties can be determined with sufficient accuracy. We shall illustrate the procedure in human biophoton signals emitted from dorsal and palm sides of the hand. The human hand is selected as an in-vivo sample because it is easily measurable, it is without a substrate (no sample substrate interactions), its life time is much larger than the measuring time and the subject can provide feedback while measurements are performed.

Biophoton signals are usually detected with broadband photo multiplier tubes (**Figure 1(a)**) and have signal to noise ratio of around one, which necessitates background noise correction to the properties of the series of observed (*obs*) signal to obtain the properties of actual signal (*sig*) and makes the determination of spectral decomposition in human photon signal difficult. Experiments are performed by detecting spontaneous signals in intervals of 3 min by counting photons in 3600 contiguous intervals of 50 ms (bin size). The outcomes consitute a series of integer photon counts (0,1,2...) for bin size of 50 ms (**Figure 1(b)**).We then combine neighbouring bins together and form series of series with bin sizes that are integral multiples of 50 ms (*obs*) (**Figure 1(c)**). Similar series of series are generated with background noise (*bg*) in order to make background correction. The subscripts *obs*, *bg* and *sig* are added, both to the series and the properties, of observed, background noise and actual signals. The properties of a series are equated to those of its signal. This amounts to assuming that the series contains outcomes of repeated measurements of signal

strength (ergodicity). The measured series determine the properties of background and observed signals. The signal properties are obtained from them by assuming that signal and background noise produce photons independently and no interference occurs in their detections. Our analysis requires photon count distribution, P, which is the set of probabilities of detecting different numbers of photons n = 0,1,2... for the bin size, Δ (**Figure 1(c)**). From it we obtain mean signal strength, k, and variance, V (**Figure 1(d)**). Signal properties (*sig*) are obtained from measured quantities by the following equations [7]:

$$k_{obs} = k_{sig} + k_{bg} \qquad (1)$$

$$V_{obs} = V_{sig} + V_{bg} \qquad (2)$$

An important intrinsic property of a signal is k_{sig}. It increases linearly with bin size in a series indicating that signal strength expressed in counts/s is the same in all series of signal. A nearly unchanging value of signal strength over macroscopic interval points towards a coherent mechanism for the origin of the signal [8]. V_{sig} is different in different time series of a signal. In a classical signal, it merely determines the ensemble fluctuations in the signal strength and is not considered an intrinsic property. In contrast, in quantum signals, it is an intrinsic property and carries information about the signal. The existence of signal specific information in V_{sig} provides evidence of quantum coherence. In-depth analysis of this quantity has been performed in other studies [9]. Here we shall restrain ourselves to the analysis of variance normalised by signal strength (V_{sig}/k_{sig}) at different bin sizes and show that information is easily extracted from its attributes. The normalised variance is called Fano Factor [10],

$$F = \frac{V_{obs} - V_{bg}}{k_{obs} - k_{bg}} \qquad (3)$$

Fano Factor of a signal is different in its series at different bin sizes. It fluctuates around a point value in a classical signal but around a curve in a quantum signal. The curve contains signal specific information. In human biophoton signals, the curve is nearly a straight line (with a small curvature). The intercept and slope therefore characterize the curve. They are properties of signal and we identify them as holistic attributes of the biological object emitting the signal.

Figure 2 depicts the Fano Factor for 100 bin sizes in three signals: background noise (BG), spontaneous biophoton signal from palm side of a hand (SE) (and 3rd interval of signal emitted in response to stimulation of 500 mM hydrogen peroxide (H_2O_2) (3rd int, see Section 3). The intercepts of Fano Factor in the respective signals are 2.01, 1.31 and 1.01. The slope of Fano Factor is ill determined.

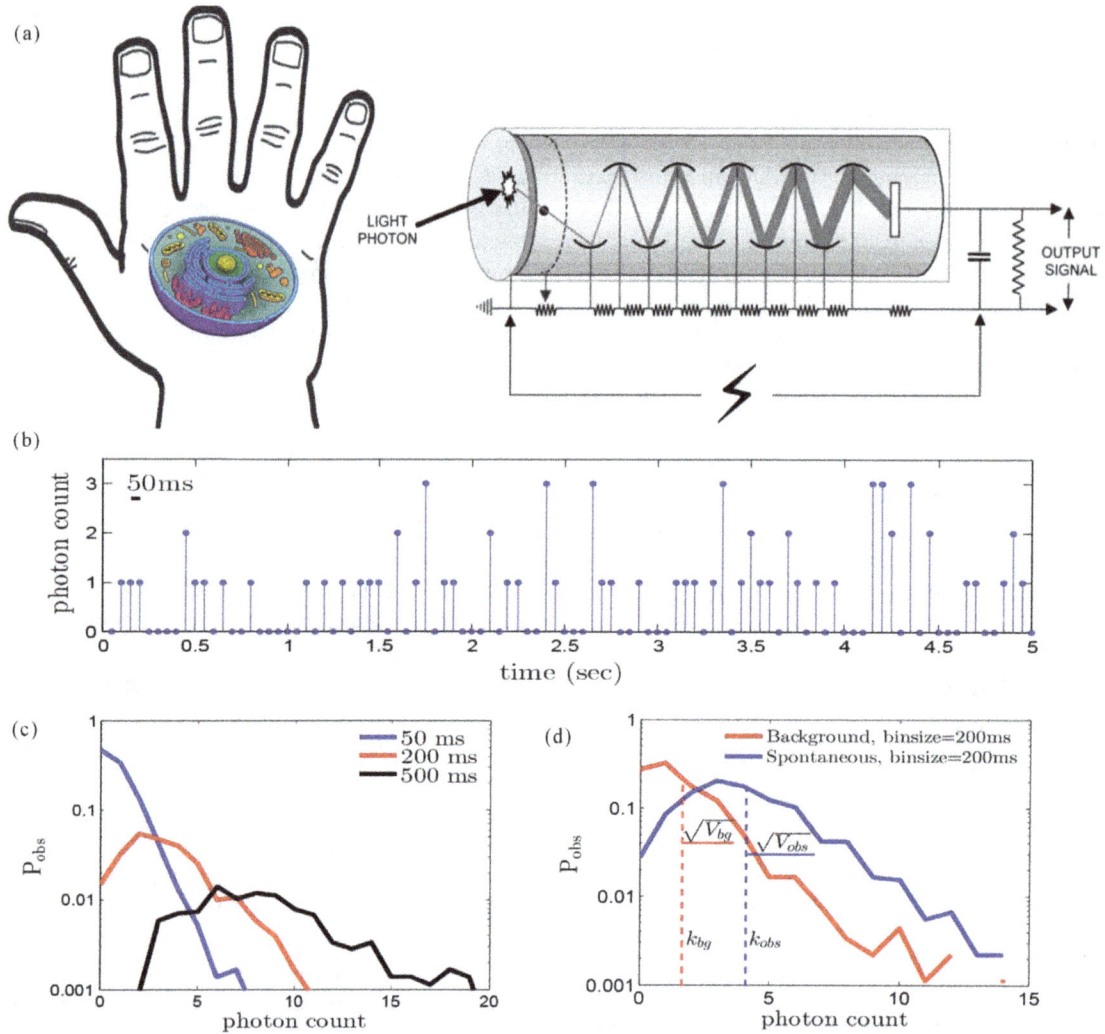

Figure 1. (a) Experimental setup: Human hands photo-emission is detected with photomultilier tubes; (b) Raw photon signal: Photo counts in 50 ms bin size; (c) Probability distributions: P_{obs} for original bin size (50 ms) and grouped bin sizes (200, 500 ms); (d) Background and spontaneous signal properties: We use observed and background means (k_{obs}, k_{bg}) and variances (V_{obs}, V_{bg}) to determine the properties of biophoton signals.

In a parallel study, we also analysed Fano Factor of 10 background noise and 60 spontaneous biophoton signals of 15 human subjects measured over a period of 30 min with two different photo multipliers tubes [11]. The intercept was around 2 and the slope was nearly zero in background signals. The intercept was around 1 in most biophoton signals but was also less than 1 in a few signals. The slope was usually positive and small. It was well determined among four subjects emitting relatively stronger signals. A Fano Factor less than one is a strong indicator of quantum coherence. The Fano Factor curve was below one in two weak biophoton signals for many bin sizes but the small value of signal strength diminishes its reliability.

The indication of quantum coherence in quantum optics is obtained from the value of second order correlation coefficient $g^{(2)}(0)$. One can show [12] that its rela-tion to Fano Factor at zero bin size is given by

$$\left[g^{(2)}(0) - 1 \right] = \frac{V_{sig} - k_{sig}}{k_{sig}^2} \quad (4)$$

The right hand side of Equation (4) is to be extrapo-lated towards its value when bin size tends to zero.

The value of $\left[g^{(2)}(0) - 1 \right]$ in respective signals (BG, SE, 3rd int) are 2.57, 0.17 and 0.029 for bin size of 50 ms and 0.026, 0.016 and 0.0003 at bin size of 5 s (**Figure 2**). Its value in two of the signals (SE, 3rd int) is much small-ler than in background noise, an indication of quantum coherence.

3. Quantum Coherence of Signals Emitted in Response to Stimulation

Additional information about quantum coherence in the

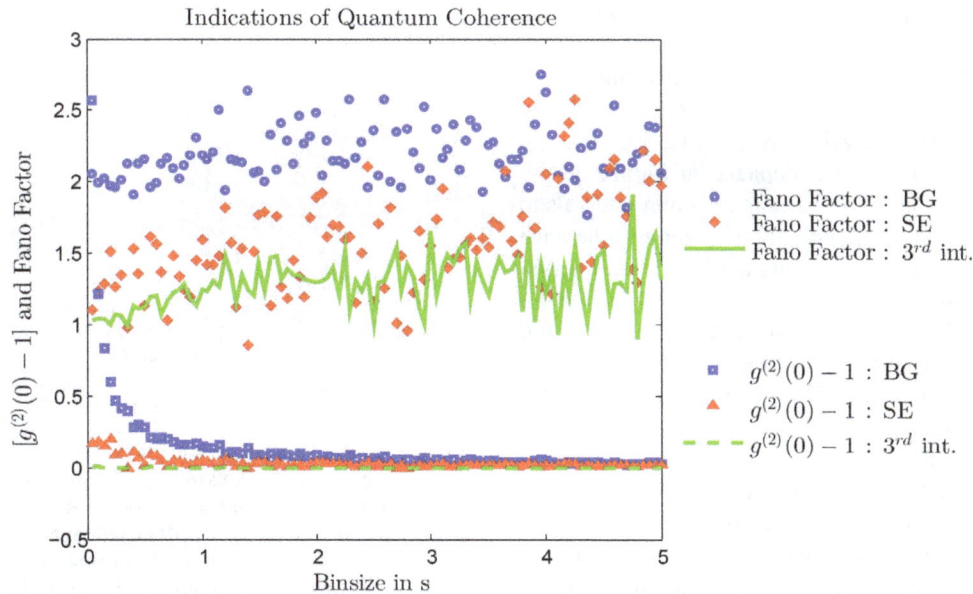

Figure 2. Fano Factor and [$g^{(2)}(0)$−1] at different bin sizes: Two factors pointing to the possibility of classical or quantum signal are depicted at 100 bin sizes for the background noise (BG), spontaneous biophoton signal (SE) and 3rd 3 min interval emitted from the palm side in response to stimulation of 500 mM of H_2O_2 (3rd int, see Section 3). For the smallest of bin size, a value of [$g^{(2)}(0)$−1] less than or nearly 0 points to a strong quantum component of the signal.

living system is provided by the photon signals emitted in response to small physical and chemical stimulations. The most extensively studied stimulation is exposure of a living system to light triggering the emission of a photon signal with the twin features of photons in the visible range and non-exponential decay [13]. These twin features again indicate coherence of photon signal and of biomolecules. The response signals have been called stimulated or light induced biophoton signals.

Investigations with the light induced biophoton signals have remained confined to models that aim to explain decay shape and extract strength parameters [10], and do not explicitly address the problem of coherence and its nature. The model analysed here addresses these important issues and is henceforth called quantum model [14, 15]. The quantum model does so explicitly by assigning an evolving quantum squeezed state to every response signal [16]. In light induced response signals of human subjects, the decay is obervable for less than a second, which is too small for verifying quantum coherence. Luckily however, human subjects respond to chemical stimulation by H_2O_2 on the skin by emitting photon signals with above mentioned twin features. These response signals are measurable for a much longer duration, which permits the verification of quantum coherence. When a small amount of mild concentration H_2O_2 (500 mM) is applied on human skin, the skin immediately starts emitting a response signal that decays continuously with decreasing decay rate [17-19] for the duration of nearly an hour (**Figure 3**). One can determine the statistical properties of the decay signal by dividing it in 3 min intervals

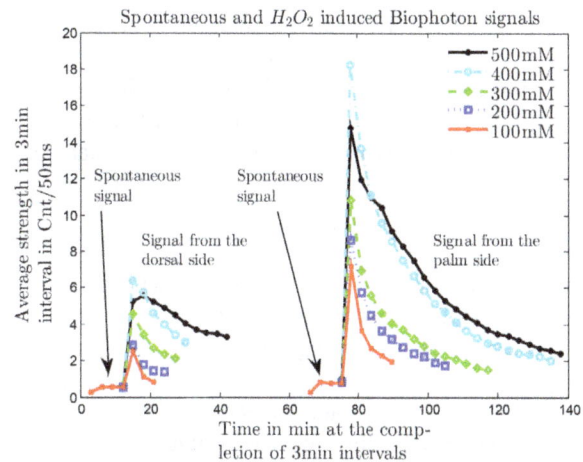

Figure 3. Decay of response signals: The strength of visible range photon signal emitted by a human subject in response to stimulation of skin by H_2O_2 is depicted for five concentrations of the chemical. Only one concentration was used on a portion of skin on the dorsal and palm sides of the left hand in one day. The signals were detected within 2 s of the applying of chemical. Background noise and observed spontaneous signals emitted prior to stimulation are also depicted on the figure.

during which its strength is nearly constant. The decay nature of the signal can be ignored in each 3 min interval. The photon count distribution (P) can then be used to ascertain the quantum coherence of the signal in the interval. The quantum coherence of response signal can be ascertained through 3 min intervals that scan the entire signal.

We measured ten response signals emitted within 2 s of applying 500 μl of five concentrations of H_2O_2 (100 mM - 500 mM) on an area of nearly 30 cm^2 of the skin at the palm and dorsal sides of the left hand of a subject. Ninety-eight 3 min intervals were detected. The average strength in these intervals is depicted in **Figure 3**. We studied the behaviour of variance in all 3 min intervals to check if it indicated the possibility of quantum coherence. The signal decayed steeply during the first 3 min interval in all signals and in the subsequent interval in two intense signals. The decay in these twelve intervals could not be neglected, thereby preventing the determination of their statistical properties. The remaining eighty-six intervals indicated the possibility of quantum coherence. In **Figure 2**, we also depicted its characteristics for the interval with the highest signal strength (3rd int).

The long duration of response signal is suitable for-checking the robustness of signal specific parameters to change in the bin size. The parameters of valid description have to be robust. The checking of robustness brings out the absence of exponential decay character in response signals and points towards the validity of the quantum model. We present two models which use different functional forms for $n(t)$, where $n(t) \cdot \Delta t$ is the number of photons detected in a small interval Δt around t.

One model has a functional form which shows exponential decay character and is taken to be the sum of two exponential decay terms, for definiteness, but can also have more terms,

$$n(t) = S_o + S_1 e^{-\lambda_1 t} + S_2 e^{-\lambda_2 t} \qquad (5)$$

It has five parameters S_o; λ_1; S_1; λ_2 and S_2. They specify strength of background noise, slow decay constant, strength of slow decay, fast decay constant and strength of fast decay, respectively. The parameter S_o is not a property of signal and expected to be same in all signals. This model embraces a classical description [3].

The functional form of $n(t)$ in the quantum model [15] is

$$n(t) = B_o + \frac{B_1}{(t + t_o)} + \frac{B_2}{(t + t_o)^2} \qquad (6)$$

which has four parameters B_o; B_1; B_2 and t_o. The background noise contribution, S_2, is included in B_o.

The nine parameters of the two models were estimated for each of the ten response signals with bin sizes varying from 50 ms to 3 min. The parameters B_o; B_1 and t_o remained same for all bin sizes whereas the other parameters varied significantly with bin sizes. **Figure 4** depicts the contributions of B_1; B_2 and S_2 to the signal at $t = 0$ along with t_o and λ_2 in the most intense response signal. The contribution of the B_2 term is less than 1% and it further decreases for larger t which,

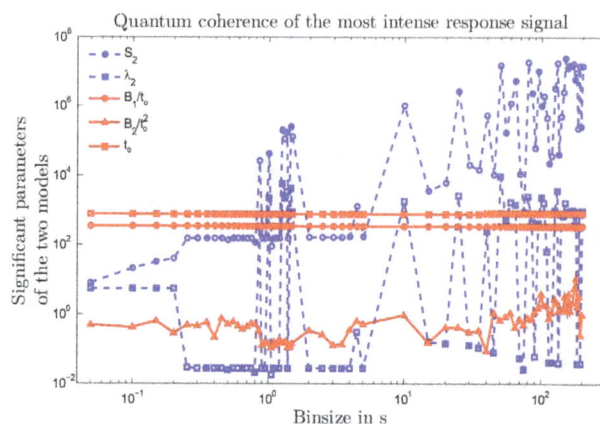

Figure 4. Robustness of the parameters of the quantum model: The contributions of B_1; B_2 and S_2 at $t = 0$ in the signal emitted in response to 500 mM of H_2O_2 from the palm side of left hand are depicted against bin size. The figure also depicts the values of parameters t_o and λ_2. These parameters provide the dominant contribution to the signal and are correctly estimated. S_1 and λ_1 are not depicted in order to avoid the clumsiness while the values of B_o and S_o are too small for depiction in the same figure. B_1; t_o and B_o are robust and the contribution of B_2 is less than 1% at all bin sizes.

probably, makes it ill determined as well as non-robust. Conversely, the contribution of B_o is insignificant at $t = 0$ but becomes significant at larger t which, probably, makes it well determined and robust. In the classical model, the dominant contribution to the signal comes from S_2 and λ_2. The figure (**Figure 4**), illustrates how the quantum based model provides the best picture of the decay. Similar figures of other response signals of this subject as well as two other subjects measured by us convey the same message.

4. A Quantum Framework to Understand the Living System?

Our analysis points towards statistical time coordination in fluctuations of spontaneously emitted photons. The classical interpretation of fluctuations is devoid of fundamental information. Statistical time coordination establishes their role in manifesting overall coordination, balance or equilibrium of the emitting system. Fano Factor brings out the coordination and quantifies it.

The holistic nature of the characteristics suggests the possibility of their correlation with other holistic features of human subjects e.g. with some qualitative aspects of health. If such a correlation is found then, their measure-ability makes those aspects quantitative and measurable.

It is suspected that other characteristics, such as quantum optics squeezed state index [20,21,16], individually or in combination can identify and measure physiological, pathological and psychological aspects of human health. The suspicion needs confirmation, it is planned to perform non-invasive measurements of few minutes in subjects recuperating from illnesses.

Determining the quantum state of a biophoton signal is a definite proof of its quantum coherence as well as the biomolecules implicated in its emission. Quantum biophoton signal can only be emitted by an assembly of biomolecules in a definite quantum state [9]. The confirmation can transform biophoton signals into potent clinical parameters [22].

Response signals manifested the coordination of human subject during oxidative stress. Even mild oxidative stress does not elicit a linear one dimensional response from human subject. Perhaps, it is true in other stresses encountered inadvertently and interventions made for managing health. The variation of signal strength from 11.1 to 0.84 counts/50 ms in different intervals showed the resilience of the quantum picture. The quantum mechanism is not overwhelmed with the abundance of oxidising molecules and continues operating efficiently. The study opens up new vistas of human response to explore and comprehend. This gives credence to the scenario of quantum coherence envisaged by Fröhlich [23] and searched by Popp [13]. It also presents enigmatic biophoton signal into a rich source of information.

REFERENCES

[1] F. A. Popp, "Some Essential Questions of Biophoton Research and Probable Answers," In: F. A. Popp, K.-H. Li and Q. Gu, Eds., *Recent Advances in Biophoton Research and Its Applications*, World Scientific Pub Co., Inc., 1992, pp. 1-46. doi:10.1142/9789814439671_0001

[2] G. Vitiello, "My Double Unveiled: The Dissipative Quantum Model of Brain (Advances in Consciousness Research)," John Benjamins Publishing Company, Amsterdam, 2001.

[3] V. Weisskopf and E. Wigner, "Berechnung der naturelichen linienbreite auf Grund der diracschen lichttheorie," *Zeitschrift für Physik*, Vol. 63, No. 1-2, 1930, pp. 54-73. doi:10.1007/BF01336768

[4] R. P. Bajpai, "Quantum Coherence of Biophotons and Living Systems," *Indian Journal of Experimental Biology*, Vol. 41, No. 5, 2003, pp. 514-527.

[5] J. Perina, "Coherence of Light," Springer, Berlin, Heidelberg, 1985.

[6] R. Bajpai, "Coherent Nature of the Radiation Emitted in Delayed Luminescence of Leaves," *Journal of Theoretical Biology*, Vol. 198, No. 3, 1999, pp. 287-299. doi:10.1006/jtbi.1999.0899

[7] E. Van Wijk, R. Van Wijk, R. Bajpai and J. van der Greef, "Statistical Analysis of the Spontaneously Emitted Photon Signals from Palm and Dorsal Sides of Both Hands in Human Subjects," *Journal of Photochemistry and Photobiology B: Biology*, Vol. 99, No. 3, 2010, pp. 133-143. doi:10.1016/j.jphotobiol.2010.03.008

[8] R. P. Bajpai, "The Physical Basis if Life," In: F.-A. Popp,

and L. Beloussov, Eds., *Integrative Biophysics, Biophotonics*, Kluwer Academic Publishers, Dordrecht, 2003, pp. 439-465. doi:10.1007/978-94-017-0373-4_13

[9] R. Bajpai, "Squeezed State Description of Spectral Decompositions of a Biophoton Signal," *Physics Letters A*, Vol. 337, No. 4, 2005, pp. 265-273. doi:10.1016/j.physleta.2005.01.079

[10] U. Fano, "Ionization Yield of Radiations. II. The Fluctuations of the Number of Ions," *Physical Review*, Vol. 72, No. 1, 1947, pp. 26-29. doi:10.1103/PhysRev.72.26

[11] R. Bajpai, E. Van Wijk, R. Van Wijk and J. van der Greef, "Attributes Characterizing Ultraweak Photon Signals of Human Subjects," *Journal of Photochemistry and Photobiology*, Submitted 2013.

[12] D. Walls and G. J. Milburn, "Quantum Optics," Springer, Berlin, Heidelberg, 2008, pp. 29-55. doi:10.1007/978-3-540-28574-8_3

[13] F. Popp, "On the Coherence of Ultraweak Photonemission, from Living Tissues," In: C. W. Kilmister, Ed., *Disequilibrium and Self-Organisation Mathematics and Its Applications*, Reidel, Dordrecht, 1986, pp. 207-230.

[14] R. P. Bajpai, S. Kumar and V. A. Sivardasan, "Frequencystable Damped Oscillator Model of Biophoton Emission," *Frontier Perspectives*, Vol. 6, No. 2, 1997, pp. 9-16.

[15] R. Bajpai, S. Kumar and V. Sivadasan, "Biophoton Emission in the Evolution of a Squeezed State of Frequency Stable Damped Oscillator," *Applied Mathematics and Computation*, Vol. 93, No. 2-3, 1998, pp. 277-288. doi:10.1016/S0096-3003(97)10117-5

[16] H. P. Yuen, "Two-Photon Coherent States of the Radiation Field," *Physical Review A*, Vol. 13, No. 6, 1976, pp. 2226-2243. doi:10.1103/PhysRevA.13.2226

[17] A. Rastogi and P. Pospisil, "Ultra-Weak Photon Emission as a Non-Invasive Tool for Monitoring of Oxidative Processes in the Epidermal Cells of Human Skin: Comparative Study on the Dorsal and the Palm Side of the Hand," *Skin Research and Technology*, Vol. 16, No. 3, 2010, pp. 365-370.

[18] M. Havaux, "Spontaneous and Thermoinduced Photon Emission: New Methods to Detect and Quantify Oxidative Stress in Plants," *Trends in Plant Science*, Vol. 8, No. 9, 2003, pp. 409-413. doi:10.1016/S1360-1385(03)00185-7

[19] A. Rastogi and P. Pospisil, "Effect of Exogenous Hydrogen Peroxide on Biophoton Emission from Radish Root Cells," *Plant Physiology and Biochemistry*, Vol. 48, No. 2-3, 2010, pp. 117-123. doi:10.1016/j.plaphy.2009.12.011

[20] F. A. Popp, B. Ruth, W. Bahr, J. Böhm, P. Grass, G. Grolig, M. Rattemeyer, H. G. Schmidt and P Wulle, "Emission of Visible and Ultraviolet Radiation by Active Biological Systems," Collective Phenomena 3, Gordon and Breach Science Publishersh, 1981, pp. 187-214.

[21] X. Shen, F. Liu and X. Y. Li, "Experimental Study on Photocount Statistics of the Ultraweak Photon Emission from Some Living Organisms," *Experientia*, Vol. 49, No. 4, 1993, pp. 291-295. doi:10.1007/BF01923404

[22] R. P. Bajpai and M. Drexel, "Effect of Colorpuncture on

Spontaneous Photon Emission in a Subject Suffering from Multiple Sclerosis," *Journal of Acupuncture and Meridian Studies*, Vol. 1, No. 2, 2008, pp. 114-120.

[23] H. Froehlich, "Quantum Mechanical Concepts in Biology," In: M. Marais, Ed., *Theoretical Physics and Biology* (*Proceedings of the* 1*st International Conference on Theoretical Physics and Biology*, Versailles, 1967), North Holland, Amsterdam, 1969, pp. 13-22.

11

Ergogenic Capacity of a 7-Chinese Traditional Medicine Extract in Aged Mice

Jian-Rong Zhou[1], Mohamed Aly M. Morsy[2], Kiyoshi Kunika[3],
Kazumi Yokomizo[1], Takeshi Miyata[1]

[1]Department of Presymptomatic Medical Pharmacology, Faculty of Pharmaceutical Sciences, Sojo University, Kumamoto, Japan
[2]Department of Pharmacology, Faculty of Medicine, Minia University, Minya, Egypt
[3]Division of Science and Medicine, Institute of International Kampo Co. Ltd., Nihonmatsu, Japan
Email: zhoujr@ph.sojo-u.ac.jp

ABSTRACT

The ergogenic properties of a 7-Chinese traditional medicine water extract (*Ligustrum lucidum ait*, LLA), which is composed of the essences of *Lycii fructus, Crataegi fructus, Phyllanthi fructus, Chrysanthemi flos, Coicis semen, Ganoderma lucidum*, and *Zizyphi fructus*, were studied using aged mice. Mice were chronically (one month) administered LLA (0.1% and 1%) in the drinking water. Mice pre-treated with LLA showed a good appetite; however, they exhibited a lower rate of body weight increase compared to control mice. In mice subjected to the rotarod test, 1% LLA treatment provided effective adaption to fatigue and significantly increased the duration of mice on the rotarod. In locomotor activity test, 1% LLA potentiated mice mobility and significantly increased rearing behavior. In the antioxidant experiment, 1% LLA treatment significantly increased superoxide dismutase activity in the spleen and liver glutathione levels. These findings suggest that LLA may be utilized as an antifatigue agent, which may function through its antioxidant activity.

Keywords: Antifatigue; Antioxidant; Chinese Traditional Medicine

1. Introduction

A 7-Chinese traditional medicine water extract (*Ligustrum lucidum ait*, LLA) has been used for more than thirty years in China and Japan, and is composed of the essences of *Lycii fructus* from *Lycium chinense* Miller, *Crataegi fructus* from *Crataegus cuneata* Siebold et Zuccarini, *Phyllanthi fructus* from *Phyllanthus emblica* L., *Chrysanthemi flos* from *Chrysanthemum morifolium*, *Zizyphi fructus* from *Zizyphus jujuba* Miller var. inermis Rehd, *Ganoderma lucidum*, and *Coicis semen* from *Coix lacryma-jobi* L. var. mayuen Stapf. In an *in vitro* experiment with aged mice, it was demonstrated that at a lower concentration LLA could act as a co-stimulator with mitogens, whereas at a higher concentration it was able to act as an immunosuppressive agent [1]. In a clinical study, Chien *et al.* reported that after administration of LLA, IL-2 levels increased and decreased levels of lymphocyte transformation returned to normal levels in aged volunteers. Follow-up medical examinations showed that inspiration (100%), good appetite (95%), sexual (35%) and sound sleep (95%) were the general clinical manifestations [1]. We are interested in the improved general clinical manifestations following LLA treatment; however, it is still unknown whether the underlying pharma-cological mechanism involves immunomodulation and/or other pathways.

The main nutrient compositions of LLA are listed in **Table 1**, and the most important thing is that LLA contains a variety of components with antioxidant activities, such as Lycium, Crataegus, Emblica, and Ganoderma, and their antioxidant activities have been well described. It has been reported that polysaccharides from *Lycium chinense*, a component of LLA, improved superoxide dismutase (SOD) activity in damaged rat testes, and its antioxidant activities were comparable to the normal antioxidant, vitamin C [2,3]. An increasing number of reports have also suggested that Ganoderma, which has multiple health benefits for a broad range of conditions (from arthritis to cancers), has antioxidant properties as a free radical scavenger [4,5]. Furthermore, it was found that Emblica, another component of LLA, had a higher content of vitamin C, accounting for 45% - 70% of the antioxidant activity [6]. Dicaffeoylquinic acids from Chrysanthemi Flos and six phenolic compounds from Coicis Semen showed potent DPPH radical scavenging activity [7,8]. These may contribute greatly to the antioxidant property of LLA.

Although LLA has a significant folk history in China

Table 1. Mean values of the nutrient composition (amino acid, mineral, vitamine and sugar content) for 100 g LLA extract.

Amino acid	Mean (mg/100 g)	Mineral	Mean (/100 g)
Arginine	52	Sodium (Na)	113.00 mg
Lysine	9	Phosphorous (P)	24.60 mg
Histidine	11	Iron (Fe)	0.84 mg
Phenylanine	6	Calcium (Ca)	13.50 mg
Tyrosine	7	Potassium (K)	295.00 mg
Leucine	20	Magnesium (Mg)	16.10 mg
Isoleucine	8	Chlonium (Cl)	85.00 mg
Methionine	2	Copper (Cu)	48.00 µg
Valine	16	Zinc (Zn)	231.00 µg
Alanine	94	Sulfur (S)	0.01 g
Glycine	12		
Proline	178		
Glutamic acid	156	**Vitamine**	**Mean (/100 g)**
Serine	66	Vitamine B1	0.05 mg
Threonine	31	Vitamine B2	0.07 mg
Aspartic acid	269	Vitamine B6	55.00 µg
Tryptophan	6	Folic acid	11.00 µg
Cystine	11	Patoten acid	0.16 mg
		Biotin	4.30 µg
Mean (g/100 g)		Niacin	0.96 mg
Sugar content	10.80		

and Japan, further scientific investigation of LLA-induced effects is required, as it is important to provide an evidence-based supplement. Therefore, we investigated the antifatigue effect of LLA in aged mice using open-field and rotarod tests, and assessed whether its mechanism of action is related to its antioxidant activity.

2. Materials and Methods

2.1. Animals

Male ddY mice (SPF grade), 60 weeks old, were obtained from Kyudo Co., Ltd. (Fukuoka, Japan). Mice were housed under the following controlled conditions: temperature (24°C ± 2°C), humidity (50% ± 10%) and a 12-hour light/dark cycle (7:00 a.m. to 7:00 p.m.). Food and water were available *ad libitum*. There was a one-week adaptation period, after which the mice were administered either water or 0.1% or 1% LLA. All experiments were conducted in strict accordance with the

Guidelines of the Japanese Pharmacological Society for the Care and Use of Laboratory Animals.

2.2. Materials

LLA was prepared and provided by the International Kampo Institute (Nihonmatsu, Japan). SOD Assay Kit-WST and total GSH Quantification Kits were purchased from Dojindo (Kumamoto, Japan). Other agents were obtained as follows: bovine erythrocyte SOD (Sigma, St. Louis, MO, USA); pentobarbital sodium (Dainippon Sumitomo Pharma, Osaka, Japan); sucrose (Nacalai Tesque, Kyoto, Japan). LLA (0.1% and 1%) were prepared in water.

2.3. Assay of Antifatigue Endurance Activity Using Rotarod Test

Either LLA (0.1% or 1%) or water (control group) was administered from water pots for one month. First, the mice were placed on a rotarod (Ugo Basile, Comerio VA, Italy) to induce fatigue for 30 min at 16 rpm. Fatigued mice were again placed on the rotarod (40 rpm) and the riding time (the time before the mice fell off the rod) was determined.

2.4. Assay of Spontaneous Locomotor Activity Using the Open-Field Test

The locomotor behavior of mice was measured as previously reported [9]. Briefly, the mice were put into an acrylic cage (30 × 36 × 17 cm) 30 min before the locomotion determination. Lines were drawn on the bottom of the cage, dividing it into nine rectangles. Locomotor activity was evaluated as the ambulation behavior (the number of times a mouse crossed a section) and the rearing behavior (rearing number) during the 5-minute observation period.

2.5. Assay of Antioxidant Activity Using SOD and GSH Kits

After one-month LLA administration, mice were sacrificed by decapitation, and blood and tissues were collected. For SOD determination, tissue samples were homogenized in sucrose buffer (0.25 M sucrose, 10 mM Tris, 1 mM EDTA, pH 7.4). The homogenates were centrifuged at 10,000 × g for 15 min at 4°C and supernatants were collected. Bovine erythrocyte SOD was used as the standard. For total GSH determination, serum was mixed with 5% 5-sulfosalicylic acid solution. The mixture was centrifuged at 8000 × g for 10 min at 4°C and the supernatant was collected. Tissue samples were homogenized in 5% 5-sulfosalicylic acid solution. The homogenates were centrifuged at 8000 × g for 10 min at 4°C, and the supernatants were collected. SOD and total

GSH activities were determined in triplicate with colorimetric assays, following the manufacturer's instructions. For tissues, SOD and total GSH were expressed as units per mg protein and μM per mg protein relative to the standards, respectively. Protein concentration was measured using the Bradford method.

2.6. Statistical Analysis

Each value represents the mean ± SEM for 5 - 6 mice. The data were statistically evaluated using student's t-test. Probability (p) values less than 0.05 were considered to be statistically significant.

3. Results

3.1. Changes in Food Intake and Weight

The LLA group consumed more food than the control group (**Figure 1(a)**), while the rate of body weight increase in the LLA group showed a decreasing tendency after 15 days of administration (**Figure 1(b)**).

3.2. Extension of Rotarod Riding Time

We studied the antifatigue effect of LLA on aged mice using the rotarod test. As shown in **Figure 2**, the rotarod riding time in the LLA group was increased 2.8 ± 1.6 and 6.7 ± 1.4 times on the 20th and 30th day of administration, respectively. The time measured on the 30th day was significantly longer ($p < 0.05$) compared to the control mice.

3.3. Excitory Effects on Spontaneous Locomotor Behavior

As shown in **Figure 3**, ambulation and rearing behaviors in the LLA group for 5 min were 45.4 ± 11.2 and 25.5 ± 5.5 counts, respectively, and those of the control group were 20.4 ± 6.6 and 7.5 ± 2.3 counts, respectively. LLA induced an increase in ambulation and rearing behaviors in mice, and the increase in rearing behavior was significant ($p < 0.05$).

3.4. Antioxidant Activity

To determine whether the supplementation of LLA demonstrates ergogenic performance by improving the oxidant status in mice, we assessed the SOD and total GSH activities of LLA in aged mice serum and tissues.

As shown in **Figure 4(a)**, the spleen SOD level was elevated significantly by LLA; level was 1.6 ± 0.1 and 2.4 ± 0.2 units/mg protein in the control and LLA groups, respectively. The testes SOD level in LLA mice showed an increasing tendency; the level was 6.0 ± 1.0 and 10.8 ± 2.9 units/mg protein in the control and LLA groups, respectively. On the other hand, there were no significant

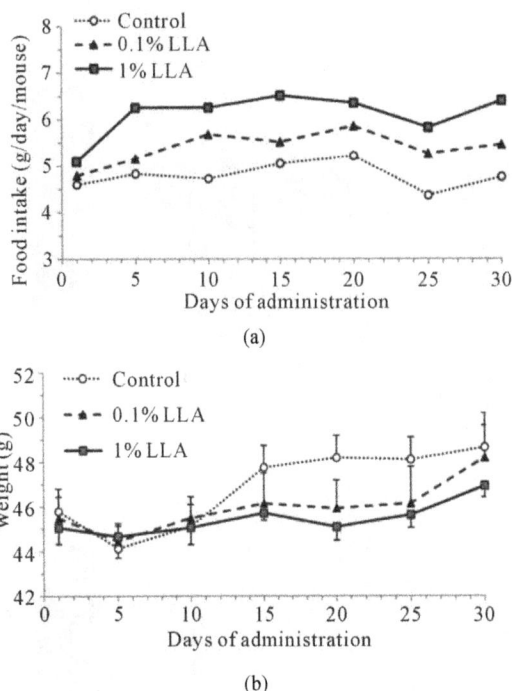

(a)

(b)

Figure 1. Effects of LLA supplementation (versus the control group receiving water) on food intake and weight in aged mice. LLA (1%) and water (control group) were administered from water pots for one month. Food and water were available *ad libitum* (n = 5).

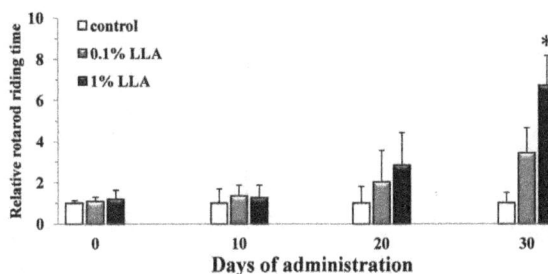

Figure 2. Chronic intake of LLA extends rotarod riding time in aged mice. Data are means ± SEM (n = 4 - 5). *p < 0.05, significantly different from the control.

differences in brain, liver and kidney SOD levels between the control and LLA groups. The serum SOD level was 25.7 ± 11.7 and 27.5 ± 4.9 units/ml in the control and LLA groups, respectively (data not shown).

For total GSH activity, LLA significantly increased liver GSH levels (**Figure 4(b)**) in the control (0.1 ± 0.02 μM/mg protein) and LLA (0.2 ± 0.02 μM/mg protein) groups. However, there were no significant differences in the total GSH levels of serum and other tissues between the two groups (data not shown).

4. Discussion

In the present study, chronic administration of LLA demonstrated an ergogenic property, possibly mediated

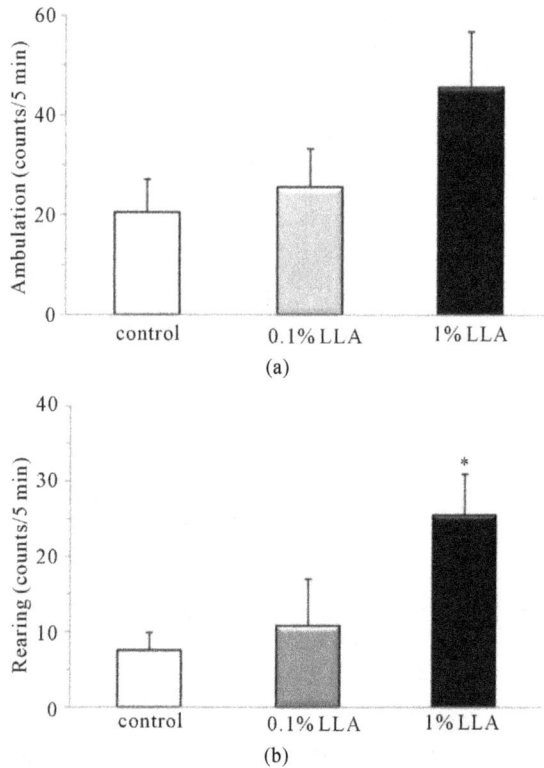

Figure 3. Effects of LLA treatment on spontaneous loco-motor activity. Data are means ± SEM (n = 4 ~ 5). *p < 0.05, significantly different from the control.

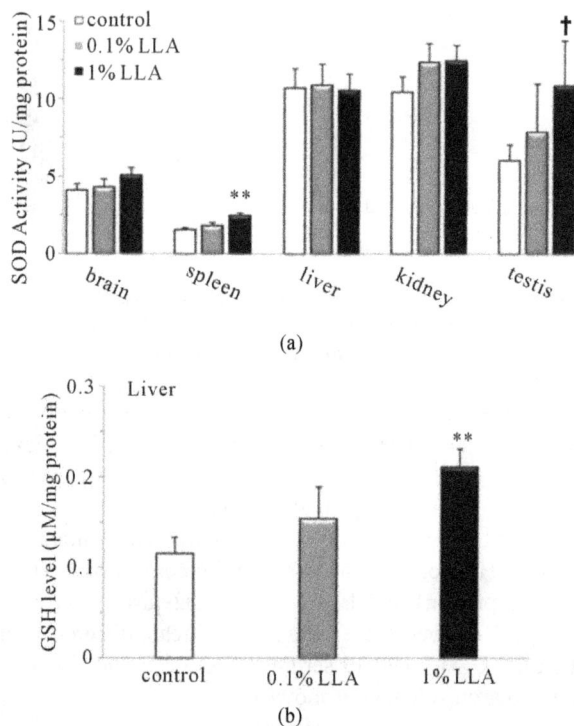

Figure 4. Antioxidant activity in tissues from aged mice after chronic intake of LLA. Data are means ± SEM (n = 4 ~ 5). **p < 0.01, significantly different from the control. †p < 0.1, tendency differing from control.

by functioning in an antioxidative system.

In the *in vivo* experiment, aged mice had a good appetite following LLA treatment (**Figure 1**). Preliminary clinical studies also suggest LLA supplementation had appetizing effects. Despite the increased food intake, the rate of increase in body weight of LLA mice was not as high as that of control mice. This may be important effect for humans, since the trend of increasing rates of obesity appears to be unwavering, and the most effective, currently available, treatment for severe obesity is obesity surgery. It has been reported that *Crataegus fructus*, one of the components in LLA, markedly reduces food intake, body weight, brown and white adipose tissue weights (in hamsters), as well as improving dyslipidemia or obesity [10]. Our results also support this finding of LLA in the active control of behaviors that balance energy intake and expenditure.

In the present study, there was an extending effect in the LLA group on rotarod duration time (**Figure 2**). After 20 days of treatment, aged mice were able to remain on the rotarod 2.8 times longer than aged controls, while the duration time after 30 days of treatment was prolonged 6.7 times ($p < 0.05$). The rotarod test not only measures effects on muscular endurance and antifatigue but also sensorimotor coordination and flexibility. Thus, the increased ability of aged mice to remain on the rotarod indicates that LLA may play a role in improving fatigueand flexibility. Our data also noted behavioral changes in aged mice administered LLA (**Figure 3**). LLA treatment resulted in higher spontaneous locomotor activity; the rearing and ambulation behaviors in aged mice were increased 3.4 and 2.2 times, respectively, than in the control mice, suggesting LLA had an excitation effect on the locomotor behavior of mice. Thus, the results from the rotarod and open-field tests provide controlled *in vivo* evidence of the ergogenic property of LLA. Interestingly, Ganoderma, one of components in LLA, has been reputed to increase youthful vigor and vitality since ancient times. However, it has been reported decreased levels of spontaneous motor activity in a D-galactose mouse-aging model after treatment with *Lycium barbarum* [11]. These observations suggest that the increased motor activity, as a result of LLA administration, may not simply be produced through the additive effects of the seven components of LLA. Thus the interaction of these components may be worthy of further study.

In the present study, chronic LLA intake caused a significant augmentation of SOD activity in aged mice spleen and an increasing tendency in testes (**Figure 4(a)**). Reduction in intracellular antioxidant activities, including SOD, GSH, catalase and glutathione-*S*-transferase, caused by fatigue has been reported in a mouse model [12,13]. An increase in mouse spleen and testes SOD following chronic LLA intake may play a role in defense against oxidative fatigue stress. Strenuous exercise can result in a dramatic increase in oxygen consumption in the body. Furthermore, it has been reported that strenuous exercise can result in increased reactive oxygen species (ROS) [14-16]. Increased ROS production accelerates muscle fatigue in rat [17], canine [18,19] and mouse [20] models. Thus, chronic administration of LLA may be able to protect aged mice from fatigue-induced oxidative stress.

However, no significant changes in SOD levels in the brain, liver and kidney of aged mice were detected after 4 weeks of LLA supplementation. This indicates that the augmented action of LLA on SOD may be tissue-dependent. In addition, there were no significant changes in serum SOD and GSH levels in aged mice with chronic LLA intake.

On the other hand, chronic supplementation with LLA resulted in a significant GSH activity augmentation in aged mouse liver. GSH is an integral oxidant scavenger, which protects cells and tissues from oxidative damage [21]. It is suggested that increased GSH levels enable detoxification of ROS, which are responsible for exercise-induced protein oxidation, leading to the prevention of fatigue. Thus, LLA administration may improve antioxidant status and delay exercised-induced muscle fatigue. It has also been reported that Crataegus, one of the seven components of LLA, is rich in polyphenols and its extracts inhibit LDL oxidation [22]. Furthermore, it was found that pre-treatment with Crataegus prevented the depletion of reduced GSH content in the liver of CCl_4-injected rats [23], while Ganoderma extract was able to protect the liver from superoxide-induced hepatic damage [24]. Therefore, identification of which component is responsible for the antioxidant property may be needed.

It is suggested that the antifatigue effect of LLA supplementation might be related to antioxidant activity. The antifatigue effect of LLA may be related to the central nervous system, as it potentiates the locomotor activity of the mice. Further study is needed to elucidate the details of the mechanisms involved.

In summary, the present findings suggest that improved ergogenic capacity and alleviated fatigue by LLA supplementation, as demonstrated using the rotarod exercise model, might be due in part to the protective effect against exercise-induced oxidative stress. Thus, LLA most likely functions as an antioxidant agent to improve ergogenic capacity.

5. Acknowledgements

We wish to thank International Friendship Trade Co. Ltd., Japan, for donating LLA. We also thank Dr. Pernilla Berin for providing language help.

REFERENCES

[1] Y. K. Chien, Y. H. Liu and D. G. Massey, "Interleukin-3 and Anti-Aging Medication: A Review," *Journal of Hawaii Medicine*, Vol. 49, No. 5, 1990, pp. 160-165.

[2] Q. Luo, Y. Cai, J. Yan, M. Sun and H. Corke, "Lycium Barbarum Polysaccharides: Protective Effects against Heat-Induced Damage of Rat Testes and H_2O_2 Induced DNA Damage in Mouse Testicular Cell and Beneficial Effect on Sexual Behavior and Reproductive Function of Hemicastrated Rats," *Life Science*, Vol. 79, No. 7, 2006, pp. 613-621. doi:10.1016/j.lfs.2006.02.012

[3] X. M. Li, Y. L. Ma and X. J. Liu, "Effect of the Lycium Barbarum Polysaccharides on Age-Related Oxidative Stress in Aged Mice," *Journal of Ethnopharmacology*, Vol. 111, No. 3, 2007, pp. 504-511. doi:10.1016/j.jep.2006.12.024

[4] T. M. Zhu, Q. Chang, L. K. Wong, F. S. Chong and R. C. Li, "Triterpene Antioxidant from *Ganoderma lucidum*," *Phytother Research*, Vol. 13, No. 6, 1999, pp. 529-531. doi:10.1002/(SICI)1099-1573(199909)13:6<529::AID-PTR481>3.0.CO;2-X

[5] S. Wachtel-Galor, B. Tomlinson and I. F. Benzie, "*Ganoderma lucidum* ('Lingzhi'), a Chinese Medicinal Mushroom: Biomarker Responses in a Controlled Human Supplementation Study," *The British Journal of Nutrition*, Vol. 91, No. 2, 2004, pp. 263-269. doi:10.1079/BJN20041039

[6] P. Scartezzini, F. Antogononi, M. A. Raggi, F. Poli and C. Sabbioni, "Vitamin C Content and Antioxidant Activity of the Fruit and of the Ayurvedic Preparation of Emblica Officinalis Gaertn," *Journal of Ethnopharmacology*, Vol. 104, No. 1, 2006, pp. 113-118. doi:10.1016/j.jep.2005.08.065

[7] C. C. Kuo, W. Chiang, G. P. Liu, Y. L. Chien, J. Y. Chang, C. K. Lee, S. L. Huang, M. C. Shin and Y. H. Kuo, "2,2'-Diphenyl-1-Picrylhydrazyl Radical Scavenging Active Components from Adlay (Coix Lachryma-Jobi L. var. Ma-Yuen Stapf) Hulls," *Journal of Agriculture Food Chemistry*, Vol. 50, No. 21, 2002, pp. 5850-5855. doi:10.1021/jf020391w

[8] H. J. Kim and Y. S. Lee, "Identification of New Dicaffeoylquinic Acids from Chrysanthemum Morifolium and Their Antioxidant Activities," *Planta Medica*, Vol. 71, No. 9, 2005, pp. 871-876. doi:10.1055/s-2005-873115

[9] H. Oku, Y. Ueda and Y. K. Ishiguro, "Antipruritic Effects of the Fruits of Chaenomeles Sinensis," *Biological and Pharmaceutical Bulletin*, Vol. 26, No. 7, 2003, pp. 1031-1034. doi:10.1248/bpb.26.1031

[10] D. H. Kuo, C. H. Yeh, P. C. Shieh, K. C. Cheng, F. A. Chen and J. Cheng, "Effect of Shanzha, a Chinese Herbal Product, on Obesity and Dyslipidemia in Hamsters Receiving High-Fat Diet," *Journal of Ethnopharmacology*, Vol. 124, No. 3, 2009, pp. 544-550. doi:10.1016/j.jep.2009.05.005

[11] H. B. Deng, D. P. Cui, J. M. Jiang, Y. C. Feng, N. S. Cai and D. D. Li, "Inhibiting Effects of Achyranthes Bidentata Polysaccharide and Lycium Barbarum Polysaccharide on Nonenzyme Glycation in D-Galactose Induced Mouse Aging Model," *Biomedical and Environmental*

Sciences, Vol. 16, No. 3, 2003, pp. 267-275.

[12] A. Singh, P. S. Naidu, S. Gupta and S. K. Kulkama, "Effect of Natural and Synthetic Antioxidants in a Mouse Model of Chronic Fatigue Syndrome," *Journal of Medicinal Food*, Vol. 5, No. 4, 2002, pp. 211-220. doi:10.1089/109662002763003366

[13] Y. You, J. Park, H. G. Yoon, Y. H. Lee, K. Hwang, J. Lee, K. Kim, K. W. Lee, S. Shim and W. Jun, "Stimulatory Effects of Ferulic Acid on Endurance Exercise Capacity in Mice," *Bioscience, Biotechnology, and Biochemistry*, Vol. 73, No. 6, 2009, pp. 1392-1397. doi:10.1271/bbb.90062

[14] K. J. Davies, A. T. Quintanilha, G. A. Brooks and L. Packer, "Free Radicals and Tissue Damage Produced by Exercise," *Biochemical and Biophysical Research Communication*, Vol. 107, No. 4, 1982, pp. 1198-1205. doi:10.1016/S0006-291X(82)80124-1

[15] M. J. Jackson, R. H. Edwards and M. C. Symons, "Electron Spin Resonance Studies of Intact Mammalian Skeletal Muscle," *Biochimica et Biophysica Acta*, Vol. 847, No. 2, 1985, pp. 185-190. doi:10.1016/0167-4889(85)90019-9

[16] D. M. Bailey, B. Davies, I. S. Young, M. J. Jackson, G. W. Davison, R. Isaacson and R. S. Richardson, "EPR Spectroscopic Detection of Free Radical Outflow from an Isolated Muscle Bed in Exercising Humans," *Journal of Applied Physiology*, Vol. 94, No. 5, 2003, pp. 1714-1718.

[17] M. B. Reid, K. E. Haack, K. M. Franchek, P. A. Valberg, L. Kobzik and M. S. West, "Reactive Oxygen in Skeletal Muscle I. Intracellular Oxidant Kinetics and Fatigue *in Vitro*," *Journal of Applied Physiology*, Vol. 7, No. 5, 1992, pp. 1797-1804.

[18] E. Nashawati, A. Dimarco and G. Supinski, "Effects Pro-duced by Infusion of a Free Radical-Generating Solution into the Diaphragm," *The American Review of Respiratory Disease*, Vol. 147, No. 1, 1993, pp. 60-65. doi:10.1164/ajrccm/147.1.60

[19] G. Supinski, D. Nethery, D. Stofan and A. DiMarco, "Effect of Free Radical Scavengers on Diaphragmatic Fatigue," *American Journal of Respiratory and Critical Care Medicine*, Vol. 155, No. 2, 1997, pp. 622-629.

[20] J. K. Barclay and M. Hansel, "Free Radicals May Contribute to Oxidative Skeletal Muscle Fatigue," *Canadian Journal of Physiology and Pharmacology*, Vol. 69, No. 2, 1991, pp. 279-284. doi:10.1139/y91-043

[21] T. P. Dalton, Y. Chen, S. N. Schneider, D. W. Nebert and H. G. Shertzer, "Genetically Altered Mice to Evaluate Glutathione Homeostasis in Health and Disease," *Free Radical Biology & Medicine*, Vol. 37, No. 10, 2004, pp. 1511-1526. doi:10.1016/j.freeradbiomed.2004.06.040

[22] C. Quettier-Deleu, G. Voiselle, J. C. Fruchart, P. Duriez, E. Teissier, F. Bailleul, J. Vasseur and F. Trotin, "Hawthorn Extracts Inhibit LDL Oxidation," *Die Pharmazie*, Vol. 58, No. 8, 2003, pp. 577-581.

[23] K. T. Ha, S. J. Yoon, D. Y. Choi, D. W. Kim, J. K. Kim and C. H. Kim, "Protective Effect of Lycium Chinese Fruit on Carbon Tetrachloride-Induced Hepatotoxicity," *Journal of Ethnopharmacology*, Vol. 96, No. 3, 2005, pp. 529-535. doi:10.1016/j.jep.2004.09.054

[24] Y. H. Shieh, C. F. Liu, Y. K. Huang, J. Y. Yang, I. L. Wu, C. H. Lin and S. C. Li, "Evaluation of the Hepatic and Renal-Protective Effects of *Ganoderma lucidum* in Mice," *The American Journal of Chinese Medicine*, Vol. 29, No. 3-4, 2001, pp. 501-507.

12

One-Month-Old Female Baby with Symmetrical Hydrocephalus: Treatment Option

**Muhammad Shakil Ahmad Siddiqui[1,2], Khan Usmanghani[2*], Ejaz Mohiuddin[2],
Laeequr Rahman Malik[2]**

[1]Rafah-e-Aam Dawakhana Ajmali (Clinics) and Rafah-e-Aam Herbal Laboratories, Karachi, Pakistan
[2]Faculty of Eastern Medicine, Hamdard University, Karachi, Pakistan
Email: *ugk_2005@yahoo.com

ABSTRACT

A female infant, named Anum 1.8 kg was born on 9th August 2007 at Jinnah Postgraduate Medical Centre (JPMC) with a big head, Occipitofrontal Circumference (OFC) 36 cm. She was admitted on 29th August 2007 and was discharged on 5th September 2007 from Jinnah Postgraduate Medical Centre after the management of moderate birth asphyxia. Cranial ultrasound revealed moderate Hydrocephalus (symmetrical) with prominent third ventricle. Treatment and its effectiveness have been discussed.

Keywords: Hydrocephalus; Meningocele; Herbal Treatment

1. Introduction

Hydrocephalus is a condition where there is an excessive accumulation of cerebrospinal fluid (CSF) under pressure and at times under no pressure resulting from impaired formation and absorption of CSF. Hydrocephalus may be of two (2) types; it may be communicating (obstructive) where there is an obstruction of the ventricular system of the brain or it may be non-communicating obstructive where there is an obstruction to the flow of CSF within ventricular system. Dorsal meningocele was operated on 3rd September 2007 at Department of Neurosurgery, Jinnah Postgraduate Medical Centre (JPMC), Karachi.

2. Case Presentation

A term female infant of one month old (**Figure 1**) was born with a big head that was not noticed earlier in-utero (**Figure 2**). There she had convulsions and mild fever after the delivery of the baby. No abnormalities were noted except for the mucous vaginal discharge which is not unusual for a female baby.

The baby was delivered through cesarean section history at Zainab Panjwani Memorial Hospital, Nishtar Road, Karachi. On delivery the baby neither cried immediately nor did she suck. She was just found to be a small baby with a big head and dorsal region of her spine showed a sac like projection identified as meningocele. After birth the APGAR score was 2 and 4 at first and

fifth minutes respectively. The case under study belongs to congenital hydrocephalus.

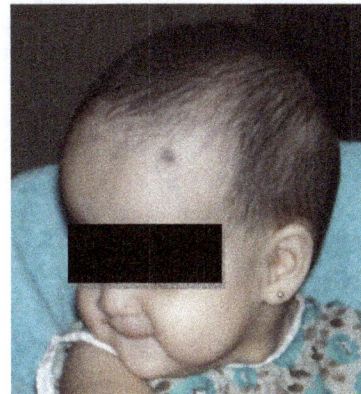

Figure 1. Hydrocephalus baby.

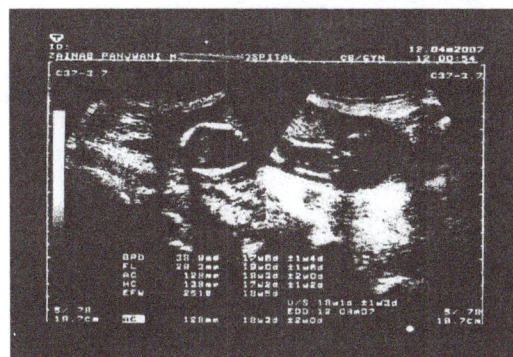

Figure 2. Ultrasound of Fetus at 18th week.

*Corresponding author.

On examination, anterior and posterior fontanelle were widen and full looking like water melon, dark brown silky hair, impaired up gaze, with abnormal head shape and large forehead, but dilatation of scalp veins and hypertonic lower extremities and the face was broadened. No other abnormal features were seen. The eyes showed setting sun sign with visible sclera above the iris. Intracranial pressure was high and nystegmus was observed.

Anthropometric measurement,

Occipitofrontal Circumference 35 cm,

(normal 32 - 35 cm conclusion, Hydrocephalus)

Length 49 cm,

Weight 2.19 kg.

One systemic examination of the central nervous system, the baby was alert with partial sucking reflex and a positive glabellar reflex, rooting reflex, grasp reflex, both hand and plantar, stepping, biceps, triceps, knee, ankle, tendon and moro reflexes. The muscle tone was hypertonic.

The diagnosis was made after, cranial ultrasound scan (US) revealing huge hydrocephalus with bilateral ventriculomegally merging into one probably due to atresia of the aqueduct of sylvius. The six days later and before the discharge, the Ultra-Sound scan was repeated showing the restriction of brain cortical growth due to fluid compression.

During stay in the ward the baby was given inj vitamin K, syp ampicillin, twice a day and syp augmentin and syp ponston once a day for four days. Moreover, the baby was kept warm with daily monitor of the respiratory rate, heart rate, and temperature and measuring of OFC. The treatment of hydrocephalus is to pass a shunt for the CSF fluid to drain into the peritoneum (ventrricoloperitoneal shunting). The parents were advised to consider adopting this procedure for which they refused, taking the responsibility themselves.

2.1. Ultrasound of Skull

Rt. Lat ventricle: 1.6
Rt. Hemisphere: 3.8
Left Ventricle: 1.6
Left Hemisphere: 3.7
3rd Ventricle: 1.1 × 0.7 cm
4th Ventricle: Not Dilated.

2.2. Impression: Moderate Hydrocephalus (Symmetrical)

Ultrasound of Skull:
Normal both Hemispheres
No abnormal lateral or 4th Ventricular Dilatation seen
Prominent 3rd ventricle measure 1.0 × 0.4 cm
No intra Ventricular Hemorrhages seen
No Midline shift seen

Normal Cerebellum and choroid plexus
Resistive Index of cerebral vessels is normal
MRI of Dorsal Spine (Full Study)
Sequences: T1 W1 sagittal and axial images were obtained.

2.3. Findings

There is a focal area of abnormal signal intensity which is seen in the subcutaneous region of the upper back. This is communicating with the spinal canal in the dorsal region through a defect in the posterior bony element in the upper dorsal spinal region. CSF is noted within the lesion. Minimal extension of cord tissue is also noted in this region. Findings are consistent with a dorsal meningomyelocele.

No tumor mass is seen.

Conusmedullaris terminates at D12-L1.

2.4. Impression

There is a focal area of abnormal signal intensity which is seen in the subcutaneous region of the upper back. This is communicating with the spinal canal in the dorsal region through a defect in the posterior bony element in the upper dorsal spinal region. CSF is noted within the lesion. Minimal extension of cord tissue is also noted in this region. Findings are consistent with a dorsal meningomyelocele.

2.5. Hydrocephalus Herbal Formulation

The patient was brought by the family members to Hakim Muhammad Shakil Ahmad Siddiqui at Rafah-e-Aam Dawakhana Ajmali (Clinics) and Rafah-e-Aam Herbal Laboratories for consultation. After reviewing the case thoroughly the patient was prescribed the herbal medicine as follows. Formulation I: Afteemoon (*Cuscuta reflexa* herb) 20 mg, Berg Gaozaban (*Borage officinalis* leaf) 20 mg, Bisfaij (*Polypodium vulgare* Linn root) 20 mg, Kabab Chini (*Piper cubeba* fruit) 20 mg, Ushba (*Sarsaparilla indica* herb) 20 mg, Chob Chini (*Smilax chinensis* root) 30 mg, Gluemundin (*Sphaeranthus indicus*) Aqueous ext. 20 mg.

Formulation II: Gule Surkh (*Rosa demascena* flower) 30 mg, Sandal safed (*Santalum album* wood) 30 mg, Sandal surkh (*Pterocarpus santalinus* wood) 30 mg, Senna (*Cassia senna* leaf) 40 mg, Post Balela (*Terminalia belerica* fruit coat) 10 mg, Sumbultib (*Nardostachys jatamansi* root) 10 mg, Haleela Siyah (*Terminalia chebula* unripe fruit) 6 mg, Post Haleela Zard (*Terminalia chebula* half ripe fruit coat) 6 mg.

For associated symptoms the herbal dosage form design included Laooq Khiyar Shanber for constipation, Ghutti (Saunf, Ajowain, Podina and Ilachi) for indigestion, Sherbet Katan and Diya Quza for cough, Shobi

Lehsan and Nukhsa Sobi, for otitis, and Laooq Sapistan and Nukhsa Nazla for cold and rhinitis.

The treatment was started on 20 September 2007 and continued up to 11 October 2008. During the treatment the following clinical features were observed. Weight gain 7.5 kg. Setting sun sign showed improvement, there was no vomiting or fits and the baby showed improvement of normal growth. The monitoring of clinical features exhibited mild improvement between 20 September to 11 October 2007, Moderate improvement was seen between 12 October 2007 till 10 December 2007, and complete improvement was seen by 11 October 2008.

3. Discussion

Peach [1] has specified that the congenital hydrocephalus produces brain atrophy hence week prognosis and mental retardation is observed with the passage of time. Therefore, it is advisable to observe carefully all other system manifestation of the body along with nervous system manifestation. In this respect the CT scan and ultra sound scan should be useful tool to monitor multi-organ damage.

We had constantly monitored the patients over a period of 5 years with prescribed dosage form design of composite mixture of herbal drugs as specified in the text. However for other sign and symptoms of associated disorder beside the prescribed medicine, other herbal drugs were also administered to wipe out the malaise. As such the stunting of the baby patients was refused by the parents; therefore the patient was carefully monitored and overall performance was improved. The patients showed no mental retardation but otherwise the child is very much active and study performance is over all is good.

So indirectly it can be inferred that the different herbal drugs prescribed showed the synergistic effects both on mental and body faculties and that hydrocephalus effects was not noticeable. The herbal formulations were selected on the bases to expel cerebrospinal fluid and to expand the ventricles to reduce the pressure. However, it is very difficult to pin point the mechanism by which these herbal drugs have brought about the positive and beneficent effect on the hydrocephaly. However in this child, there was a possibility of mental retardation and delayed mile stone due to brain cortical growth failure were nullified by the use of prescribed herbal medication. The overall effects of prescribed herbal medication could be assigned as neuro degenerative disease and neuronal dysfunction treatment. As such neuro degenerative disease and neuronal dysfunction has been treated by herbal medicine and the composition comprised of *Angelica sinensis*, *Ligusticum chuanxiong*, *Polygonum sibricum*, *Carthamus tinctorius*, *Astragalus mebrananaceus*, *Glycyrrhiza uralensis*. This is given in United State Patent Xia, Patent No: US7, 416, 747 B2, date of patent: August 26, 2008. In addition drugs such as Isosorbide which produces hyperosmotic diuresis and those as such Aacetazolamide which decrease the secretion of Cerebrospinal Fluid (CSF) may be treated as temporary management of clinical situation for the treatment of hydrocephalus [2].

REFERENCES

[1]   B. A. Peach, "Malformation: Morphogenesis," *Archives of Neurology*, Vol. 12, No. 5, 1955, pp. 527-535. doi:10.1001/archneur.1965.00460290083009

[2]   R. Raza and Q. Anjum, *Journal of the Pakistan Medical Association*, Vol. 55, No. 11, 2005, pp. 502-507.

13

PEONIES: Comparative Study by Anatomy and TLC of Three Traditional Chinese Medicinal Plants

F. El Babili[1*], M. El Babili[2], I. Fouraste[3], C. Chatelain[1]
[1]Faculté des Sciences Pharmaceutiques, Laboratoire de BOTANIQUE, Toulouse, France
[2]Université Claude Bernard, Lyon I, Institut Michel Pacha, La Seyne sur Mer, France
[3]Faculté des Sciences Pharmaceutiques, Laboratoire de Pharmacognosie, Toulouse, France
Email: *fatiha.el-babili@univ-tlse3.fr

ABSTRACT

Anatomical and TLC study of three Chinese peonies were conducted to make a comparative analysis. Peonies (*Paeonia suffruticosa* (tree peony), *Paeonia lactiflora* (Chinese peony) and *Paeonia veitchii* (Chinese peony)) are traditionally used on the Qinghai-Tibet Plateau in China. Recent studies have shown that the peonies have different pharmacological activities and clinical applications. To distinguish these three species of peonies and ensure the safety and effectiveness in their use, the microscopic characteristics and chromatographic profile of their roots and the corresponding powder were studied. Plant materials sectioned and stained and the raw powder were studied with an optical microscope using standard techniques in microscopy. The results of microscopic features and TLC were described and illustrated. The three species have different microscopic characteristics and TLC profiles, which allow us to distinguish them. In fact, with the help of features semi-quantitative and qualitative, an identification key was developed in our work and illustrated with photos and a table. The aim of our work was to show that the optical microscopy and related techniques provide a achievable practicality, which can be applied without ambiguity to the authentication of species peonies.

Keywords: *Peonies*; Microscopic Identification; TLC; *P. suffructicosa*; *P. lactiflora*; *P. vetchii*

1. Introduction

Peonies are herbaceous perennials belonging to the family Paeoniaceae which consists of 96 species worldwide, mainly distributed in the alpine regions of Asia and Europe. China is a major production area of peonies, containing 73 species, 2 subspecies and 7 varieties. There are 3 species in Paeoniaceae that are used in traditional Chinese medicine (TCM) under the general heading of "Peony": *Paeonia suffruticosa* (tree peony), *Paeonia lactiflora* (Chinese peony) and *Paeonia veitchii* (Chinese peony). These three species of Chinese peonies are perennials and can reach heights of up to nine meters (the tree peony is a bit more). They have alternate and elliptic leaves and smooth edges worn smooth by stems bearing two or more flowers. The large flowers of the peony Chinese may have a range of colors and generally have a diameter of 4 - 6 cm. The roots of all peonies are large, straight and firm and have an easily separable bark revealing an under layer powder during its removal [1].

Peonies have provided useful drugs and attractive ornamental flowers for over 3000 years in China and at least 500 years in Europe [1]. For millennia, the peony root has been used to treat wounds, fungal infections and spasmodic pain in TCM. Recently, the peony root has received increasing attention in research, mainly in Japan and China. In Europe, the peony has also long been used, particularly for spasmodic [2].

There are three drugs produced from the Chinese peonies used in traditional Chinese medicine [3]. *P. lactiflora* roots without bark provide "Baishao" or "*Radix paeoniae alba*", referred to below as white peony. In fact, the root without bark of these same three plants provides "baishao" (white peony), although most often this medicine is derived from *P. lactiflora*.

The root bark of *P. veitchii* (and sometimes *P. lactiflora*) roots provides "Aba" or "*Radix paeoniae rubra*", also called red peony.

P. suffruticosa bark of root provides "Mudanpi" or "*Cortex Paeonia moutan*", referred to below as tree peony. The color designation does not refer to the flowers of

---

*Corresponding author.

these plants (which are most commonly pink, red, purple, or white) but refer to the color of the root after processing.

Several studies suggest that red and white peonies can be beneficial for people suffering from atherosclerosis and/or hypertension [3-5]. These 2 peonies are traditionally used in Asia to treat people with chronic viral hepatitis [6,7]. Their biochemical analysis showed the presence of paeniflorine, a sedative alkaloid, analgesic and anticonvulsifiant, which could explain the ancient practice of "big medicine". *P. officinalis* also contains paenol, known for its analgesic, antispasmodic and anti-inflammatory [8].

To solve the problem of identifying these three species, which are often difficult to distinguish because of their great similarity, the microscopic and TLC analysis is simple, economical and reliable. For reasons of safety, efficacy and quality control, we have developed a TLC and microscopic identification technique, systematic and detailed for the three species studied. Our study thus demonstrates that optical microscopy supplied by TLC allows authentication of the 3 studied peonies in a simple, not expensive and unambiguous way.

2. Materials and Methods

2.1. Plant Material

Samples of root washers or fragmented and powders have been provided by European Pharmacopeia:

Paeonia lactiflora Pall (*Radix paeoniae alba* or Chinese phonetic name: Baishao);

Paeonia veitchii Lynch (*Radix paeoniae rubra* or Chinese phonetic name: Aba);

Paeonia suffructicosa Andr. (*Cortex paeonia moutan* or Chinese phonetic name: Mudanpi).

2.2. Preparing Slides

Observations are based on microscopic studies of sectioned and stained material of tissues Transverse sections are prepared with a sliding microtome (MSE) and stained in alun carmine-green combination or *Mirande* reagent [9] during 2 to 3 minutes then washed with water. Following staining, the transverse sections are mounted on glass slides using glycerine gel. Powder observations were made using *Chloral hydrate solution* R. [10]. Observations were made with a LEICA Microsystems DMLB microscope, and pictures were taken with Digital Camera Power Shot S40 CANON photo-micrographic system. For the description we have used some help books [11,12].

2.3. Comparative Study of Three Species of Peonies

2.3.1. Anatomical Analysis

The dry materials were divided into appropriate sizes.

Samples of root, rhizome were sectioned on a microtome in slices thick. Mid regions of stem and the most mature region of the root and rhizome available were taken. Tissues were stained by alun carmine-green combination or *Mirande* reagent and finally mounted on glass slides using glycerine gel for observation. Some sections were not stained so that idioblasts and other deposits would not be destroyed or otherwise altered during processing. The samples of crude drug were powdered. Ten different slides from the same powder were observed. Microchemical reactions were applied with lactic reagent or Gazet reagent to study powders in order to reveal lignified elements such as wood fibres, sclerenchyma and calcium oxalate crystals. All representative microscopic features were recorded by colour photography.

2.3.2. TLC Analysis

An aliquot of methanol solution of *Paeonia suffructicosa* Andr., *Paeonia veitchii* Lynch, *Paeonia lactiflora* Pall. (101.28, 100.04 and 79.98 28 mg/mL, respectively, 40 μL) was directly deposited (as spots or bands) onto the TLC plates. TLC plates were developed in a presaturated solvent chamber with toluene-ethyl acetate-formic acid-methylene chloride (10:12:6:12) as developing reagents until the solvent front reached 1 cm from the top of plates. The developed TLC plates were then removed from the chamber, and allowed to air-dry for 30 min. Each TLC plate was then monitored under UV light at 254 and 366 nm.

3. Results

3.1. Anatomical Analysis [Table 1]

3.1.1. Paeoniae Alba (Baishao) [Photos 1-12]

The transverse section of the root, almost circular, stained with alun carmine-green combination or Mirande reagent shows various characteristic elements from the outer to the inner side:

Cork shows a very broad, well developed zone composed of 8 - 10 layers of elongated tangentially reddish-brown cells with suberized walls. Cork tears in places giving rise to a kind of cones. Cork cambium is composed of 2 - 3 layers of more or less collapsed meristematic cells. Phelloderm consists of single-layered cells. Cortical parenchyma consists of numerous layers of elongated thin-walled cells, scattered air-spaces and is invaded by calcium oxalate crystals and numerous thick walled fibres, singly or grouped, with a narrow lumen, in its outermost area.

Phloem occupies unless than 13 % of the transverse section. Each phloem patch contains small groups of sieve tubes, parenchyma and a few fibres separated by medullary rays. Cambium is a distinct zone of 2 - 3 layers of small meristematic cells. Xylem is a broad radiate

Table 1. Key authentication and comparison parameters of the three species of Chinese paeony.

Cell specification	*P. lactiflora* (alba)	*P. veitchii* (rubrae)	*P. suffructicosa* (moutan)
Root transverse section General view	almost circular	almost circular	almost circular
Scale bar	100 μm	235.29 μm	133.3 μm
cork	150 μm	<100 μm	250 μm
Cortical parenchyma	Occupying less than 1/3	Occupying up to 1/3	Occupying almost 1/2
Lignified fibres thick walled	112.5 μm large; 150 μm long Isolated or grouped; Present only in cortex	Absent	27.5 μm large grouped present in all parenchyma
calcium oxalate crystals	11 - 35 μm in diameter	20 - 25 μm	25 - 33 μm
Vascular bundle ⇨ Xylem	⇨ Xylem rays (fibres and parenchyma alternately arranged)	⇨ Xylem rays (10 - 30 rows of fibres and parenchyma alternately arranged)	⇨ narrow
⇨ phloem	⇨ narrow	⇨ narrow	⇨ Large (rays 1 - 3 cells wide)
Starch	Masses of gelatinized starch grains fairly abundant	Simple starch granules	14 μm Abundant starch grains in parenchymatous cells

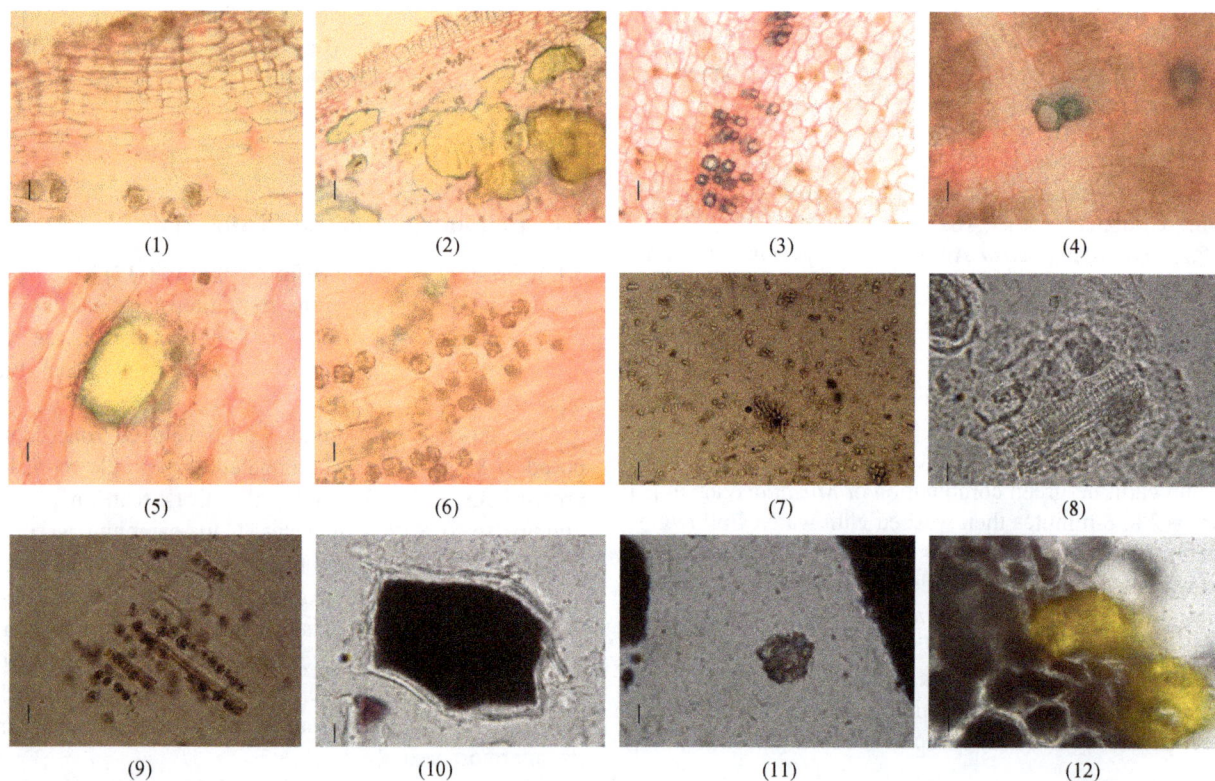

Photos 1-12. Paeonia alba (*Paeonia lactiflora* Pall.): (1)-(5): transverse sections and (7)-(12): ground powder. Scale bars: (1): 104.1 μm; (2): 54.3 μm; (3): 25 μm; (4): 29.6 μm; (5): 20.83 μm; (6): 250 μm; (7): 25 μm; (8): 19.2 μm; (9): 9.85 μm; (10): 8.07 μm; (11): 9.2 μm. (1) cork; (2) fibers; (3) vascular bundle; (4) vessels; (5) thick walled fibre; (6) calcium oxalate crystals; (7) general view; (8) spiral trachea of wood; (9) bundle surrounded by rows of calcium oxalate crystals; (10) gelatinized starch grains masses in parenchyma cell; (11) calcium oxalate crystal; (12) grouped fibres.

zone, composed of wedge-shaped xylem patches consisting of radially elongated groups of spiral trachea and wood parenchyma. Each xylem patch is separated from its neighbour by large starchy medullary rays. Pith is completely resolved at its centre.

Clusters calcium oxalate crystals and masses of gelatinized starch grains are numerous in parenchyma cells, occurring always in the regions of cortex, phloem, xylem and pith.

Powder

Examined under a microscope in the lactic R reagent, the **Baishao** powder, reddish brown, shows reddish-brown cells with suberized walls of cork, elongated thin-walled cells of parenchyma, calcium oxalate crystals and numerous thick walled fibres, spiral trachea of wood and masses of gelatinized starch grains in parenchyma cells.

3.1.2. *Paeoniae rubra* (Aba) [Photos 13-22]
The transverse section of the root, almost circular, stained with alun carmine-green combination or Mirande reagent shows various characteristic elements from the outer to the inner side:

Cork tears in places. Phelloderm consists of single-layered cells. Cortical parenchyma consists of numerous layers of elongated thin-walled cells, separated by intercellular spaces and invaded by starch granules. There are no thick walled fibres.

Occupying unless than 25% of the transverse section, phloem is composed of sieve tube and phloem cells. Each phloem patch contains small groups of sieve tubes, parenchyma and a few fibres and formed shaped cones separated by medullary rays. Cambium, distinct, is constituted of 2 - 3 distinct layers of small meristematic cells. Xylem is a broad radiate zone, composed of wedge-shaped xylem patches consisting of radially elongated groups of spiral trachea and wood parenchyma. Each xylem patch is separated from its neighbour by narrow starchy medullary rays. Phloem and the medullar parenchyma are invaded by calcium oxalate crystals. Pith is completely reduced to its center.

Powder

Examined under a microscope in the lactic R reagent, the **Aba** powder, slightly brown, shows reddish-brown cells with suberized walls of cork, elongated thin-walled cells of parenchyma invaded by starch grains, calcium oxalate crystals and spiral trachea of wood.

3.1.3. *Paeonia moutan* (Mudanpi) [Photos 23-34]
The transverse section of the root, almost circular, stained with alun carmine-green combination or Mirande reagent shows various characteristic elements from the outer to the inner side:

Cork shows a very broad, well developed zone composed of 12 - 16 layers of tangentially-elongated, red-

dish-brown cells with suberized walls. Phelloderm consists of single-layered cells. Cortex consists of numerous rows of elongated thin-walled cells, separated by intercellular spaces and invaded by calcium oxalate crystals scattered in whole zone. Its innermost zone is totally starchy. Lignified fibres thick walled, singly or grouped in 2 - 4, with a narrow lumen are present in a small amount especially in the phloem area.

Phloem is occupying up to 50% - 60% of the transverse section. Phloem is organized in alternating zone with Liberian cell walls thickened and non-thickened.

Cambium is not distinct. Xylem is a broad radiate zone composed of vessels and wood parenchyma. Each xylem patch is separated from its neighbour by large starchy medullary rays.

Powder

Examined under a microscope in the lactic R reagent, the **Mudanpi** powder, reddish brown, shows reddish-brown cells with suberized walls of cork, elongated thin-walled cells of parenchyma, calcium oxalate crystals, starch grains, lignified fibres thick walled, singly or grouped in 2 - 4, with a narrow lumen and spiral trachea of wood.

3.2. TLC Analysis

Methanol solutions of *Paeonia suffructicosa* Andr., *Paeonia veitchii* Lynch, *Paeonia lactiflora* Pall. were monitored by a TLC (**Figure 1**) method to highlight the chemical differences of these 3 extracts and to confirm botanical differentiation because this method gives quick access for detection and localization of compounds in complicated plant extracts.

4. Discussion

The comparative microscopic observations of plant organs, tissues and crude drug powder of the three species of peonies indicate that many of these anatomical characteristics are homologous. Accordingly, we drew up a generalized description to account for these similarities:

Cork tending to peel off; developed parenchyma, with scattered large intercellular air-spaces; numerous calcium oxalate crystals; parenchyma tissue cells filled with starch grains, but usually distinct; the vascular bundles, developed in root, open collateral type. However, different species possess the unique micro structural characteristics. The anatomy and micro-morphology of peonies also reflect the high degree of diversity, which can be taken as the identifying standard of peonies. The characteristics in **Table 1** are a summary of key authentication and comparison parameters of these three species, in the present study.

Paeonia suffruticosa by its durability, excellent resistance to extreme climates (it supports cold as heat,

(13)   (14)   (15)   (16)   (17)

(18)   (19)   (20)   (21)   (22)

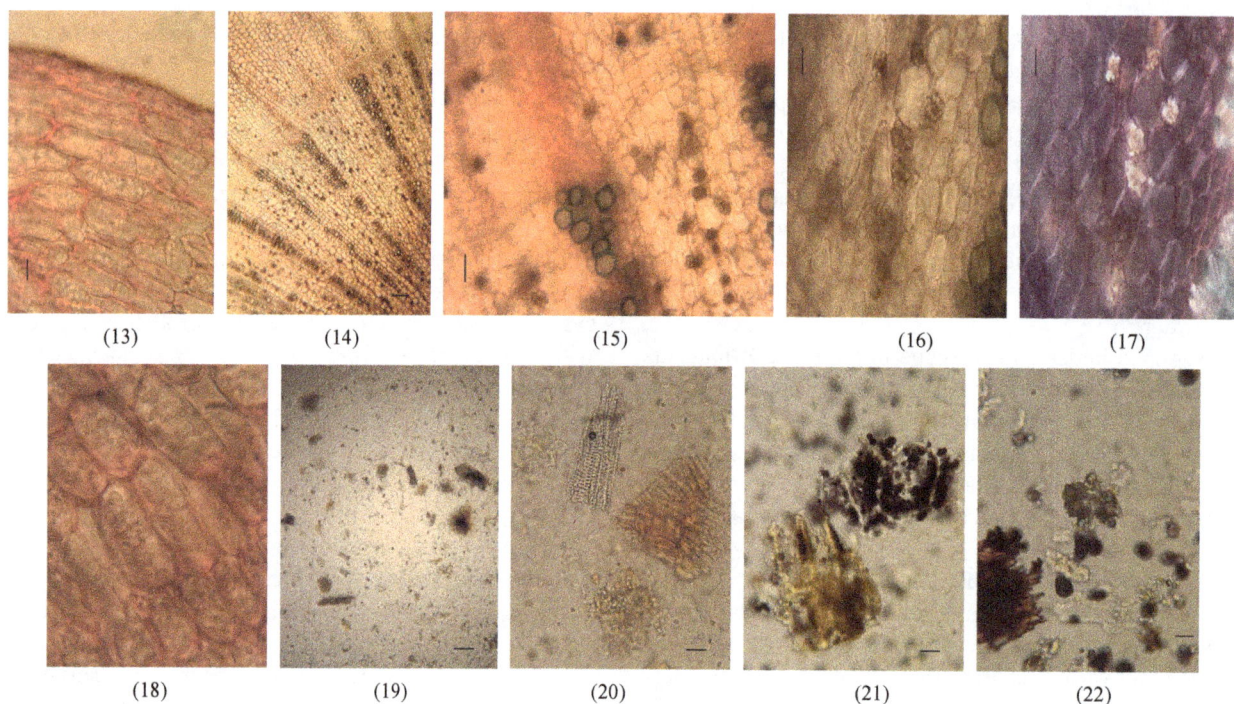

Photos 13-22. *Paeonia rubrae (Paeonia veitchii* Lynch). (12)-(17): transverse sections and (18)-(21): ground powder. *Scale bars*—(13) 53.57 μm; (14) 222.2 μm; (15) 28.57 μm; (16) 16 μm; (17) 16 μm; 18: 27.17 μm; (19) 250 μm; (20) 25 μm; (21) 21.87 μm;l (22) 8.33 μm. (13) thin cork; (14) cortical parenchyma; (15) cambial zone and vascular bundles; (16) calcium oxalate crystals under light; (17) calcium oxalate crystals under polarized light; (18) starch in parenchyma cells; (19) general view; (20) spiral trachea of wood and cork; (21) starch grains in parenchyma cell; (22) calcium oxalate crystal.

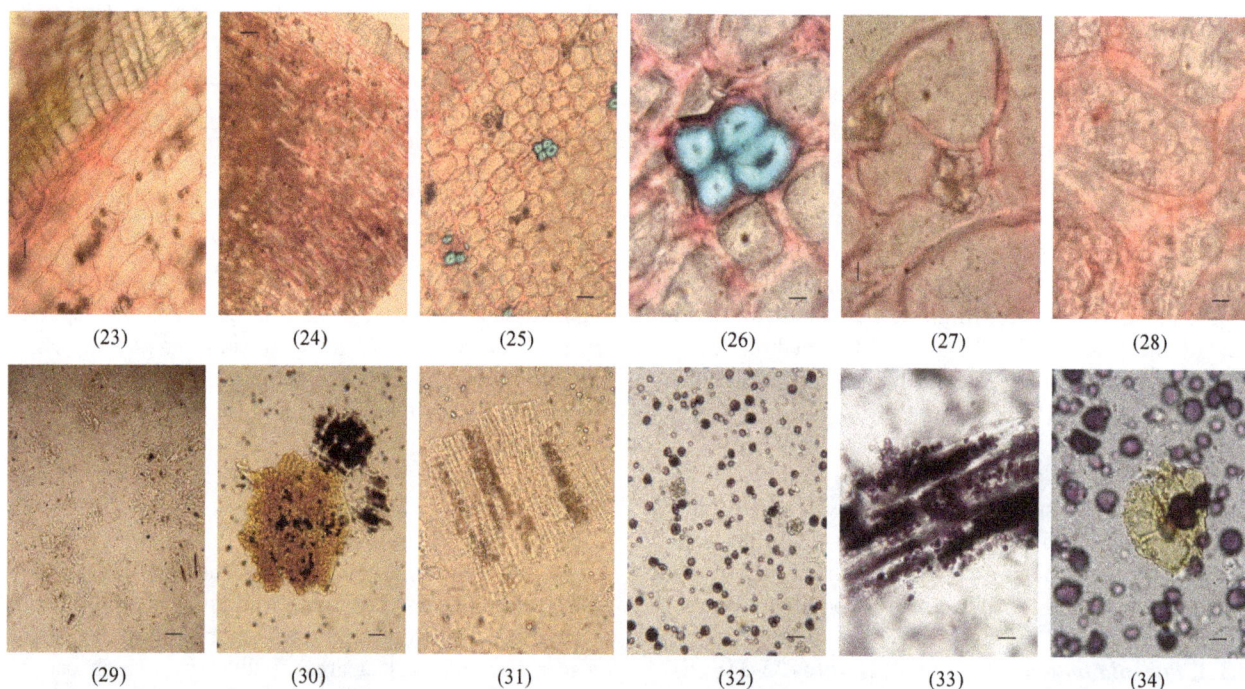

(23)   (24)   (25)   (26)   (27)   (28)

(29)   (30)   (31)   (32)   (33)   (34)

Photos 23-34. *Paeonia mountan (Paeonia suffructicosa* Andr.). (23)-(28): transverse sections; and (29)-(34): ground powder. *Scale bars*—(23) 37.71 μm; (24) 153.85 μm; (25) 50 μm; (26) 11.46 μm; (27) 11 μm; (28): 8 μm; (29) 314.3 μm; (30) 46.66 μm; (31) 47.22 μm; (32) 25 μm; (33) 35 μm; (34) 11.66 μm. (23) cork; (24) cortical parenchyma; (25) grouped fibres in parenchyma; (26) fibres; (27) calcium oxalate crystals; (28) starch in parenchyma cells; (29) general view; (30) cells with suberized walls of cork; (31) spiral trachea of wood with calcium oxalate crystal; (32) starch grains and calcium oxalate crystals; (33) starchy parenchyma; (34) lignified fibre thick walled.

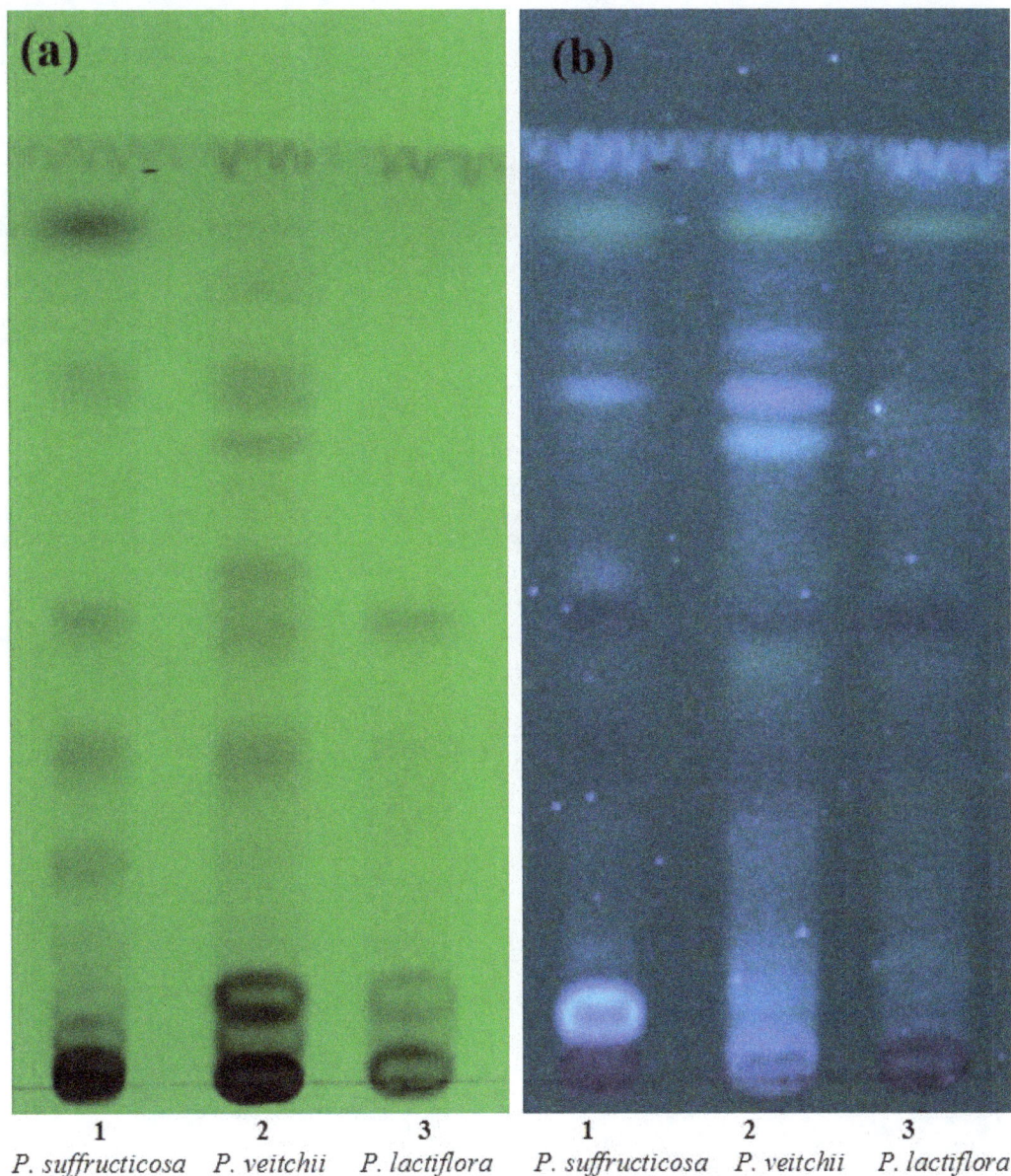

Figure 1. TLC plates visualized (A) under UV 254 nm, and (B) under UV 366 nm. 40 μl of methanol extract of *Paeonia suffructicosa* Andr. (1), *Paeonia veitchii* Lynch (2), *Paeonia lactiflora Pall.* (3) were applied as bands on TLC layers respectively.

drought and humidity) is a very interesting herb.

Indeed, the peonies have a very strong ability to survive in a hostile environment (cold, hypoxia, etc.). The microscopic comparison of three species shows that their structures are closely related to specific functions to adapt to their environment. For example, large quantities of idioblasts are not only important in resistance to drought and physiological cold, but also play an important role in resistance to ultraviolet rays and in protecting plants against damage. In addition, because of the characteristics of air and soil in the highlands, the peonies have developed a wood to withstand strong winds. Consequently, a microscopic analysis of the internal structure of peonies can contribute greatly to our understanding of

adaptation strategies to environmental extremes. Through the comparative study of the anatomy and micromorphology of three species, we hope to ensure their safety and efficacy.

A bio-guided phytochemical study will be underway to characterize the components and identify those that are biologically and chemically active (antioxidants, inhibitor of XO, anti-MCF7) extracts TLC.

REFERENCES

[1] S. Foster and C. X. Yue, "Herbal Emissaries: Bringing Chinese Herbs to the West," Healing Arts Press, Rochester, 1992, pp. 200-207.

[2]   M. Blumenthal, "The Complete German Commission E Monographs: Therapeutic Guide to Herbal Medicines," Integrative Medicine Communications, Newton, 1998, p. 364.

[3]   D. Bensky, A. Gamble and T. Kaptchuk, "Chinese Herbal Medicine Materia Medica," Revised Edition, Eastland Press, Seattle, 1993, pp. 70-71,277-278,331-332.

[4]   J. Liu, "Effect of Paeonia Obovata 801 on Metabolism of Thromboxane B2 and Arachidonic Acid and on Platelet Aggregation in Patients with Coronary Heart Disease and Cerebral Thrombosis," *Chung Hua I Hsueh Tsa Chih*, Vol. 63, 1983, pp. 477-481.

[5]   T. L. Guo and X. W. Zhou, "Clinical Observations on the Treatment of the Gestational Hypertension Syndrome with Angelica and Paeonia Powder," *Chung Hua I Hsueh Tsa Chih*, Vol. 6, 1986, pp. 714-716,707.

[6]   D. G. Yang, "Comparison of Pre- and Post-Treatment Hepatohistology with Heavy Dosage of Paeonia Rubra on Chronic Active Hepatitis Caused Liver Fibrosis," *Chung Hua I Hsueh Tsa Chih*, Vol. 14, 1994, pp. 207-209,195.

[7]   C. B. Wang and A. M. Chang, "Plasma Thromboxane B2 Changes in Severe Icteric Hepatitis Treated by Traditional Chinese Medicine—Dispelling the Pathogenic Heat from Blood, Promoting Blood Circulation and Administrating Large Doses of Radix Paeoniae—A Report of 6 Cases," *Chung Hua I Hsueh Tsa Chih*, Vol. 5, 1985, pp. 326-328,322.

[8]   B. Boullard, "Dictionnaire des Plantes Médicinales du Monde: Réalités & Croyances," Estem, 2001.

[9]   R. Mirande, "Sur le Carmin Aluné et son Emploi, Combiné avec celui du vert D'iode, en Histologie végétale," *CR Academic Science*, Vol. 170, 1920, pp. 197-199.

[10] "European Pharmacopoeia (in Force)," Maison Neuve Moulins, les Metz.

[11] A. Speranza and G. L. Calzoni, "Atlas de la structure des plantes," Belin, 2005, pp. 125-203.

[12] Z. Y. Chen, Y. T. Chen and D. H. Wang, "HPLC Determination of Salidroside in the Roots of Rhodiola Plants," *China Journal of Chinese Materia Medica*, Vol. 11, 2006, pp. 939-941.

14

Anti-Hyperglycemic Effect of Single Administered Gardeniae Fructus in Streptozotocin-Induced Diabetic Mice by Improving Insulin Resistance and Enhancing Glucose Uptake in Skeletal Muscle

Qing Yu[1], Tatsuo Takahashi[1], Masaaki Nomura[2], Shinjiro Kobayashi[1*]

[1]Department of Clinical Pharmacy, Faculty of Pharmaceutical Sciences, Hokuriku University,
3-Ho Kanagawa-Machi, Kanazawa, Japan

[2]Department of Education Center of Clinical Pharmacy, Faculty of Pharmaceutical Sciences,
Hokuriku University, 3-Ho Kanagawa-Machi, Kanazawa, Japan

Email: *s-kobayashi@hokuriku-u.ac.jp

ABSTRACT

The mechanisms of Gardeniae Fructus (GF) for anti-hyperglycemic action were demonstrated in streptozotocin (STZ)-diabetic mice. Six hours after single intraperitoneal administration of GF (300 mg/kg) or H_2O into 3 hour-fasted STZ-diabetic mice, glucose and insulin tolerances were assessed by intraperitoneal glucose (1.5 g/kg) tolerance test (IPGTT) and intraperitoneal insulin (0.65 U/kg) tolerance test (IPITT), respectively. Effects of GF on insulin signaling pathways in soleus muscle such as glucose uptake, expression of glucose transporter 4 (GLUT4) in the plasma membrane and phosphorylation of Akt (P-Akt) in cytosolic fraction were examined in STZ-diabetic mice. In IPGTT test, GF significantly accelerated clearance of exogenous glucose and its glucose-lowering action was greater than H_2O-treated control in STZ-diabetic mice. GF also promoted an exogenous glucose-increased insulin level in STZ-diabetic mice. In IPITT test, GF decreased glucose level to the greater extent than H_2O-treated control in STZ-diabetic mice. Furthermore, GF significantly decreased high HOMA-IR in STZ-diabetic mice from 21.6 ± 2.4 to 12.4 ± 1.9 (mg/dl × μU/ml). These results implied that GF improved insulin resistance in STZ-diabetic mice. GF increased glucose uptake of soleus muscle 1.5 times greater than H_2O-treated control in STZ-diabetic mice. GF enlarged insulin (10 nmol/ml)-increased glucose uptake to 1.8 time-greater. Correspondingly, GF increased expression of GLUT4 in the plasma membrane of soleus muscle to 1.4 time-greater, and P-Akt in the cytosolic fraction of soleus muscle to 1.9 time-greater than those in H_2O-treated control. In conclusion, the improvement of GF on insulin resistance is associated with the repair of insulin signaling via P-Akt, GLUT4 and glucose uptake pathway in soleus muscle of STZ-diabetic mice.

Keywords: Gardeniae Fructus (GF); Streptozotocin (STZ); Soleus Muscle; Insulin Resistance; Glucose Uptake; Glucose Transporter 4 (GLUT4); Phosphorylation of Akt (P-Akt)

1. Introduction

It has been reported by the World Health Organization that there will be 366 million cases of diabetes by the year 2030. Diabetes mellitus is a problem to perplex the world [1]. Diabetes mellitus is a group of metabolic diseases marked by hyperglycemia, which arises from abnormal insulin secretion and/or peripheral insulin resistance [2]. Insulin plays an important role in maintaining whole body glucose homeostasis by stimulating the transport of glucose into peripheral tissues, such as skeletal and cardiac muscles and white and brown adipose tissues [3]. Insulin resistance is defined as a reduced responsiveness of insulin on a target cell or a whole organ [4], which results in reducing insulin-mediated glucose utilization in peripheral tissues, accompanying glucose intolerance and insulin intolerance [5]. Insulin resistance is not only the major pathophysiological condition of type 2 diabetes (non-insulin-dependent diabetes mellitus) [6], but also present in type 1 diabetes (insulin-dependent diabetes mellitus) [7].

*Corresponding author.

Impaired glucose uptake in skeletal muscle is present in insulin resistance diabetes [8]. The rate-limiting step in muscle glucose uptake is the transmembrane transport of glucose mediated by glucose transporter 4(GLUT4). GLUT4, a protein stored in intracellular vesicles, plays a pivotal role in regulating insulin-stimulated glucose transport into skeletal muscle and adipose tissue [9,10]. The conditional depletion of GLUT4 caused insulin resistance and chronic hyperglycemia [11]. In a diabetic state, reduced expression of GLUT4 causes impairment of insulin signaling pathway in skeletal muscle and stimulates glucose production in the liver [12]. It has been reported that GLUT4 can be activated by phosphatidylinositol 3-kinase (PI-3)/Akt insulin signaling pathway in peripheral tissues. Concretely, under the stimulation of insulin, glucose uptake is induced by phosphorylation and activation of Akt which lead the translocation of GLUT4 from intracellular storage particles to the cellular surface for glucose uptake [13]. Skeletal muscle accounts for nearly 40% of body mass and is the most important tissue for glucose utilization. Skeletal muscle plays an important role in regulating insulin sensitivity [14]. Hence glucose uptake in skeletal muscle is an important target for anti-hyperglycemia.

Streptozotocin (STZ) has been commonly used to induce models of Type 1 and Type 2 diabetes. According to the dosages used, STZ is producing mild to severe types of diabetes by either single intravenous or intraperitoneal injection [15]. STZ-diabetic mice have the features such as polydipsia, polyphagia, polyuria, dyslipidemia and hyperglycemia [4,16,17]. Insulin resistance is also observed in STZ-induced diabetic rats [18].

In the recent year, plant-based medicines have gained advance of the treatment of metabolic diseases such as diabetes [19]. Gardeniae Fructus (GF) is a traditional Chinese medicine, which has alleviating effect on cytotoxicity [20], antioxidant activity [21] and protective action on pancreatitis [22]. We have also reported [23,24] that GF composed in Bofutsushosan alleviates the abnormal glucose/lipid metabolism in STZ-diabetic mice. In the present study, we sought to investigate the mechanisms of single administered GF for anti-hyperglycemic action in STZ-diabetic mice. The effects of GF on glucose tolerance, insulin tolerance, glucose uptake in soleus muscle, the expression of GLUT4 in the plasma membrane and P-Akt in cytosolic fraction of soleus muscle will be unveiled in STZ-diabetic mice.

2. Materials and Methods

2.1. Preparation of STZ-Diabetic Mice

Fed male mice (ddY strain; 4 weeks of age; 16 - 20 g; Japan SLC, Shizuoka, Japan) were injected with a single dose (150 mg/kg) of STZ (Sigma, St. Louis, MO, USA)

in saline into the tail vein. STZ-diabetic mice (7 weeks of age; blood glucose over 450 mg/dl) were used for experiments at 3 weeks after the injection of STZ. Age-matched normal male mice (ddY strain; 7 weeks of age) were used in the control experiments. These mice were given by CRF-1 (Oriental Yeast Co., Tokyo, Japan) and water ad libitum and kept at 25°C - 26°C with lights on from 7 a.m. to 7 p.m. The Ethics Review Committee for Animal Experimentation of Hokuriku University approved the experimental protocol.

2.2. Preparation and Administration of Drug

GF was purchased from Tsumura Co. (Tokyo) and extracted in 10 volumes of distilled water with an automatic extractor "Torobi" (Tochimoto, Osaka, Japan) for 1 hour. A water extract of GF was filtered through a mesh (No. 42, Sanpo, Tokyo), lyophilized with a freeze-drier (DF-03G, ULVAC, Tokyo), and stored at 4°C [25,26]. A dosage of 300 mg/kg GF solution or H_2O were singly administered intraperitoneally (0.1 ml/10g body weight) into 3 hour-fasted STZ-diabetic mice. Because GF significantly lowered blood glucose levels in STZ-diabetic mice at the dosage of 300 mg/kg in the previous study [23,24], we used only 300 mg/kg GF in this study to research the mechanism of GF for anti-hyperglycemic action.

2.3. Measurement of Glucose, Insulin, Triglyceride and Cholesterol Levels in Serum

Blood was collected from the neck vein plexus of STZ-diabetic mice before and 6 hours after single administration of GF or H_2O. Blood samples were centrifuged at 8000 rpm at 25°C for 5 min. Glucose level of the supernatant was measured by the glucose oxidase method with a serum glucose monitor set (MEDISAFE MINI, Terumo, Tokyo). Serum insulin level was measured with a mouse ELISA kit for insulin (Morinaga, Yokohama, Japan). Serum triglyceride and cholesterol levels were measured with ELISA kits for triglyceride and cholesterol (Wako, Osaka), respectively.

2.4. Determination of Glucose Tolerance and Insulin Tolerance

Six hours after treated with GF or H_2O, glucose tolerance in STZ-diabetic mice was assessed by intraperitoneal (*ip*) glucose tolerance test (IPGTT). After a bolus of glucose (1.5 g/kg, 30% solution, *ip*) was injected, blood was collected sequentially from the neck vein at time intervals of 0, 30, 60, 90 and 120 min and tested serum glucose and insulin levels.

To evaluate insulin tolerance, intraperitoneal insulin tolerance test (IPITT) was performed. A bolus of insulin

(0.65 U/kg, *ip*) was injected and blood was taken sequentially from the neck vein at time intervals of 0, 30, 60, 90 and 120 min and tested serum glucose level.

2.5. Determination of Insulin Resistance by Homeostasis Model Assessment of Insulin Resistance (HOMA-IR) Analysis

HOMA-IR analysis was used to assess insulin resistance in STZ-diabetic mice. After over-night fasting, values for HOMA-IR were calculated from the values of fasting serum glucose (mg/dl) and fasting serum insulin (μU/ml) by using the following formula: HOMA-IR = fasting glucose value (mg/dl) × fasting insulin value (μU/ml)/405 [27].

2.6. Assay for 2-Deoxy-D-Glucose Uptake

Six hours after treated with GF or H_2O, soleus muscles isolated from STZ-diabetic mice or normal mice were dissected out respectively, and incubated for 30 min at 35°C in 2 ml of Krebs-Henseleit buffer (KHB) containing 0.1% bovine serum albumin (BSA), 32 mM mannitol, and 8 mM glucose in the presence or absence of insulin (10 nmol/ml) under the condition of 95% O_2/5% CO_2. All muscles were transferred to 2 ml of KHB containing 0.1% BSA and 40 mM mannitol in the presence or absence of insulin (10 nmol/ml) for 10 min at 29°C to wash out glucose. Muscles were then incubated for 10 min in 2 ml KHB containing 1 mM 2-[^{3}H]-Deoxy-D-glucose (2-DG) (2.25 μCi/mmol), 39 mM [^{14}C] mannitol (8.5 μCi/mmol) and 1% BSA at 29°C under 95% O_2/5% CO_2. Insulin was added to KHB when insulin was present in the previous incubations. The muscles were processed by lysing in 0.5 N NaOH for 1 hour at 60°C with shaking. Muscle extracts (100 μl) were placed in scintillation vials containing 4 ml of scintillation liquid (Triton X-100: methylbenzene, 1:2) and counted in liquid scintillation counter with channels present for simultaneous [^{3}H] and [^{14}C] counting. The amount of each isotope present in the samples was determined and used to calculate the intracellular concentration of 2-DG [28].

2.7. Western Blot Analysis

The plasma membrane and cytosolic fractions were prepared from soleus muscles as described previously [29]. Briefly, 6 hours after treated with GF or H_2O, soleus muscles of STZ-diabetic mice were dissected out and chopped into pieces as small as possible with scissors. Muscles (100 mg) was homogenized with 3 volumes of buffer A (10 mM Tris at pH 7.8, 10 mM KCl, 1.5 mM $MgCl_2$, 1 mM phenylmethylsulfonyl fluoride , 0.5 mM dithiothreitol (DTT), 5 μg/ml aprotinin and 10 μg/ml leupeptin) containing 0.1% Nonidet P-40, and passed through a 22-gauge needle three times. The homogenate

was centrifuged at 1000 × g for 10 min at 4°C. The pellet was resuspended in buffer A and centrifuged at 1000 × g for another 10 min at 4°C. Plasma membrane fraction was obtained by resuspending the resulting pellet in buffer A containing 1.0% (v/v) Nonidet P-40, and centrifuged at 10,000 × g for 20 min at 4°C.

To obtain the cytosolic fraction, soleus muscles were homogenized in buffer A and lysed with buffer B(10 mM Tris at pH 8, 150 mM NaCl, 1.0% (v/v) Nonidet P-40, 0.5% (w/v) sodium deoxycholate, 0.1% (w/v) sodium dodecyl sulfate (SDS), 0.5 mM DTT, 1 mM phenylmethylsulfonylfluoride, 5 μg/ml aprotinin and 10 μg/ml leupeptin), and centrifuged at 16,000 × g for 20 min at 4°C. The supernatant was referred as the cytosolic fraction.

After the proteins of the plasma membrane and the cytosolic fractions of soleus muscle had been respectively separated by 8% SDS-polyacrylamide gel electrophoresis (SDS-PAGE), they were transferred to PDVF membranes and blocked for 1 hour with 1% (w/v) nonfat dry milk in TBST (10 mM Tris at pH 7.6, 150 mM NaCl and 0.1% Tween-20). The plasma membrane fraction was incubated with the primary antibody of GLUT4 (G4048, SIGMA-ALDRICH Co., Tokyo), and the cytosolic fraction was incubated with the primary antibodies of Akt (9272, Cell Signaling Technology Co., Tokyo) or phospho-Akt (Ser 473) (9271, Cell Signaling Technology Co., Tokyo) for over night at 4°C. The membranes were further incubated respectively with secondary antibody (7074s, Cell Signaling Technology Co., Tokyo) for 1 hour at room temperature. The antibody-bound proteins were detected by fluorescence assay with an ECF Western Blotting Kit (GE Healthcare; Little Chalfont, Buckinghamshire, UK), and bands were analyzed using a Typhoon 9410 imaging analyzer (GE Healthcare; Little Chalfont, Buckinghamshire, UK).

2.8. Statistical Analyses

All values were expressed as means ± S.E.M. Differences between group data were evaluated by unpaired *t*-test at $P = 0.05$ or 0.01. A value of $P < 0.05$ was considered statistically significant.

3. Results

3.1. Characteristics of STZ-Diabetic Mice

To confirm the characteristics of our STZ-diabetic model, body weight, levels of serum glucose, insulin, triglyceride and cholesterol, and HOMA-IR index were compared with those in normal mice (**Table 1**). Mice injected with a single dose (150 mg/kg) of STZ displayed significantly increased serum glucose level (915.4 ± 55.0 mg/dl) when compared to normal mice. The insulin level of STZ-diabetic mice was significant lower (299.0 ± 31.6

Table 1. The different characteristics between normal mice and STZ-diabetic mice.

	Normal mice	STZ-diabetic mice
Body weight (g)	37.5 ± 0.3	34.9 ± 0.3[**]
Serum Glucose (mg/dl)	129.8 ± 2.9	915.4 ± 55.0[**]
Serum Insulin (pg/ml)	1024.2 ± 64.2	299.0 ± 31.6[**]
Serum Triglyceride (mg/dl)	100.2 ± 5.2	187.3 ± 10.3[**]
Serum Cholesterol (mg/dl)	135.4 ± 3.7	183.2 ± 4.8[**]
HOMA-IR(mg/dl × μU/ml)	1.9 ± 0.3	21.6 ± 2.4[**]

Body weight, serum glucose, serum insulin, serum triglyceride and serum cholesterol in 3 hour-fasted mice, and HOMA-IR were measured in STZ-diabetic and age-matched normal mice. Values represent means ± S.E.M. of 4-31 data. [**]$P < 0.01$: Significantly different from normal mice.

pg/ml) than that of normal mice. STZ-diabetic mice also showed significantly high levels of triglyceride (187.3 ± 10.3 mg/dl) and cholesterol (183.2 ± 4.8 mg/dl) compared to normal mice. Using serum glucose and insulin concentrations in mice fasted over night, HOMA-IR was calculated. HOMA-IR of STZ-diabetic mice was 11.3 time-greater increased compared to that of normal mice. STZ-diabetic mice showed increased levels of serum glucose, triglyceride, cholesterol and HOMA-IR, and decreased level of serum insulin.

3.2. Effect of GF on Glucose Tolerance

Effect of GF on glucose tolerance was examined in STZ-diabetic mice. After glucose loading, the levels of serum glucose (**Figure 1(a)**) and serum insulin (**Figure 1(b)**) were measured in normal mice, GF-treated and H$_2$O-treated STZ-diabetic mice. There was a significant increased in serum glucose level from 773.6 ± 94.1 to 1217.6 ± 119.1 mg/dl at 30 min after glucose loading, and continually increased to 1296.4 ± 86.5 mg/dl at 60 min. High glucose level reached a plateau and was not changed from 60 min to 120 min. Glucose level in GF-treated STZ-diabetic mice increased from 498.0 ± 48.7 to 882.5 ± 149.2 mg/dl at 30 min after glucose loading, and then quickly reduced in a time-dependent manner during 30 min to 120 min. At 120 min after glucose loading, the glucose level lowered significantly from 882.5 ± 149.2 to 631.3 ± 90.8 mg/dl in GF-treated STZ-diabetic mice. This pattern of glucose-lowering action in GF-treated STZ-diabetic mice was similar to that of normal mice (**Figure 1(a)**). GF-treated STZ-diabetic mice showed better control of glucose than H$_2$O-treated control after glucose loading.

After glucose loading, the level of insulin in GF-treated STZ-diabetic mice was significantly increased at 30 min (**Figure 1(b)**). Although increased level of insulin in GF-treated diabetic mice was smaller than that in normal mice, this increasing pattern of insulin in GF-treated diabetic mice was similar to that in normal mice.

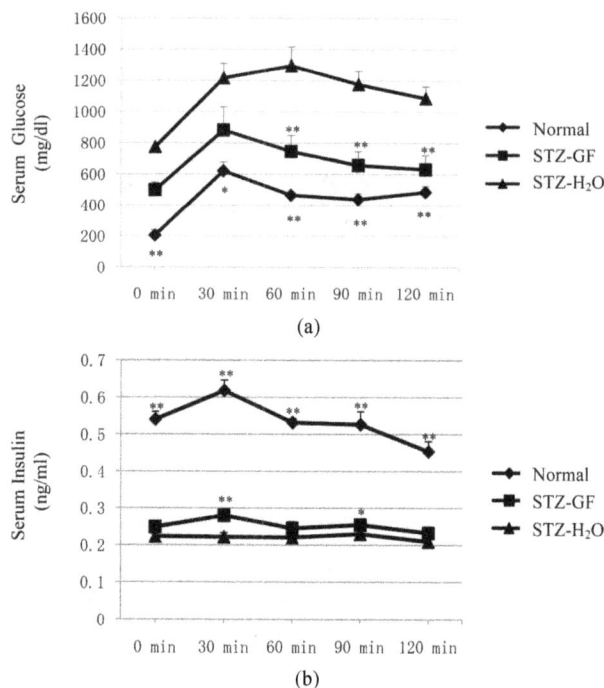

Figure 1. Effects of GF on serum glucose level (a) and serum insulin level (b) in STZ-diabetic mice after loading a bolus of glucose. GF was treated for 6 hours into 3 hour-fasted STZ-diabetic mice. After loading a bolus of glucose (1.5 g/kg), blood was collected sequentially from the neck vein at intervals of 0, 30, 60, 90 and 120 min and measured serum glucose level and serum insulin level. Values represent means ± S.E.M. of 4-7 data. [*]$P < 0.05$, [**]$P < 0.01$: Significantly different from H$_2$O-treated STZ-diabetic mice.

In contrast, insulin level in H$_2$O-treated STZ-diabetic mice was not changed after glucose loading. GF stimulated insulin release after exogenous glucose loading.

3.3. Effect of GF on Insulin Tolerance

Effect of GF on insulin tolerance was examined in STZ-diabetic mice. After loading a bolus of insulin (0.65 U/kg), insulin-induced changes of glucose level were measured in normal mice, GF-treated and H$_2$O-treated STZ-diabetic mice (**Figure 2**). The serum glucose level of GF-treated STZ diabetic mice decreased significantly from 30 min to 120 min after insulin loading. However, serum glucose level was only decreased at 30 min in normal mice but was not influenced in H$_2$O-treated STZ-diabetic mice during incubation times. GF significantly decreased serum glucose in STZ-diabetic mice in the presence of insulin.

3.4. Effect of GF on HOMA-IR

Effect of GF on HOMA-IR was examined in STZ-diabetic mice. HOMA-IR analysis was used to assess insulin resistance in normal mice, GF-treated and H$_2$O-treated STZ-diabetic mice (**Figure 3**). Values for HOMA-IR were

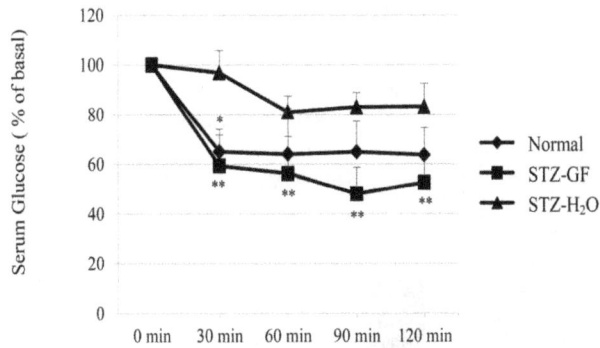

Figure 2. Effect of GF on serum glucose level in STZ-diabetic mice after loading a bolus of insulin. GF was treated for 6 hours in 3 hour-fasted STZ-diabetic mice. After loading a bolus of insulin (0.65 U/kg), blood was collected sequentially from the neck vein at intervals of 0, 30, 60, 90 and 120 min and measured serum glucose level. Values represent means ± S.E.M. of 4-5 data. $^*P < 0.05$, $^{**}P < 0.01$: Significantly different from H_2O-treated STZ-diabetic mice.

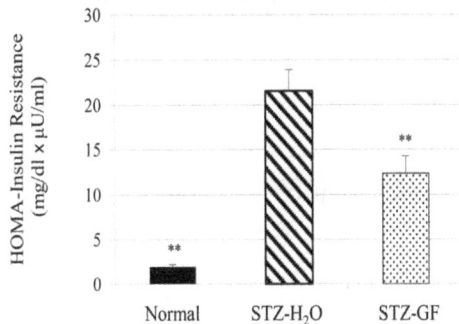

Figure 3. Effect of GF on values of HOMA-IR in STZ-diabetic mice. HOMA-IR was calculated from glucose (mg/dl) and insulin (μU/ml) levels, using the following formula: HOMA = fasting glucose (mg/dl) x fasting insulin (μU/ml) / 405. Values represent means ± S.E.M. of 4-22 data. $^{**}P < 0.01$: Significantly different from H_2O-treated STZ-diabetic mice.

calculated from the values of serum glucose (mg/dl) and serum insulin (μU/ml) in mice fasted over night. HOMA-IR in STZ-diabetic mice was about 11.3 time-greater than that in normal mice. However, HOMA-IR in GF-treated STZ-diabetic mice was significantly smaller than that in H_2O-treated control. GF improved insulin resistance in STZ-diabetic mice.

3.5. Effect of GF on 2-Deoxy-D-Glucose Uptake in Soleus Muscle

Effect of GF on uptake of 2-DG was measured in soleus muscle of STZ-diabetic mice. 2-DG uptake in soleus muscle of H_2O-treated STZ-diabetic mice was significantly lower than that of normal mice. After treated with GF, GF increased 2-DG uptake 1.5 time-greater than control of H_2O-treated STZ-diabetic mice (**Figure 4**). GF promoted basal 2-DG uptake in soleus muscle of STZ-

diabetic mice.

Insulin (10 nmol/ml) significantly increased 2-DG uptake of soleus muscle1.4 times and 1.3 times greater in normal and GF-treated STZ-diabetic mice, respectively. Whereas insulin did not affect 2-DG uptake of soleus muscle in H_2O-treated STZ-diabetic mice. Compared to H_2O-treated control, GF increased 2-DG uptake 1.8 time-greater with insulin in STZ-diabetic mice (**Figure 4**). GF promoted insulin-induced 2-DG uptake in soleus muscle of STZ-diabetic mice.

3.6. Effect of GF on Expression of GLUT4 to the Plasma Membrane in Soleus Muscle

Effect of GF on GLUT4 expression in plasma membrane was measured in soleus muscle of STZ-diabetic mice. After treatment of GF for 3 hours in STZ-diabetic mice, GF significantly increased GLUT4 expression in plasma membrane fraction 1.1 time-greater than that in H_2O-treated control. After its treatment for 6 hours, GF significantly increased GLUT4 expression 1.4 time-greater (**Figure 5**). GF increased GLUT4 expression in plasma membrane of soleus muscle in STZ-diabetic mice in an incubation time-dependent manner.

3.7. Effect of GF on Phosphorylation of Akt (P-Akt) in Soleus Muscle

Effect of GF on the P-Akt in cytosolic fraction of soleus muscle was measured in STZ-diabetic mice. After treatment of GF for 3 hours in STZ-diabetic mice, GF significantly increased ratio of P-Akt to Akt in cytosolic fraction of soleus muscle 1.4 time-greater. After its treatment for 6 hours, GF significantly increased ratio of P-Akt to Akt in the cytosolic fraction 1.9 time-greater (**Figure 6**).

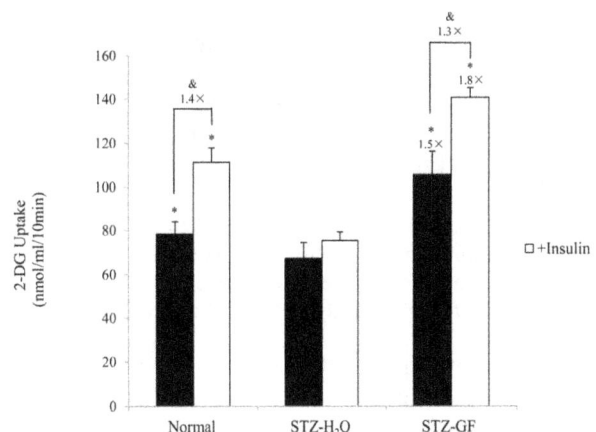

Figure 4. Effect of GF on 2-DG uptake in soleus muscle of STZ-diabetic mice. Soleus muscles were incubated for 10 min in 2-DG with or without insulin (10 nmol/ml). 2-DG uptake was normalized to tissue weight. Values represent means ± S.E.M. of 3 data. $^*P < 0.05$: Significantly different from H_2O-treated STZ-diabetic mice. $^\&P < 0.05$: Significantly different from without insulin.

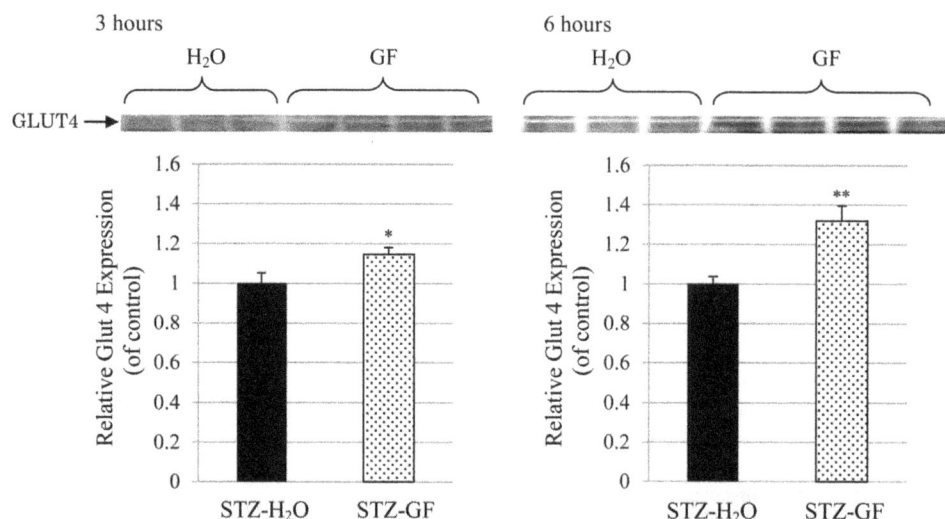

Figure 5. Effect of GF on GLUT4 expression in the plasma membrane of soleus muscle in STZ-diabetic mice. GF was treated in 3 hour-fasted STZ-diabetic mice for 3 hours (left) and 6 hours (right). The protein levels of GLUT4 in plasma membrane fraction of soleus muscle were detected by western blotting analysis. Values represent means ± S.E.M. of 6-12 data. $^*P < 0.05$, $^{**}P < 0.01$**: Significantly different from H₂O-treated STZ-diabetic mice.**

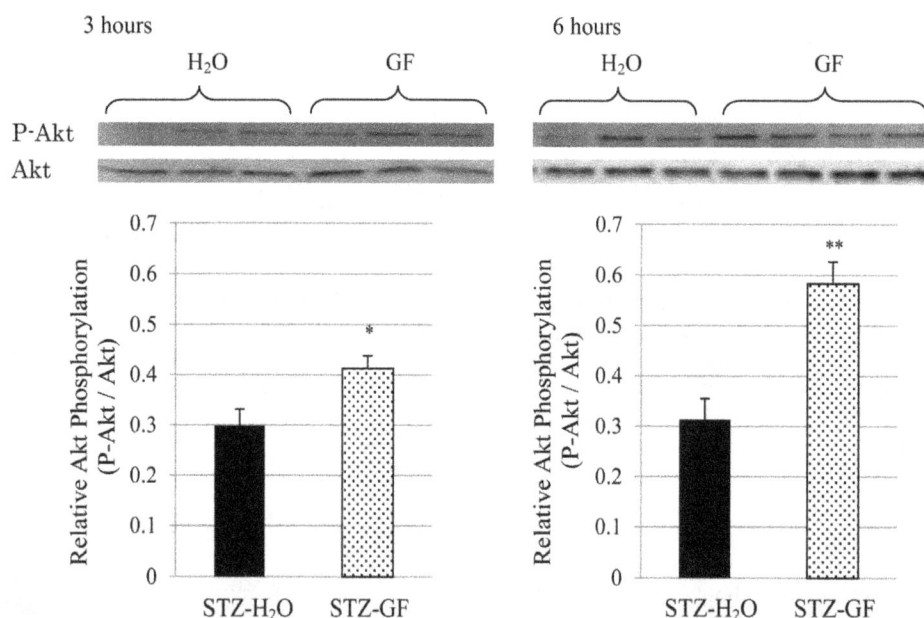

Figure 6. Effect of GF on proportion of P-Akt in Akt in cytosolic fraction of soleus muscle in STZ-diabetic mice. GF was treated in 3 hour-fasted STZ-diabetic mice for 3 hours (left) and 6 hours (right). The protein levels of Akt and P-Akt in cytosolic fraction of soleus muscle were detected by western blotting analysis. Values represent means ± S.E.M. of 4 - 6 data. $^*P < 0.05$, $^{**}P < 0.01$**: Significantly different from H₂O-treated STZ-diabetic mice.**

GF significantly increased relative Akt phosphorylation in soleus muscle of STZ -diabetic mice in an incubation time-dependent manner.

4. Discussion

GF has long been used in traditional Chinese medicine [30] and alleviates the abnormal glucose/lipid metabolism in STZ-diabetic mice [23,24]. The present study demonstrated mechanisms of GF for anti-hyperglycemic

action in STZ-diabetic mice. Single administrated GF to STZ-diabetic mice improved glucose level after glucose loading, as observed in the IPGTT (**Figure 1**). GF accelerated clearance of exogenous glucose, and significantly lowered serum glucose level in STZ-diabetic mice. GF also reduced insulin intolerance in STZ-diabetic mice as observed in the IPITT (**Figure 2**). After insulin loading, GF potentiated insulin-induced decrease in serum glucose level in STZ-diabetic mice, demonstrating that GF improved insulin sensitivity in STZ-diabetic mice. STZ-diabetic mice increased HOMA-IR, another insulin resistance index (**Table 1**). GF significantly reduced HOMA-IR in STZ-diabetic mice (**Figure 3**), supporting that GF improve insulin resistance of diabetic mice.

Effect of GF on insulin resistance for 2-DG uptake was investigated in soleus muscle of STZ-diabetic mice. Insulin did not affect 2-DG uptake in soleus muscle of STZ-diabetic mice. However, GF increased both basal 2-DG uptake without insulin and insulin-induced 2-DG uptake to soleus muscle. The effect of GF on insulin-induced 2-DG uptake was greater than that on basal 2-DG uptake (**Figure 4**). These results demonstrate that GF improves resistance of insulin for 2-DG uptake in the soleus muscle of STZ-diabetic mice. The uptake of 2-DG is closely associated with expression of GLUT4 in plasma membrane of soleus muscle. GF increased expression of GLUT4 in the plasma membrane of diabetic soleus muscle in a treatment time-dependent manner (**Figure 5**). GF may enhance expression of GLUT4 in plasma membrane to improve insulin sensitivity for glucose uptake in STZ-diabetic mice. These effects of GF on GLUT4 expression and 2-DG uptake are a novel and intriguing finding in STZ-diabetic mice. Moreover, GF increased proportion of phosphorylated Akt in cytosolic fraction of soleus muscle (**Figure 6**). From these results, GF-increased phosphorylation of Akt may have a key role for translocation of GLUT4 to plasma membrane and for improvement of insulin resistance for glucose uptake in diabetic soleus muscle. Ma et al. reported that genipin, an aglycone of geniposide which was a main bioactive compound of GF, activated IRS-1, PI3-K and P-Akt, and resulted in GLUT4 translocation and glucose uptake in C_2C_{12} myotubes [31].

Our previous study demonstrated that GF had anti-hyperglycemic action but did not change serum insulin level when GF was treated in 3 hour-fasted STZ-diabetic mice for 6 hours [23,24]. However, GF significantly increased serum insulin level at 30 min after glucose (1.5 g/kg) loading in IPGTT test (**Figure 1(b)**). It implied that GF did not directly stimulate insulin secretion like sulfonylurea. The effect of GF on release of insulin was under the stimulation of high exogenous glucose in STZ-diabetic mice. Possible mechanism of GF maybe associated with one or some factors, which restrict insulin secretion in the presence of glucose.

Mitochondrial uncoupling proteins (UCPs) are present in the mitochondrial inner membrane, which dissipate the proton gradient by allowing the re-entry of protons into the mitochondrial matrix during oxidative ATP generation, resulting in the uncoupling of the respiratory chain and heat production [32]. It has been reported that UCP2 and UCP3 gene expressions were increased in skeletal muscle in STZ-diabetic rat, while UCP1, UCP2 and

UCP3 gene expressions were reduced in brown adipose tissue of these rats [33]. UCP2 negatively regulates glucose-stimulated insulin secretion in type 2 diabetes models through altering the yield of ATP synthesis from glucose [34,35]. UCP3 is suggested to limit the product of reactive oxygen species (ROS) by mediating mechanism of mild uncoupling, diminishing super oxide production [36]. Genipin is an inhibitor of UCP2 and increased insulin secretion by pancreatic β cell under the stimulation of glucose [37]. Genipin inhibited UCP3 to increase levels of ROS and ATP, activated IRS-1, PI3-K and downstream signaling pathway, resulting in GLUT4 translocation and increased glucose uptake in C_2C_{12} myotubes [31]. It is also reported that geniposide activates the glucagon-like peptide-1 receptor (GLP-1R) to improve glucose stimulated insulin secretion in INS-1 cells [38].

5. Conclusion

Single administered GF improved insulin resistance and showed anti-hyperglycemic action in STZ-diabetic mice. The improving action of GF on insulin resistance was coupled to reduced glucose intolerance, improved insulin tolerance, reduced HOMA-IR, and the potentiation of insulin signaling pathway via P-Akt, GLUT4 and glucose uptake in soleus muscle of STZ-diabetic mice.

REFERENCES

[1] S. Wild, G. Roglic, A. Green, R. Sicree and H. King, "Global Prevalence of Diabetes: Estimates for the Year 2000 and Projections for 2030," *Diabetes Care*, Vol. 27, No. 5, 2004, pp. 1047-1053. http://dx.doi.org/10.2337/diacare.27.5.1047

[2] M. F. White, "Insulin Signaling in Health and Disease," *Science*, Vol. 302, No. 5651, 2003, pp. 1710-1711. http://dx.doi.org/10.1126/science.1092952

[3] T. Haruta, A. J. Morris, D. W. Rose, J. G. Nelson, M. Mueckler and J. M. Olefsky, "Insulin-Stimulated GLUT4 Translocation Is Mediated by a Divergent Intracellular Signaling Pathway," *The Journal of Biological Chemistry*, Vol. 270, No. 47, 1995, pp. 27991-27994.

[4] C. Rerup and F. Tarding, "Streptozotocin and Alloxan-Diabetes in Mice," *European Journal of Pharmacology*, Vol. 7, No. 1, 1969, pp. 89-96. http://dx.doi.org/10.1016/0014-2999(69)90169-1

[5] M. H. Shanik, Y. Xu, J. Skrha, R. Dankner, Y. Zick and J. Roth, "Insulin Resistance and Hyperinsulinemia: Is Hyperinsulinemia the Cart or the Horse?" *Diabetes Care*, Vol. 31, Suppl. 2, 2008, pp. 262-268.

[6] C. George, A. Lochner and B. Huisamen, "The efficacy of Prosopis Glandulosa as Antidiabetic Treatment in Rat Models of Diabetes and Insulin Resistance," *Journal of Ethnopharmacology*, Vol. 137, No. 1, 2011, pp. 298-304. http://dx.doi.org/10.1016/j.jep.2011.05.023

[7] O. Pedersen and H. Beck-Nielsen, "Insulin Resistance and Insulin-Dependent Diabetes Mellitus," *Diabetes Care*,

Vol. 10, No. 4, 1987, pp. 516-523.

[8] A. Zisman, O. D. Peroni, E. D. Abel, M. D. Michael, F. Mauvais-Jarvis, B. B. Lowell, J. F. Wojtaszewski, M. F. Hirshman, A. Virkamaki, L. J. Goodyear, C. R. Kahn and B. B. Kahn, "Targeted Disruption of the Glucose Transporter 4 Selectively in Muscle Causes Insulin Resistance and Glucose Intolerance," *Nature Medicine*, Vol. 6, No. 8, 2000, pp. 924-928. http://dx.doi.org/10.1038/78693

[9] J. E. Pessin, D. C. Thurmound, J. S. Elmendorf, K. J. Coker and S. Okada, "Molecular Basis of Insulin-Stimulated GLUT4 Vesicle Trafficking. Location! Location! Location!" *The Journal of Biological Chemistry*, Vol. 274, No. 5, 1999, pp. 2593-2596.

[10] N. J. Bryant, R. Govers and D. E. James, "Regulated Transport of the Glucose Transporter GLUT4," *Nature Reviews Molecular Cell Biology*, Vol. 3, No. 4, 2002, pp. 267-277. http://dx.doi.org/10.1038/nrm782

[11] J. K. Kim, A. Zisman, J. J. Fillmore, O. D. Peroni, K. Kotani, P. Perret, H. Zong, J. Dong, C. R. Kahn, B. B. Kahn and G. I. Shulman, "Glucose Toxicity and the Development of Diabetes in Mice with Muscle-Specific Inactivation of GLUT4," *The Journal of Clinical Investigation*, Vol. 108, No. 1, 2001, pp. 153-160.

[12] I. T. Nizamutdinova, Y. C. Jin, J. I. Chung, S. C. Shin, S. J. Lee, H. G. Seo, J. H. Lee, K. C. Chang and H. J. Kim, "The Anti-Diabetic Effect of Anthocyanins in Streptozotocin-Induced Diabetic Rats through Glucose Transporter 4 Regulation and Prevention of Insulin Resistance and Pancreatic Apoptosis," *Molecular Nutrition & Food Research*, Vol. 53, No. 11, 2009, pp. 1419-1429. http://dx.doi.org/10.1002/mnfr.200800526

[13] P. H. Ducluzeau, L. M. Fletcher, G. I. Welsh and J. M. Tavaré, "Functional Consequence of Targeting Protein Kinase B/Akt to GLUT4 Vesicles," *Journal of Cell Science*, Vol. 115, No. 14, 2002, pp. 2857-2866.

[14] M. Ueda, S. Nishiumi, H. Nagayasu, I. Fukuda, K. Yoshida and H. Ashida, "Epigallocatechingallate Promotes GLUT4 Translocation in Skeletal Muscle," *Biochemical and Biophysical Research Communications*, Vol. 377, No. 1, 2008, pp. 286-290. http://dx.doi.org/10.1016/j.bbrc.2008.09.128

[15] A. Junod, A. E. Lambert, L. Orci, R. Pictet, A. E. Gonet and A. E. Renold, "Studies of the Diabetogenic Action of Streptozotocin," *Proceedings of the Society for Experimental Biology and Medicine*, Vol. 126, No. 1, 1967, pp. 201-205. http://dx.doi.org/10.3181/00379727-126-32401

[16] J. Movassat and B. Portha, "Beta-Cell Growth in the Neonatal Goto-Kakisaki Rat and Regeneration after Treatment with Streptozotocin at Birth," *Diabetologia*, Vol. 42, No. 9, 1999, pp. 1098-1106. http://dx.doi.org/10.1007/s001250051277

[17] M. S. Gokhale, D. H. Shah, Z. Hakim, D. D. Santani and R. K. Goyal, "Effect of Chronic Treatment with Amlodipine in Non-Insulin-Dependent Diabetic Rats," *Pharmacological Research*, Vol. 37, No. 6, 1998, pp. 455-459. http://dx.doi.org/10.1006/phrs.1998.0319

[18] R. W. Gelling, G. J. Morton, C. D. Morrison, K. D. Niswender, M. G. Myers Jr., C. J. Rhodes and M. W. Schwartz, "Insulin Action in the Brain Contributes to Glu-

cose Lowering during Insulin Treatment of Diabetes," *Cell Metabolism*, Vol. 3, No. 1, 2006, pp. 67-73. http://dx.doi.org/10.1016/j.cmet.2005.11.013

[19] P. K. Mukherjee, K. Maiti, K. Mukherjee, P. J. Houghton, "Leads from Indian Medicinal Plants with Hypoglycemic Potentials," *Journal of Ethnopharmacology*, Vol. 106, No. 1, 2006, pp. 1-28. http://dx.doi.org/10.1016/j.jep.2006.03.021

[20] R. Jagadeeswaran, C. Thirunavukkarasu, P. Gunasekaran, N. Ramamurty and D. Sakthisekaran, "*In Vitro* Studies on the Selective Cytotoxic Effect of Crocetin and Quercetin," *Fitoterapia*, Vol. 71, No. 4, 2000, pp. 395-399. http://dx.doi.org/10.1016/S0367-326X(00)00138-6

[21] T. H. Tseng, C. Y. Chu, J. M. Huang, S. J. Shiow and C. J. Wang, "Crocetin Protects against Oxidative Damage in rat Primary Hepatocytes," *Cancer Letters*, Vol. 97, No. 1, 1995, pp. 61-67. http://dx.doi.org/10.1016/0304-3835(95)03964-X

[22] W. S. Jung, Y. S. Chae, D. Y. Kim, S. W. Seo, H. J. Park, G. S. Bae, T. H. Kim, H. J. Oh, K. J. Yun, R. K. Park, J. S. Kim, E. C. Kim, S. Y. Hwang, S. J. Park and H. J. Song, "Gardenia Jasminoides Protects against Cerulein-Induced Acute Pancreatitis," *World Journal of Gastroenterology*, Vol. 14, No. 40, 2008, pp. 6188-6194. http://dx.doi.org/10.3748/wjg.14.6188

[23] Q.Yu, M. Yasuda, T. Takahashi, M. Nomura, N. Hagino and S. Kobayashi, "Effects of Bofutsushosan and Gardeniae Frutus on Diabetic Serum Parameters in Streptozotocin-Induced Diabetic Mice," *Chinese Medicine*, Vol. 2, No. 4, 2011, pp. 130-137. http://dx.doi.org/10.4236/cm.2011.24022

[24] Q. Yu, T. Takahashi, M. Nomura, M. Yasuda, K. Obatake-Ikeda and S. Kobayashi, "Effects of Single Administered Bofutsushosan-Composed Crude Drugs on Diabetic Serum Parameters in Streptozotocin-Induced Diabetic Mice," *Chinese Medicine*, Vol. 4, No. 1, 2013, pp. 24-31. http://dx.doi.org/10.4236/cm.2013.41005

[25] N. Nakashima, I. Kimura, M. Kimura and H. Matsuura, "Isolation of Pseudoprototimosaponin AIII from Rhizomes of *Anemarrhena asphodeloides* and Its Hypoglycemic Activity in Streptozotocin-Induced Diabetic Mice," *Journal of Natural Products*, Vol. 56, No. 3, 1993, pp. 345-350. http://dx.doi.org/10.1021/np50093a006

[26] T. Miura, H. Toyoda, M. Miyake, E. Ishihara, M. Usami and K. Tanigawa, "Hypoglycemic Action of Stigma of *Zea mays* L. in Normal and Diabetic Mice," *Natural Medicines*, Vol. 50, No. 5, 1996, pp. 363-365.

[27] D. R. Matthews, J. P. Hosker, A. S. Rudenski, B. A. Naylor, D. F. Treacher and R. C. Turner, "Homeostasis Model Assessment: Insulin Resistance and Beta-Cell Function from Fasting Plasma Glucose and Insulin Concentrations in Man," *Diabetologia*, Vol. 28, No. 27, 1985, pp. 412-419. http://dx.doi.org/10.1007/BF00280883

[28] P. A. Hansen, E. A. Gulve, B. A. Marshall, J. Gao, J. E. Pessin, J. O. Holloszy and M. Mueckler, "Skeletal Muscle Glucose Transport and Metabolism Are Enhanced in Transgenic Mice Overexpressing the Glut4 Glucose Transporter," *The Journal of Biological Chemistry*, Vol. 270, No. 4, 1995, pp. 1679-1684.

[29] N. T. Dang, R. Mukai, K. Yoshida and H. Ashida, "D-Pinitol and Myo-Inositol Stimulate Translocation of Glucose Transporter 4 in Skeletal Muscle of C57BL/6 Mice," *Bioscience, Biotechnology, and Biochemistry*, Vol. 74, No. 5, 2010, pp. 1062-1067. http://dx.doi.org/10.1271/bbb.90963

[30] S. Miyasita, "A Historical Study of Chinese Drugs for the Treatment of Jaundice," *The American Journal of Chinese Medicine* (*Garden City NY*), Vol. 4, No. 3, 1976, pp. 239-243.

[31] C. J. Ma, A. F. Nie, Z. J. Zhang, Z. G. Zhang, L. Du, X. Y. Li and G. Ning, "Genipin Stimulates Glucosetransport in C_2C_{12} Myotubes via an IRS-1 and Calcium-Dependent Mechanism," *The Journal of Endocrinology*, Vol. 216, No. 3, 2013, pp. 353-362.

[32] H. Aquila, T. A. Link and M. Klingenberg, "The Uncoupling Protein from Brown Fat Mitochondria Is Related to the Mitochondrial ADP/ATP Carrier. Analysis of Sequence Homologies and of Folding of the Protein in the Membrane," *The EMBO Journal*, Vol. 4, No. 9, 1985, pp. 2369-2376.

[33] H. Kageyama, A. Suga, M. Kashiba, J. Oka, T. Osaka, T. Kashiwa, T. Hirano, K. Nemoto, Y. Namba, D. Ricquier, J. P. Giacobino and S. Inoue, "Increased Uncoupling Protein-2 and -3 Gene Expressions in Skeletal Muscle of STZ-Induced Diabetic Rats," *The Federation of European Biochemical Societies Letters*, Vol. 440, No. 3, 1998, pp. 450-453. http://dx.doi.org/10.1016/S0014-5793(98)01506-3

[34] C. B. Chan, D. De Leo, J. W. Joseph, T. S. McQuaid, X. F. Ha, F. Xu, R. G. Tsushima, P. S. Pennefather, A. M. Salapatek and M. B. Wheeler, "Increased Uncoupling Protein-2 Levels in Beta-Cells Are Associated with Impaired Glucose-Stimulated Insulin Secretion: Mechanism of Action," *Diabetes*, Vol. 50, No. 6, 2001, pp. 1302-1310. http://dx.doi.org/10.2337/diabetes.50.6.1302

[35] C. Y. Zhang, G. Baffy, P. Perret, S. Krauss, O. Peroni, D. Grujic, T. Hagen, A. J. Vidal-Puig, O. Boss, Y. B. Kim, X. X. Zheng, M. B. Wheeler, G. I. Shulman, C. B. Chan and B. B. Lowell, "Uncoupling Protein-2 Negatively Regulates Insulin Secretion and Is A Major Link between Obesity, Beta Cell Dysfunction, and Type 2 Diabetes," *Cell*, Vol. 105, No. 6, 2001, pp. 745-755. http://dx.doi.org/10.1016/S0092-8674(01)00378-6

[36] K. S. Echtay, T. C. Esteves, J. L. Pakay, M. B. Jekabsons, A. J. Lambert, M. Portero-Otini, R. Pamplona, A. J. Vidal-Puig, S. Wang, S. J. Roebuck and M. D. Brand, "A Signaling Role for 4-Hydroxy-2-nonenal in Regulation of Mitochondrial Uncoupling," *The EMBO Journal*, Vol. 22, No. 16, 2003, pp. 4103-4110. http://dx.doi.org/10.1093/emboj/cdg412

[37] C. Y. Zhang, L. E. Parton, C. P. Ye, S. Krauss, R. Shen, C. T. Lin, J. A. Porco Jr. and B. B. Lowell, "Genipin Inhibits UCP2-Mediated Proton Leak and Acutely Reverses Obesity- and High Glucose-Induced Beta Cell Dysfunction in Isolated Pancreatic Islets," *Cell Metabolism*, Vol. 3, No. 6, 2006, pp. 417-427. http://dx.doi.org/10.1016/j.cmet.2006.04.010

[38] L. X. Guo, Z. N. Xia, X. Gao, F. Yin and J. H. Liu, "Glucagon-Like Peptide 1 Receptor Plays a Critical Role in Geniposide-Regulated Insulin Secretion in INS-1 cells," *Acta Pharmacologica Sinica*, Vol. 33, No. 2, 2012, pp. 237-241. http://dx.doi.org/10.1038/aps.2011.146

15

Hepatoprotective Diterpenoids Isolated from *Androgaphis paniculata*

Wen-Wan Chao[1]*, Bi-Fong Lin[2]*#

[1]Department of Nutrition and Health Sciences, School of Healthcare Management,
Kainan University, Taipei, Taiwan
[2]Department of Biochemical Science and Technology, College of Life Science,
National Taiwan University, Taipei, Taiwan
Email: *bifong@ntu.edu.tw, d91623701@ntu.edu.tw, wwchao@mail.knu.edu.tw

ABSTRACT

Androgaphis paniculata (Burm.f.) Nees (Acanthaceae), a plant widely used as traditional herbal medicine in many countries, has drawn attention of the researchers in recent years. Its major constituents are diterpenoids and flavonoids. This article reviews the anti-hepatotoxic effects of *A. paniculata* extract and derivative compounds, such as andrographolide, the major active compound, most studied for its bioactivities. Neoandrographolide shows anti-inflammatory and anti-hepatoxic properties. 14-deoxy-11,12-didehydroandrographolide and 14-deoxyabdrographolide have immunostimulatory, anti-atherosclerotic, and anti-hepatotoxic activities. The hepatoprotective activities include 1) inhibiting carbontetrachloride (CCl_4), tert-butylhydroperoxide (t-BHP)-induced hepatic toxicity; 2) acting as cytochrome P450 enzymes (CYPs) inducers; 3) modulating glutathione (GSH) content; 4) influence glutathione S-transferase (GSTP) activity and phosphatidylinositol-3-kinase/Akt (PI3k/Akt) pathway; 5) synergistic effect with anti-cancer drugs induced apoptosis contributing to the bioactivities of *A. paniculata* extracts and isolated bioactive compounds. The articles reviewed suggest that the above compounds could be candidates for research and development as potential hepatoprotective drugs.

Keywords: *Androgaphis paniculata*

1. Cytochrome P450 Enzymes and Liver Function

Cirrhosis may result from chronic metabolizing of xenobiotics including drugs, toxins, and chemical carcinogens in the liver. The cytochrome P450 enzymes (CYPs) are known as a superfamily of haemoproteins with a unique spectrophotometric absorbance peak at 450 nm when reduced by a reducing agent and bound by carbon monoxide [1]. Anti-hepatotoxic enzymes include cytochrome P450s (P450) super-family, or normalizing the levels of marker enzymes for the liver function test, such as glutamate pyruvate transaminase (GPT), glutamate oxaloacetate transaminase (GOT), alkaline phosphatase (ALP) and acid phosphatase (ACP) [2]. Phase I and phase II biotransformation enzymes are involved in the metabolic activation and detoxification of various carcinogens. Phase I enzymes convert xenobiotics to active intermediates and phase II enzymes catalyze the conjugation of these active intermediates with endogenous cofactors to increase their water solubility and facilitate their excretion through urine or bile. Glutathione S-transferase (GST) is one of phase II enzymes [3].

P450s, CYP1A1 and CYP1A2 have been shown to be the major enzymes in the metabolism of potential procarcinogens such as polycyclic aromatic hydrocarbons (PAHs) and aryl and heterocyclic arylamines. CYP1A1 is expressed constitutively in several extrahepatic tissues. But, while CYP1A1 expression has been demonstrated in liver after inducer treatment, CYP1A2 is constitutively and inducibly expressed only in the liver. CYP1B1 is a relatively new member of family 1 which is constitutively expressed in steroidogenic tissues, but is not detected in liver, kidney and lung [4]. Cytochrome P450 2C19 (CYP2C19), is a major hepatic CYP isoform involved in metabolism of many clinical drugs such as *S*-mephenytoin [5]. Human cytochrome P450s are concentrated in the liver, the major isoforms include CYP 1A2 (13%), CYP 2C9 and 2C19 (20%), CYP 2E1 (7%), CYP 2A6 (4%), CYP 2D6 (2%) and CYP 3A4 (30%). The 5 CYP isoforms 3A4, 2D6, 2C9, 1A2 and 2C19 account for almost 70% of all drug clearance [6].

---

*WWC and BFL searched the literature and drafted the manuscript. All authors read and approved the final version of the manuscript.
#Corresponding author.

2. Bioactive Constituents from *Andrographis paniculata*

Andrographis paniculata (Burm.f.) Nees (Acanthaceae) has been used as a traditional medicine in Taiwan, China, India and Thailand [7-9]. In traditional Chinese medicine, it is an important cold property herb used for antipyretic properties. And it is commonly used to prevent and treat the common cold [10].

A. *paniculata* contains diterpenes, lactones and flavonoids. Flavonoids mainly exist in the root, but also can be isolated from the leaves. The leaves contain two bitter lactone andrographolides, and kalmeghin. Active compounds extracted with ethanol or methanol from the whole plant, leaf and stem of *A. paniculata* include over 20 diterpenoids and over 10 flavonoids [11-13]. The active constituents of *A. paniculata* are diterpene lactones, including andrographolide, 14-deoxy-11,12-didehydroandrographolide, neoandrographolide and 14-deoxyandrographolide (**Figure 1**). Andrographolide is the most active and important compound of the plant [14-19]. Neoandrographolide shows anti-inflammatory and anti-hepatoxic properties. 14-deoxy-11,12-didehydroandrographolide and 14-deoxyabdrographolide have immunostimulatory, anti-atherosclerotic, and anti-hepatotoxic activities. Two flavonoids identified as 5,7,2',3'-tetramethoxyflavanone and 5-hydroxy-7,2',3'-trimethoxyflavone were also isolated from the whole plant. Extracts of the plant have been reported to exhibit a wide range of biological activities of therapeutic effects such as anti-inflammation, anti-cancer, immunomodulation, anti-infection, anti-hepatotoxicity, anti-atherosclerosis, anti-hyperglycemic effect and anti-oxidation [20].

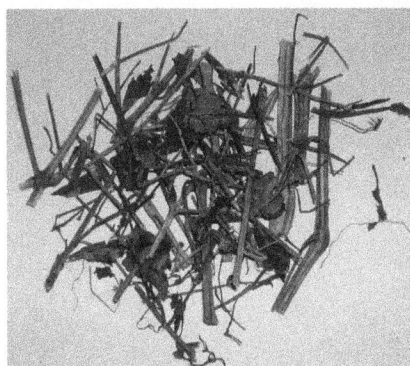

Andrographis paniculata

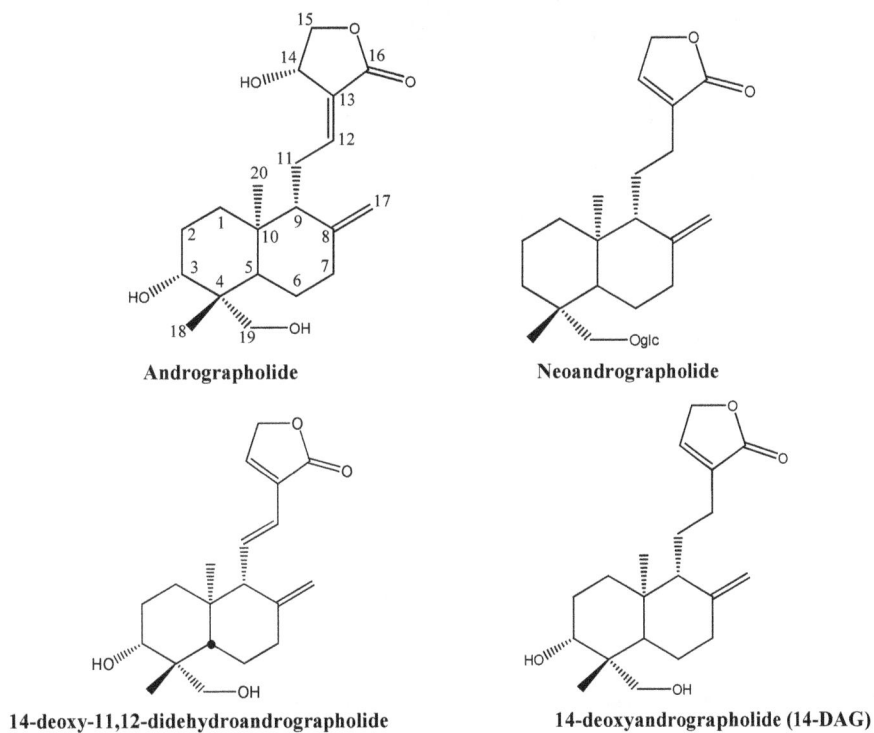

Andrographolide

Neoandrographolide

14-deoxy-11,12-didehydroandrographolide

14-deoxyandrographolide (14-DAG)

Figure 1. Chemical structures of the active compound for *Andrographis paniculata.*

Table 1. Anti-hepatotoxic mechanisms of *A. paniculata* and its bioactive compounds.

Pharmacological properties	References
1. Against CCl$_4$ and tBHP	
Kalmegh leaf extract ↓ CCl$_4$ (5 ml/kg) induced hepatic toxicity	[22]
Andrographolide, andrographiside and neoandrographolide (100 mg/kg, *i.p.*) ↓ CCl$_4$ or tBHP induced hepatic toxicity in serum MDA, GPT, ALP contents in mice	[25]
A.paniculata methanol extract ↓ CCl$_4$ induced plasma lipid peroxidation, ALT and AST contents	[26]
Andrographolide ↓ acetaminophen induced liver damage in rats	[27,28]
Andrographolide prevents CCl$_4$ induced acute liver injury via ↑ HO-1 and ↓TNF-α in mice	[29]
A. paniculata (100 - 200 mg/kg) ↓ paracetamol induced hepatotoxicity in mice	[30]
2. Act as CYPs inducers	
A. paniculata extract ↑ mouse hepatic CYP1A1 and CYP2B	[31]
Andrographolide ↑ CYP1A1 and CYP1A2 mRNA expression levels	[32]
Andrographolide ↑ CYP1A1 and CYP1B1 mRNA expression	[33]
A. paniculata 60% ethanol extract or andrographolide ↓ CYP3A, CYP2C9 *in vitro* and CYP2C11 *in vivo*	[34,35]
Andrographolide plus 3-MC synergistically ↑ CYP1 family gene in male B6 mice	[36]
14-deoxy-11,12-didehydroandrographolide and andrographolide ↓ CYP1A2, CYP2D6 and CYP3A4 expression in HepG2 cells	[37]
A. paniculata ethanol and methanol extracts ↓ CYP3A4, CYP2C9; andrographolide ↓ CYP3A4	[38]
Andrographolide and 14-deoxy-11,12-didehydroandrographolide co-treatment with BNF ↑ CYP1A1 expression; but, neoandrographolide co-treatment with BNF ↓ CYP1A1 expression	[39]
Andrographolide (1, 10, 100 μM) ↓ CYP3A4 mRNA and protein levels in Caco-2 cells	[40]
3. Modulate GSH content	
Andrographolide interaction with GSH ↑ BNF induced CYP1A1 mRNA expression in B6 mouse	[41]
A. paniculata ethanol extracts ↓ CYP2C19 activity	[42]
4. Influence GSTP activity and PI3k/Akt pathway	
A. paniculata ethanol, EtOAc extracts and andrographolide ↑ GSTP expression in rat primary hepatocytes	[43]
Andrographolide ↑ GSTP expression is mediated by the PI3k/Akt pathway	[44]
5. Synergistic effects with anti-cancer drugs	
Andrographolide and 5-FU combination treatment ↑ apoptosis in SMMC-7721 cells	[45]
Andrographolide combined with D-penicillamine ↓ copper toxicosis	[46]
Andrographolide (50, 100, 200 mg/kg, *i.p.*) ↓ serum ALT, AST, TNF-α, IL-1β and Bax, cytochrome c in BDL SD rats	[47]
Andrographolide ↑ doxorubicin induced apoptosis via ↓ STAT3 pathway in HepG2 cell	[48]
14-DAG ↓ TNF-α mediated apoptosis in primary rat hepatocytes	[49]
Andrographolide ↑ BSO improved the inhibition of tumor growth in nude mice bearing xenografted Hep3B	[50]
Andrographolide ↓ Con A induced liver injury	[54]

3. *A. Paniculata* and Pure Compounds Anti-Hepatotoxic Mechanisms (Table 1)

3.1. Against Carbontetrachloride (CCl₄) and Tert-Butylhydroperoxide (t-BHP)

It is well known that CCl₄ is converted by cytochrome P450 mixed function oxygenases in smooth endoplasmic reticulum of liver into toxic metabolite, mainly trichloromethyl radical (CCl₃•). In the presence of oxygen this free radical can induce peroxidation of lipids on target cells resulting in extensive damage [21]. Choudhury and Poddar reported that oral administration of kalmegh leaf extract (500 mg/kg) or its bitter compound, andrographolide (5 mg/kg), to adult male albino rats produced no significant change in nicotinamide adenine dinucleotide phosphate (NDAPH)-induced hepatic microsomal lipid peroxidation. The data suggests that kalmegh leaf has greater protective effect on carbontetrachloride (5 ml/kg)-induced hepatic toxicity than andrographolide [22].

t-BHP has often been used as a model to investigate the mechanism of cell injury initiated by acute oxidative stress [23]. t-BHP can be metabolized to free radical intermediates by cytochrome P450 (in hepatocytes) or hemoglobin (in erythrocytes), which can subsequently initiate lipid peroxidation [24] and affect cell integrity. Pretreatment of mice with andrographolide, andrographiside and neoandrographolide (100 mg/kg, *i.p.*) reduced CCl₄ or t-BHP-induced malondialdehyde (MDA) levels and release of GPT and ALP in the serum, as effective as the known hepatoprotective agent silymarin [25]. Oral treatment of rats with the *A. paniculata* methanol extract followed by CCl₄ administration restored plasma lipid peroxidation, alanine transaminase (ALT) and aspartate transaminase (AST) levels [26]. Oral or *i.p.* pretreatment with andrographolide was also protective against galactosamine-induced liver damage in rats. On the other hand, protection was also observed when rats were treated with andrographolide post acetaminophen challenge and on an *ex vivo* preparation of isolated rat hepatocytes by increasing the viability of the hepatocytes after parcacetamol-induced toxicity [27,28]. Ye *et al.* demonstrated that andrographolide prevents acute liver injury induced by CCl₄ via induction of heme oxygenase-1 (HO-1) and inhibition of an inflammatory response such as tumor necrosis factor-α (TNF-α) production in mice [29]. Oral administration of *A. paniculata* (100 - 200 mg/kg) exerted a significant dose dependent protection against paracetamol-induced hepatotoxicity in mice [30].

3.2. The Role of *A. paniculata* as CYPs Inducers

A crude extract of *A. paniculata* induce mouse hepatic cytochrome P450 isoforms CYP1A1 and CYP2B via increases in ethoxyresorufin *O*-dealkylase (EROD) and pentoxyresorufin *O*-dealkylase activities [31]. Andrographolide, a single substance extracted from *A. paniculata*, was further demonstrated to significantly up-regulate the CYP1-A1 and CYP1A2 mRNA expression, as did the CYP1A inducers such as benzanthracene and β-naphthoflavone [32]. Andrographolide significantly induced the expression of CYP1A1 and CYP1B1 mRNAs in a concentration-dependent manner, and also synergistically induced CYP1-A1 expression with the typical CYP1A inducers [33].

In addition, the *A. paniculata* 60% ethanol extract or andrographolide may cause herb-drug interactions through CYP3A and CYP2C9 inhibition *in vitro* or CYP2C11 inhibition *in vivo* [34,35]. A synergistically enhanced the expression of CYP1 family gene after andrographolide plus 3-methylcholanthrene (3-MC, a polycyclic aromatic hydrocarbon) treatment in male B6 mice. They demonstrated that a male hormone associated system to have a positive role in the synergistic effect [36]. 14-deoxy-11, 12-didehydroandrographolide and andrographolide have been shown to inhibit CYP1A2, CYP2D6 and CYP3A4 expressions in HepG2 cells [37]. *A. paniculata* ethanol and methanol extracts inhibited CYP3A4 and CYP2C9 activities more than aqueous and hexane extracts. On the other hand, andrographolide was found to weakly inhibit CYP3A4 activity [38]. Molecular docking analysis data supported that andrographolide and 14-deoxy-11,12-didehydroandrographolide induced CYP1A1 expression or co-treatment with CYP1A1 inducer (β-naphthoflavone, BNF) showed a synergistic increase expression of CYP1A1. In contrast, neoandrographolide suppressed BNF induced CYP1A1 expression [39]. Qiu *et al.* study the herb-drug interactions in combination therapy. They demonstrated that andrographolide (1, 10, 100 μM) significantly down regulates the mRNA level and protein level of CYP3A4 in Caco-2 cells [40].

3.3. The Modulatory Effect on Glutathione (GSH) Content

GSH is abundant in liver cells and a major protective factor against oxidative stress. Andrographolide interaction with GSH significantly enhanced the BNF inducible CYP1A1 mRNA expression in C57BL/6 mouse hepatocytes [41]. Pan *et al.* reported that *A. paniculata* ethanol extract weakly inhibited CYP 2C19 activity [42].

3.4. Influence Glutathione S-Transferase (GSTP) Activity and Phosphatidylinostol-3-Kinase/Akt (PI3k/Akt) Pathway

The π class of GST (GSTP) belongs to the cytosolic class. GSTP is not expressed in healthy liver but it is increased in both chemically induced and spontaneously arising precancerous lesions and hepatomas in experimental carcinogenesis studies [3]. Induction of drug-metabolizing enzymes is considered to be an adaptive response to a cytotoxic environment. The *A. paniculata* ethanol extract, EtOAc extract and andrographolide induce the expression of GSTP, a phase II biotransformation enzymes involved in detoxification of various classes of environmental carcinogens, in rat primary hepatocytes [43]. Furthermore, they also demonstrated that andrographolide induced GSTP expression is mediated by the PI3K/Akt pathway in SD rat primary hepatocytes [44].

3.5. The Role in Apoptosis Pathway

The combination of andrographolide and anti-cancer drug 5-fluorouracil (5-FU) could enhance the apoptosis in hapatocellular carcinoma (SMMC-7721) cells through a caspase-8 dependent mitochondrial pathway involving p53, Bax, cytochrome c, caspase-9 and caspase-3 [45]. Copper accumulation within the hepatocyte results in oxidative stress and promotes apoptosis. One study demonstrated that andrographolide combined with D-penicillamine could decrease caspase-8 activation and upstream events of caspase-3 activation and inflammatory cytokines production for treatment of copper toxicosis [46]. Bile duct ligation (BDL) could induce hepatic fibrosis. The BDL SD rats treated with andrographolide (50, 100, 200 mg/kg, *i.p.*) significantly reduced serum ALT, AST, TNF-α and interleukin-1β (IL-1β) levels and Bax, cytochrome c [47]. Zhou *et al.* reported that andrographolide promoted anti-cancer drug doxorubicin-induced apoptosis in HepG2 cell, indicating that andrographolide enhances cancer cells to anticancer drug doxorubicin *via* signal transducers and activators of transcription-3 (STAT3) pathway suppression [48]. 14-deoxyandrographolide (14-DAG), a bioactive compound of *A. paniculata*, was shown to protective on TNF-α-mediated apoptosis. Pre-treatment of primary rat hepatocytes with 10 nM 14-DAG accentuated microsomal Ca-ATPase activity through induction of NO/cGMP pathway and desensitizes hepatocytes to TNF-α-mediated apoptosis through the release of tumor necrosis factor receptor 1 (TNFR1) [49]. In nude mice bearing xenografted Hep3B tumors, buthionine sulfoximine (BSO, an inhibitor of cellular GSH biosynthesis) improved the inhibition of tumor growth by andrographolide [50]. Concanavalin A (Con A)-induced hepatitis model was widely used for the investigation of immune mediated acute liver injury [51-53]. Shi and coworkers demonstrated that andrographolide attenuated Con A-induced liver injury through reducing oxidative stress and inhibited hepatocyte apoptosis [54].

4. Conclusion

The major compounds andrographolide, neoandrographolide, 14-deoxy-11,12-didehydroandrographolide and 14-deoxyandrographolide of *A. paniculata* are most well studied for both bioactivities and functional mechanisms. They exert anti-hepatotoxic actions, such as 1) inhibiting CCl$_4$,

t-BHP induced hepatic toxicity; 2) acting as CYPs inducers; 3) modulating GSH content; 4) influencing GSTP activity and PI3k/Akt pathway; 5) synergistic effects with anti-cancer drugs inducing apoptosis are suggested to be the bioactivities of *A. paniculata* extracts and isolated active compounds. With more *in vitro* and *in vivo* studies, the *A. paniculata* extracts and purified active compounds might be developed into potential anti-hepatotoxic drug that warrant further research and development in the future.

REFERENCES

[1] F. J. Gonzalez, "The Molecular Biology of Cytochrome P450s," *Pharmacological Reviews*, Vol. 40, No. 4, 1988, pp. 243-288.

[2] P. K. Singha, S. Roy and S. Dey, "Protective Activity of Andrographolide and Arabinogalactan Proteins from *Andrographis paniculata* Nees. against Ethanol Induced Toxicity in Mice," *Journal of Ethnopharmacology*, Vol. 111, No. 1, 2007, pp. 13-21. doi:10.1016/j.jep.2006.10.026

[3] J. D. Hayes, J. U. Flanagan and I. R. Jowsey, "Glutathione Transferases," *Annual Review of Pharmacology and Toxicology*, Vol. 45, 2005, pp. 51-88. doi:10.1146/annurev.pharmtox.45.120403.095857

[4] M. Iwanari, M. Nakajima, R. Kizu, K. Hayakawa and T. Yokoi, "Induction of CYP1A1, CYP1A2 and CYP1B1 mRNAs by Nitropolycyclic Aromatic Hydrocarbons in Various Human Tissue Derived Cells: Chemical-, Cytochrome p450 Isoforms-, and Cell Specific Differences," *Archives of Toxicology*, Vol. 76, No. 5-6, 2002, pp. 287-298. doi:10.1007/s00204-002-0340-z

[5] P. J. Wedlund, "The CYP2C19 Enzyme Polymorphism," *Pharmacology*, Vol. 61, No. 3, 2000, pp. 174-183. doi:10.1159/000028398

[6] T. Shimada, H. Yamazaki, M. Mimura, Y. Inui and F. P. Guengerich, "Interindividual Variations in Human Liver Cytochrome P450 Enzymes Involved in the Oxidation of Drugs, Carcinogens and Toxic Chemicals: Studies with Liver Microsomes of 30 Japanese and 30 Caucasians," *Journal of Pharmacology and Experimental Therapeutics*, Vol. 270, No. 1, 1994, pp. 414-423.

[7] B. Kligler, C. Ulbricht, E. Basch, C. D. Kirkwood, T. R. Abrams, M. Miranda, K. P. Singh Khalsa, M. Giles, H. Boon and J. Woods, "*Andrographis paniculata* for the Treatment of Upper Respiratory Infection: A Systematic Review by the Natural Standard Research Collaboration," *Explore*, Vol. 2, No. 1, 2006, pp. 25-29. doi:10.1016/j.explore.2005.08.008

[8] M. Roxas and J. Jurenka, "Colds and Influenza, a Review of Diagnosis and Conventional, Botanical and Nutritional Considerations," *Alternative Medicine Review*, Vol. 12, No. 1, 2007, pp. 25-48.

[9] A. S. Negi, J. K. Kumar, S. Luqman, K. Sbanker, M. M. Gupta and S. P. S. Kbanuja, "Recent Advances in Plant Hepatoprotectives: A Chemical and Biological Profile of Some Important Leads," *Medicinal Research Reviews*,

Vol. 28, No. 5, 2008, pp. 746-772.
doi:10.1002/med.20115

[10] D. D. Caceres, J. L. Hancke, R. A. Burgos and G. K. Wikman, "Prevention of Common Colds with *Andrographis paniculata* Dried Extract: A Pilot Doudle-Blind Trial," *Phytomedicine*, Vol. 4, 1997, pp. 101-104.

[11] H. Y. Cheung , C. S. Cheung and C. K. Kong, "Determination of Bioactive Diterpenoids from *Andrographis paniculata* by Micellar Electrokinetic Chromatography," *Journal of Chromatography A*, Vol. 930, No. 1-2, 2001, pp. 171-176. doi:10.1016/S0021-9673(01)01160-8

[12] T. Matsuda, M. Kuroyanagi, S. Sugiyama, K. Umehara, A. Ueno and K. Nishi, "Cell Differentiation Inducing Diterpenes from *Andrographis paniculata* Nees.," *Chemical & Pharmaceutical Bulletin*, Vol. 42, No. 6, 1994, pp. 1216-1225. doi:10.1248/cpb.42.1216

[13] N. Pholphana, N. Rangkadilok, S. Thongnest, S. Ruchirawat, M. Ruchirawat and J. Satayavivad, "Determination and Variation of Three Active Diterpenoids in *Andrographis paniculata* (Burm.f.) Nees," *Phytochemical Analysis*, Vol. 15, No. 6, 2004, pp. 365-371. doi:10.1002/pca.789

[14] P. H. Kishore, M. V. Reddy, M. K. Reddy, D. Gunasekar, C. Caux and B. Bodo, "Flavonoids from *Andrographis lineate*," *Phytochemistry*, Vol. 63, No. 4, 2003, pp. 457-461. doi:10.1016/S0031-9422(02)00702-1

[15] J. Li, W. Huang, H. Zhang, X. Wang and H. Zhou, "Synthesis of Andrographolide Derivatives and Their TNF-Alpha and IL-6 Expression Inhibitory Activities," *Bioorganic & Medicinal Chemistry Letters*, Vol. 17, No. 24, 2007, pp. 6891-6894. doi:10.1016/j.bmcl.2007.10.009

[16] W. Parichatikanond, C. Suthisisang, P. Dhepakson and A. Herunsalee, "Study of Anti-Inflammatory Activities of the Pure Compounds from *Andrographis paniculata* (burm.f.) Nees and Their Effects on Gene Expression," *International Immunopharmacology*, Vol. 10, No. 11, 2010, pp. 1361-1373. doi:10.1016/j.intimp.2010.08.002

[17] W. W. Chao, Y. H. Kuo, W. C. Li and B. F. Lin, "The Production of Nitric Oxide and Prostaglandin E_2 in Peritoneal Macrophages Is Inhibited by *Morus alba, Angelica sinensis* and *Andrographis paniculata* Ethyl Acetate Fraction Extracts," *Journal of Ethnopharmacology*, Vol. 122, No. 1, 2009, pp. 68-75. doi:10.1016/j.jep.2008.11.029

[18] W. W. Chao, Y. H. Kuo, S. L. Hsieh and B. F. Lin, "Inhibitory Effects of Ethyl Acetate Extract of *Andrographis paniculata* on NF-κB Trans-Activation Activity and LPS-Induced Acute Inflammation in Mice," *eCAM*, Vol. 2011, 2011, p. 254531.

[19] W. W. Chao, Y. H. Kuo and B. F. Lin, "Anti-Inflammatory Activity of New Compounds from *Andrographis paniculata* by NF-κB Trans-Activation Inhibition," *Journal of Agricultural and Food Chemistry*, Vol. 58, No. 4, 2010, pp. 2505-2512. doi:10.1021/jf903629j

[20] W. W. Chao and B. F. Lin, "Isolation and Identification of Bioactive Compounds in *Andrographis paniculata* (Chuanxinlian)," *Chinese Medicine*, Vol. 5, 2010, p. 17. doi:10.1186/1749-8546-5-17

[21] R. O. Recknagel, "Carbon Tetrachloride Hepatotoxicity: Status Quo and Future Prospects," *Trends in Pharmacological Sciences* Vol. 4, 1983, pp. 129-131. doi:10.1016/0165-6147(83)90328-0

[22] B. R. Choudhury and M. K. Poddar, "Andrographolide and Kalmegh (*Andrographis paniculata*) Extract: *In Vivo* and *in Vitro* Effect on Hepatic Lipid Peroxidation," *Methods & Findings in Experimental & Clinical Pharmacology*, Vol. 6, No. 9, 1984, pp. 481-485.

[23] G. F. Rush, J. R. Gorski, M. G. Ripple, J. Sowinski, P. Bugelski and W. R. Hewitt, "Organic Hydroperoxide-Induced Lipid Peroxidation and Cell Death in Isolated Hepatocytes," *Toxicology and Applied Pharmacology*, Vol. 78, No. 3, 1985, pp. 473-483. doi:10.1016/0041-008X(85)90255-8

[24] J. Hogberg, S. Orrenius and P. J. O'Brien, "Further Studies on Lipid-Peroxide Formation in Isolated Hepatocytes," *European Journal of Biochemistry*, Vol. 59, No. 2, 1975, pp. 449-455. doi:10.1111/j.1432-1033.1975.tb02473.x

[25] A. Kapil, I. B. Koul, S. K. Banerjee and B. D. Gupta, "Antihepatotoxic Effects of Major Diterpenoid Constituents of *Andrographis paniculata*," *Biochemical Pharmacology* Vol. 46, No. 1, 1993, pp. 182-185. doi:10.1016/0006-2952(93)90364-3

[26] G. A. Akowuah, I. Zhari, A. Mariam and M. F. Yam, "Absorption of Andrographolides from *Andrographis paniculata* and Its Effect on CCl_4-Induced Oxidative Stress in Rats," *Food and Chemical Toxicology*, Vol. 47, No. 9, 2009, pp. 2321-2326. doi:10.1016/j.fct.2009.06.022

[27] S. S. Handa and A. Sharma, "Hepatoprotective Activity of Andrographolide against Galactosamine and Paracetamol Intoxication in Rats," *Indian Council of Medical Research*, Vol. 92, 1990, pp. 284-292.

[28] P. K. Visen, B. Shukla, G. K. Patnaik and B. N. Dhawan, "Andrographolide Protects Rat Hepatocytes against Paracetamol Induced Gamage," *Journal of Ethnopharmacology*, Vol. 40, No. 2, 1993, pp. 131-136. doi:10.1016/0378-8741(93)90058-D

[29] J. F. Ye, H. Zhu, Z. F. Zhou, R. B. Xiong, X. W. Wang, L. X. Su and B. D. Luo, "Protective Mechanism of Andrographolide against Carbon Tetrachloride Induced Acute Liver Injury in Mice," *Biological and Pharmaceutical Bulletin*, Vol. 34, No. 11, 2011, pp. 1666-1670. doi:10.1248/bpb.34.1666

[30] R. Nagalekshmi, A. Menon, D. K. Chandrasekharan and C. K. K. Nair, "Hepatoprotective Activity of *Andrographis paniculata* and *Swertia Chirayita*," *Food and Chemical Toxicology*, Vol. 49, No. 12, 2011, pp. 3367-3373. doi:10.1016/j.fct.2011.09.026

[31] K. Jarukamjorn, K. Don-in, C. Makejaruskul, T. Laha, S. Daodee, P. Pearaksa and B. Sripanidkulchai, "Impact of *Andrographis paniculata* Crude Extract on Mouse Hepatic Cytochrome P450 Enzymes," *Journal of Ethnopharmacology*, Vol. 105, No. 3, 2006, pp. 464-467. doi:10.1016/j.jep.2005.11.024

[32] A. Jaruchotikamol, J. Kanokwan, S. T. S. Wanna, K. Yuki and N. Nobuo, "Strong Synergistic Induction of CYP1A1 Expression by Andrographolide plus Typical CYP1A Inducers in Mouse Hepatocytes," *Toxicology and Applied*

Pharmacology, Vol. 224, No. 2, 2007, pp. 156-162. doi:10.1016/j.taap.2007.07.008

[33] W. Chatuphonprasert, K. Jarukamjorn, S. Kondo and N. Nemoto, "Synergistic Increases of Metabolism and Oxidation Reduction Genes on Their Expression after Combined Treatment with a CYP1A Inducer and Andrographolide," *Chemico-Biological Interactions*, Vol. 182, No. 2-3, 2009, pp. 233-238. doi:10.1016/j.cbi.2009.09.001

[34] D. Pekthong, H. Martin, C. Abadie, A. Bonet, B. Heyd, G. Mantion and L. Richert, "Differential Inhibition of Rat and Human Hepatic Cytochrome P450 by *Andrographis paniculata* Extract and Andrographolide," *Journal of Ethnopharmacology*, Vol. 115, No. 3, 2008, pp. 432-440. doi:10.1016/j.jep.2007.10.013

[35] D. Pekthong, N. Blanchard, C. Abadie, A. Bonet, B. Heyd, G. Mantion, A. Berthelot, L. Richert and H. Martin, "Effects of *Andrographis paniculata* Extract and Andrographolide on Hepatic Cytochrome P450 mRNA Expression and Monooxygenase Activities after *in Vivo* Administration to Rats and *in Vitro* in Rat and Human Hepatocyte Cultures," *Chemico-Biological Interactions*, Vol. 179, No. 2-3, 2009, pp. 247-255.

[36] K. Jarukamjorn, S. Kondo, W. Chatuphonprasert, T. Sakuma, Y. Kawasaki and N. Nemoto, "Gender-Associated Modulation of Ineucible CYP1A1 Expression by Andrographolide in Mouse Liver," *European Journal of Pharmaceutical Sciences*, Vol. 39, No. 5, 2010, pp. 394-401. doi:10.1016/j.ejps.2010.01.009

[37] J. P. Ooi, M. Kuroyanagi, S. F. Sulaiman, T. S. T. Muhammad and M. L. Tan, "Andrographolide and 14-Deoxy-11, 12-Didehydroandrographolide Inhibit Cytochtome P450s in HepG2 Hepatoma Cells," *Life Sciences*, Vol. 88, No. 9-10, 2011, pp. 447-454. doi:10.1016/j.lfs.2010.12.019

[38] Y. Pan, B. A. Abd-Rashid, Z. Ismail, R. Ismail, J. W. Mak, P. C. K. Pook, H. M. Er and C. E. Ong, "*In Vitro* Determination of the Effect of Andrographis Paniculata Extracts and Andrographolide on Human Hepatic Cytochrome P450 Activities," *Journal of Natural Medicines*, Vol. 65, No. 3-4, 2011, pp. 440-447. doi:10.1007/s11418-011-0516-z

[39] W. Chatuphonprasert, T. Remsungnen, N. Nemoto and K. Jarukamjorn, "Different AhR Binding Sites of Diterpenoid Ligands from Andrographis Paniculata Caused Differential CYP1A1 Induction in Primary Culture in Mouse Hepatocytes," *Toxicology in Vitro*, Vol. 25, No. 8, 2011, pp. 1757-1763. doi:10.1016/j.tiv.2011.09.004

[40] F. Qiu, X. L. Hou, K. Takahashi, L. X. Chen, J. Azuma and N. Kang, "Andrographolide Inhibits the Expression and Metabolic Activity of Cytochrome P450 3A4 in the Modified Caco-2 Cells," *Journal of Ethnopharmacology*, Vol. 141, No. 2, 2012, pp. 709-713. doi:10.1016/j.jep.2011.09.002

[41] S. Kondo, W. Chatuphonprasert, A. Jaruchotikamol, T. Sakuma and N. Nemoto, "Cellular Glutathione Content Modulates the Effect of Andrographolide on β-Naphtho-Flavone Induced CYP1A1 mRNA Expression in Mouse Hepatocytes," *Toxicology*, Vol. 280, No. 1-2, 2011, pp. 18-23. doi:10.1016/j.tox.2010.11.002

[42] Y. Pan, B. A. Abd-Rashid, Z. Ismail, R. Ismail, J. W. Mak, P. C. K. Pook, H. M. Er and C. E. Ong, "*In Vitro* Modula-

tory Effects of *Andrographis paniculata*, *Centella asiatica* and *Orthosiphon stamineus* on Cytochrome P450 2C19 (CYP2C19)," *Journal of Ethnopharmacology*, Vol. 133, No. 2, 2011, pp. 881-887. doi:10.1016/j.jep.2010.11.026

[43] K. T. Chang, C. K. Lii, C. W. Tsai, A. J. Yang and H. W. Chen, "Modulation of the Expression of the π Class of Glutathione *S*-Transferase by *Andrographis paniculata* Extracts and Andrographolide," *Food and Chemical Toxicology*, Vol. 46, No. 3, 2008, pp. 1079-1088. doi:10.1016/j.fct.2007.11.002

[44] C. Y. Lu, C. C. Li, C. K. Lii, H. T. Yao, K. L. Liu, C. W. Tsai and H. W. Chen, "Andrographolide Induced Pi Class of Glutathione *S*-Transferase Gene Expression via PI3K/ AKt Pathway in Rat Primary Hepatocytes," *Food and Chemical Toxicology*, Vol. 49, No. 1, 2011, pp. 281-289. doi:10.1016/j.fct.2010.10.030

[45] L. Yang, D. Wu, K. Luo, S. Wu and P. Wu, "Andrographolide Enhances 5-Fluorouracil-Induced Apoptosis via Caspase-8 Dependent Mitochondrial Pathway Involving p53 Participation in Hepatocellular Carcinoma (SMMC-7721) Cells," *Cancer Letters*, Vol. 276, No. 2, 2009, pp. 180-188. doi:10.1016/j.canlet.2008.11.015

[46] D. N. Roy, G. Sen, K. D. Chowdhury and T. Biswas, "Combination Therapy with Andrographolide and D-Penicillamine Enhanced Therapeutic Advantage over Monotherapy with D-Penicillamine in Attenuating Fibrogenic Response and Cell Death in the Periportal Zone of Liver in Rats during Copper Toxicosis," *Toxicology and Applied Pharmacology*, Vol. 250, No. 1, 2011, pp. 54-68. doi:10.1016/j.taap.2010.09.027

[47] T. Y. Lee, K. C. Lee and H. H. Chang, "Modulation of the Cannabinoid Receptors by Andrographolide Attenuates Hepatic Apoptosis Following Bile Duct Ligation in Rats with Fibrosis," *Apoptosis*, Vol. 15, No. 8, 2010, pp. 904-914. doi:10.1007/s10495-010-0502-z

[48] J. Zhou, C. N. Ong, G. M. Hur and H. M. Shen, "Inhibition of the JAK-STAT3 Pathway by Andrographolide Enhances Chemosensitivity of Cancer Cells to Doxorubicin," *Biochemical Pharmacology*, Vol. 79, No. 9, 2010, pp. 1242-1250. doi:10.1016/j.bcp.2009.12.014

[49] D. N. Roy, S. Mandal, G. Sen, S. Mukhopadhyay and T. Biswas, "14-Deoxyandrographolide Desensitizes Hepatocytes to Tumour Necrosis Factor-Alpha Induced Apoptosis through Calcium Dependent Tumour Necrosis Factor Receptor Superfamily Member 1A Release via the NO/cGMP Pathway," *British Journal of Pharmacology*, Vol. 160, No. 7, 2010, pp. 1823-1843. doi:10.1111/j.1476-5381.2010.00836.x

[50] L. Ji, K. Shen, P. Jiang, G. Morahan and Z. Wang, "Critical Roles of Cellular Glutathione Homeostasis and JNK Activation in Andrographolide Mediated Apoptotic Cell Death in Human Hepatoma Cells," *Molecular Carcinogenesis*, Vol. 50, No. 8, 2011, pp. 580-591. doi:10.1002/mc.20741

[51] G. Tiegs, J. Hentschel and A. Wendel, "A T Cell Dependent Experimental Liver Injury in Mice Inducible by Concanavalin A," *The Journal of Clinical Investigation*, Vol. 90, No. 1, 1992, pp. 196-203.

doi:10.1172/JCI115836

[52] Z. L. Wang, X. H. Wu, L. F. Song, Y. S. Wang, X. H. Hu, Y. F. Luo, Z. Z. Chen, J. Ke, X. D. Peng, C. M. He, W. Zhang, L. J. Chen and Y. Q. Wei, "Phosphoinostide 3 Kinase Gamma Inhibitor Ameliorates Concanavalin A Induced Hepatic Injury in Mice," *Biochemical and Biophysical Research Communications*, Vol. 386, No. 4, 2009, pp. 569-574. doi:10.1016/j.bbrc.2009.06.060

[53] D. H. Adams, C. Ju, S. K. Ramaiah, J. Uetrecht and H. Jaeschke, "Mechanisms of Immune Mediated Liver Injury," *Toxicological Sciences*, Vol. 115, No. 2, 2010, pp. 307-321. doi:10.1093/toxsci/kfq009

[54] G. Shi, Z. Zhang, R. Zhang, X. Zhang, Y. Lu, J. Yang, D. Zhang, Z. Zhang, X. Li and G. Ning, "Protective Effect of Andrographolide against concanavalin A Induced Liver Injury," *Naunyn-Schmiedeberg's Archives of Pharmacology*, Vol. 385, No. 1, 2012, pp. 69-79. doi:10.1007/s00210-011-0685-z

Abbreviations

CYPs: cytochrome P450 enzymes;
GPT: glutamate pyruvate transaminase;
GOT: glutamate oxaloacetate transaminase;
ALP: alkaline phosphatase;
ACP: acid phosphatase;
GST: Glutathione S-transferase;
PAHs: polycyclic aromatic hydrocarbons;
CCl_4: carbontetrachloride;
tBHP: tert-butylhydroperoxide;
NDAPH: nitotinamide adenine dinucleotide phosphate;
MDA: malondialdehyde;
ALT: alanine transaminase;
AST: aspartate transaminase;
HO-1: heme oxygenase-1;

TNF-α: tumor necrosis factor-α;
3-MC: 3-methylcholanthrene;
BNF: β-naphthoflavone;
GSH: glutathione;
GSTP: glutathione S-transferase;
PI3k/Akt: phosphatidylinositol-3-kinase/Akt;
5-FU: 5-fluorouracil;
BDL: Bile duct ligation;
IL-1β: interleukin-1β;
STAT3: signal transducers and activators of transcription-3;
14-DAG: 14-deoxyan-drographolide;
TNFR1: tumor necrosis factor receptor 1;
BSO: buthionine sulfoximine;
Con A: concanavalin A

16

A Review of the Potential Issues of Pollution Caused by the Mineral Elements, Mercury, Lead and Arsenic, Its Possible Impacts on the Human Beings and the Suggested Solutions

Yau Lam[1], Cho Wing Sze[1], Yao Tong[1], Tzi Bun Ng[2], Pang Chui Shaw[3], Yanbo Zhang[1]
[1]School of Chinese Medicine, The University of Hong Kong, Hong Kong, China
[2]The School of Biomedical Sciences and School of Life Science, The University of Hong Kong, Hong Kong, China
[3]The School of Biochemistry and Faculty of Science, The Chinese University of Hong Kong, Hong Kong, China
Email: ybzhang@hkucc.hku.hk

ABSTRACT

Objective: This paper mainly discusses and summarises the potential issues of pollution caused by the Mineral elements, Mercury, Lead and Arsenic, its possible impacts on the human beings and the suggested solutions. **Methods:** This paper is prepared by reviewing the latest academic literatures. **Result:** First, this article discusses two aspects including the effects of Mercury, Lead and Arsenic on the Chinese herbal medicine and the potential issues of causing the environmental pollution. And then further study its toxicity effects and the side impacts on the human bodies in order to realize the actual circumstances people are encountering nowadays. This paper will also the corresponding its treatment method of reviews. Hope this will provide a valuable reference. **Conclusion:** Theses issues caused by the Mineral elements are prominent nowadays, thus the ongoing researches on the impacts of pollution and the possible solutions are regarded as highly valued in order to conserve the natural environment and meanwhile safeguard the well beings of people and the future offspring.

Keywords: Mineral Elements; Arsenic; Lead; Mercury

1. Introduction

With the continuous development of the science, more and more serious pollutions stem from Mineral elements, including arsenic, lead, mercury, cadmium, nickel, copper and zinc, fierce, and sources etc. The sources of pollutions are very broad, factors including environment, food and drugs. This paper mainly discusses three Mineral elements, Mercury, Lead and Arsenic. The focuses are mainly on the basis of environment and drugs. We can also realize the extent of harm of the heavy metals on the human health and the feasible methods in resolving the health impacts.

2. Pollution of Mercury, Lead and Arsenic

Rapid economic development in countries and concern for both the environment and protection against pollutants is increasing. Identification of sources of contaminants and evaluation of current environmental status are essential to environmental pollution management. Mining and metallurgical activities these anthropogenic Mineral elements from the contaminated areas into the environment. Harmful Mineral elements included Mercury, Lead and Arsenic. Lead is used in many industries, including lead smelting and processing, the manufacturing of batteries, pigments, solder, plastics, cable sheathing, ammunition, ceramics, and battery recycling. It was the most common Mineral elements contaminant [1-3]. Arsenic contamination in the arises due to human activities like mining, combustion, and pesticide application. As indicated by the presence of pyrite, hydrous ferric oxide, organic matter, clay minerals, fracture surfaces, and high permeable (moldic) zones. Arsenic was present in all of the stratigraphic units at low concentrations, close to the global average for as in limestone of 2.6 mg/kg. The highest As concentration was 69 mg/kg [4,5]. Mercury was common Mineral elements in home contamination. If you broken thermostats or from the accidental or intentional spilling or sprinkling of elemental mercury. Because it can easily trapped in porous surfaces such as plaster or stucco interiors, carpeting or cracks between tile or wood floors. So it may persist in an indoor environment for several years. There are many publications in the scientific literature addressing this issue, including several excellent reviews. This type of contamination is a public health issue worldwide. In particular the ongoing catastrophic problems in Bangladesh and West Bengal have been front-page stories in newspapers and scientific journals [6-9].

Toxic contaminant release; toxic substances can follow different environmental pathways and accumulate in environmental soil and elevated concentrations of toxic metals. Metals are persistent in soils for a longer time after their introduction, and most metals do not undergo microbial or chemical degradation. Such as deforestation and soil erosion, inevitably resulted in environmental degradation in the surrounding seas induced historical soil and groundwater pollution by Mineral elements. That is a worldwide problem (**Tables 1** and **2**).

3. Traditional Chinese Medicine and Proprietary Chinese Medicines in Mineral Elements of Arsenic, Mercury and Lead

In recent years, the total number of people using traditional Chinese herbal medicine is vast and steadily increasing in East Asian countries and Chinese society. The industrial output value of traditional Chinese herbal medicine has also continued to expand rapidly across the world since the year 2000 [43]. Thereafter, the united states studies show, that approximately 14.8 billion USD were spent in 2007 on non-mineral, non-vitamin natural products, most of which consisted of herbal medicines,

Table 1. Comparisons of the concentrations of trace metals in urban soils of different cities in China (mg·kg^{-1}).

Chinese provinces and cities	Pb	Hg	As	Reference
		Soils pollution		
Beijing	25.5 - 208	n.d	n.d	[10]
Changchun	19.7 - 378	0.026 - 1.43	6.1 - 67.7	[11,12]
(Jilin)	28.8	0.037	8.0	[13]
Changsha	7.80 - 413	0.050 - 1.29	2.49 - 79.8	[13]
(Hunan)	29.7	0.12	15.7	[13]
Chongqing	13.5 - 53.9	0.049 - 0.89	4.12 - 18.9	[14]
(Sichuan)	30.9	0.061	10.4	[14]
Fuzhou	22.8 - 1072	0.020 - 6.24	1.39 - 42.2	[15]
(Fujian)	41.3	0.093	6.30	[15]

The chart above indicates the distribution status of lead, mercury and arsenic in the soil of both provinces and cities of China. The results show that the distribution of lead element in the soil of provinces is higher than that of cities; conversely, the distribution of arsenic in the soil of cities is higher than that of provinces; the discrepancy is much less for the content of mercury in the soil of both provinces and cities.

Table 2. Concentration of several elements (mg·kg^{-1}) found in sediments collected in different estuaries of the world.

Around the world in Estuary	Pb	As	Reference
	Pollution of Estuary		
1. Medway (UK)	67	14	[16]
2. Thames (UK)	63	15	[17]
3. Odiel-Tinto (Spain)	523	278	[18]
4. Nerbioi-Ibaizabal	21 - 445	0.6 - 220	[19]
5. Krka (Croatia)	11	n.d	[20]
6. St Lucie (Florida)	2.8 - 23	n.d	[21]
7. Vigo (Spain)	57	n.d	[22]
8. Mersey (UK)	65	n.d	[23]
9. Hudson (New York)	81	n.d	[24]
10. Pearl River (China)	16 - 93.3	n.d	[25]
11. Severn (UK)	50 - 68	n.d	[26]
12. Tagus (Portugal)	65 - 200	n.d	[27]
13. Ulla (Spain)	57 - 58	n.d	[28]
14. Marabasco (Mexico)	2 - 18	n.d	[29]
15. Pontevedra (Spain)	37 - 144	n.d	[30]
16. Ennore Creek (India)	32	n.d	[31]
17. Tamaki (New Zeeland)	51 - 122	n.d	[32]
18. Pearl River Estuary (China)	59.4	n.d	[33]
19. Shenzhen Bay (China)	46.0	n.d	[34]
20. Jiaozhou Bay (China)	30.9	n.d	[35]
21. Quanzhou Bay (China)	34.3 ± 16.9	n.d	[36]
22. Western Xiamen Bay (China)	50.0	n.d	[37]
23. New York Harbor (USA)	109 - 136	n.d	[38]
24. Bremen Harbor (Germany)	122	n.d	[39]
25. Izmir Harbor (Turkey)	97	n.d	
26. Boston Harbor (USA)	86	n.d	[40]
27. Marine Sediment Quality Primary standard criteria	60	n.d	[41]
28. Marine Sediment Quality Secondary standard criteria	130	n.d	[41]
29. Sediment guideline for effects range-low (ERL)	46.7	n.d	[42]
30. South China Sea (China)	23.6 ± 8.9	n.d	[42]

The above chart indicates the extent of air pollution triggered by lead and arsenic in different countries. The results show that the extent of air pollution triggered by the elements in the countries such as United States, China and India are different. There is less data obtained for the analysis of arsenic element. Based on all available information, the extent of pollution triggered by lead is higher than that of arsenic.

up from an estimated total of 6.6 billion USD spent ten years previously but several studies have shown that CHMs and other botanical supplements may be contaminated with minerals and metals 15, also in some cases at toxic levels. Much of what has been reported regarding potentially worrisome contamination in herbal medicines relates to patent or proprietary medicines [44-46].

We learned that Proprietary Chinese Medicines can produce Mineral elements poisoning and that physicians need to take patient histories carefully, being aware of the possible side effects of herbal medicines. In traditional Chinese medicine, mercury and arsenic is part of some preparations. In which "calomel" (mercury chloride) or "hydrargyri oxydum rubrum" (mercury oxide) and it contains 10% cinnabar HgS (mercury sulfide) of An-Gong-Niu-Huang Wan (AGNH）[47]. Also that arsenic including arsenolite, orpiment (mainly containing As_2S_3), realgar (mainly containing As_4S_4), arsenolite and arsenic trioxide (mainly containing As_2O_3) [48]. It has long been used in traditional medicine for treating various diseases but in some cases at toxic levels [49].

3.1. Orpiment, Realgar and Arsenic Stone Toxicity of Mineral Elements

Arsenical preparations have been used by many physicians in the treatment of malignant diseases, such as leukemia, Hodgkin's disease, pernicious anemia and non-malignant diseases, such as psoriasis, pemphigus, eczema, and asthma for centuries [50]. Recent studies prove that realgar is used to counteract toxicity, kill parasites, and cure malaria [51]. Also that orpiment nanoparticles can inhibit the telomerase activity of K562 cells, which may be an important mechanism in the anticancer effect of orpiment nanoparticles [52,53]. In fact, it is a known human carcinogen producing a series of organic cancers and has many other profound toxic effects following short-term or long-term exposure [54]. In which, arsenolite and arsenic trioxide are highly toxic compared to orpiment and realgar. Short-term toxicity of As_2O_3 is the major concern in the use of this agent against malignancies, and at least three sudden deaths have been reported [55]. To ensure the safe use of mineral arsenicals, identifying them accurately is necessary (**Table 3**).

3.2. An-Gong-Niu-Huang Wan (AGNH) Toxicity of Mineral Elements (Mercury)

An-Gong-Niu-Huang Wan (AGNH) is a patent traditional Chinese medicine for brain disorders. The medicine containing cinnabar is insoluble, has very low bioavailability and thus is poorly absorbed from the gastrointestinal tract. In study display, long-term administration (>30 days) of cinnabar at doses above 100 mg/kg

also produced mercury poisoning [56]. In addition, heating cinnabar results in release of mercury vapor, which in turn can produce toxicity similar to inhalation of these vapors [57]. The cinnabar which contains 96% mercuric sulfide (HgS), Mercury binds to other elements, such as chlorine, sulfur, or oxygen, to form inorganic mercurous ($Hg_1þ$) or mercuric ($Hg_2þ$) salts, such as mercury sulfide (HgS, purified from cinnabar), mercurous chloride (Hg_2Cl_2, also called calomel) and mercuric chloride ($HgCl_2$) [58]. In which ethyl mercury ($C_2H_5Hgþ$) is the major component of thimerosal. Mercuric oxide was once used as a disinfectant and antiseptic agent [59]. Other preparations containing mercury are still used as antibacterials [60] but dimethyl mercury [$(CH_3)2Hg$] is the most toxic mercurial [61]. The abuse of cinnabar leading to intoxication of Hg in infants has been reported so these uses have largely been replaced by safer therapies [62,63] (**Table 4**).

3.3. Mineral Elements of Hongdan (Pb₃O₄) and Lead

Hongdan is the official term for red lead (Pb_3O_4) according to the pharmacopeia of traditional Chinese medicine. In addition to its use in traditional medicine, Hongdan is widely used in paint and in the battery industry as a raw or additive material. Also, used for superstitious purposes (by low income families in China) as a cultural

Table 3. Effect of metallic element to human health (Hg), (As) and (Pb) [65,66].

Diseases	Toxic metals potentially involved in etiology	Reference
Allergy	Hg	[67,68]
Autism	Hg	[69]
Parkinson's disease	Hg, Pb, As	[70,71]
Poisoning and anemia	Pb	[72]
Diabetes	As	[71]

The above chart indicates that the lead, mercury and arsenic poisoning could cause certain diseases among which Parkinson's disease is the common disease which could be caused by all three of the elements.

Table 4. Hg (10 mg/kg) for 10 weeks on liver, kidney, cerebral and cerebellar injury of male and female [72].

	Cerebral	Cerebellar	Liver	Kidney
	Cortex	Cortex		
Male	15 µg/g	21 µg/g	112 µg/g	180 µg/g
Female	9 µg/g	18 µg/g	80 µg/g	140 µg/g

The above chart indicates that mercury could cause damages of Cerebral cortex, cerebellar cortex, liver and kidney for both males and females. Overall, the damages to males are more serious than that to females.

powder to ward off bad luck by daubing. Use to traditional medicine, Though most qualified physicians are aware of its potential toxicity, most traditional medicine practitioners are not certificated to practice. In April 2009, the national Food and Drug Administration responded to the report and launched a campaign nationwide. Until now, China as a suggestion to prohibit the use of Hongdan as a remedy [64].

4. Lead, Mercury and Arsenic Poisoning and Its Treatment Method

Lead (Pb), mercury (Hg) and arsenic (As) are metals ranked among the top ten most toxic substances, summarized as follows [73].

4.1. The Toxicity of Lead

We defined high lead content to be >1.5 mcg/serving. The early European Pharmacopoeia has issued a draft monograph herbal drugs, proposing the limits for Mineral elements in herbal drugs: 5 mg·kg^{-1} for lead, furthermore, the European Commission has established the lead limits in food supplements of America [74,75].

After that, in America, California criteria for acceptable lead levels of <1.5 mcg/serving of natural calcium supplement.

Lead is mainly divided into two kinds of structure: Inorganic and organic. Inorganic and organic forms of lead are absorbed through the lungs and gastrointestinal tract; in occupational settings, exposure through inhalation is more common, whereas in the general population, it is largely through ingestion. And organic lead compounds may also be absorbed through the skin [76]. Excretion is primarily via the kidneys, and the half-life of lead in the blood is about 30 days. If high lead is taken up in the blood and deposited in soft tissues (brain, liver, kidney, bone marrow) and bone up to 94% of the body burden of lead is in bone, where it has a half-life of years to decades [77]. A clinical report showed, ordinary people may include abdominal pain, anorexia, nausea and constipation, headache, joint and muscle pain, difficulties with concentration and memory, sleep disturbances, anemia with basophilic stippling, peripheral neuropathy and nephropathy [78]. Among adults, the potential implications of low-level lead exposure are most relevant to women of child-bearing age, as lead is especially harmful to developing nervous systems of fetuses and children and passes through the placenta and breast milk [79-81]. As lead accumulates in bones and is mobilized into circulation during periods of increased bone turnover (particularly in women during periods of pregnancy, lactation, and menopause). Calcium deficiency increases lead absorption and lead retention, and is a risk factor for increased maternal lead transfer. In which, Methyl mercury crosses the placenta and reaches the fetus, and is concentrated in the fetal brain at least 5 to 7 times that of maternal blood [82-86]. Prenatal methyl mercury exposure at high levels can induce widespread damage to the fetal brain. Given birth to infants with severe developmental disabilities, raising initial concerns for mercury as a developmental toxicant. The child's brain and nervous system equally susceptible to its effect of lead [87].

4.2. The Toxicity of Mercury

Mercury is known to produce toxicity of Mineral elements. The European Pharmacopoeia has issued a draft monograph Herbal drugs, proposing the following limits for heavy metals in herbal drugs: 0.1 mg·kg^{-1} for mercury. Furthermore, the European Commission has established the mercury limits in food supplements [88]. Mercury is mainly divided into two kinds of structure: Inorganic and organic. It is distributed primarily to the central nervous system and the kidneys. Elimination is through the urine and feces. The half-life of elemental and inorganic mercury in the blood is 40 - 60 days, and the half-life of organic mercury in the blood is about 70 days. Signs and symptoms of mercury toxicity vary with the form of mercury and route of exposure [89]. In which, inhalation of high concentrations of elemental mercury vapor also damages the lungs, skin, eyes, and gingival. Chronic exposure to elemental mercury vapor primarily affects the central nervous system. Major symptoms include a fine tremor, psychological changes (e.g., increased excitability), and gingivitis. Other symptoms can include insomnia, loss of appetite, irritability, depression, headache, short-term memory loss, and muscle wasting [90]. Symptoms of acute exposure include cough, dyspnea, chest pain, nausea, vomiting, diarrhea, fever, and a metallic taste in the mouth. If the exposure is great enough, these symptoms can progress to interstitial pneumonitis, renal injury, increased blood pressure and heart rate, and pulmonary edema [91]. In which, the woman developed a variety of symptoms, including pain and tingling in one hand, abdominal pain and bloating, diarrhea and constipation, increased bruising, varicose veins and fatigue. In the fetus, organic mercury disrupts the cytoarchitecture of the developing brain and has been associated with neuropsychological changes after birth [92].

4.3. The Toxicity of Arsenic

Arsenic is a poison since ancient times. It is a geogenic water menace affecting millions of people all over the world and is regarded as the largest mass poisoning in history. Moreover, it has been used as a Chinese herbal medicine and proprietary Chinese medicines for many centuries [93]. In force since 1 July 2009, shows national and regional limits for arsenic and toxic metals in various types of herbal products proposed by the WHO [94]. Therefore, removal and recovery of arsenic from contaminated water and effective and safe use of mineral arsenicals has attracted more and more attention. Arsenic occurs in the environment in several chemical forms, showing different toxicological characteristics. Organic forms of arsenic are rarely significant in ground water, however, the inorganic forms: arsenite (AsO_3^{3-}) and arsenate (AsO_3^{3-}) are often found in this kind of water. Permanent arsenic intake leads to chronic intoxication. Dosages much lower than this have been associated with a variety of adverse health effects including mild symptoms such as throat irritation, nausea, and more serious signs of intoxication such as anaemia, liver injury, skin injury, renal failure, encephalopathy and a gastrointestinal bleeding [95]. Prenatal exposure to arsenic is associated with later life health effects in adults [96-98]. Toxic metal exposures in utero and during childhood may result in significant health effects including, low birth weight, reduced fetal growth and reproductive and cognitive deficits in adolescents [99-101]. Results in the appearance of diverse types of cancer, such as hyperkeratosis, lung, and skin cancer.Increased mortality and increased risk [102,103]. Once the report display, the Vietnamese pills have caused a classic case of fatal arsenic poisoning in Vietnam [104].

5. Determination of Lead, Mercury and Arsenic

5.1. Determination of Lead

The lead pollution comes mainly from environmental factors. Asia and America same affected by pollution [105]. In China, the powder was analyzed in a chemistry laboratory in Guangzhou Center for Disease Control. There use to flame atomic absorption spectrometry (FAAS, Zeeman-5000, Hitachi Limited, Japan) and use to situ XRF for structure determination of lead. In addition, China specializing in lead poisoning treatment. The BLLs were measured again by graphite furnace atomic absorption spectrometry with Zeeman back-ground correction (GFAAS; Thermo Elemental, Solaar MQZ) in the hospital [106]. The lead structure included: $Pb(NO_3)_2$; $Pb(C_2H_5)_4$; $PbCO_3$; $PbSiO_3$; $PbCrO_4$; PbO_2; PbO (litharge); PbO (massicot) *et al.* [107]. Based on the sample analysis using inductively coupled plasma mass spectrometry (ICP-MS) [108].

In USA of El Paso and TX have been used synchrotron-based XAFS (X-ray absorption fine structure) to identify and quantify the major Pb species present in airborne PM collected so. It can bulk technique that provides structural information at the molecular level about a given element in a sample and hence used to environ-mental testing. If you visited the family to investigate the source of lead exposure used to a portable X-ray fluorescence analyzer (XRF, Innov-α 4000, Innov-X System Company, Woburn, MA) was used to screen the indoor environment, household products, drinking water and food [109]. Hence, in lead poisoning treatment use of (GFAAS); in the pharmaceutical analysis and the environmental pollution can be used on X-ray fluorescence spectrometry [110].

5.2. Determination of Mercury

Several techniques are currently available in the determination of mercury and these include cold vapor atomic absorption/fluorescence spectrometry (CV-AAS/AFS), gas and liquid chromatography (GC/LC) and inductively coupled plasma with either atomic emission spectrometry (ICP-AES) or mass spectrometry (ICP-MS), etc. [111, 112]. Laboratory studies revealed, urine specimens were analyzed for inorganic mercury using an automated flow injection mercury system (FIMS) that uses cold vapor atomic absorption spectrometry and Urine specimens were analyzed for total mercury using inductively coupled plasma mass spectrometry (ICP-MS) [113-115]. CVG technique has some merits such as high sensitivity, wide linear dynamic range, low noise level, fast analysis speed, ease of operation, and low cost [116]. However, the drawbacks are also serious and remarkable. This sample pre-treatment step is time-consuming. moreover potential losses of the volatile mercury species in the sample may also occur and quite often also the major source of contamination, Furthermore, still some difficulties exist in the analysis of mercury in some TCM drugs because of its extremely low concentrations following the interferences caused by the complex sample matrices and the wide change in matrix composition from sample to sample [117]. Comparing with other technique, the thermolysis atomic absorption method provides an attractive alternative in mercury analysis, because of its direct solid sampling without pre-treatment, which eliminates tedious sample digestion or derivatization steps commonly used in conventional methods. The method is rapid, typically requiring only 4 min to complete a total mercury analysis. Moreover, the method provides high sensitivity, low detection limit and outstanding background correction capability utilizing Zeeman-effect. In this study, our objective is to develop and apply this technique to investigate the content of mercury and the preliminary species in several TCM drug products for quality assessment and regulatory purposes [118,119].

5.3. Determination of Arsenic

Determination of arsenic in many methods including:

X-ray diffraction analysis [120]; Hydride generation (HG), liquid chromatography (LC), gas chromatography (GC) and capillary electrophoresis (CE) are commonly being utilized for the separation of as species. However, the advantage of HG method is that it can easily be connected to various detection systems like ICP-MS, AAS, ETAAS, ICPAES, AFS, and ICP-MS [121-123]. The most commonly analyzed species are As(III), As(V), MMAA, DMAA, arsenocholine (AsC), arsenobetaine (AsB) or TMAs+ (tetramethylarsonium ion-Me$_4$As+), TMAO (trimethylarsine oxide—Me$_3$AsO), arsenosugars, phenylarsonic acid (PAS) and metaloproteins [124].

The commonly used to Hydride generation of HG-AAS method, because of Hydride generation is a well-known technique for the determination of As at trace levels, which consists of the reaction of As compounds with sodium tetrahydroborate in acidic medium to produce various arsines (AsH3) [125]. As for example, As(III) and As(V) give AsH3, MMAA gives monomethylarsine (MMA-CH3AsH2) and DMAA produces dimethylarsine (DMA-(CH3)2AsH). Also, the AAS combined with HG is widely used for As speciation included, As(III) and As(V) [126,127]. It has been specific advantages included, selectivity, sensitivity, efficiency, rapidity and detection limit (DL), in addition, often combined with high performance liquid chromatography. The use of HPLC-HG-AAS enabled the elimination of interference and the highly sensitive determination of As(V) [128].

After that, the macroscopic and microscopic features are given in detail. In study display, that modern microscopic technique is a simple, fast, effective, low cost, and the results are in agreement with ICP-MS analysis. The authentication results for arsenolite and arsenic trioxide same are confirmed by ICP-MS analysis. But there are a lot of problems included inductively coupled plasma atomic emission spectrometry (ICPAES) [129], inductively coupled plasma mass spectrometry (ICP-MS) [130-134], graphite furnace atomic absorption spectrometry (GFAAS) [135], hydride generation atomic absorption spectrometry (HGAAS) [136], and hydride generation atomic fluorescence spectrometry (HG-AFS) [137]. These methodologies are often laboratory-based and time-consuming and may lead to large capital cost for multi-sample analysis and its major drawback is that these methods are unable to distinguish between As(III) and As(V) in the analyzed samples.

Recent studies, a novel hyphenated technique, a microfluidic chip-based capillary electrophoresis (μchip-CE) hydride generation (HG) system was interfaced with a microwave induced plasma optical emission spectrometry (MIP-OES) to provide two inorganic arsenic species separation capabilities. The detection limits for As(III) and As(V) are 3.9 and 5.4 ng·mL^{-1}, at the moment the microchip system requires manual filling with background buffer and sample. Further improvements of the features of μCE-HG-MIP-OES may lie in the use of aminiaturized MIP at atmospheric pressure and miniaturized and portable spectrometer because toxic of hevy metal As(V) is much higher than that of As(III) [138,139]. There are few proposed methods to the direct determination of As(V), without pretreatment of samples. Today, a colorimetric method using the molybdenum blue complex has been developed for the sensitive de- termination of As(V) [140].

6. Conclusion

Based on the research conducted in this article, it is apparent that the pollutions of heavy metal stem from a variety of cause. It could devastate the health of wildlife and human beings, especially to the pregnant females and the fetus. The impact on the mental growth could prolong from the new born to the childhood and result in an irreparable jeopardy. As a matter of fact, many might have acknowledged that heavy metal pollutions are inevitable by-products during the exploration and development of society, therefore, in-depth study of the methods in resolving the heavy metal pollution is an important subject. In the future, in addition to enhance heavy metal to detection, also should consider the mineral traditional Chinese medicine on dosage and use method and the related problems, ensure the safety of medication.

7. Acknowledgements

This study was supported by Funding from Innovation and Technology Support Programme, the Government of the Hong Kong Special Administrative Region No. ITS/313/11 and Seed Funding Programme for Basic Research from The Hong Kong University No. 201111159043.

REFERENCES

[1] Y. W. Chiang, R. M. Santos, K. Ghyselbrecht, V. Cappuyns, J. A. Martens, R. Swennen, T. Van Gerven and B. Meesschaert, "Strategic Selection of an Optimal Sorbent Mixture for in-Situ Remediation of Heavy Metal Contaminated Sediments: Framework and Case Study," *Journal of Environmental Management*, Vol. 105, 2012, pp. 1-11.

[2] A. Fischbein, "Occupational and Environmental Exposure to Lead," In: W. N. Rom, Ed., *Environmental and Occupational Medicine*, 3rd Edition, Lippincott-Raven, Philadelphia, 1998, pp. 973-996.

[3] T. S. Bowers, B. D. Beck and H. S. Karam, "Assessing the Relationship between Environmental Lead Concentrations and Adult Blood Lead Levels," *Risk Analysis*, Vol. 14, No. 2, 1994, pp. 183-189.

[4] A. A. Carbonell-Barrachina, M. A. Aarabi, R. D. Delaune, R. P. Gambrell and J. W. H. Patrick, "Arsenic in Wetland

Vegetation: Availability, Phytotoxicity, Uptake and Effects on Plant Growth and Nutrition," *Science of the Total Environment*, Vol. 217, No. 3, 1998, pp. 189-199.

[5]   T. Pichler, R. Price, O. Lazareva and A. Dippold, "Determination of Arsenic Concentration and Distribution in the Floridan Aquifer System," *Journal of Geochemical Exploration*, Vol. 111, No. 3, 2011, pp. 84-96.

[6]   L. H. Zayas and P. O. Ozuah, "Mercury Use in Espiritismo: A Survey of Botanicas," *American Journal of Public Health*, Vol. 86, No. 1, 1996, pp. 111-112. doi:10.2105/AJPH.86.1.111

[7]   Association of Toxic Substances and Disease Registry (ATSDR), "Toxicological Profile for Mercury (Update)," Department of Health and Human Services, Atlanta, 2006. http://www.atsdr.cdc.gov/toxprofiles/tp46.html

[8]   M. Amini, K. C. Abbaspour, M. Berg, L. Winkel, S. J. Hug, E. Hoehn, H. Yang and C. A. Johnson, "Statistical Modeling of Global Geogenic Arsenic Contamination in Groundwater," *Environmental Science & Technology*, Vol. 42, No. 10, 2008, pp. 3669-3675.

[9]   M. F. Ahmed, S. Ahuja, M. Alauddin, S. J. Hug, J. R. Lloyd, A. Pfaff, T. Pichler, C. Saltikov, M. Stute and A. van Geen, "Ensuring Safe Drinking Water in Bangladesh. Science," 2006. doi:10.1126/science.1133146

[10] T. B. Chen, Y. M. Zheng, M. Lei, Z. C. Huang, H. T. Wu and H. Chen, "Assessment of Heavy Metal Pollution in Surface Soils of Urban Parks in Beijing, China," *Chemosphere*, Vol. 60, No. 4, 2005, pp. 542-551.

[11] Z. P. Yang, W. X. Lu, Y. Q. Long and X. R. Liu, "Prediction and Precaution of Heavy Metal Pollution Trend in Urban Soils," *Urban Environment and Urban Ecology*, Vol. 23, No. 3, 2010, pp. 1-4.

[12] P. Guo, Z. L. Xie, J. Li, C. L. Kang and J. H. Liu, "Relationships between Fractionations of Pb, Cd, Cu, Zn and Ni and Soil Properties in Urban Soils of Changchun City," *Chinese Geographical Science*, Vol. 15, No. 2, 2005, pp. 179-185.

[13] T. Zhou, C. Z. Xi, T. G. Dai and D. Y. Huang, "Comprehensive Assessment of Urban Geological Environment in Changsha City," *Guangdong Trace Elements Science (In Chinese)*, Vol. 15, No. 6, 2008, pp. 32-38.

[14] Z. P. Li, Y. C. Chen, X. C. Yang and S. Q. Wei, "Assessment of Potential Ecological Hazard of Heavy Metals in Urban Soils in Chongqing City," *Journal of Southwest Agricutral University Natural Science (in Chinese)*, Vol. 28, No. 2, 2006, pp. 227-230.

[15] T. Chen, X. M. Liu, M. Z. Zhu, K. L. Zhao, J. J. Wu and J. M. Xu and P. Huang, "Identification of Trace Element Sources and Associated Risk Assessment in Vegetable Soils of the Urban-Rural Transitional Area of Hangzhou, China," *Environmental Pollution*, Vol. 151, No. 1, 2008, pp. 67-78.

[16] K. L. Spencer, "Spatial Variability of Metals in the Inter-Tidal Sediments of the Medway Estuary, Kent, UK," *Marine Pollution Bulletin*, Vol. 44, No. 9, 2002, pp. 933-944.

[17] M. J. Attrill and R. M. Thomes, "Heavy Metal Concentrations in Sediment from the Thames Estuary, UK," *Ma-*

rine Pollution Bulletin Vol. 30, No. 11, 1995, pp. 742-744.

[18] J. Gonzalez-Perez, J. de Andres, L. Clemente, J. Martin and F. Gonzalez-Vila, "Organic Carbon and Environmental Quality of Riverine and Off-Shore Sediments from the Gulf of Cadiz, Spain," *Environmental Chemistry Letters*, Vol. 6, No. 1, 2008, pp. 41-46.

[19] S. Fdez-Ortiz de Vallejuelo, G. Arana, A. de Diego and J. M. Madariaga, "Risk Assessment of Trace Elements in Sediments: The Case of the Estuary of the NerbioiIbaizabal River (Basque Country)," *Journal of Hazardous Materials*, Vol. 181, No. 1-3, 2010, pp. 565-573.

[20] E. Prohic and G. Kniewald, "Heavy Metal Distribution in Recent Sediments of the Krka River Estuary—An Example of Sequential Extraction Analysis," *Marine Chemistry*, Vol. 22, 1987, pp. 279-297.

[21] M. Zhang, Z. He, P. Stoffella, D. Calvert, X. Yang and P. Sime, "Concentrations and Solubility of Heavy Metals in Muck Sediments from the St. Lucie Estuary, USA," *Environmental Geology*, Vol. 44, No. 1, 2003, pp. 1-7.

[22] M. A. Rubio and F. Nombela, "Geochemistry of Major and Trace Elements in Sediments of the Ria de Vigo (NW Spain): An Assessment of Metal Pollution," *Marine Pollution Bulletin*, Vol. 40, No. 11, 2000, pp. 968-980.

[23] D. Harland and A. T. Wither, "The Distribution of Mercury and Other Trace Metals in the Sediments of the Mersey Estuary over 25 Years 1974-1998," *Science of the Total Environment*, Vol. 253, No. 1-3, 2000, pp. 45-62.

[24] J. Feng, H. Kirk, B. J. Cochran, D. J. Lwiza and B. Hirschberg, "Distribution of Heavy Metal and PCB Contaminants in the Sediments of an Urban Estuary: The Hudson River," *Marine Pollution Reseach*, Vol. 45, No. 1, 1998, pp. 69-88.

[25] L. Carman, Z. Xiang-Dong, W. Gan and L. Onyx, "Trace Metal Distribution in Sediments of the Pearl River Estuary and the Surrounding Coastal Area, South China," *Environmental Pollution*, Vol. 147, No. 2, 2007, pp. 311-323.

[26] S. Duquesne, L. C. Newton, L. Giusti, S. B. Marriott, H. J. Stark and D. J. Bird, "Evidence for Declining Levels of Heavy-Metals in the Severn Estuary and Bristol Channel UK and Their Spatial Distribution in Sediments," *Environmental Pollution*, Vol. 143, No. 2, 2006, pp. 187-196.

[27] S. Franc. A. C. Vinagre, I. C. ador and H. N. Cabrl, "Heavy Metal Concentrations in Sediment, Benthic Invertebrates and Fish in Three Salt Marsh Areas Subjected to Different Pollution Loads in the Tagus Estuary (Portugal)," *Marine Pollution Bulletin*, Vol. 50, No. 9, 2005, pp. 998-1003.

[28] R. Prego and A. Cobelo-Garcia, "Twentieth Century Overview of Heavy Metals in the Galician Rias (NW Iberian Peninsula)," *Environmental Pollution*, Vol. 121, No. 3, 2003, pp. 425-452.

[29] A. J. Marmolejo-Rodriguez, R. Prego, A. Meyer-Willerer, E. Shumilin and A. Cobelo-Garcia, "Total and Labile Metals in Surface Sediments of the Tropical River-Estuary System of Marabasco (Pacific Coast of Mexico): Influence of an Iron Mine," *Marine Pollution Bulletin*, Vol. 55, No.

10-12, 2007, pp. 459-468.

[30] N. Fernandez, J. Bellas, J. Lorenzo and R. Beiras, "Complementary Approaches to Assess the Environmental Quality of Estuarine Sediments," *Water, Air, and Soil Pollution*, Vol. 189, No. 1-4, 2008, pp. 163-177.

[31] M. Jayaprakash, M. P. Jonathan, S. Srinivasalu, S. Muthuraj, V. Ram-Mohan and N. Rajeshwara-Rao, "Acid-Leachable Trace Metals in Sediments from an Industrialized Region (Ennore Creek) of Chennai City, SE Coast of India: An Approach towards Regular Monitoring, Estuarine Coast," *Estuarine, Coastal and Shelf Science*, Vol. 76, No. 3, 2008, pp. 692-703. doi:10.1016/j.ecss.2007.07.035

[32] G. Abrahim and R. Parker, "Assessment of Heavy Metal Enrichment Factors and the Degree of Contamination in Marine Sediments from Tamaki Estuary, Auckland, New Zealand," *Environmental Monitoring and Assessment*, Vol. 136, No. 1-3, 2008, pp. 227-238. doi:10.1007/s10661-007-9678-2

[33] F. Liu, W. Yan, W. Z. Wang, S. C. Gu and Z. Chen, "Pollution of Heavy Metals in the Pearl River Estuary and Its Assessment of Potential Ecological Risk," *Marine Environmental Science*, Vol. 21, No. 3, 2002, pp. 34-38.

[34] X. Huang, X. Li, W. Yue, L. Huang and Y. Li, "Accumulation of Heavy Metals in the Sediments of Shenzhen Bay, South China," *Environmental Science (in Chinese with English Abstract)*, Vol. 24, No. 4, 2003, pp. 144-149.

[35] X. D. Xu, Z. H. Lin and S. Q. Li, "The Studied of the Heavy Metal Pollution of Jiaozhou Bay," *Marine Sciences (in Chinese with English Abstract)*, Vol. 29, No. 1, 2005, pp. 48-53.

[36] R. L. Yu, X. Yuan, Y. H. Zhao, G. R. Hu and X. L. Tu, "Heavy Metal Pollution in Intertidal Sediments from Quanzhou Bay, China," *Journal of Environmental Sciences*, Vol. 20, No. 6, 2008, pp. 664-669. doi:10.1016/S1001-0742(08)62110-5

[37] L. P. Zhang, X. Ye, H. Feng, Y. H. Jing, O. Y. Tong, X. T. Yu, R. Y. Liang, C. T. Gao and W. Q. Chen, "Heavy Metal Contamination in Western Xiamen Bay Sediments and Its Vicinity, China," *Marine Pollution Bulletin*, Vol. 54, No. 7, 2007, pp. 974-982. doi:10.1016/j.marpolbul.2007.02.010

[38] USEPA-Region II, USACE-New York District, USDOE-BNL, "Fast Track Dredged Material Decontamination Demonstration for the Port of New York and New Jersey," 1999.

[39] A. Filibeli and R. Yilmaz, "Dredged Material of Izmir Harbor: Its Behavior and Pollution Potential," *Water Science and Technology*, Vol. 32, No. 2, 1995, pp. 105-113. doi:10.1016/0273-1223(95)00575-8

[40] M. H. Bothner, T. B. Buchholtz and F. T. Manheim, "Metal Concentrations in Surface Sediments of Boston Harbor—Changes with Time," *Marine Environmental Research*, Vol. 45, No. 2, 1998, pp. 127-155. doi:10.1016/S0141-1136(97)00027-5

[41] CSBTS (China State Bureau of Quality and Technical Supervision), "Marine Sediment Quality," Standards Press of China, Beijing, 2002.

[42] L. Zhu, J. Xu, F. Wang and B. Lee, "An Assessment of Selected Heavy Metal Contamination in the Surface Sediments from the South China Sea before 1998," *Journal of Geochemical Exploration*, Vol. 108, No. 1, 2011, pp. 1-14. doi:10.1016/j.gexplo.2010.08.002

[43] G. D. Du, "White Paper on China's Drug Supervision," 2008. http://news.xinhuanet.com/english/2008-07/18/content_8 567067_4.htm

[44] R. L. Nahin, P. M. Barnes, B. J. Stussman and B. Bloom, "Costs of Complementary and Alternative Medicine (CAM) and Frequency of Visits to CAM Practitioners: United States, 2007," *National Health Statistic Reports*, Vol. 30, No. 18, 2009, pp. 1-14.

[45] D. M. Eisenberg, R. B. Davis, S. L. Ettner, S. Appel, S. Wilkey and M. van Rompay, "Trends in Alternative Medicine Use in the United States, 1990-1997—Results of a Follow-Up National Survey," *The Journal of the American Medical Association*, Vol. 280, No. 18, 1998, pp. 1569-1575. doi:10.1001/jama.280.18.1569

[46] S. J. Eric, C. A. C. Shugeng, A. B. Littlefield, A. J. Craycroft, R. Scholten, T. Kaptchuk, Y. L. Fu, W. Q. Wang, Y. Liu, H. B. Chen, Z. Z. Zhao, J. Clardy, A. D. Woolf and D. M. Eisenberg, "Heavy Metal and Pesticide Content in Commonly Prescribed Individual Raw Chinese Herbal Medicines," *Science of the Total Environment*, Vol. 409, No. 20, 2011, pp. 4297-4305.

[47] J. Liu, Y. F. Lu, Q. Wu, R. Goyer and M. P. Waalkes, "Mineral Arsenicals in Traditional Medicines: Orpiment, Realgar, and Arsenolite," *Pharmacology*, Vol. 326, No. 2, 2008, pp. 363-368. doi:10.1124/jpet.108.139543

[48] J. Liu, J. Z. Shi, L. M. Yu, R. A. Goyer and M. P. Waalkes, "Mercury in Traditional Medicines: Is Cinnabar Toxicologically Similar to Common Mercurials?" *Experimental Biology and Medicine*, Vol. 233, No. 7, 2008, pp. 810-817. doi:10.3181/0712-MR-336

[49] R. B. Saper, R. S. Phillips, A. Sehgal, N. Khouri, R. B. Davis and J. Paquin, "Lead, Mercury, and Arsenic in US- and Indian-Manufactured Ayurvedic Medicines Sold via the Internet," *The Journal of the American Medical Association*, Vol. 300, No. 8, 2008, pp. 915-923. 2008. doi:10.1001/jama.300.8.915

[50] Y. F. Lu, Q. Wu, W. Miao, J. S. Shi and J. Liu, "Evaluation of Hepatotoxicity Potential of Cinnabar-Containing. An-Gong-Niu-Huang Wan, a Patent Traditional Chinese Medicine," *Regulatory Toxicology and Pharmacology*, Vol. 60, No. 2, 2011, pp. 206-211. doi:10.1016/j.yrtph.2011.03.007

[51] A. Hamzah, C. W. Beh, S. B. Sarmani and J. Y. Liow, "Abugassa Studies on Elemental Analysis of Chinese Traditional Herbs by Neutron Activation Technique and Their Mutagenic Effect," *Journal of Radioanalytical and Nuclear Chemistry*, Vol. 259, No. 3, 2004, pp. 499-503.

[52] L. I. Qin, C. Chu, Y. Q. Wang, H. B. Chen, L. I. Ping and Z. Z. Zhao, "Authentication of the 31 Species of Toxic and Potent Chinese Materia Medica by Microscopic Technique Assisted by ICP-MS Analysis, Part 4: Four Kinds of Toxic and Potent Mineral Arsenical CMMs," *Microscopy Research and Technique Journal*, Vol. 74,

No. 1, 2011, pp. 1-8.

[53] A. M. Evens, M. S. Tallman and R. B. Gartenhaus, "The Potential of Arsenic Trioxide in the Treatment of Malignant Disease: Past, Present, and Future," *Leukemia Research*, Vol. 28, No. 9, 2004, pp. 891-900. doi:10.1016/j.leukres.2004.01.011

[54] Chinese Pharmacopoeia Commission, "Pharmacopoeia of the People's Republic of China," People's Medical Publishing House, Beijing, 2005.

[55] M. Lin, Z. Y. Wang and D. S. Zhang, "Preparation of As_2S_3 Nanoparticles and Their Therapeutic Effect on liver Cancer SMMC-7721 Cells," *Journal of Southeast University (Natural Science Edition)*, Vol. 2, No. 36, 2006, pp. 298-302.

[56] M. Lin and D. S. Zhang, "Effect of Orpiment Nanoparticles on Telomerase Activity in K562 Cell Line," *Journal of the Medical Sciences*, Vol. 11, No. 6, 2007, pp. 5-7.

[57] K. Cooper, B. Noller, D. Connell, J. Yu, R. Sadler, H. Olszowy, G. Golding, U. Tinggi, M. R. Moore and S. Myers, "Public Health Risks from Heavy Metals and Metalloids Present in Traditional Chinese Medicines," *Journal of Toxicology and Environmental Health A*, Vol. 70, No. 19, 2007, pp. 1694-1699. doi:10.1080/15287390701434885

[58] P. Westervelt, R. A. Brown, D. R. Adkins, H. Khoury, P. Curtin, D. Hurd, S. M. Luger, M. K. Ma, T. J. Ley and J. F. Dipersio, "Sudden Death among Patients with Acute Promyelocytic Leukemia Treated with Arsenic Trioxide," *Blood*, Vol. 98, No. 2, 2001, pp. 266-271. doi:10.1182/blood.V98.2.266

[59] A. Liang, J. Wang, B. Xue, C. Li, T. Liu, Y. Zhao, C. Cao and Y. Yi, "Study on Hepatoxicity and Nephrotoxicity of Cinnabar in Rats," *Zhongguo Zhong Yao Za Zhi*, Vol. 34, No. 3, 2009, pp. 312-328.

[60] J. Liu, J. Z. Shi, L. M. Yu, A. R. Goyer and M. P. Waalkes, "Mercury in Traditional Medicines: Is Cinnabar Toxicologically Similar to Common Mercurials?" *Journal of Experimental Biology and Medicine*, Vol. 233, No. 7, 2008, pp. 810-817.

[61] C. D. Klaassen, "Heavy Metals and Heavy-Metal Antagonists," In: J. G. Hardman, L. E. Limbird and A. G. Gilman, Eds., *The Pharmacological Basis of Therapeutics*, McGraw-Hill, New York, 2001, pp. 1851-1876.

[62] Agency for Toxic Substances and Disease Registry, "Toxicological Profile for Mercury (Update)," Agency for Toxic Substances and Disease Registry, Atlanta, 1999.

[63] J. F. Risher, H. E. Murray and G. R. Prince, "Organic Mercury Compounds: Human Exposure and Its Relevance to Public Health," *Toxicology and Industrial Health*, Vol. 18, No. 3, 2002, pp. 109-160. doi:10.1191/0748233702th138oa

[64] G. Z. Lin, F. Wu, C. H. Yan, *et al.*, "Childhood Lead Poisoning Associated with Traditional Chinese Medicine: A Case Report and the Subsequent Lead Source Inquiry," *Clinica Chimica Acta*, Vol. 413, No. 13-14, 2012, pp. 1156-1159. doi:10.1016/j.cca.2012.03.010

[65] G. C. Fang, Y. L. Huang and J. H. Huang, "Study of Atmospheric Metallic Elements Pollution in Asia during 2000-2007," *Journal of Hazardous Materials*, Vol. 180, No. 1-3, 2010, pp. 115-121. doi:10.1016/j.jhazmat.2010.03.120

[66] J. D. Marth, "A Unified Vision of the Building Blocks of Life," *Nature Cell Biology*, Vol. 10, No. 9, 2008, pp. 1015-1016. doi:10.1038/ncb0908-1015

[67] B. Rowley and M. Monestier, "Mechanisms of Heavy Metal-Induced Autoimmunity," *Molecular Immunology*, Vol. 42, No. 7, 2005, pp. 833-838. doi:10.1016/j.molimm.2004.07.050

[68] K. M. Pollard, P. Hultman and D. H. Kono, "Toxicology of Autoimmune Diseases," *Chemical Research in Toxicology*, Vol. 23, No. 3, 2010, pp. 455-466.

[69] S. Bernard, A. Enayati, H. Roger, T. Binstock and L. Redwood, "The Role of Mercury in the Pathogenesis of Autism," *Molecular Psychiatry*, Vol. 7, No. 2, 2002, pp. S42-S43. doi:10.1038/sj.mp.4001177

[70] J. M. Gorell, C. C. Johnson, B. A. Rybicki, E. L. Peterson, G. X. Kortsha, G. G. Brown and R. J. Richardson, "Occupational Exposures to Metals as Risk Factors for Parkinson's Disease," *Neurology*, Vol. 48, No. 3, 1997, pp. 650-658. doi:10.1212/WNL.48.3.650

[71] J. Shu, J. A. Dearing, A. P. Morse, L. Yu and N. Yuan, "Determining the Sources of Atmospheric Particles in Shanghai, China, from Magnetic and Geochemical Properties," *Atmospheric Environment*, Vol. 35, No. 15, 2001, pp. 2615-2625. doi:10.1016/S1352-2310(00)00454-4

[72] C.-F. Huang, S.-H. Liu and S. Y. Lin-Shiaub, "Neurotoxicological Effects of Cinnabar (a Chinese Mineral Medicine, HgS)," *Toxicology and Applied Pharmacology*, Vol. 224, No. 2, 2007, pp. 192-201. doi:10.1016/j.taap.2007.07.003

[73] R. J. Huang, Z. X. Zhuang, Y. Tai, X. R. Wang and F. S. C. Lee, "Direct Analysis of Mercury in Traditional Chinese Medicines Using Thermolysis Coupled with On-Line Atomic Absorption Spectrometry," *Talanta*, Vol. 68, No. 3, 2006, pp. 728-734. doi:10.1016/j.talanta.2005.05.014

[74] B. J. Alloway, "The General Monograph Herbal Drugs (1433)," *Pharmeuropa*, Vol. 20, No. 2, 2008, pp. 302-303.

[75] Commission Regulation (EC) No. 629/2008 Amending Regulation (EC) No. 1881/2006 of 19 December 2006, "Setting Maximum Levels for Certain Contaminants in Foodstuffs," *Official Journal of the European Union*, Vol. 173, No. 51, 2008, pp. 6-9.

[76] T. I. Lidsky and J. S. Schneider, "Neurotoxicity in Children: Basic Mechanisms and Clinical Correlates," *Brain*, Vol. 126, No. 1, 2003, pp. 5-19. doi:10.1093/brain/awg014

[77] Agency for Toxic Substances and Disease Registry (ATSDR), "Toxicological Profile for Lead [Draft]," Public Health Service, US Department of Health and Human Services, Washington DC, 2005. www.atsdr.cdc.gov/toxprofiles

[78] US Centers for Disease Control and Prevention (CDC), "Third National Report on Human Exposure to Environmental Chemicals," Atlanta, 2005.

www.cdc.gov/exposurereport/3rd/default.htm

[79]　A. Menke, P. Muntner, V. Batuman, E. K. Silbergeld and E. Guallar, "Blood Lead below 0.48 Micromol/l (10 microg/dl) and Mortality among US Adults," *Circulation*, Vol. 114, No. 13, 2006, pp. 1388-1394. doi:10.1161/CIRCULATIONAHA.106.628321

[80]　D. C. Bellinger, "Very Low Lead Exposures and Children's Neurodevelopment," *Current Opinion in Pediatrics*, Vol. 20, No. 2, 2008, pp. 172-177. doi:10.1097/MOP.0b013e3282f4f97b

[81]　C. D. Carrington and P. M. Bolger, "An Assessment of the Hazards of Lead in Food," *Regulatory Toxicology and Pharmacology*, Vol. 16, No. 3, 1992, pp. 265-272. doi:10.1016/0273-2300(92)90006-U

[82]　A. Gomaa, H. Hu, D. Bellinger, *et al.*, "Maternal Bone Lead as an Independent Risk Factor for Fetal Neurotoxicity: A Prospective Study," *Pediatrics*, Vol. 110, Part 1, 2002, pp. 110-118. doi:10.1542/peds.110.1.110

[83]　S. DeMichele, "Nutrition of Lead," *Comparative Biochemistry and Physiology B-Biochemistry & Molecular Biology*, Vol. 78, No. 3, 1984, pp. 401-408.

[84]　M. J. Heard and A. C. Chamberlain, "Effect of Minerals and Food on Uptake of Lead from the Gastrointestinal Tract in Humans," *Human & Experimental Toxicology*, Vol. 1, No. 4, 1982, pp. 411-415. doi:10.1177/096032718200100407

[85]　K. M. Six and R. A. Goyer, "Experimental Enhancement of Lead Toxicity by Low Dietary Calcium," *Journal of Laboratory and Clinical Medicine*, Vol. 76, No. 6, 1970, pp. 933-942.

[86]　Y. Cheng, W. C. Willett, J. Schwartz, D. Sparrow, S. Weiss and H. Hu, "Relation of Nutrition to Bone Lead and Blood Lead Levels in Middle-Aged to Elderlymen. The Normative Aging Study," *American Journal of Epidemiology*, Vol. 147, No. 12, 1998, pp. 1162-1174. doi:10.1093/oxfordjournals.aje.a009415

[87]　T. W. Clarkson, "The Three Modern Faces of Mercury," *Environmental Health Perspectives*, Vol. 110, No. S1, 2002, pp. 11-23. doi:10.1289/ehp.02110s111

[88]　S. A. Counter and L. H. Buchanan, "Mercury Exposure in Children: A Review," *Toxicology and Applied Pharmacology*, Vol. 198, No. 2, 2004, pp. 209-230. doi:10.1016/j.taap.2003.11.032

[89]　I. Kosalec, J. Cvek and S. Tomic, "Contaminants of Medicinal Herbs and Herbal Products," *Archives of Industrial Hygiene and Toxicology*, Vol. 60, No. 4, 2009, pp. 485-501. doi:10.2478/10004-1254-60-2009-2005

[90]　US Centers for Disease Control and Prevention (CDC), "Third National Report on Human Exposure to Environmental Chemicals," 2005. www.cdc.gov/exposurereport/3rd/default.htm

[91]　Association of Toxic Substances and Disease Registry (ATSDR), "Toxicological Profile for Mercury (Update)," Department of Health and Human Services, Atlanta, 2006. http://www.atsdr.cdc.gov/toxprofiles/tp46.html

[92]　J. H. Roberts, "Metal Toxicity in Children, Training Manual on Pediatric Environmental Health: Putting It into Practice," 2005.

http://www.cehn.org/cehn/trainingmanual/manual-front.html

[93]　W. H. Miller, H. M. Schipper, J. S. Lee, J. Singer and S. Waxman, "Mechanisms of Action of Arsenic Trioxide," *Cancer Research*, Vol. 62, No. 14, 2002, pp. 3893-3903.

[94]　World Health Organization (WHO), "WHO Guidelines for Assessing Quality of Herbal Medicines with Reference to Contaminants and Residue," WHO, Geneva, 2007.

[95]　B. Liu, X. Lv, D. Wang, Y. Xu, L. Zhang and Y. Li, "Adsorption Behavior of As(III) onto Chitosan Resin with As(III) as Template Ions," *Journal of Applied Polymer Science*, Vol. 125, No. 1, 2012, pp. 246-253. doi:10.1002/app.35528

[96]　M. Vahter, "Health Effects of Early Life Exposure to Arsenic," *Basic & Clinical Pharmacology & Toxicology*, 102, No. 2, 2008, pp. 204-211. doi:10.1111/j.1742-7843.2007.00168.x

[97]　E. J. Tokar, W. Qu and M. P. Waalkes, "Arsenic, Stem Cells, and the Developmental Basis of Adult Cancer," *Toxicological Sciences*, Vol. 120, No. S1, 2011, pp. S192-S203. doi:10.1093/toxsci/kfq342

[98]　M. P. Waalkes and J. Liu, "Early-Life Arsenic Exposure: Methylation Capacity and Beyond," *Environmental Health Perspectives*, Vol. 116, No. 3, 2008, pp. A104-A104. doi:10.1289/ehp.11276

[99]　K. L. Huyck, M. L. Kile, G. Mahiuddin, Q. Quamruzzaman, M. Rahman, *et al.*, "Maternal Arsenic Exposure Associated with Low Birth Weight in Bangladesh," *Journal of Occupational and Environmental Medicine*, Vol. 49, No. 10, 2007, pp. 1097-1104. doi:10.1097/JOM.0b013e3181566ba0

[100]　R. Quansah and J. J. K. Jaakkola, "Paternal and Maternal Exposure to Welding Fumes and Metal Dusts or Fumes and Adverse Pregnancy Outcomes," *International Archives of Occupational and Environmental Health*, Vol. 82, No. 4, 2009, pp. 529-537. doi:10.1007/s00420-008-0349-6

[101]　J. Thompson and J. Bannigan, "Cadmium: Toxic Effects on the Reproductive System and the Embryo," *Reproductive Toxicology*, Vol. 25, No. 3, 2008, pp. 304-315. doi:10.1016/j.reprotox.2008.02.001

[102]　J. Liaw, G. Marshall, Y. Yuan, C. Ferreccio, C. Steinmaus, *et al.*, "Increased Childhood Liver Cancer Mortality and Arsenic in Drinking Water in Northern Chile," *Cancer Epidemiology Biomarkers & Prevention*, Vol. 17, No. 8, 2008, pp. 1982-1987. doi:10.1158/1055-9965.EPI-07-2816

[103]　J. Liu and M. P. Waalkes, "Liver Is a Target of Arsenic Carcinogenesis," *Toxicological Sciences*, Vol. 105, No. 1, 2008, pp. 24-32. doi:10.1093/toxsci/kfn120

[104]　A. Anzblau and R. Lilis, "Acute Arsenic Intoxication from Environmental Arsenic Exposure," *Archives of Environmental Health: An International Journal*, Vol. 44, No. 6, 1989, pp. 385-390. doi:10.1080/00039896.1989.9935912

[105]　W. H. Mielke and S. Zahran, "The Urban Rise and Fall of Air Lead (Pb) and the Latent Surge and Retreat of Societal Violence," *Environment International*, Vol. 43, 2012,

pp. 48-55. doi:10.1016/j.envint.2012.03.005

[106] J. A. Menezes-Filho, G. F. de S. Viana and C. R. Paes, "Determinants of Lead Exposure in Children on the Outskirts of Salvador, Brazil," *Environmental Monitoring and Assessment*, Vol. 184, No. 4, 2012, pp. 2593-2603. doi:10.1007/s10661-011-2137-0

[107] E. Nicholas, W. J. C. Pingitore Jr., A. M. A. Beata and M. J. J. Reynoso, "Urban Airborne Lead: X-Ray Absorption Spectroscopy Establishes Soil as Dominant Source," *The Smithsonian/NASA Astrophysics Data System*, Vol. 4, No. 4, 2009, p. e5019.

[108] L. Luo, B. Chu, Y. Li, T. Xu, X. Wang, J. Yuan, J. Sun, Y. Liu, Y. Bo, X. Zhan, S. Wang and L. Tang, "Determination of Pb, As, Cd and Trace Elements in Polluted Soils near a Lead-Zinc Mine Using Polarized X-Ray Fluorescence Spectrometry and the Characteristics of the Elemental Distribution in the Area," *X-Ray Spectrometry*, Vol. 41, No. 3, 2012, pp. 133-143. doi:10.1002/xrs.2364

[109] G. Z. Lin, F. Wu, C. H. Yan, K. Li and X. Y. Liu, "Childhood Lead Poisoning Associated with Traditional Chinese Medicine: A Case Report and the Subsequent Lead Source Inquiry," *Clinica Chimica Acta*, Vol. 413, No. 13-14, 2012, pp. 1156-1159. doi:10.1016/j.cca.2012.03.010

[110] H. Bae, "Reducing Environmental Risks by Information Disclosure: Evidence in Residential Lead Paint Disclosure Rule," *Journal of Policy Analysis and Management*, Vol. 31, No. 2, 2012, pp. 404-431. doi:10.1002/pam.21600

[111] F. Barbosa, C. D. Palmer, F. J. Krug, P. J. Parsons and J. Anal, "Determination of Total Mercury in Whole Blood by Flow Injection Cold Vapor Atomic Absorption Spectrometry with Room Temperature Digestion Using Tetramethylammonium Hydroxide," *Atomic Spectroscopy*, Vol. 19, No. 8, 2004, pp. 100-1005. doi:10.1039/b400315b

[112] S. Q. Tao, S. F. Gong, L. Xu and J. C. Fanguy, "Mercury Atomic Absorption by Mercury Atoms in Water Observed with a Liquid Core Waveguide as a Long Path Absorption Cell," *Analyst*, Vol. 129, No. 4, 2004, pp. 342-346. doi:10.1039/b400426d

[113] L. P. Yu and X. P. Yan, "Flow Injection On-Line Sorption Preconcentration Coupled with Cold Vapor Atomic Fluorescence Spectrometry and On-Line Oxidative Elution for the Determination of Trace Mercury in Water Samples," *Atomic Spectroscopy*, Vol. 25, No. 3, 2004, pp. 145-153.

[114] G. Centineo, E. B. Gonzalez and A. Sanz-Medel, "Multi-Elemental Speciation Analysis of Organometallic Compounds of Mercury, Lead and Tin in Natural Water Samples by Headspace-Solid Phase Microextraction Followed by Gas Chromatography-Mass Spectrometry," *Journal of Chromatography A*, Vol. 1034, No. 1-2, 2004, pp. 191-197. doi:10.1016/j.chroma.2004.01.051

[115] H. P. Chen, D. C. Paschal, D. T. Miller and J. D. C. Morrow, "Determination of Total and Inorganic Mercury in Whole Blood by On-Line Digestion with Flow Injection," *Atomic Spectroscopy*, Vol. 19, 1998, pp. 176-179.

[116] P. J. Parsons, C. D. Palmer, K. L. Caldwell and R. L. Jones, "Determination of Total Mercury in Urine by Inductively Coupled Plasma Mass Spectrometry (ICP-MS)," Royal Society of Chemistry, London, 2005.

[117] S. H. Rogers, N. Jeffery, S. Kieszak, P. Fritz, H. Spliethoff, D. Christopher, P. J. P. Parsons, E. Daniel, K. K. Caldwell, G. Eadon and C. Rubin, "Mercury Exposure in Young Children Living in New York City," *Journal of Urban Health: Bulletin of the New York Academy of Medicine*, Vol. 85, No. 1, 2007, pp. 39-51.

[118] W. B. Zhang, Z. F. Su, X. F. Chu and X. A. Yang, "Evaluation of a New Electrolytic Cold Vapor Generation System for Mercury Determination by AFS," *Talanta*, Vol. 80, No. 5, 2010, pp. 2106-2112. doi:10.1016/j.talanta.2009.11.016

[119] X. R. Wang, Z. X. Zhuang, D. H. Sun, J. X. Hong, X. H. Wu, F. S. C. Lee, F. S. C. Lee, M. S. Yang and H. W. Leung, "Trace Metals in Traditional Chinese Medicine: A Preliminary Study Using ICP-MS for Metal Determination and as Speciation," *Atomic Spectroscopy*, Vol. 20, No. 3, 1999, p. 86.

[120] S. Scholupov, S. Pogarev, V. Ryzhov, N. Mashyanov and A. Stroganov, "Zeeman Atomic Absorption Spectrometer RA-915+ for Direct Determination of Mercury in Air and Complex Matrix Samples," *Fuel Processing Technology*, Vol. 85, No. 6-7, 2004, pp. 473-485. doi:10.1016/j.fuproc.2003.11.003

[121] R. J. Huang, Z. X. Zhuang, R. F. Huang, X. R. Wang and F. S. C. Lee, "Direct Analysis of Mercury in Traditional Chinese Medicines Using Thermolysis Coupled with On-Line Atomic Absorption Spectrometry," *Talanta*, Vol. 68, No. 3, 2006, pp. 728-734. doi:10.1016/j.talanta.2005.05.014

[122] J. G. Tian, Y. Lu, J. G. Zhou, T. B. Gao, Q. T. Zheng and D. C. Chen, "The Powder X-Ray Diffraction Analysis of Mineral Drug Realgar with Its Associated Minerals," *Chinese Journal of Clinical Pharmacy*, No. 2, 1998, pp. 86-89.

[123] H. Jiang, Y. H. Zhang, J. H. Ding, S. T. Shi, P. Xue, S. Gao, H. Z. Gong and G. F. Sun, "Determination of As(III) Content in Realgar by HPLCHG-AFS," *Chemical Research*, Vol. 19, 2008, pp. 67-69.

[124] G. Li, Y. K. Cheng, C. G. Huang, K. R. Li and Q. A. Wu, "Analysis on the Mineral Chinese Medicine Realgar," *Nanjing Shidan Xue Bao (Natural Science Edition)*, Vol. 31, 2008, pp. 63-67.

[125] L. W. Zhang, Y. H. Xie, S. L. Dong, Y. Y. Zhang and G. H. Su, "Researches on Arsenic and Its Appearance Analysis in Chinese Medicines (Review)," *Clinical Pharmacy*, Vol. 11, 2008, pp. 578-581.

[126] S. Latva, M. Hurtta, S. Peraniemi and M. Ahlgren, "Separation of Arsenic Species in Aqueous Solutions and Optimization of Determination by Graphite Furnace Atomic Absorption Spectrometry," *Analytica Chimica Acta*, Vol. 418, No. 1, 2000, pp. 11-17. doi:10.1016/S0003-2670(00)00947-8

[127] J. Dedina and D. L. Tsalev, "Hydride Generation Atomic Absorption Spectrometry," Wiley, Chichester, 1995.

[128] P. Carrero, A. Malave, J. L. Burguera, M. Burguera and C. Rondon, "Determination of Various Arsenic Species by

Flow Injection Hydride Generation Atomic Absorption Spectrometry: Investigation of the Effects of the Acid Concentration of Different Reaction Media on the Generation of Arsines," *Analytica Chimica Acta*, Vol. 438, No. 1-2, 2001, pp. 195-204. doi:10.1016/S0003-2670(01)00796-6

[129] W. E. Gan, W. B. Zhang and X. Q. Lin, "Electrochemical Hydride Generation Atomic Fluorescence Spectrometry for the Simultaneous Determination of Arsenic and Antimony in Chinese Medicine Samples," *Analytica Chimica Acta*, Vol. 539, No. 1-2, 2005, pp. 335-340. doi:10.1016/j.aca.2005.03.050

[130] H. M. Anawara, "Arsenic Speciation in Environmental Samples by Hydride Generation and Electrothermal Atomic Absorption Spectrometry," *Talanta*, Vol. 88, No. 28, 2012, pp. 30-42. doi:10.1016/j.talanta.2011.11.068

[131] G. Pearson and G. Greenway, "A Highly Efficient Sample Introduction System for Interfacing Microfluidic Chips with ICP-MS," *Journal of Analytical Atomic Spectrometry*, Vol. 22, No. 6, 2007, pp. 657-662. doi:10.1039/b702624b

[132] X. D. Tian, Z. X. Zhuang, B. Chen and X. R. Wang, "Movable Reduction Bed Hydride Generation System as an Interface for Capillary Zone Electrophoresis and Inductively Coupled Plasma Atomic Emission Spectrometry for Arsenic Speciation Analysis," *Analyst*, Vol. 123, No. 5, 1998, pp. 899-903. doi:10.1039/a707452b

[133] Y. Liu and V. Lopez-Avila, "On-Line Microwave-Induced Helium Plasma Atomic Emission Detection for Capillary Zone Electrophoresis," *Journal of High Resolution Chromatography*, Vol. 16, No. 12, 1993, pp. 717-720. doi:10.1002/jhrc.1240161209

[134] H. Matusiewicz and M. Ślachciński, "Method Development for Simultaneous Multielement Determination of Hydride Forming Elements (As, Bi, Ge, Sb, Se, Sn) and Hg by Microwave Induced Plasma-Optical Emission Spectrometry Using Integrated Continuous-Microflow Ultrasonic Nebulizer-Hydride Generator Sample Intro-

duction System," *Microchemical Journal*, Vol. 95, No. 2, 2010, pp. 213-221. doi:10.1016/j.microc.2009.12.004

[135] H. Matusiewicz and B. Golik, "Determination of Major and Trace Elements in Biological Materials by Microwave Induced Plasma Optical Emission Spectrometry (MIP-OES) Following Tetramethylammonium Hydroxide (TMAH) Solubilization," *Microchemical Journal*, Vol. 76, No. 1-2, 2004, pp. 23-29. doi:10.1016/j.microc.2003.10.007

[136] K. Jankowski and A. Jackowska, "Spectroscopic Diagnostics for Evaluation of the Analytical Potential of Argon + Heliummicrowave-Induced Plasma with Solution Nebulization," *Journal of Analytical Atomic Spectrometry*, Vol. 22, No. 9, 2007, pp. 1076-1082. doi:10.1039/b705288j

[137] H. Matusiewicz and M. Ślachciński, "Development of a New Hybrid Technique for Inorganic Arsenic Speciation Analysis by Microchip Capillary Electrophoresis Coupled with Hydride Generation Microwave Induced Plasma Spectrometry," *Microchemical Journal*, Vol. 102, 2012, pp. 61-67.

[138] Q. J. Song, G. M. Greenway and T. McCreedy, "Interfacing a Microfluidic Electrophoresis Chip with Inductively Coupled Plasma Mass Spectrometry for Rapid Elemental Speciation," *Journal of Analytical Atomic Spectrometry*, Vol. 19, No. 7, 2004, pp. 883-887. doi:10.1039/b401657b

[139] H. Matusiewicz and M. Ślachciński, "Interfacing a Microchip-Based Capillary Electrophoresis System with a Microwave Induced Plasma Spectrometry for Copper Speciation," *Central European Journal of Chemistry*, Vol. 9, No. 5, 2011, pp. 896-903. doi:10.2478/s11532-011-0079-6

[140] H. Matusiewicz and M. Ślachciński, "Interfacing a Microchip-Based Capillary Electrophoresis System with a Microwave Induced Plasma Spectrometry for Copper Speciation," *Central European Journal of Chemistry*, Vol. 9, No. 5, 2011, pp. 896-903.

17

Studies on the Degranulation of RBL-2H3 Cells Induced by Traditional Chinese Medicine Injections[*]

Jia-Ming Tang[#], Jiong Liu, Wenbin Wu

Laboratory Animal Center, Shanghai University of Traditional Chinese Medicine, Shanghai, China

Email: tangjiaming@hotmail.com

ABSTRACT

Aims: To study RBL-2H3 cell degranulation phenomena induced by some TCMIs through cell morphological and ultra-structural observation, released enzyme activity and establish RBL-2H3 cell degranulation test indicated by β-hexosaminidase activity as a method to evaluate TCMIs at nonclinical stage. **Methods:** RBL-2H3 cells were used to study the degranulation by co-culture with positive control C48/80 and some TCMIs through morphological and ultra-structure observation, β-hexosaminidase activity detection. RBL-2H3 cell degranulation test was established to detect β-hexosaminidase activity caused by 17 kinds of TCMIs and their ingredients. The cytotoxicity effect of some TCMIs on both RBL 2H3 and BRL cells was measured by CCK-8 assay. **Results:** Toluidine blue staining and ultra-structure of electronic microscope observation of treated RBL-2H3 cells showed degranulation morphologically. Detection of β-hexosaminidase activity in the supernatant of treated cells showed some TCMIs had elevated enzyme release rates. Further analysis of the ingredients and compound in Tanreqing injection and Shengmai injection showed Scutellaria baicalensis Georgi in Tanreqing injection, Red ginseng and Fructus Schisandrae Chinensis in Shengmai injection were responsible to the degranulation of RBL-2H3 cells. Osmotic pressures and pH influenced RBL-2H3 degranulation. High Osmotic pressure of Tanreqing injection and low pH of chlorogenic acid at 2.5 and 5.0 mmol/L congcentration might be responsible to high β-hexosaminidase activity. Most of the TCMIs inducing degranulation had cytotoxicity effect for both RBL-2H3 and BRL cells, but some TCMIs inducing degranulation had no cytotoxicity effect. **Conclusion:** Some TCMIs can induce degranulation of RBL-2H3 cells; RBL-2H3 cell degranulation test can be used in non-clinical stage to detect the risk causing anaphylactoid reactions. Osmotic pressures and pH influenced RBL-2H3 degranulation, and they should be measured before testing. The mechanism of degranulation caused by some TCMIs is cytotoxic, and some are non-cytotoxic and may be through exicytosis.

Keywords: Traditional Chinese Medicine Injection (TCMI); RBL-2H3 Cells; Degranulation; β-Hexosaminidase; Anaphylactoid Reaction

1. Introduction

In recent years, with the widespread use of Traditional Chinese Medicine injections (TCMIs), the adverse reactions reported increased gradually [1,2]. Adverse reactions may be caused by many reasons, but allergic reactions are generally considered to be more frequent, more harmful side effects. Based on clinical reports analysis, some cases of the allergic reactions may actually belong to the class of anaphylactoid reactions. The clinical symptoms of both Type I allergic reactions and anaphylactoid reactions are similar and related to the mast cell (MC) degranulation, and MCs are the final effector cells of type I allergic reactions and anaphylactoid reactions. An important mechanism differentiating anaphylactoid reactions from allergic reactions is that in the former with no immune system involved, and the drugs directly stimulate MCs or basophils to degranulate, or activate the complement bypass through MBL pathway, producing C3a and C4a *in vivo*, the latter stimulate MCs or basophils to degranulate and release some bioactive media, such as histamine and leukotriene, causing systemic or local pathophysiological reaction, such as allergic shock, bronchospasm and skin rash *et al.* [3,4].

Currently the detection techniques and methods of immunotoxicity safety evaluations for TCMIs are based on "Technical Guidelines for Studies of Chinese Medicine & Natural Drug Immunotoxicity (Allergic and light allergic reaction) [5]". There is no specific detection techniques and methods available to evaluate anaphylactoid reactions caused by TCMIs in non-clinical stage. But recent

[*]Author contribution: Prof. Tang Jiaming designed and wrote the paper Liu Jiong performed the experiments and analyzed the results statistically.

[#]Correspondence author.

reports showed that some TCMIs and their cosolvent (Tween 80) can cause degranulation of RBL-2H3 cells *in vitro* [6,7] and mast cells *in vivo* [8].

In this study, in order to establish techniques and methods for detecting anaphylactoid reactions, we investigated RBL-2H3 cell degranulation phenomena induced by some TCMIs through cell morphological and ultrastructural observation, released enzyme activity detection, and established the RBL-2H3 cell degranulation test to detect β-hexosaminidase activity induced by some TCMI, then discussing the degranulation mechanism and some influence factors related to this test.

2. Materials and Methods

2.1. Cells

RBL-2H3 cell line (Wistar rat basophilic leukemia cell line), and BRL cell line (Buffalo rat liver cells) were purchased from the cell bank of the Chinese Academy of Sciences. RBL-2H3 cell line was cultured in MEM medium containing 10% fetal calf serum and 100 U/ml penicillin and 100 ug/ml streptomycin, and BRL cell line was cultured in high glucose DMEM medium containing 15% fetal calf serum and 100 U/ml penicillin and 100 ug/ml streptomycin. The 2 cell lines were incubated in a humidified incubator at 37°C, 5% CO_2. When the cells covered approximately 80% of the bottom area of culture flask, passage could be done by ratio of 1:3.

2.2. Reagents

The positive control chemical C48/80 (Compound 48/80) was purchased from Sigma Company, and diluted with sterilized normal saline to 1mg/ml as stock solution. Tyrode's buffer (pH 7.4, NaCl 7.5972 g, $MgCl_2$ 0.2033 g, KCl 0.3728 g, $CaCl_2$ 0.1554 g, glucose 1.0 g, dissolved in 1000 ml distilled water). Cell Counting kit (CCK-8, Japan Institute of Chemistry Colleagues). β-hexosaminidase substrate (1 mmol/L 4-nitroPhenyl-N-acetyl-β-D-glucosaminide diluted with 0.05 mol/L citrate buffer, pH 4.5), purchased from sigma company. Reaction stop solution (100 mmol/L Na_2CO_3, 100 mmol/L $NaHCO_3$ buffer, pH 10.7). 17 kinds of Traditional Chinese Medicine Injections (TCMI) were obtained from Shanghai institute for food and drug control, which included Ciwujia injection, Danhong injection, Danshen injection, Danxiangguanxin injection, Dengzhanhua injection, Gualoupi injection, Guanxinning injection, Huangqi injection, Mailuoning injection, Qingkailing injection, Shengmai injection, Shenmai injection, Shuxuening injection, Tanreqing injection, Xiangdan injection, Yinxing injection and Yinzhihuang injection. The 8 kind ingredients of TCMI were kindly given by manufacturer. Chlorogenic acid was purchased from National Institutes

for Food and Drug Control.

2.3. Morphological Study by Toluidine Blue Staining

RBL-2H3 cells (1×10^5/well) in 48-well plates after 24 h culture were washed with HBSS(GIBCO), and divided into 4 groups: negative control group, positive control group, TCMI group and total enzyme activity group, 5 wells for each group. TCMI group was cultured by adding 500 μl of diluted TCMIs, negative group by adding an equal volume of Tyrode's buffer, positive control group by adding an equal volume of C48/80 solution, the total enzyme group by adding an equal volume of 10% Triton X-100 at 37°C for 1 h for interaction with cells, then the supernatant was taken into sterile 1.5 ml eppendorf tube. After centrifuging at 2000 r/min for 10 min, the supernatant was drawn for β-hexosaminidase activity assay, and the remaining cells in 48-well plates were used for staining with toluidine blue. The cells in the wells were fixed by adding 200 μl of 100% methanol for 30 min, then discarded the fixative, stained with 200 μl of 0.5% of toluidine blue dye for 30 - 45 min, the stained cells were observed under microscope.

2.4. Ultra-Structural Study by Electronic Microscope Observation

RBL-2H3 cells in 25 cm^2 culture flask (3.0×10^6/flask) after 24 h culture were washed three times with Tyrode's buffer. The flasks were divided into the negative control group, positive control group (C48/80, 50 μg/ml) and Qingkailing group (1:5 diluted), then drugs were added and incubated at 37°C for 1 h. The culture flasks were washed three times with Tyrode's buffer, and cells were collected by scraping cells with a rubber scraper into 1.5 ml eppendorf tube, centrifugated at 2000 r/min for 8 min. Then, the cell pellets were fixed in 2.5% glutaraldehyde solution followed by osmium tetroxide, embedded in Araldite, cut into ultra-thin slices, stained with Lead citrate and uranyl acetate. The ultra-thin slices were examined under electron microscope.

2.5. β-Hexosaminidase and Tryptase Activity Assays

For detecting β-hexosaminidase activity, 100 μl of the supernatant of each group was added into 96-well plate, plus 100 μl of substrate, 5 wells for each test solution, plus 5 wells for the background solution. The mixture was incubated at 37°C for 90 min, then 150 μl of stop solution was added to stop the reaction. The absorbance at 405 nm (*OD*) of each well was measured. The percentage of enzyme release was calculated using the following formula:

β-hexosaminidase release rate$(\%)$

$$= \frac{OD_{\text{supernatant}} - OD_{\text{background}}}{OD_{\text{Triton}\,X-100} - OD_{\text{blank}}} \times 100\%$$

For detecting tryptase activity, 100 μl of the supernatant of each group was added into 96-well plate, plus 30 μl of 0.1 mol/L Tris-HCl (pH 7.4), 20 μl of BAPNA substrate, The mixture was incubated at 37°C for 30 min, then add 50 μl of 30% acetic acid to terminate the reaction. The absorbance at 405 nm (OD) of each well was measured. Trypsin was used as standard for standard curve.

tryptase release rate$(\%)$

$$= \frac{OD_{\text{supernatant}} - OD_{\text{background}}}{OD_{\text{trypsin}} - OD_{\text{blank}}} \times 100\%$$

2.6. Measurement of IC50 of TCMIs on RBL-2H3 and BRL Cells by CCK-8 Assay

RBL-2H3 and BRL cells were seeded at 4×10^4/well in 96-well plate (100 μl/well). After 24 h culture, the wells were divided into blank group, negative control group, C48/80 group (80, 50, 30, 10, 8, 5, 2.5 μg/ml) and TCMI group (dilution 1:2, 1:4, 1:8, 1:16, 1:32, 1:64, 1:128), 5 wells for each group. TCMI group was cultured by adding diluted TCMI 100 μl, negative group and blank group by adding an equal volume of Tyrode's buffer, C48/80 group by adding an equal volume of C48/80 solution at 37°C for 1 h for interaction with cells, abandoned the supernatant, then added 100 μl of 10% CCK-8 reagent diluted with Tyrode's buffer containing 5% fetal bovine serum, continued to incubate at 37°C for 1 h. The OD values were measured with the microplate reader at absorbance 450 nm.

Inhibition rate calculated$(\%)$

$$= \frac{1 - \text{drug group }OD}{\text{control }OD} \times 100\%$$

and calculated IC_{50} by using GraphPad Prism 5.0 version (IC_{50} expressed as the reciprocal dilution).

2.7. Measurement of Osmotic Pressure Values and pH Values of Testing Samples

Measurement of osmotic pressure of testing samples was taken by using Fiske^R Mocro-osmometer, the results were recorded as mOsm/kg, and measurement of pH values was taken by using pH-meter.

2.8. Statistical Analysis

All data were reported as means ± standard deviation (SD). Statistical significance was analyzed using one way ANOVA. Values of $P < 0.05$ were considered statistically significant.

3. Results

3.1. Morphological Observations on the Degranulation of RBL-2H3 Cells Induced by TCMIs

3.1.1. Toluidine Blue Staining

RBL-2H3 cells in negative control stained with toluidine blue were shown pleomorphic or spindle-shaped, full cytoplasm dyed deep blue, with clearly visible nucleus. While in C48/80 group, after contacting with drugs for 1 h, the normal spindle cells became round cells or tadpole-shaped cells, with cytoplasm disappeared; in Qingkailing group though still showing as spindle cells, but the cytoplasm of all cells was lightly stained, some cells were vacuolated (**Figure 1**). The different degrees of morphological degranulation also could be seen in some other TCMIs, such as Shenmai injection, Tanreqing Injection, and Yinxing injection.

3.1.2. Ultra-Structural Changes

Under electron microscopy, it was found that the normal RBL-2H3 cells differed in size, with cell membranes intact and many microvilli on them. In the cytoplasm were full of dense granules varying in size and density and some expanded endoplasmic reticulums, and nucleuses were lobulated. In cells treated with C48/80, most of the membrane microvilli disappeared, with the membrane inward hollow. The granules in the cytoplasm reduced significantly, and cell endoplasmic reticulum extreme expanded, showing vacuolated. In Qingkailing injection treated cells, the membrane microvilli disappeared, and the granules in the cytoplasm reduced, with the membrane

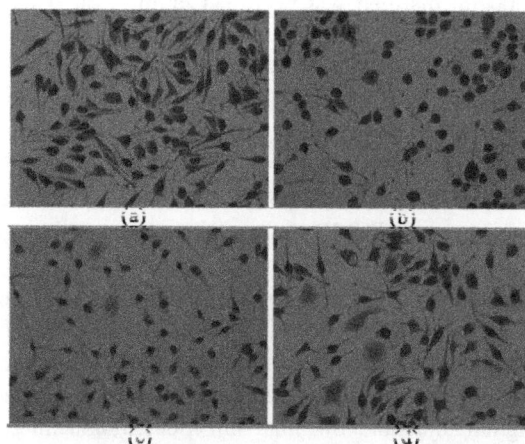

Figure 1. (a) normalRBL-2H3 cells; **(b)** RBL-2H3 cells treated with C48/80; **(c)** RBL-2H3 cells treated with Qingkailing injection; **(d)** RBL-2H3 cells treated with Shengmai injection. Magnification: ×200.

uncomplete and inward hollow, endoplasmic reticulum extreme expanded, vesicles and vacuole shape structure increasing, showing typical characteristics of degranulation (**Figure 2**).

3.2. β-Hexosaminidase and Tryptase Release Rates Induced by C48/80

Induced by C48/80 at different concentrations (1.25, 2.5, 5, 10, 20 mg/ml) and different time (15, 30, 45, 60 min), the changes of β-hexosaminidase and tryptase release rates from RBL-2H3 were shown in **Figure 3**. When C48/80 concentration was at 10 - 20 mg/ml, and reaction time in 45 - 60 min, β-hexosaminidase release rates were relatively high, while no tryptase activity was shown in this test system, therefore 60 min reaction time for detecting β-hexosaminidase activity was chosen duration experiment thereafter.

3.3. β-Hexosaminidase Release Rate Induced by TCMIs

With the dilution of 1:10 and 1:20, 17 kings of TCMIs reacted with RBL-2H3 cells respectively for 1 h, then β-hexosaminidase activity in supernatant was determined. As shown in **Table 1**, the β-hexosaminidase release rate in control group was about 10%, while the release rate in positive control reached to 27%. The effects of 17 kinds of TCMIs on inducing RBL-2H3 cells to release β-hexosaminidase were quite different, the degranulations of induced RBL-2H3 cells were stronger in Shenmai injection, Yinxing injection, Guanxinning injection, Tanreqing injection, Dengzhanhua injection, Qingkailing injection, shengmai injection and Mailuoning injection,

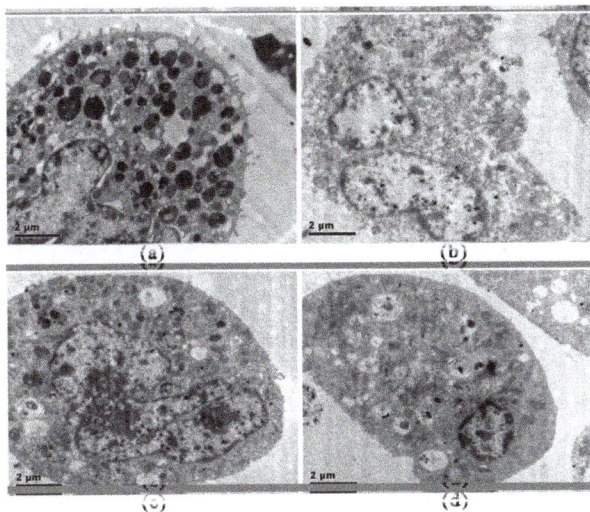

Figure 2. (a) normal RBL-2H3 cell; (b) RBL-2H3 cells treated with C48/80; (c) RBL-2H3 cells treated with Qingkailing injection; (d) RBL-2H3 cells treated with Qingkailing injection, showing uncomplete and inward hollow membrane.

Table 1. β-hexosaminidase release rate of RBL-2H3 cells induced by some TCMIs $(\bar{x} \pm s)$.

TCMIs	n	β-hexosaminidase release rate (%)	
		1:10	1:20
Control	5	9.96 ± 2.74	
C$_{48/80}$ (20 μg/ml)	5	26.71 ± 21.93	
Ciwujia injection	5	10.03 ± 8.31	14.76 ± 7.02
Danhong injection	5	8.26 ± 3.21	8.80 ± 4.22
Danshen injection	5	−9.55 ± 21.70	4.70 ± 12.75
Danxiangguanxin injection	5	−47.52 ± 2.67	−43.15 ± 0.35
Dengzhanhua injection	5	32.37 ± 18.42	22.58 ± 12.96
Gualoupi injection	5	9.57 ± 4.86	8.70 ± 9.10
Guanxinning injection	5	29.49 ± 10.23	31.65 ± 4.47
Huangqi injection	5	0.53 ± 0.22	1.36 ± 0.13
Mailuoning injection	5	61.21 ± 3.47[*]	66.15 ± 3.44[*]
Qingkailing injection	5	58.90 ± 11.60[*]	13.13 ± 22.02
Shengmai injection	5	24.11 ± 9.51	20.33 ± 8.65
Shenmai injection	5	45.04 ± 2.97[*]	44.71 ± 2.58[*]
Shuxuening injection	5	−9.81 ± 8.23	6.18 ± 3.52
Tanreqing injection	5	64.11 ± 32.34[*]	66.34 ± 7.52[*]
Xiangdan injection	5	11.70 ± 1.74	12.12 ± 3.31
Yinxing injection	5	81.37 ± 16.13[*]	77.90 ± 7.86[*]
Yinzhihuang injection	5	12.91 ± 1.09	11.12 ± 3.47

Note: compared with negative control, [*]$P < 0.05$.

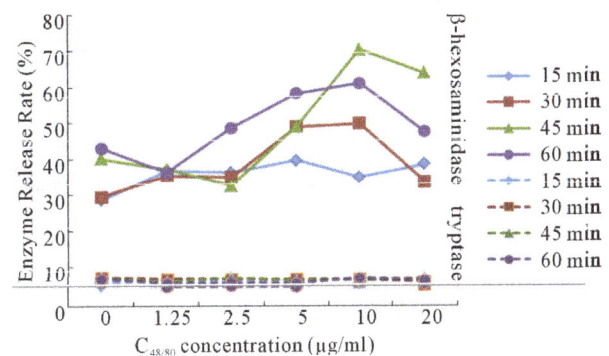

Figure 3. β-hexosaminidase release rates induced by C48/80.

the release rates in all of them were over 20%. Compared with the negative control, the release rates in most of them were statistically significant difference ($P < 0.05$), while the release rates in Huangqi injection, Danxiangguanxin injection, Danshen injection, Xiangdan injection, Ciwujia injection, Shuxuening injection, Yinzhihuang Injection, Danhong injection and Gualoupi injection were below 20%, and there were no statistically different when compared with negative control.

3.4. β-Hexosaminidase Release Rates Induced by Each Ingredients of Tanreqing Injection and Shengmai Injection

Each ingredient of Tanreqing injection and Shengmai injection (the final dilutions were equal to 1:10 and 1:20 of each injection) was taken to react with RBL-2H3 cells for 1 h, then the release rates of β-hexosaminidase in supernatant were determined. As shown in **Table 2**, the ingredients Scutellaria baicalensis of Tanreqing injection, and the ingredients Red ginseng and Schisandra Chinensis of Shengmai injection could induce the degranulationof RBL-2H3 cells obviously, the release rates were over 20%, and had significant statistically when compared with the negative control.

3.5. The Cytotoxicity Effect of 17 Kinds of TCMIs on RBL-2H3 and BRL Cells

The values of half inhibitory concentration (IC_{50}) of 17 kinds of TCMIs were determined on RBL-2H3 and BRL cells by CCK-8, the results expressed by the reciprocal of

Table 2. The effect of ingredients on the release rates of β-hexosaminidase of RBL-2H3 cells.

Group	n	β-hexosaminidase release rates (%)	
		1:10	1:20
Control	5	10.02 ± 3.48	
$C_{48/80}$ (20 µg/ml)	5	28.81 ± 8.80	
Tanreqing's ingredients			
Beer gall powder	5	6.54 ± 9.32	1.35 ± 0.61
Honeysuckle	5	7.08 ± 2.04	9.24 ± 1.39
Goat horn	5	6.07 ± 4.52	15.47 ± 13.75
Scutellaria baicalensis Georgi	5	$71.01 \pm 36.27^*$	42.82 ± 37.94
Weeping forsythia	5	2.08 ± 1.02	4.23 ± 1.84
Shengmai's ingredients			
Fructus Schisandrae Chinensis	5	34.34 ± 4.25	37.71 ± 9.61
Ophiopogon japonicus	5	6.87 ± 3.87	3.25 ± 1.66
Red ginseng	5	32.43 ± 18.05	22.36 ± 3.81

Note: compared with negative control, $^*P < 0.05$.

dilution (**Table 3**). If the $IC_{50} \leq 0.1$ (1:10 dilution) is determined as cytotoxic, then the 5 kinds of TCMIs, Xiangdan, Mailuoning, Guanxinning, Tanreqing and Qingkailing, had toxicity on both RBL-2H3 and BRL cells. However, the toxicity (IC_{50}) on RBL-2H3 cells was relatively stronger than that on BRL cells, indicating that these 5 kinds of TCM injections inducing RBL-2H3 cell degranulation is in part due to cytotoxicity. The Yinxing injection had no toxicity on both RBL-2H3 and BRL cells, but the release rate of β-hexosaminidase was high, suggesting that Yinxing injection induce RBL-2H3 cell degranulation by non-cytotoxic way.

3.6. Correlation Analysis on IC50 Values between RBL-2H3 and BRL Cells

The correlation analysis has been done on IC_{50} values of 17 kinds of TCM injections, and the $|r|$ value is about 0.61, suggesting that a little cytotoxicity correlation exists between the two cell lines.

Table 3. The IC50 values of RBL-2H3 and BRL cells caused by some TCM injections.

TCMIs	Degranulation*	IC_{50}	
		RBL-2H3	BRL
Ciwujia injection	—	>0.5	0.72
Danhong injection	—	0.2	0.25
Danshen injection	—	0.12	0.13
Danxiangguanxin injection	—	0.24	0.12
Dengzhanhua injection	+	>0.5	>0.5
Gualoupi injection	—	0.16	>0.5
Guanxinning injection	+	0.006	0.07
Huangqi injection	—	0.16	>0.5
Mailuoning injection	+++	0.05	0.05
Qingkailing injection	++	0.03	0.05
Shengmai injection	+	>0.5	>0.5
Shenmai injection	++	0.002	>0.5
Shuxuening injection	—	>0.5	0.38
Tanreqing injection	+++	0.008	0.03
Xiangdan injection	—	0.04	0.1
Yinxing injection	++++	>0.5	>0.5
Yinzhihuang injection	—	0.17	0.7

Note: $^+$indicates the release rates of β-hexosaminidase between 21% - 40%; $^{++}$between 41% - 60%, $^{+++}$between 61% - 80%, $^{++++}$higher than 81%.

3.7. Measurement of Osmotic Pressures and pH Values of 17 Kinds of TCMIs

In order to exclude the influence of some factors on the release rate of β-hexosaminidase, the osmotic pressures and pH values of 15 kinds of TCMIs was measured. The results showed that the osmotic pressures of the most of the TCMI samples were within the normal range (290 mOsm·kg^{-1} ± 20%), while the osmotic pressures of Tanreqing injection was 45% higher than that of normal saline (**Table 4**), which showed high release rate of β-hexosaminidase, indicating that high osmotic pressure of testing sample may destroy RBL-2H3 cells, thus releasing the enzyme.

3.8. Measurement of β-Hexosaminidase Release Rates, Osmotic Pressures and pH Values of Chlorogenic Acid

The different concentrations of chlorogenic acid were

Table 4. Relation between osmotic pressure, pH and release rates of β-hexosaminidase.

TCMIs (dilution 1:10)	Osmotic pressure (mOsm/kg)*	pH	β-hexosaminidase release rate**
Ciwujia injection	258$^{(-)}$	5.2	–
Danshen injection	217$^{(--)}$	5.05	–
Dengzhanhua injection	286	ND	+
Huangqi injection	274	6.65	–
Danhong injection	259$^{(-)}$	5.37	–
Danxiangguanxin injection	300	ND	–
Gualoupi injection	245$^{(-)}$	5.91	–
Guanxinning injection	286	5.75	+
Mailuoning injection	ND	ND	+++
Qingkailing injection	298	7.07	++
Shenmai injection	233$^{(-)}$	5.44	++
Shengmai injection	270	6.71	+
Shuxuening injection	347$^{(+)}$	5.35	–
Tanreqing injection	419$^{(++++)}$	7.17	+++
Yinzhihuang injection	248$^{(-)}$	5.76	–
Normal saline	291	7.10	ND
Tyrode's buffer	283	7.14	–

Note: * "+" or "–" indicates the Osmotic pressure is higher or lower than 10% of normal saline. ** "+" indicates the release rates of β-hexosaminidase between 21%-40%, "++" between 41%-60%, "+++" between 61%-80%, "++++" higher than 81%. ND: not done.

taken to react with RBL-2H3 cells for 1 h, then the release rates of β-hexosaminidase in supernatant were determined. As shown in **Table 5**, the release rates of β-hexosaminidase in supernatant rised as the concentrations of chlorogenic acid increased. There were significant statistically in 2.5 and 5.0 mmol/L group, but when the concentration of chlorogenic acid reach 10 mmol/L, the release rate drop sharply.

The osmotic pressures of different concentrations of Chlorogenic acid was almost the same, but the pH values was very low, and decreased as the concentration increased.

3.9. Influence of Sample pH on the Release Rate of β-Hexosaminidase

In order to explore whether the low pH could cause degranulation of RBL-2H3, we adjust the pH values of Tyrode's buffer to 2.5, 3.0, 3.5, 4.0, 4.5, 5.0, 5.5, 6.0, 6.5, 7.0 respectively as test samples. The results showed that when the pH of test sample between 3.0 and 3.5, the release rate of β-hexosaminidase increase to above 50%, then drop to 10% at pH 4.0 afterward (**Figure 4**).

3.10. Comparison of Chlorogenic Acid Samples between pH Unadjusted and pH Adjusted to 7.0

Chlorogenic acid was diluted to the concentration of

Table 5. The relation between osmotic pressure, pH and release rates of β-hexosaminidase.

Chlorogenic acid	Osmotic pressure (mOsm/kg)*	pH	β-hexosaminidase release rate**
0.63 mmol·L^{-1}	285	3.74	25.23 ± 2.87
1.25 mmol·L^{-1}	285	3.55	–40.19 ± 4.54
2.5 mmol·L^{-1}	283	3.34	53.45 ± 4.27
5.0 mmol·L^{-1}	285	3.15	40.74 ± 6.77
10.0 mmol·L^{-1}	285	2.92	–29.82 ± 8.14

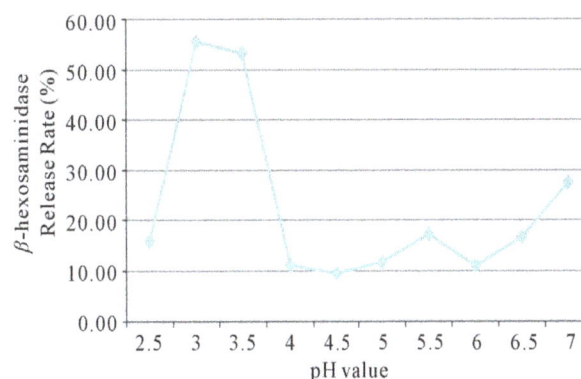

Figure 4. A model of RBL-2H3 degranulation caused by different pH values of Tyrode's buffer.

0.625, 1.25, 2.5, 5.0 and 10 mmol/L, which included pH unadjusted and pH adjusted to 7.0 in each concentration, then cocultured with RBL-2H3 cells. The results showed that all the pH adjusted chlorogenic acid did not cause β-hexosaminidase release, while chlorogenic acid at 2.5 and 5.0 mmol/L which pH were not adjusted showed high β-hexosaminidase release rate above 40%, at which concentration, the pH values were 3.34 and 3.15 (**Figure 5**), indicating that RBL-2H3 cell degranulation is not caused by chlorogenic acid, but by low pH.

4. Discussion

TCMIs are a new type of preparation (including solution type and powder type) made from single or multi-ingredients Chinese drugs or natural drugs by using modern science and technology. It can be used clinically by intramuscular injection, intravenous injection or infusion, point injection and other routes of administration into the body to treat certain diseases. Because this new preparation has the advantages of rapid effecting, stronger efficacy, and easy to use, applying traditional Chinese medicine to the field of clinical emergency and severe cases become a reality. This has important theoretical and practical significance for the development of traditional Chinese medicine.

However, TCMIs also appear likely to endanger their survival and development problem. That is, in the clinical practice, some adverse reactions occur, and even endanger the lives of patients, while in preclinical safety evaluation almost all TCMIs have been found no significant positive results by using authorized routine methods.

From the reports of "Adverse Drug Reaction Information Bulletin" published by SFDA, many cases showed adverse events with TCMIs at the first time treated. Some scholars have noted the relationship between adverse reaction and TCMIs, and try to establish some methods as indicators to detect anaphylactoid reactions *in vitro* and *in vivo*, and to clarify the mechanism of anaphylactoid reactions caused by TCMIs. It was reported that several TCMIs could cause RBL-2H3 cell significant

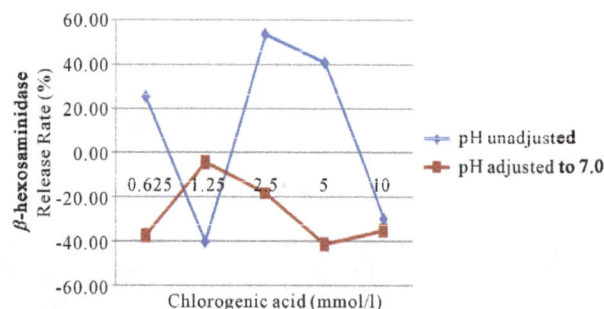

Figure 5. Comparison of chlorogenic acid samples between pH unadjusted and pH adjusted to 7.0.

degranulation *in vitro*, and increase the level of β-hexosaminidase in supernatant [6,7]. ZHANG *et al.* found that cosolvent Tween-80 and RBL-2H3 cell line co-culture *in vitro* could be result in RBL-2H3 degranulation, and there was a clear dose-effect relationship [9]. Therefore, it is essential to establish reliable, stable, and sensible methods as indicators to evaluate the potential anaphylactoid reaction caused by TCMIs in non-clinical stage.

Our results show that some TCMIs do cause degranulation of RBL-2H3 cells by the evidences of cell morphological examination (toluidine blue staining) and ultra-structral observation (electronic microscope observation) , but it is difficult to quantificat the results and to be objective endpoint by toluidine blue staining, and the electronic microscope observation cannot used as routine examination.

Detecting the bio-active materials released from mast cells or basophiles, such as histamine, leukotriene, β-hexosaminidase and tryptase, is common methods for allergic reactions and anaphylactoid reactions. Our results show that β-hexosaminidase activity is a good indicator for RBL-2H3 degranulation, because this method is simple, stable, and reproducible. Although the color of some TCMIs may interfere with the results, it can be solved by adding background controls. We found little tryptase activity in the supernatant could be detected, which may be attributed to the lower enzyme activity in the granules of RBL-2H3 cells themselves. Therefore, the tryptase activity does not a sensitive indicator for detecting RBL-2H3 cell degranulation.

Our results shown that some TCMIs could induce RBL-2H3 degranulation by detecting β-hexosaminidase activity, while others not. Calculated according to the release rate, Yinxing injection, Tanreqing injection, and Mailuoning injection were considered as the strong inducer, and Qingkailing Injection, Shenmai injection as medium, while Guanxinning injection and Shengmai injection as weak inducer. The other 10 kinds of TCMIs could not induce RBL-2H3 degranulation.

To further explore which ingredient caused RBL-2H3 degranulation, we used each ingredient of Tanreqing injection and Shengmai injection to detect their effect on RBL-2H3 cell degranulation. It was found that among the 5 kind ingredients in Tanreqing injection, only Scutellaria baicalensis Georgi was the strong inducers, while the other 4 ingredients were not; among the 3 kind ingredients in Shengmai injection, red ginseng and Fructus Schisandrae Chinensis were the weak inducers, while Ophiopogon japonicus was not, suggesting this method can be used for analyze which ingredients induce RBL-2H3 cell degranulation.

The results of RBL-2H3 cell degranulation test can be interfered with the physical-chemical characteristics of tested samples, such as osmotic pressure and pH. In most of the TCMIs osmotic pressure and pH have been adjusted to allowable value range before marketing. In the testing system, after dilution, the osmotic pressure and pH values of test samples were within the normal ranges, but in this study Tanreqing injection was found that its osmotic pressure value was as high as 419 mOsm/kg, about 44.5% higher than normal osmotic pressure. Therefore its high osmotic pressure was regarded to be the cause of high β-hexosaminidase release rate.

Chlorogenic acid is a compound existing in many Chinese herbs, such as *Lonicera* and *Forsythia et al.* It is regarded as allergen causing type I allergic reactions and anaphylactoid reactions [10-12]. We found that chlorogenic acid at 2.5 mmol/L to 5.0 mmol/L could induce RBL-2H3 degranulation, and below these concentration, the enzyme release rate drop sharply. This result is almost in correspondence with the report written by Huang [12]. In order to exclude the other factors causing degranulation, we tested the osmotic pressures and pH values of these concentrations. It was found that the osmotic pressure values at 1.25 mmol/L, 2.5 mmol/L, and 5.0 mmol/L were within the normal range, while the pH values at these concentrations were very low, 3.55, 3.34, 3.14 respectively. In order to study whether the low pH itself could cause RBL-2H3 cell degranulation, we adjusted the pH of Tyrode's buffer from 2.5 to 7.0 respectively as samples adding to the test system. The results showed that pH 3.0 to 3.5 could cause β-hexosaminidase activity increases, this pH range was just in correspondence with the pH of chlorogenic acid 2.5 mmol/L and 5.0 mmol/L concentration. For the reason why no β-hexosaminidase activity pH below 3.0, the explanation is pH below 3.0 can inhibit the activity of the enzyme, so that no enzymatic reaction occurs. In order to further prove that low pH of chlorogenic acid induce RBL-2H3 cell degranulation, we adjusted the pH of different concentration of chlorogenic acid to 7.0 or so. The results showed that β-hexosaminidase activity in different concentration of chlorogenic acid after adjusted was not obviously increased, indicating that chlorogenic acid compound itself can not cause mast cells degranulation.

Since the concentration of chlorogenic acid in some TCMIs are very low (about 0.04 - 0.08 mg/ml in Dengzhanxixin injection) [13,14], about one twentieth of the test concentration causing degranulation, furthermore both Weeping Forsythia and Honeysuckle contain chlorogenic acid, but did not cause enzyme release, therefore the chlorogenic acid seems unlike to cause mask cell degranulation *in vivo*.

Finally, in order to answer the question that whether or not the degranulation of RBL-2H3 is caused by cytotoxicity, we determined the IC_{50} values of both RBL-2H3 and BRL cells. BRL cells are normal rat liver cells and have no degranulation function structurally. It was found that half of tested TCMIs (4/8) causing RBL-2H3 degranulation had cytotoxic effect for both RBL-2H3 and BRL cells, and it seemed that according to the values of IC^{50} RBL-2H3 cells were more sensitive than BRL cells, though the level of cytotoxic effect determined by IC_{50} was not in correspondence with the enzyme activity. Some TCMIs had no cytotoxic effect and degranulation, and 3 kinds of TCMIs had obvious degranulation but no cytotoxic effect, suggesting that the degranulation caused by these TCMIs occurs through exicytosis.

The adverse reactions mainly include allergic reactions and anaphylactoid reactions. It is advocated to establish techniques and methods for detecting both of them simultaneously at non-clinical stage, thus reducing the risk of occurrence of adverse reactions clinically. The relation between the degranulations of RBL-2H3 cells *in vitro* and clinical occurrence of adverse reactions caused by some TCMIs remains further study.

5. Acknowledgements

This study was supported by the Important New Drug Innovation Project, Ministry of Science & Technology (No. 2009ZX09502-002). Authors are grateful to Prof. Lu Xiong, who observed and analyzed electronic microscope pictures, and Director J. I. Shen, Department of Chinese Medicine, Shanghai institute for food and drug control, vice general manager Liu Shaoyong, Shanghai Kaibao Pharmaceutical Co., LTD., who provided testing samples of TCMIs.

REFERENCES

[1] L. Q. Zhu, Y. G. Xu, P. Wang, Z. Y. Gao and Y. Y. Chen, "Analysis on Cause of ADR Associated with Tranditional Chinese Medicine Injections," *China Parmacy*, Vol. 18, No. 3, 2007, pp. 215-217.

[2] Y. Q. Zhu and X. H. Hong, "Analysis of Adverse Drug Reaction of Traditional Chinese Medicinal Injection," *Lishizhen Medicine and Materia Medica Research*, Vol. 18, No. 4, 2007, pp. 1004-1006.

[3] H. D. Schlumberger, "Pseudo-Allergic Reactions to Drugs and Chemicals," *Ann Allergy*, Vol. 51, No. 2, 1983, pp. 317-324.

[4] M. M. Fisher and B. A. Baldo, "Diagnosis and Investigation of Acute Anaphylactoid Reactions to Anesthetic Drugs," *International Anesthesiology Clinics*, Vol. 23, No. 3, 1985, pp. 161-173.

[5] Project Group, "Technical Guidelines for Studies of Chinese Medicine & Natural Drug Immunotoxicity (Allergic and light allergic reaction)," 2005.
http://ishare.iask.sina.com.cn/f/16123642.html

[6] X. Luo, Q. Wang, L. Zhou, Y. Dong and Y. P. Jiang, "Effect of Several Traditional Chinese Medicine Injections on Degranulation in RBL-2H3 Cells," *Traditional*

Chinese Drug Research & Clinical Pharmacology, Vol. 20, No. 6, 2009, pp. 506-510.

[7]   W. H. Huang and X. Luo, "The Influence of Qingkailing Injection on the Degranulation of RBL-2H3 Cells," *Journal of Guiyang College of Traditional Chinese Medicine*, Vol. 32, No. 4, 2010, pp. 80-82.

[8]   A. H. Liang, C. Y. Li, T. Liu, C. Y. Cao, R. Hao, Y. Yi, J. Guo, H. Yang, H. Yi, Z. Wang and Z. F. Ma, "Animal Models and Methodologies for Evaluation of Chinese Herbal Injection-Induced Pseudoanaphylactoid Reactions," *World Science and Technology/Modernization of Traditional Chinese Medicine and Materia Medica*, Vol. 12, No. 6, 2010, pp. 998-1004.

[9]   J. Zhang, P. Li, Y. K. Li and L. D. Li, "Effect of Tween-80 on the Degranulation of RBL-2H3 Cells," *Modern Immunology*, Vol. 29, No. 3, 2009, pp. 240-245.

[10] Z. He, H.-H. Qu, X.-Q. Wang, Y. Zhao, Y.-F. Li, L.-N. Hu, J.-Q. Lu and Q.-G. Wang, "Allergenicity of Chlorogenic Acid as Hapten," *Journal of Beijing University of Traditional Chinese Medicine*, Vol. 33, No. 10, 2010, pp. 667-680.

[11] X. D. Wu, H. R. Yang, D. S. Lin, J. Zhang, F. Luo and X. P. Xu, "Comprehensive Research and Evaluation of Chlorogenic Acid Allergy," *Chinese Journal of Chinese Materia Medica*, Vol. 35, No. 24, 2010, pp. 3357-3361.

[12] F.-H. Huang, X.-Y. Zhang, L.-Y. Zhang, Q. Li, B. Ni, X. L. Chen and A. Jun, "Mast Cell Degranulation Induced by Chlorogenic Acid," *Acta Pharmacologica Sinica*, Vol. 31, No. 7, 2010, pp. 849-854.

[13] W. B. Shui, Q. He, J. J. Xu and Y. Y. Cheng, "Concentration Measurement of Chlorogenic Acid and Scutellarin in Denzhan-Xixin Injection," *China Journal of Chinese Materia Medica*, Vol. 33, No. 4, 2008, pp. 458-459.

[14] Q. R. Yan and S. Q. Wang, "Concentration Measurement of Chlorogenic Acid in Honeysuckle Flower," *Hunan Journal of Traditional Chinese Medicine*, Vol. 21, No. 6, 2005, pp. 74-75.

18

In Vitro Characterization of the Efficacy and Safety Profile of a Proprietary *Ajuga turkestanica* Extract

**José M. Zubeldia[1*], Aarón Hernández-Santana[1], Miguel Jiménez-del-Rio[1],
Verónica Pérez-López[1], Rubén Pérez-Machín[2], José Manuel García-Castellano[3]**

[1]Polinat S. L. Taibique 4, Polígono Industrial Las Majoreras, Las Palmas, Spain
[2]Molecular Oncology Group (G-OncoMol) Research Unit, University Hospital of Gran Canaria,
Canary Health and Research Foundation Barranco de la Ballena, Las Palmas, Spain
[3]Department of Orthopaedic Surgery, Complejo Hospitalario Universitario Insular, Las Palmas, Spain
Email: *jose@polinat.com

ABSTRACT

Ajuga turkestanica, an herbaceous flowering species in the mint family, has been traditionally used in Turkey and Uzbekistan for heart disease, muscle aches and stomach problems. Due to its high levels of phytoecdysteroids (particularly the characteristic C-11-hydroxylated Turkesterone), anabolic properties have also been reported. The aim of our study was to screen for early signs of efficacy and safety of a proprietary *Ajuga turkestanica* extract (ATE) using *in vitro* models. C_2C_{12} mouse myotube cell line was used to study potential effects on viability and gene modulation. Cell viability was evaluated with different concentrations [0.2 - 200 ppm (mg/L)] of ATE. Gene modulation was assessed by quantitative polymerase chain reaction (qRT-PCR) after 6 h incubation (ATE vs. the androgenic anabolic steroid methandrostenolone). Total androgenic activity was measured using the A-SCREEN bioassay. Ultra-high performance liquid chromatography analysis showed good correlation between the phytochemical profile of the native plant and our ATE. C_2C_{12} mouse myotube cells treated with ATE experienced no significant loss of viability (concentrations 0.2 - 200 ppm, 1 - 24 hs, $p > 0.05$). qRT-PCR array analysis showed significant ($p < 0.05$) down regulation of Caspase-3 (2-fold) and Myostatin (4-fold). The extract showed no androgenic activity within the dose range used. Our results indicate the potential for an ATE to support muscle mass without typical androgenic side effects of synthetic anabolic drugs.

Keywords: Ecdysteroids; *Ajuga turkestanica*; Turkesterone; Caspase 3; Myostatin; Androgenic Activity; Sarcopenia

1. Introduction

The genus Ajuga (Labiatae) is comprised of more than 40 species widely distributed in temperate regions of both hemispheres and contains at least three classes of potentially bioactive compounds: clerodane diterpenes, phytoecdysteroids and iridoid glycosides. *Ajuga turkestanica* (Regel) Briq is a perennial herb growing mainly in Central Asia known as a rich source of bioactive substances and used by local people to treat heart diseases, muscle and stomach aches [1]. With regards to phytoecdysteroids several bioactive compounds have been isolated including turkesterone, 20-hydroxyecdysone (20-HE), cyasterone, cyasterone 22-acetate, ajugalactone, ajugasterone B, α-ecdysone and ecdysone 2,3-monoacetonide [2,3]. A characteristic feature of *Ajuga turkestanica* is the presence of the C11-hydroxylated turkesterone, which has not been observed in other species of the same genus [4].

Ecdysteroids are polyhydroxylated ketosteroids with long carbon side chains. These steroid hormones control moulting and reproduction in arthropods, but their role in plants is less well known as they do not elicit any of the classical plant hormone responses [5]. Plants may use ecdysteroids as a chemical defense against insects by disrupting their hormonal balance and moulting process [6]. The discovery of these steroid molecules in 1966 in several plant species led to their availability in large amounts for pharmacologic studies in search of safer more specific insecticides. While showing no signs of toxicity, ecdysteroids had other possible beneficial effects that could support their use in folk medicine such as immunomodulation, antiarrythmic, hepatoprotective, or antidiabetes effects [7-10].

Ecdysteroids are structurally different from mammalian steroids, and they are not expected to bind to vertebrate steroid receptors. However, anabolic effects have been reported in vertebrates: increased growth in mice, rats, sheep, or pigs, and increased physical performance without training in rats with increased synthesis of myofibrillar proteins [11].

The potential for any substance to increase protein synthesis in muscle by-passing secondary effects common with steroid synthetic drugs may be an attractive approach for important health issues such as sarcopenia, a condition in which subjects have progressive generalized loss of skeletal muscle mass and function. It has been associated with adverse outcomes such as falls, mobility limitations, incident disability, and fractures in the elderly [12]. It is also associated with insulin resistance in both non-obese and obese individuals and abnormal blood glucose levels in obese individuals, especially in those younger than 60 years of age [13]. Finally, sarcopenia plays a key role in the development of cachexia, a syndrome occurring at terminal stages of cancer, chronic heart or kidney failure, or AIDS [14]. Proposed treatments include testosterone supplementation, which would require close monitoring of androgenic side effects such as prostate hypertrophy [15].

The aim of our study was to initially screen a proprietary *Ajuga turkestanica* extract (ATE), rich in ecdysteroids for early signs of efficacy (increase/protection of muscle mass) and safety (lack of androgenic activity).

2. Materials and Methods

2.1. Chemicals and Materials

HPLC grade acetonitrile and methanol were purchased from Merck (Spain). Water was purified and deionized by a Milli-Q ultrapure water system. Turkesterone and 20-hydroxyecdysone (20-HE) reference standards were obtained from Chromadex (Irvine, USA). Methandrostenolone, a commercially available synthetic anabolic steroid, and 17β-Estradiol (E2) were purchased from Sigma-Aldrich (Spain). Methyltrienolone (R1881), a non-me- tabolizable synthetic anabolic steroid, was provided from Perkin Elmer (Spain).

2.2. Plant Extraction

Ajuga turkestanica was collected in Uzbekistan. The dried whole plant (1 kg) was extracted in a percolator at room temperature using 10 L of 85% ethanol in water for 2 hs. The liquid fraction was removed and the whole process was repeated. The two liquid fractions (20 L) were combined and ethanol was removed in vacuo before freeze-drying (Telstar Cryodos benchtop freezedrier). Samples were vacuum sealed in plastic bags and stored at room temperature inside a dessicator.

2.3. Chromatography

Ajuga turkestanica whole dried plant (finely ground) or powdered extract (0.1 g) was diluted in methanol (25 ml) and sonicated for 15 min at room temperature. The solution was filtered through a 0.2 μm syringe filter (Micron Analytical, Spain) before analysis by ultra high performance liquid chromatography (UPLC). UPLC analysis was performed on a Waters Acquity H-Class UPLC system coupled to a photodiode array detector (PDA). Separation was carried out on an Acquity C18 BEH column (Waters, 100 × 2.1 mm, 1.7 μm). The mobile phase consisted of ultrapure water (A) and acetonitrile (B). The following linear gradient was used: 0 - 5 min, 10% - 50% B; 5 - 6 min, 50% - 100% B, 6 - 8 min, 100% B. Each run was followed by an equilibration period of 2 min. The flow rate was 0.5 ml/min and the injection volume 1 μL. The column temperature was 50°C and the detection wavelength was set to 245 nm.

2.4. Gene Expression Study

A mouse skeletal muscle cell line, C_2C_{12} (American Type Culture Collection, UK), was cultured in Dulbecco's Modified Eagle's Medium (DMEM) with high glucose (Thermo Fisher Scientific, Spain) supplemented with 10% fetal bovine serum (Lonza Group, Switzerland), 2 mM glutamine, 100 units/ml penicillin and 100 μg/ml streptomycin. Cells between passages 3 and 10 were seeded at a density of 10,000 cells per cm^2. Cells were grown for 48 hs until they reached 80% - 90% confluence. To induce myogenic differentiation, the medium was replaced with differentiation medium, DMEM supplemented with 2% horse serum (PAA Laboratories, Austria) [11,16]. After 10 days the myoblasts had fused into multinucleated myotubes. Cells were maintained at 37°C in a humidified 5% CO_2 incubator and medium was changed every other day.

Cell viability after ATE treatment was determined using the Presto Blue cell viability kit (Invitrogen, Spain) following the manufacturer's instructions. C_2C_{12} cells were plated and differentiated to myotubes into 96-well plates. After differentiation, the culture medium was replaced with DMEM containing various concentrations of ATE (0.2 - 200 ppm) for 1, 3, 6 and 24 hours. Before Presto Blue kit reagents were added, the medium was removed and cells were washed with PBS. The cells were incubated with Presto Blue for 20 min at 37°C. Fluorescence was measured on a MX3005P Q-PCR System (Agilent Technologies, Spain) using a Cy3 filter set on plate read mode.

For RNA extraction, C_2C_{12} cells were plated and differentiated to myotubes into 12-wells plates. After differentiation, cells were incubated with 20 ppm ATE (approx. 1 μM total ecdysteroids) or 1 μM methandrostenolone for 6 h. RNA was then extracted using an All Prep RNA/Protein Kit (Qiagen, Spain). Total RNA was quantified using a fluorometric method with Quant-iT kit (Invitrogen, Spain). RNA was stored at −80°C until further use. cDNA was reverse-transcribed from the RNA extract using RT^2 First Stand cDNA kit and we used a RT^2 Profiler PCR Array to analyze a panel of 84 genes involved in skeletal muscle development and disease (Qiagen, Spain). Quantitative real-time RT-PCR was carried out using a SYBR-Green/ROX detection in a MX3005P Q-PCR System. Samples were heated at 95°C for 10 min, followed by a second stage composed of 15 sec at 95°C, 1 min at 60°C which was repeated 40 times and third stage for dissociation curve composed of 1 min at 95°C, 30 sec at 55°C and 30 sec at 95°C.

To analyze the PCR-array data, an MS-Excel sheet with macros was downloaded from the manufacturer's website (http://www.sabiosciences.com). This program calculated relative gene expression and statistical significance.

2.5. Androgenic Study

MCF-7-AR1 cells were kindly provided by Nicolas Olea from Granada University, Spain. The MCF-AR1 cells result from stably transfected MCF-7 human breast cancer cell with a full human AR 27. The MCF-7-AR1 cell line was grown routinely in a humidified atmosphere of 5% CO$_2$ at 37°C in Dulbecco's modified Eagle's Medium (DMEM) without phenol red containing 10% fetal bovine serum (FBS) supplemented with 2 mM glutamine, 100 units/ml penicillin, 100 μg/ml streptomycin, 15 mM HEPES and 4.2 mM sodium bicarbonate (FBS-DMEM) (Lonza Group, Switzerland). Cells become proliferative quiescent when transferred into the same Culture medium but supplemented with 10% charcoal-dextran-treated FBS (CD-FBS, steroid free) (Thermo Fisher Scientific, Spain) instead of FBS. The CD-FBS-DMEM medium was used as experimental medium. MCF-7-AR1 cells proliferate maximally in experimental medium plus 100 pM E2, and respond to androgens by decreasing their proliferation rate in a dose-dependent fashion.

To test for the potential cytotoxicity of AE on MC7-AR1, cells were trypsinized, counted and plated into 96-wells plates (NUNC) at seed density of 4000 cell per well in FBS-DMEM. After 24 hs to allow attachment, cells were treated with FBS-DMEM alone and with FBS-DMEM in the presence of a range of ATE concentrations. After incubation for five days, the FBS-DMEM was gently aspirated and the cells were trypsinized. Trypan blue exclusion test was used to count viable cells and non-viable cells. The method stains selectively non-viable cells. Briefly, a suitable cell suspension was given into a tube and 0.4% w/v of trypan blue stain was added. After mixing, solution was incubated 5 mins at room temperature. Cells were finally counted in a TC10 automated cell counter (BioRad Laboratories, Spain).

The A-Screen bioassay compares the cell number of similar inocula of MCF-7-AR1 cells growing in CD-FBS-DMEN in the absence of any estrogen and androgens (negative control), in the presence of 100 pM of E2 (estrogen control) and 100 pM of E2 plus a range of ATE concentrations. MCF-7-AR1 were trypsinized and seeded into 96-wells plate (Nunclon delta) at concentration of 6000 cell/well in experimental medium. After 24 hours to allow attachment, experimental medium with 100 pM of E2 containing the various dilutions ATE (0.1 to 100 PPM) was added into each well. Positive (100 pM E2) and negative control (CD-FBS-DMEM), as well as plant extract doses were tested six-fold. In addition, an androgen reference curve made with R1881 or methandrostenolone was set up as positive control in every experiment. After 120 hs, the assay was finished by gently removing the experimental medium and the addition of ice-cold 10% Thricloroacetic acid (wt/vol). The plates were left on ice for 30 mins, then rinsed gently 3 times with water and allowed to air dry. Cells were then stained with 0.4% sulforhodamine B (SRB) in 1% (vol/col) acetic acid for 20 mins. The bound dye was solubilized with Tris-base pH 10.6. After short shaking, absorbance was read in a MW plate reader (Biotek) at 492 nm subtracting the background measurement at 620 nm. It has been established previously that there is a direct linear relationship between cell number and the absorbance values of the Tris-SRB solution. Experimental readings were in the lineal range of the standard curve (Data not shown).

3. Results

The most abundant ecdysteroids in the *A. turkestanica* extract were quantified with UPLC-PDA. **Figure 1** shows the chemical structures and the chromatographic separation of the main bioactive compounds typically found in *Ajuga turkestanica* plant extracts and the powder extract used in this study. The ATE powder contained approximately 0.69% (w/w) turkesterone and 1.30% (w/w) 20-HE. No significant difference was observed between the *Ajuga turkestanica* plant and the corresponding powder extract, indicating that the phytochemical profile of the main bioactive compounds does not change during the extraction and preparation process. Preservation of the native constituents in the plant is essential prior to any biological testing.

To evaluate potential cytotoxicity, myotubes were treated with ATE powder at concentrations from 0.2 to 200 ppm (mg/L) for up to 24 hs and cell viability was evaluated using the Presto Blue cell viability kit. This reagent kit is a resazurin-based assay, where resazurin is converted to the fluorescent product resorufin by metabolically active cells and measured quantitatively [17].

This transformation of non-fluorescent resazurin to fluorescent resorufin is the basis for the use of this fluorometric indicator for the determination of cell viability. We did not see any significant loss of cell viability for the range of concentrations and treatment period used in this study (**Figure 2(a)**, p > 0.05).

Our ATE showed a 2-fold downregulation of caspase-3 in myotubes while the androgenic anabolic steroid methandrostenolone downregulated caspase-3 but to a lesser extent compared to the ATE (<2-fold). Myotubes treated for 6 hs with ATE showed a 4-fold down-regulation of Myostatin. Methandrostenolone treatment also downregulated myostatin to a lesser extent (<2-fold) (**Figure 2(b)**, p < 0.05).

Since androgenic activity is ultimately based on cell number end-point, it was necessary to establish whether any decrease in proliferation could be associated with a

cytotoxic effect of the extract rather than AR agonist action before the A-Screen was performed. Trypan blue dye exclusion assay was used to examine ATE-mediated cytotoxicity (expressed as non-viable cells) and to assess cell viability upon exposure to ATE in complete medium (FBS-DMEM). ATE treatment reduced both total cell number and viability of MCF7-AR1 cells in a dose-dependent manner (**Figure 3**). The results show that ATE inhibits MCF7-AR1 cell viability at very high doses (200 and 600 ppm) by inducing both a cytotoxic cell response and reducing the number of viable cells. Based on the above, the concentration of ATE used in the A-Screen assay was limited to a range of 0.1 - 100 ppm.

Results of the A-Screen test are shown in **Figure 4**. The synthetic androgen methyltrienolone (R1881) was used as the reference compound (Ca, positive control) and a dose-response curve showed that R1881 inhibited

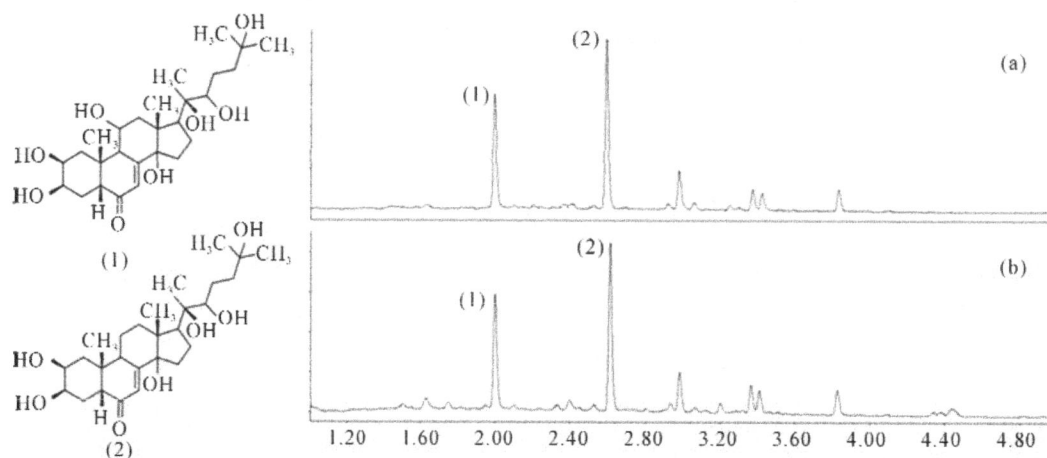

Figure 1. Chemical structures of the main bioactive compounds in *Ajuga turkestanica*: (1) turkersterone; and (2) 20-HE. **UPLC chromatograms of (a)** *Ajuga turkestanica* **whole plant; and (b) the corresponding freeze-dried powder extract (ATE) measured at 245 nm.**

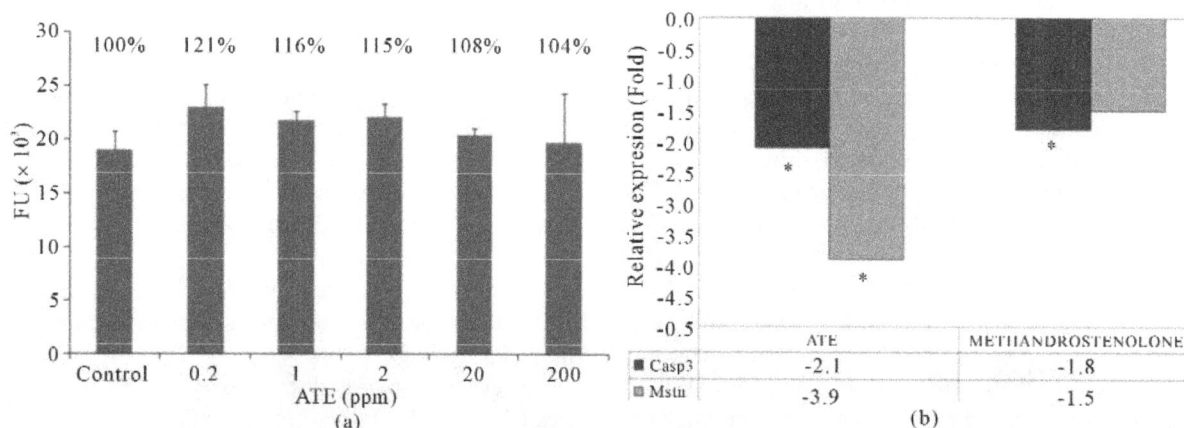

Figure 2. (a) Effect of AE treatment on C_2C_{12} muscle cell viability. Cells were cultured with media containing different concentrations of ATE (0.2 - 200 ppm) for 24 hs (n = 3). Results are expressed in fluorescence units (FU) and percentage of viability, calculated using the following equation: (FU treated/FU control) × 100; (b) Effect of ATE and methandrostenolone on Caspase-3 (Casp-3) and myostatin (Mstn) gene expression levels in C_2C_{12} muscle cells. Test groups were treated with 20 ppm of ATE for 6 hours (n = 3). *p < 0.05.

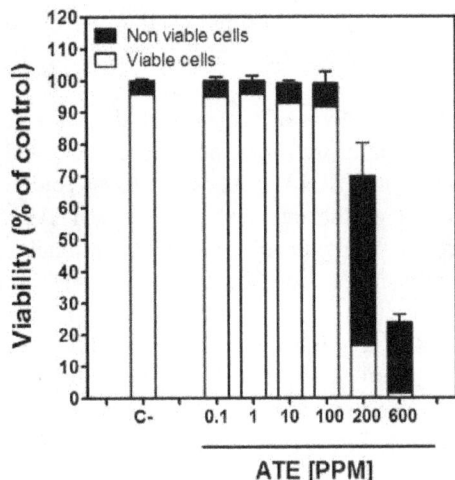

Figure 3. Effect of ATE on cell viability of MCF-7AR1 determined by trypan blue dye exclusion assay. Cells were grown for 5 days with FBS-DMEM in the presence of a range of AE concentrations (0.1 - 600 ppm). C-: FBS-DMEM only. Results are showed as fraction of viable and nonviable cells and are expressed as percentage of the negative control total (viable and non viable) cell number.

cell proliferation at very low concentrations (**Figure 4(a)**), IC50 = 20 pM). Methandrostenolone also inhibited cell proliferation at higher concentrations (**Figure 4(b)**, IC50 = 350 pM). The addition of ATE at a range of concentrations (0.1 - 100 ppm) to the culture media in the presence of E2 did not show a significant proliferative inhibition compared with the control (MCF7-AR1 cells plus E2) at doses up to 100 ppm (**Figure 4(c)**).

4. Discussion

The C_2C_{12} mouse cell line is a well-established *in vitro* model for skeletal muscle studies [18]. C_2C_{12} myoblasts may be readily differentiated into multinucleated myotubes under controlled conditions, and these cells behave in many ways like skeletal muscle fibers, contracting when stimulated and expressing characteristic muscle proteins [19,20]. In this context, C_2C_{12} myotubes were used to study cell viability and changes in modulation of genes associated with muscle skeletal, muscle development and disease upon treatment with our ATE.

Evaluation of the molecular pathways involved in the putative anabolic effect of the ecdysteroids present in the ATE suggests two possible pathways. During muscle wasting caspase-3 activation and the ubiquitin proteasome system (UPS) act synergistically to increase the degradation of muscle proteins. Activation of the former is required to convert actomyosin and myofibrils into substrates of the UPS. Caspase-3 cleaves specific 19 S proteasome subunits in C_2C_{12} muscle cells with a cell-specific activity. Caspase-3 cleaves different subunits in myoblasts and myotubes hence intervening in cell dif-

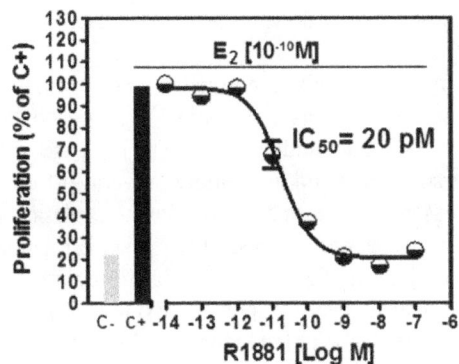

(a)

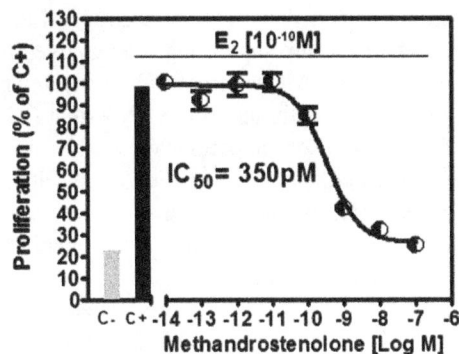

(b)

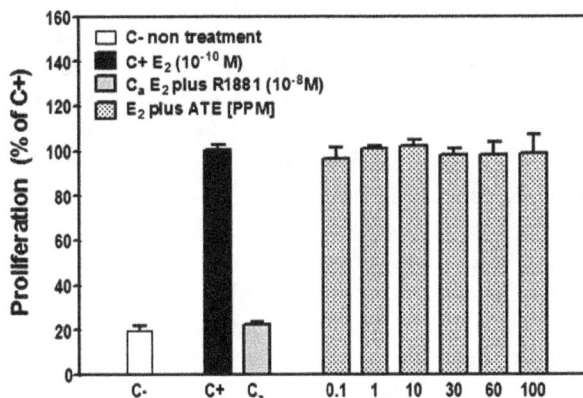

(c)

Figure 4. Androgenic activity bioassay (A-Screen): Dose-response curve to (a) methyltrienolone (R1881) and (b) methandrostenolone by MCF7-AR1 cells in the presence E2. (c) Proliferative response of E2 treated MCF7-AR1 cells to ATE in a range of concentrations (0.1 - 100 ppm). C-, non-treated; C+, E2; Ca, E2 plus R1881.

ferentiation or muscle wasting [21]. Recently, Bhatnagar and colleagues have shown that adding a caspase-3 inhibitory peptide to myotube cultures resulted in inhibition of tumor necrosis factor-like weak inducer of apoptosis (TWEAK) induced loss of myosin heavy chain and myotube diameter [22]. Our ATE showed a 2-fold down-regulation of caspase-3 in myotubes supporting its potential to protect muscle form wasting, as opposed to methandrostenolone which downregulated caspase-3 to a lesser extent (<2-fold).

Myostatin is mostly expressed in skeletal muscle and normally functions as a negative regulator of muscle growth. Upon the binding to activin type IIB receptor, this extracellular cytokine initiates several different signaling cascades resulting in the down-regulation of the important myogenesis genes. Muscle size is regulated via a complex interplay of myostatin signaling with the insulin-like growth factor 1/phosphatidylinositol 3-kinase/ Akt pathway responsible for increase in protein synthesis in muscle 14. Myostatin blockage or its natural absence leads to a significant increase in muscle mass [23]. Myotubes treated for 6 h with ATE showed a 4-fold downregulation of myostatin, supporting the putative anabolic effects of the plant. Methandrostenolone treatment also downregulated myostatin but to a lesser extent (<2-fold). These results are also compatible with other investigations. Gorelick-Feldman et al. studied the mechanism of action of ecdysteroids in murine C_2C_{12} myotubes in which a 95% ethanol-based extraction preparation provoked a 15% increase in protein synthesis.

However, when myotubes were pretreated with a Phosphatidyl Inositol 3-kinase (PI3K) inhibitor, the effect on protein synthesis was significantly reduced indicating the involvement of this particular molecular pathway [11]. Knockout of the myostatin gene has been associated with the up-regulation of proteins involved in glycolitic shift of muscle and down regulation of proteins involved in oxidative energy metabolism. Specifically, investigators have found increased expression of genes belonging to the PI3K pathway in myostatin-null mice as opposed to the wild type [24]. Hence, down-regulation of myostatin by our ATE in C_2C_{12} myotubes goes in accordance with previous published results.

Testosterone and other androgenic steroid drugs have been used in the past to increase or maintain muscle mass. These drugs act via the androgen receptors and as such have shown significant side effects that must be carefully evaluated before initiating any therapy. There is an increased risk for prostate hyperplasia and cancer in men, virilization in women, and cardiac hypertrophy and atherosclerosis for both [25]. Safer approaches have been evaluated as well. A randomized, double-blind, placebo controlled, multicenter trial was conducted to evaluate the safety and efficacy of a novel selective androgen receptor modulator (SARM). A total of 120 healthy men and postmenopausal women were evenly randomized to take placebo or 0.1, 0.3, 1 or 3 mg of SARM for 12 weeks. The incidence of adverse events was similar amongst groups with no serious events reported. Specifically, the novel compound did not have effects on sebum production or hair growth in women while eliciting a dose-dependent increase in total lean body mass,

highlighting the benefits of dissociating the anabolic and androgenic activities when a therapeutic effect is sought [26].

The anabolic effect of ecdysteroids is connected with the acceleration of translocation processes instead of the induction of new RNA synthesis. Ecdysteroids are not likely to act as the classical steroids, via cytoplasmic receptor and regulation of gene transcriptional activity. In fact, an androgen dependent development is a prerequisite before the action of ecdysteroids in rats. Using radioligand assays Báthori et al. found that none of 11 tested ecdysteroids (including turkesterone) bound significantly to estrogenic, glucocorticoid or androgenic receptors [27]. Ecdysteroids display significant structural differences from anabolic-androgenic steroid hormones, which may explain the different mechanisms of their anabolic action.

MCF7-AR1 is a human cancer-derived cell line which has been genetically engineered to over express the AR [28]. The A-Screen cell bioassay, developed to measured anti-androgenic activity using MCF7-AR1 cell number as the end point, is used to identify androgenic chemicals among environmental pollutants and it has proved to be very sensitive and reproducible assay for detecting androgenic activity [29]. This assay measures androgen-dependent inhibition of proliferation of the androgen receptor (AR)-positive human mammary carcinoma cell line, MCF7-AR1. This cell line has been stably transfected with a full human AR and expresses approximately five times more AR than wild-type cells. MCF7-AR1 cells retain the capacity to proliferate in response to estrogen treatment (E2). Androgens inhibit estrogen-induced proliferation and cells arrest in G0/G1 phase in a dose-dependent manner [28].

The A-Screen bioassay compares the cell number of similar inocula of MCF-7-AR1 cells growing in media in the absence of any estrogen and androgens (C-, negative control), in the presence of E2 (C+, estrogen control) and in the presence of E2 in combination with different concentrations of the suspected androgen (**Figure 4**). Androgenic activity of a test compound results in the inhibit-tion of cell proliferation compared to the E2 control. As expected both androgens (R1881 and Methandrostenolone) inhibited cell proliferation. However, adding ATE at a non-cytotoxic concentrations (0.1 - 100 ppm) to the media did not show a significant proliferative inhibition compared with the control (MCF7-AR1 cells plus E2) (**Figure 4(c)**). Therefore and based on these results, it was established that our ATE does not show androgenic activity within the dose range used.

In conclusion, we have shown the feasibility of obtaining a standardized *Ajuga turkestanica* extract that retains the main bioactives in a ratio similar to that of the root material. Preservation of this natural ratio is essential to maintain the synergistic effect of the different phytoactive compounds. Biological activity of the high content in ecdysteroids (and particularly turkesterone) of the ATE was demonstrated by real time qRT-PCR. Caspase-3 and Myostatin were both significantly down regulated, supporting the results by others which indicate ecdysteroids may protect against muscle waste. Results of the A-screen assay showed with high sensitivity the lack of androgenic activity of the ATE, a desired trait in developing alternative approaches for managing sarcopenia in humans. We believe further clinical work is warranted.

5. Conflict of Interests

José M Zubeldia, Aarón Hernández-Santana, Miguel Jiménez del Rio, and Verónica Pérez work for Polinat SL, the company which has developed and manufactures the *Ajuga turkestanica* extract. Jose Manuel García Castellano and Rubén Pérez Machin have no disclosures. This work was funded by Polinat SL.

REFERENCES

[1] M. H. Grace, D. M. Cheng, I. Raskin and M. A. Lila, "Neo-Clerodane Diterpenes from *Ajuga turkestanica*," *Phytochemistry Letters*, Vol. 1, No. 2, 2008, pp. 81-84. doi:10.1016/j.phytol.2008.03.004

[2] I. T. Abdukadirov, M. R. Yakubova, Kh. R. Nuriddinov, A. U. Mamatkhanov and M. T. Turakhozhaev, "Ecdysterone and Turkesterone in *Ajuga turkestanica* Determined by HLPC," *Chemistry of Natural Compounds*, Vol. 41, No. 4, 2005, pp. 475-476. doi:10.1007/s10600-005-0184-x

[3] N. Sh. Ramazanov, "Phytoecdyesteroids and Other Biologically Active Compounds from Plants of the Genus Ajuga," *Chemistry of Natural Compounds*, Vol. 41, No. 4, 2005, pp. 361-369. doi:10.1007/s10600-005-0153-4

[4] B. Z. Usmanov, M. B. Gorovits and N. K. Abubakirov, "Phytoecdysones of *Ajuga turkestanica* III. The Structure of Turkesterone," *Chemistry of Natural Compounds*, Vol. 4, No. 11, 1975, pp. 466-470.

[5] I. Machackova, M. Vagner and K. Slama, "Comparison between the Effects of 20-Hydroxyecdysone and Phytohormones on Growth and Development in Plants," *European Journal of Entomolology*, Vol. 92, No. 1, 1995, pp. 309-316.

[6] I. Soriano, I. Riley, M. Potter and W. Bowers, "Phytoecdysteroids: A Novel Defense against Plant-Parasitic Nematodes," *Journal of Chemical Ecolology*, Vol. 30, No. 10, 2004, pp. 1885-1899. doi:10.1023/B:JOEC.0000045584.56515.11

[7] H. Chiang, J. Wang and R. Wu, "Immunomodulating Effects of the Hydrolysis Products of Formosanin C and Beta-Ecdyson from Paris formosana Hayata," *Anticancer Research*, Vol. 12, No. 5, 1992, pp. 1475-1478.

[8] A. G. Kurmukov and O. A. Ermishina, "Effect of Ecdys-

[9] terone on Experimental Arrhythmias, Changes in Hemodynamics and Contractility of the Myocardium Produced by a Coronary Artery Occlusion," *Farmakol Toksikol (Moscow)*, Vol. 54, No. 1, 1991, pp. 27-29.

[9] R. Lafont and L. Dinan, "Practical Uses for Ecdysteroids in Mammals Including Humans: An Update," *Journal of Insect Science*, Vol. 3, No. 7, 2003, pp. 7-36.

[10] V. Syrov, R. Sharapova and A. Kurmukov, "Effect of Ecdysterone on the Hematopoietic Activity on the Laboratory Animals with Experimentally Anemia," *Issues in Obstetrics and Gynecology*, Vol. 1, No. 1, 1976, pp. 62-63.

[11] J. Gorelick-Feldman, D. Maclean, N. Ilic, A. Poulev, M. A. Lila, D. Cheng and I. Raskin, "Phytoecdysteroids Increase Protein Synthesis in Skeletal Muscle Cells," *Journal of Agricultural Food and Chemistry*, Vol. 56, No. 10, 2008, pp. 3532-3537. doi:10.1021/jf073059z

[12] T. Lang, T. Streeper, P. Cawthon, K. Baldwin, D. R. Taaffe and T. B. Harris, "Sarcopenia: Etiology, Clinical Consequences, Intervention, and Assessment," *Osteoporosis International*, Vol. 21, No. 4, 2010, pp. 543-559. doi:10.1007/s00198-009-1059-y

[13] P. Srikanthan, A. L. Hevener and A. S. Karlamangla, "Sarcopenia Exacerbates Obesity-Associated Insulin Resistance and Dysglycemia: Findings from the National Health and Nutrition Examination Survey III," *PLoS One*, Vol. 5, No. 5, 2010, p. e10805. doi:10.1371/journal.pone.0010805

[14] Y. Elkina, S. von Haehling, S. D. Anker and J. Springer, "The Role of Myostatin in Muscle Wasting: An Overview," *Journal of Cachexia, Sarcopenia and Muscle*, Vol. 2, No. 3, 2011, pp. 43-151.

[15] L. A. Burton and D. Sumukada, "Optimal Management of Sarcopenia," *Clinical Interventions in Aging*, Vol. 5, 2010, pp. 217-228.

[16] Y. Ohira, Y. Matsuoka, F. Kawano, A. Ogura, Y. Higo, T. Ohira, M. Terada, Y. Oke and N. Nakai, "Effects of Creatine and Its Analog, β-Guanidinopropionic Acid, on the Differentiation of and Nucleoli in Myoblasts," *Bioscience, Biotechnology, and Biochemistry*, Vol. 75, No. 6, 2011, pp. 1085-1089. doi:10.1271/bbb.100901

[17] R. E. Erb and M. H. Ehlers, "Resazurin Reducing Time as an Indicator of Bovine Semen Capacity," *Journal of Dairy Science*, Vol. 33, No. 12, 1950, pp. 853-864. doi:10.3168/jds.S0022-0302(50)91981-3

[18] S. Burattini, P. Ferri, M. Battistelli, R. Curci, F. Luchetti and E. Falcieri, "C_2C_{12} Murine Myoblasts as a Model of Skeletal Muscle Development: Morpho-Functional Characterization," *European Journal of Histochemistry*, Vol. 48, No. 3, 2004, pp. 23-33.

[19] T. Kislinger, A. O. Gramolini, Y. Pan, K. Rahman, D. H. MacLennan, A. Emili, "Proteome Dynamics during C_2C_{12} Myoblast Differentiation," *Molecular & Cellular Proteomics*, Vol. 4, No. 7, 2005, pp. 887-901. doi:10.1074/mcp.M400182-MCP200

[20] N. S. Tannu, V. K. Rao, R. M. Chaudhary, F. Giorgianni, A. E. Saeed, Y. Gao and R. Raghow, "Comparative Proteomes of the Proliferating C_2C_{12} Myoblasts and Fully Differentiated Myotubes Reveal the Complexity of the

Skeletal Muscle Differentiation Program," *Molecular & Cellular Proteomics*, Vol. 3, No. 11, 2004, pp. 1065-1082. doi:10.1074/mcp.M400020-MCP200

[21] X. H. Wang, L. Zhang, W. E. Mitch, J. M. LeDoux, J. Hu and J. Du, "Caspase-3 Cleaves Specific 19 S Proteasome Subunits in Skeletal Muscle Stimulating Proteasome Activity," *The Journal of Biological Chemistry*, Vol. 285, No. 28, 2010, pp. 21249-21257. doi:10.1074/jbc.M109.041707

[22] S. Bhatnagar, A. Mittal, S. K. Gupta and A. Kumar, "TWEAK Causes Myotube Atrophy through Coordinated Activation of Ubiquitin-Proteasome System, Autophagy, and Caspases," *Journal of Cellular Physiology*, Vol. 227, No. 3, 2012, pp. 1042-1051. doi:10.1002/jcp.22821

[23] S. J. Lee, L. A. Reed, M. W. Davies, S. Girgenrath, M. E. Goad, K. N. Tomkinson, J. F. Wright, C. Barker, G. Hermantraut, J. Holmstrom, B. Trowell, B. Gertz, M. S. Jiang, S. M. Sebald, M. Matzuk, E. Li, L. F. Liang, E. Quattlebaum, R. L. Stotish and N. M. Wolfman, "Regulation of Muscle Growth by Multiple Ligands Signaling through Activin Type II Receptors," *Proceedings of the National Academy of Science US*, Vol. 102, No. 50, 2005, pp. 18117-18122. doi:10.1073/pnas.0505996102

[24] I. Chelh, B. Meunier, B. Picard, M. J. Reecy, C. Chevalier, J. F. Hocquette and I. Cassar-Malek, "Molecular Profiles of Quadriceps Muscle in Myostatin-Null Mice Reveal PI3K and Apoptotic Pathways as Myostatin Targets," *BMC Genomics*, Vol. 10, 2009, p. 196. doi:10.1186/1471-2164-10-196

[25] T. Thum and J. Springer, "Breakthrough in Cachexia Treatment through a Novel Selective Androgen Receptor Modulator?" *Journal of Cachexia, Sarcopenia and Muscle*, Vol. 2, No. 3, 2011, pp. 121-123. doi:10.1007/s13539-011-0040-8

[26] J. T. Dalton, K. G. Barnette, C. E. Bohl, M. L. Hancock, D. Rodriguez, S. T. Dodson, R. A. Morton and M. S. Steiner, "The Selective Androgen Receptor Modulator GTx-024 (Enobosarm) Improves Lean Body Mass and Physical Function in Healthy Elderly Men and Postmenopausal Women: Results of a Double-Blind, Placebo-Controlled Phase II Trial," *Journal of Cachexia Sarcopenia Muscle*, Vol. 2, No. 3, 2011, pp. 153-161. doi:10.1007/s13539-011-0034-6

[27] M. Báthori, N. Tóth, A. Hunyadi, A. Márki and E. Zádor, "Phytoecdysteroids and Anabolic-Androgenic Steroids-Structure and Effects on Humans," *Current Medicinal Chemistry*, Vol. 15, No. 1, 2008, pp. 75-91. doi:10.2174/092986708783330674

[28] J. Szelei, J. Jimenez, A. M. Soto, M. F. Luizzi and C. Sonnenschein, "Androgen-Induced Inhibition of Proliferation in Human Breast Cancer MCF7 Cells Transfected with Androgen Receptor," *Endocrinology*, Vol. 138, No. 4, 1997, pp. 1406-1412. doi:10.1210/en.138.4.1406

[29] A. M. Soto, J. M. Calabro, N. V. Prechtl, A. Y. Yau, E. F. Orlando, A. Daxenberger, A. S. Kolok, L. J. Guillette Jr., B. le Bizec, I. G. Lange and C. Sonnenschein, "Androgenic and Estrogenic Activity in Water Bodies Receiving Cattle Feedlot Effluent in Eastern Nebraska, USA," *Environmental Health Perspectives*, Vol. 112, No. 3, 2004, pp. 346-352. doi:10.1289/ehp.6590

19

How Big Is an Acupoint?

Lei Li[1*], **To Yau**[1], **Chuen-Heung Yau**[2]
[1]School of Chinese Medicine, The University of Hong Kong, Hong Kong, China
[2]School of Chinese Medicine, Hong Kong Baptist University, Hong Kong, China
Email: llie@hku.hk

ABSTRACT

The structure and size range of an acupoint were investigated thoroughly according to the expositions of ancient classics. It was revealed that the ambiguous way of thinking by the ancient Chinese had a great impact on the formation and development of the acupoint-concept. Hence all descriptions of an acupoint's structure and size range have the characteristics of ambiguity. The structure and size range of an acupoint are determined not only by the outlook of depression and blood vessel areas, but also its relationship with other acupoints in its vicinity. The different manipulations of puncturing recorded in the *Yellow Emperor's Canon of Medicine* also show the ambiguous nature of the structure and size range of an acupoint. In theory, an acupoint has been characterized as various forms, which should not be limited to a mere round dot shape.

Keywords: Acupoint; Acupoint Structure; Acupoint Size Range

1. Introduction

How to define the size range has become a major concern when it comes to the study of an acupoint, for it is closely related to clinical applications of acupuncture therapy. However, prior to deciding the size of an acupoint, its structure first needs to be clarified. Since an acupoint is a spot for the flow of Qi and blood, reflecting symptoms of diseases, and assisting in syndrome differentiations in the treatments of pathogens, its existence has appeared to be objective, and undoubtedly has the material structure. In fact, the formation of acupoints is actually a creation of the ancient Chinese based on an ambiguous logical concept. Therefore, an acupoint's structure is not limited to shape, but is also closely related to the character of its allying function. Nowadays, with all the state-of-art science and technologies, it is still impossible to explain the actual structure of acupoints. However, that does not stop us from attempting to theoretically explain the structural ambit of acupoints through analyzing related discussions in ancient literatures and classics.

2. The Acupoint Is Relatively Hollow Stereoscopic Structure

"Acupoint" implies a hole. Most of the acupoints are located in the depressions between bones and joints or muscular interstices. Thus they structurally resemble three-dimensional hollows. As the nature of the depressions between bones and joints or muscular interstices

varies, the presumed sizes of acupoints are comparatively different.

In view of the origin of acupoints, their formations are closely related to the blood vessels. In early ancient times, acupuncture meant using a stone needle to pry out blood from the pain points of a bodily part, and an acupoint meant the location of a blood vessel where the stone needle was to be applied. The *Yellow Emperor's Canon of Medicine* includes a large number of related discussions. In The *Plain Conversation: Discussion on Treatment of Lumbago with Acupuncture*, it explained the methods for locating acupoints, for example, "Needling Jiemai (branch of Foot-Taiyin channel)", "Needling Tongyin channel (collateral of Foot-Shaoyin channel)", "Needling Yangwei channel", "Needling Feiyang channel", "Needling Sanmai", "Needling the channel inside of muscles" and etc [1]. At that time, puncturing blood vessels was equivalent to the puncturing of acupoints, and the sites of the blood vessels were exactly the sites for acupoints. In addition, from the naming of Daying (ST5), Renying (ST9), Chongyang (ST42), Taichong (LR3), Chimai (TE18) and so on, we found an obvious trace of transformation from "vessels" to "acupoints". The size of an acupoint is therefore also classified according to the appearance of blood vessels.

In the Yuan Dynasty, Dou Hangqing mentioned when defining the locations of acupoints, "At the Yang level lateral to the muscle and bone, depressions as existent; at the Ying layer between hollow and poles, corresponding to the artery [2]." In the Ming Dynasty, Xu Feng further explicated, "Yang level is where all Yang channels located, such as Hegu (LI4), Sanli (ST36) and Yanglingquan (GB34), with feeling depressions lateral to the middle bone as the real locations; Yin layer is where all Ying channels are located, such as Jimen (SP11), Wuli (LR10) and Taichong (LR3), in the middle of the muscles where arteries have to be felt, and those are the real points [3]."

Acupoints are closely related with the blood vessels, which no doubt reflected the hollow characteristics of acupoint structure.

3. The Acupoint Possess Diverse Structural Features

In modern acupuncture, acupoint is merely considered as a round dot-structure, where the distributions and measurements of 14 meridians, including Meridian points, Extra points and Ashi points over the whole body are considered as one type. In fact, this is untrue. The interstices between bones and joints, and the depressions between tendons and flesh actually come with different shapes. Acupoints located at the Large Collaterals, Small Collaterals, Floating Collaterals, arteries and other kinds of blood vessels varies in shape. Therefore, a diversified three-dimensional structure has to be seen as a distinctive character of acupoint.

For instance, Jingming (BL1) is defined in the *A-B Canon of Acupuncture and moxibution*: *chapter* 3 *section* 10 as "Lateral to the inner canthus of the eye" [4]. Here, we see that the acupoint does not locate on top of a dot; but at a long and narrow hollow between the eyeball at the inner canthus of the eye and the orbit. Hence, it is a hollow structure in narrow rectangular shape. Some newly invented names, such as Superior Jingming, Medial Jingming, Lateral Jingming, Jingguang, Dongming1, Jianming4 are simply different names to describe the same Jingming (BL1). Any acupoint located in long and narrow hollows at the medial angle of the inner canthus of the eye, and between medial wall of the orbit and the eyeball shall fall into the same category as the acupoint structure of Jingming (BL1).

Weizhong (BL40) stated as "In the popliteal fossa, as the He-Sea, found with the knee bent" (*Spiritual Pivot*: *Discussion on Acupoints*) [5], and "In the popliteal fossa, near the arterial line." (*A-B Canon of Acupuncture and moxibution*: *chapter* 3 *section* 35). This acupoint is actually located in the popliteal fossa, correlated with the politeal vein and artery in its deeper layer, and medial from Weiyang (BL39). Thus, the structure and ambit of Weizhong (BL40) have been included in a large portion of popliteal fossa, and in fact, it is a rhombus with hollow structure, especially when it comes to puncturing blood from this acupoint.

Taichong (LR3) was situated "In the depression, 2 Cun above Xingjian (LR2)" (*Spiritual Pivot*: *Discussion on Acupoints*), "2 Cun posterior to the lateral side of the big toe, or 1.5 Cun in the depression" (*A-B Canon of Acupuncture and moxibution*: *chapter* 3 *section* 31), and "Half Cun posterior to Xingjian (LR2)" (*Collective Compendium on Acupuncture and moxibution*: *chapter* 3) [6]. In fact, Taichong (LR3) is located on the dorsum of the foot, between the first and second metatarsal bones, in the depression distal to the junction of two bones, underneath the Taichong pulse (the first dorsalis pedis artery of the first metatarsal bone). Its positioning is based on the pulse of the vessel, and thus the way of measurement varies: 2 Cun above the joint, 1.5 Cun above the joint, and half Cun posterior to Xingjian (LR2). From here we can see that the complete portion of long and narrow depression on the dorsum of the foot between the first and second metatarsal bones has been interpreted as Taichong (LR3), and is under its structural ambit.

Acupoint is not limited to a round dot-shaped spatial structure. Some acupoints can be dots while some can be of any other shapes. As the location of an acupoint varies, its shape and structure also differs. Starting from the late Ming Dynasty, there was a rise of Pediatric Tuina Therapy, which created some designated acupoints, some were dots, some were in lines and some were considered to be surfaces. Of course, the creation of line-shape acupoints and surface-shape acupoints originated from the different manipulation methods of Tuina when which applied to human bodies. However, it does demonstrate that the ancients had not limited their understanding of acupoints to mere round dots.

4. The Size of an Acupoint Depend on Its Location

As each acupoint has its own shape and structure, the size range will be different from one another. Some acupoints are situated at a specific narrow position, and their structural ambits are usually not huge. Typical examples are the twelve Jing-Well points, Suliao (GV25), Ciliao (BL32), Zhangmen (LR13) and Jingmen (GB25).

However, the size of an acupoint appearing on the surface of a body may not necessarily correspond to its inner structural ambit. For instance, Dicang (ST4) is located at the angulus oris, but it is usually puncturing obliquely towards Jiache (ST6), and thus its structural ambit is not limited to the angulus oris. Another example, Yaoqi (EX-B9) is positioned 2 Cun superior to the tip of the coccyx, in the depression of the sacral angle, but it is required to puncture horizontally upwards for 2 to 3 Cun, that means its structural ambit is not limited to the depression in the sacral angle.

The size of an acupoint has been closely related to

other acupoints in its neighborhood, and this seems to be a common understanding. For example, Chengfu (BL36), Xinmen (BL37), Huantiao (GB30), Zusanli (ST36) and Chengjin (BL56) are further apart from their neighborhoods, so that their structural ambits are relatively larger. When the surrounding acupoints are larger in number, the captioned acupoint will surely be limited to a smaller ambit. For example, Shenting (GV24), Shangxing (GV23) and Meichong (BL3) are close to each other; and Yingjiao (CV7), Qihai (CV6), Shimen (CV5), Zhongzhu (KI15) and Siman (KI14) are closely located; and thus all their structural ambits are fairly limited.

Some structural ambits of acupoints have been changed from time to time. For instance, in the *A-B Canon of Acupuncture and moxibution*, Chimai (TE18) was positioned as "At the vein on the back of the ear which looks like a chicken talon", while Luxi (TE19) was placed "At the vein on the back of the ear", where both acupoints had been described "On the back of the ear" and "At the vein" as their standard measurements, and their therapeutic intents are also similar. In fact, this is a practice to split one acupoint into two based on the position of the blood vessel. Another example is Baihui (GV20), which is vertically superior to the auricular apex, at the median point on top of the head. In the *Peaceful Holy Benevolent Prescriptions*, Baihui (GV20) was positioned "At the depression in the center of the head" [7]. Since the way of puncturing this acupoint was inserting the needle horizontally along the skin, this triggered the question of puncturing the needle towards its posterior, anterior, lateral or medial sides, and the solution came with the formation of Sishencong (EX-HN1). The *Peaceful Holy Benevolent Prescriptions* had stated, "Sishencong (EX-HN1), at the four sides 1 Cun apart from Baihui (GV20)". Obviously, Sishencong (EX-HN1) is extended from Baihui (GV20), and its therapeutic intent is similar as Baihui (GV20). As a result, the original structural ambit of Baihui (GV20) is far downsized due to the creation of Sishencong (EX-HN1).

Acupoint has a multidimensional structure, and the acupoint locations make a difference in their structural ambits, yet the sizes of acupoints are vague due to the fact that there are no clear boundaries for their ambits. From the historical development point of view, the bone measurement and location of each acupoint have evolved into something concrete from ambiguity, turned into precision from roughness. Unfortunately, there is no further discussion on the deeper-layer structure of acupoints by the ancients, and thus all the size range of acupuncture points is merely a relative concept. We should not limit our recognition of an acupoint as a pure shape of round dots, there is not yet any concrete quantification of the size ranges for acupoint.

5. See the Ambiguous Nature of Acupoint's Size from Acupuncture Manipulation

In the *Spiritual Pivot*: *Application of Needles*, there are many types of puncturing and manipulation methods, revealing the ambiguity in regard to the size ranges of acupoints.

Jingci (meridian needling): "Jingci means to puncture the large channel in conjunction with the collateral." Luoci (collateral needling): "Luoci means to puncture the minute collaterals to let out blood." Fenci (separate needling): "Fenci means to puncture the gap between muscles." Maoci (leather needling): "Maoci means to puncture the skin, which contains the Fubi (floating Bi-syndrome)." Huici (extensive needling): "Huici means to puncture surround the spasm muscle, lift back and forth to relax the Jinbi (Bi-syndrome of tendon)." Zhizhenci (direct needling): "Zhizhenci means to nip up the muscle and puncture directly into it, to treat the cold disease hidden at a shallow level of a body." Shuci (transmitted needling): "Shuci means to puncture perpendicularly with fewer acupoints, and insert deeply to treat the over-abundant Qi and the severed heat." Duanci (gradual needling): "Duanci is used to treat Gubi (Bi-syndrome of bone), puncture deeply reaching the bone, shake slightly up and down the bone level." Fuci (floating needling): "Fuci means to puncture superficially surround the point to treat the cold and spasm muscles." These puncturing methods are decided upon the locations and structures of acupoints when treating different diseases.

Pangzhenci (adjacent needling): "Pangzhenci means to insert one needle perpendicularly into the affected part along with another one on the side, to fix the obstinate Bi-syndrome." Qici (multiple needling): "Qici means to insert one needle perpendicular into the affected part along with two others on the sides, to treat trivial cold with deeper penetration." Yangci (scattered needling): "Yangci means to insert one needle shallowly into the center of the affected part surrounded with four others on the sides to relieve excessive Cold-Qi (syndrome)." These are the practice based on the size ranges of acupoints when deciding on the number of needles to be used: two, three or five pieces on puncturing.

Sanci (triple needling): "The so called 'Sanci is to induce Gu-Qi (Food-Qi)' by first puncturing into the skin layer to dissipate Yang-Xie (Yang pathogen); 'Then further on to induce Yin-Xie (Yin pathogen)' by going deeper into the muscle before reaching muscular interstice; further into the muscular interstice, then Gu-Qi comes. Therefore, the book *Needling Methods* had said, 'First puncture shallowly to expel Xie-Qi (pathogens) with promoting blood circulation, then puncture deeper to discharge Yin-Xie, finally puncture the deepest to conduct Gu-Qi.' This is reason for what has been mentioned." It has indicated that the depth of puncturing is divided into three layers, namely shallow, medium and deep puncturing, in accordance to the depth of an acupoint within the skin, underneath the skin and in the muscular interstice.

Wuci: "There are five puncturing methods that correspond to Five Zang-organs. The first one is called Banci (half-needling), which punctures superficially without making any damage to the muscles, and withdraws rapidly as if pulling out hairs, to deploy the Qi from the skin, and this is the way of needling that corresponds to the lungs. The second one is called Baowenci (leopard spot needling), which punctures to the left, right, anterior and posterior of the channel level of the treated part for bloodletting, and this is the way of needling that corresponds to the heart. The third one is called Guanci (joint needling), which punctures directly to the joints on four limbs as well as the parts on distal tendons to treat Jinbi (Bi-Syndrome of tendon), and this is the way of needling that corresponds to the liver. The forth one is called Heguci (tri-directional needling), which works like a chicken talon with needles puncturing into the muscular interstices to heal Jibi (Bi-syndrome of muscle), and this is the way of needling that corresponds to the spleen. The fifth one is called Shuci (transmitted needling), which inserts and withdraws needles perpendicularly into the bone level to cure Gubi (Bi-syndrome of bone), and this is the way of needling that corresponds to the kidneys." These are the puncturing methods based on the depth of skin, muscle, channel, tendon and bone, the five layers, in response to illnesses of the lungs, heart, liver, spleen and kidneys, the five organs.

As the size ranges of acupoints and the depth of puncturing cannot be lumped under one heading, the puncturing methods also become varied.

6. Conclusion

The formation and development of acupoints have surely been influenced by the ancients' ambiguous way of thinking. The size and scope of an acupoint therefore has also been carrying such sense of ambiguity. The structure and size range of an acupoint are determined not only by the outlook of depression and blood vessel areas, but also its relationship with other acupoints in its vicinity. The different manipulations of puncturing recorded in the *Yellow Emperor's Canon of Medicine* also show the ambiguous nature of the structure and size range of an acupoint. In theory, an acupoint has been characterized as various forms, which should not be limited to a mere round dot shape. Without such understanding, an acupuncture practitioner will be limited to a large extent in clinical application and the studies on acupoints will also go into a wrong direction.

REFERENCES

[1] The Yellow Emperor's Canon of Medicine, "Plain Conversation (Copied Print)," People's Health Publishing House, Beijing, 1956.

[2] G. F. Dou, "Four Books of Avupuncture and Moxibuation," People's Health Publishing House, Beijing, 1956.

[3] F. Xu, "A Complete works in Avupuncture and Moxibuation," People's Health Publishing House, Beijing, 1958.

[4] F. M. Huang, "The A-B Canon of Acupuncture and Moxibution (Copied Print)," People's Health Publishing House, Beijing, 1956.

[5] "The Spiritual Pivot (Copied Print)," People's Health Publishing House, Beijing, 1956.

[6] R. H. Liao, "An Integration of Avupuncture and Moxibuation," Cathay Bookshop, Beijing, 1986.

[7] H. Y. Wang, Y. Wang, Q. Deng, *et al.*, "Peaceful Holy Benevolent Prescriptions," People's Health Publishing House, Beijing, 1958.

20

Effects of the Supercritical Fluid Extraction of Dahurian Angelica Root and Szechwan Lovage Rhizome on Spontaneous Hypertension Rats[*]

Yan Zhang[1#], Fenxia Gao[1], Yanjun Cao[2], Hongying Wang[2], Haijie Duan[3]

[1]The Mental Health Center of Xi'an, Xi'an, China
[2]School of Medicine, Xi'an Jiaotong University, Xi'an, China
[3]No. 5 Hospital of Xi'an, Xi'an, China
Email: [#]classicyan@gmail.com

ABSTRACT

The supercritical fluid extraction of Dahurian Angelica Root (Bai Zhi) and Szechwan Lovage Rhizome (Chuan Xiong) was named as BCC. In the study, we investigated whether BCC had effects on left ventricular hypertrophy (LVH) and myocardial fibrosis in spontaneous hypertensive rats (SHR). For SHR + BCC group, BCC (0.3 g/kg) was orally administered daily for 12 weeks. The SHR group and the Wistar Kyoto rats (WKY, normal control) group, the equal volume of 5‰ CMC-Na distilled water. After 12 weeks, left ventricle was segregated from each rat in the groups, and the left ventricle weight/body weight (LVW/BW) calculated. The volume fraction of collagen (VFC) in myocardium and the diameter of cardiac muscle cell (DCMC) were examined by histological staining. Biochemical indicators of blood sample such as Angiotensin II (Ang II), Aldosterone (ALD), Hyaluronic Acid (HA), Laminin (LN), Procollagen III (PC III) and Collagen type IV (CIV) levels were detected by using radioimmunoassay (RIA). And also NOS and iNOS levels were measured by means of ultra-violet spectroscopy (UV). The results shown that in SHR + BCC group, the LVW/BW, DCMC and VFC decreased significantly versus SHR group, the same as biochemical indicators except NOS and iNOS. All of above index was similar to WKY group. Statistically significant correlations were found among the plasma Ang II level, the mean systolic blood pressure (SBP), and the NOS level of the three groups. Our study indicates that the BCC can control the LVH and myocardial fibrosis in SHR.

Keywords: Dahurian Angelica Root; Szechwan Lovage Rhizome; LVH; Myocardial Fibrosis; SHR

1. Introduction

Hypertension is one of the most significant risk factors in the development and progression of a variety of cardiovascular diseases including cardiac hypertrophy and myocardial fibrosis. Clinical studies suggest that a high arterial pressure is associated with myocardial hypertrophy and interstitial fibrosis [1]. In the hypertensive state, a number of adaptive changes occur in heart [2] such as left ventricular hypertrophy (LVH) and myocardial interstitial fibrosis. At the same time, these structural abnormalities may play an important role in the development and maintenance of hypertension [3,4]. In addition, some studies shown that the Angiotensin II (Ang II), Aldosterone (ALD) Hyaluronic Acid (HA), Laminin (LN), Procollagen III (PC III) and Collagen type IV (CIV) levels had an increase in myocardial interstitial fibrosis [5].

The effectors/hormones of Ang II and ALD could stimulate fibroblast-mediated collagen synthesis [6,7], and Ang II additionally suppresses collagenase activity [6], which synergistically leads to myocardial collagen accumulation, induces HA, LN, PCIII, CIV increased. Recent study showed reduced NOS derived NO production contributes to the hypertrophic growth and phenoltype of cardiac muscle cells [8]. All of these changes would aggravate LVH, and exacerbate hypertension.

In clinic, some drugs such as angiotensin-converting enzyme inhibitors, angiotensin II receptor antagonists and calcium channel antagonists etc can not only decrease blood pressure, but also reverse the LVH and myocardial interstitial fibrosis. In recently years, some traditional Chinese medicines were reported to be effective against the hypertension [9]. Previous studies in our lab indicated that the Bai-Chuan capsule (BCC), a complex prescription of supercritical fluid extraction of Dahurian Angelica Root (Bai Zhi) and Szechwan Lovage Rhizome (Chuan Xiong) as a traditional Chinese medi-

[*]Effects of the supercritical fluid extraction of Dahurian Angelica Root and Szechwan Lovage Rhizome on spontaneous hypertension rats (dispensable).
[#]Corresponding author.

cine, in different dosages (0.6, 0.3 and 0.15 g/kg) could obviously reduce the blood pressures in SHR [10,11]. In this paper, we will investigate the effects of the BCC on left ventricular hypertrophy (LVH) and cardiac fibrosis as an anti-hypertensive medicine in SHR. Therefore, we treated 14-week-old male SHR with chronic hypertension, advanced LVH, and myocardial fibrosis, as well as age- and sex-matched normotensive WKY for 3 months with BCC. It was the first report about the effects of BCC on the structure of LVH and myocardial fibrosis in SHR.

2. Materials and Methods

2.1. Composition of BCC

BCC was prepared with the supercritical fluid extraction of Dahurian Angelica Root (Bai Zhi) and Szechwan Lovage Rhizome (Chuan Xiong) according to 1:1, which was provided by our lab and named as Bai-Chuan Capsule (BCC). Briefly, BCC improved in the Chinese folk medicine "Du Liang Wa", which had been used for over 1000 years in China. Prescriptions can be found in "Shi Zhai Bai Yi Xuan Fang" by Miao Wang (during the Song Dynasty) and recent drug standards issued by Beijing in 1983.

2.2. Protocol

Sixteen male SHR, age of 14 weeks, 270 - 290 g, and eight male WKY rats, age of 14 weeks, 280 - 320 g were purchased from Chengdu Da Shuo Biological Technology Co., Ltd. (Chengdu, China). Rats were housed in temperature (24°C ± 2°C) and humidity (50% ± 10%) controlled room with a 12-h on/12-h off light cycle. Solid rodent chow and autoclaved water were given ad libitum.

Animals were allowed a period of 1 week of acclimatization prior to entry into any experimental protocol. To obtain an accurate blood pressure reading, rats remained still and unperturbed throughout the measurement period. Rats were conditioned to the restraint and the warming chamber for 10 - 20 min/day of 37°C before measurements. After 1 week, 16 SHR were randomly divided into two groups: SHR group and SHR + BCC group (n = 8 equally). Eight WKY rats were the normal control group. Rats in the SHR + BCC group were intragastric administration BCC at 0.3 g/kg (equal to 11-fold of clinic dosage), which was suspended in 5 ml of 5‰ CMC-Na distilled water, once a day for 12 weeks. The WKY and the SHR control groups were administrated an equal volume of 5‰ CMC-Na distilled water.

2.3. Measuring of Systolic Blood Pressure (SBP)

The SBP was measured once a week for the first 3 weeks, and then measured fortnightly till the end of the experiment (eight times totally). After training period, SBP was measured in the morning after intragastric administration 2 hour. The maximum pressure of inflation was set 20 - 40 mmHg above anticipated SBP. The instrument was set for a maximum inflation pressure of 160 mmHg for WKY rats that were expected to have pressures in the normal range and was increased to 250 or 300 mmHg for markedly SHR rats. A typical run involved 6 repetitions of the automated inflation-deflation cycle with a 2-minute interval till Rats' pulsatory signals from the arteria caudilis were displayed steadily, then the mean of 3 readings within a 5 - 10 mmHg range was taken as SBP of rat.

2.4. Measurement of Left Ventricular Hypertrophy Ratio

Twelve weeks later, the rats were weighed and anesthetized with 20% Ethylurethanm (5 ml/kg, intraperitoneal injection). The chest cavity was rapidly opened, and the heart was removed and rinsed in two washes of ice-cold saline. Major blood vessels and connective tissue was removed, the heart blotted dry, weighed, and the LVW/BW ratio calculated. Other organ weights were determined and weight to total body weight ratios calculated.

2.5. Myocardial Histological and Morphological Assay

Part of the left ventricle, about 0.5 cm above apex cordis, was segregated, fixed in 4% paraformaldehyde, embedded in paraffin, sectioned at 4 μm, and stained with Hematoxylin-Eosin (HE) and Weigert Hematoxylin-Victoria blue'B-Ponceau. Myocardial slices, 16 of those round or similar to round were chose randomly from each group. The morphometric result for each section was the average of measurements from its volume fraction of collagen (VFC) and the diameter of cardiac muscle cell (DCMC). Because of the lack of universal consensus on the definition of myocardium VFS, animals with a >30 μm width collagen were classified as 2/severe myocardial fibrosis, 5 - 30 μm as 1/medium, and <5 μm as 0/normal myocardium. At the same time, Myocardial hypertrophy was defined DCMC >45μm as 2/severe hypertrophy, 30 - 45 μm as 1/medium, and <30 μm as 0/normal cardiac muscle cell.

2.6. Measurement of Plasma Ang II, ALD, NOS and iNOS

Blood samples from all of the subjects were obtained from abdominal aorta in the morning after overnight fasting and were collected in vacuum tubes with EDTA as an anticoagulant. After being centrifuged at 3000 rpm for 20 minutes at 4°C immediately after collection, the plasma samples were then kept frozen at −40°C until analyzed. Blood Ang II and ALD levels were measured by radioimmunoassay (RIA) with commercially available kits (Beijing North Institute of Biotechnique). NOS and iNOS levels were measured by ultraviolet spectrophotometry (UV) with NOS and iNOS assay kits (Nanjing Jiancheng Bioengineering Institute).

2.7. Measurement of Serum HA, LN, PCIII and CIV

Blood samples from all of the subjects were obtained from abdominal aorta in the morning after overnight fasting and were collected in vacuum tubes with nothing as an anticoagulant. Sera were centrifuged after standing for 4 hours at room temperature, and preserved at −20°C before assays. The serum level of HA, LN, PCIII and CIV were detected by radioimmunoassay (RIA) with commercially available kits (Beijing North biology technique institute).

2.8. Statistical Analysis

Results are expressed as the mean ± S.D. Student's t-test was used for comparison between groups. Values of $P < 0.05$ were considered statistically significant.

3. Results

3.1. Comparison of LVW/BW, Left Ventricle Morphology and Histology among Groups

At the end of the treatment, it was conspicuous in our study that LVW/BW of the untreated SHR was higher than WKY rats (2.78 ± 0.49 mg/g vs 1.93 ± 0.71 mg/g), and animals treated by BCC had significantly lower LVW/BW compared with untreated animals (2.78 ± 0.49 mg/g vs 3.35 ± 0.83 mg/g, $P < 0.01$). VFC and DCMC of untreated SHR were significantly higher than of WKY rats, but decreased in the SHR + BCC group (**Figure 1**).

Weigert Hematoxylin-Victoria blue'B-Ponceau staining showed that the VFC and numeral density of SHR was more increasing; collagen fibers in media were hyperplasic, cardiac muscle cell was hypertrophy and round (**Figures 2(A)** and **(D)**). In the BCC group (**Figures 2(B)** and **(E)**), VFC was medium, the DCMC of cardiac muscle cell was smaller than untreated SHR, and shape was approximation to WKY rats (**Figures 2(C)** and **(F)**).

3.2. Serum HA, LN, PCIII and CIV Levels

Treatment with BCC caused significantly reduction in all the level of HA, LN and CIV. The recorded levels of serum HA, LN, PCIII and CIV in WKY and SHR are shown in (**Figure 3**). HA, LN, PCIII and CIV levels in the sera from SHR with fibrotic changes were significantly higher when compared to the WKY rats and treated SHR.

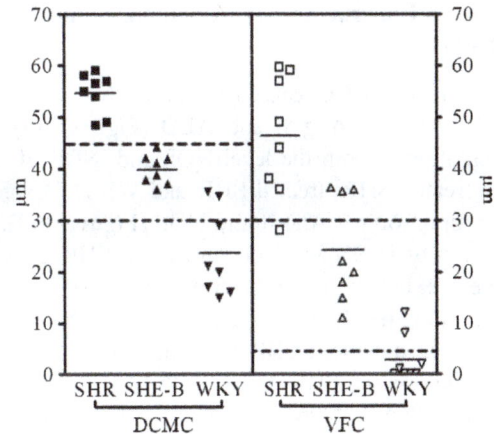

Figure 1. Photomicrographs demonstrating VFC, DCMC of SHR (SHR treated with BCC and WKY rats 12 weeks after surgery (G). 2 means severe myocardial fibrosis/severe cell hypertrophy, 1 medium, 0 normal.).

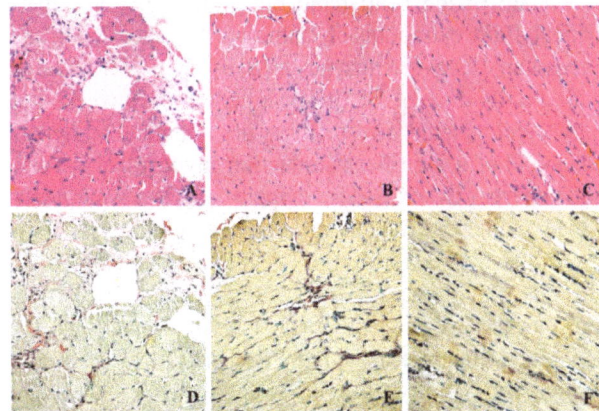

Figure 2. Heart sections of SHR staining (counterstained with HE staining (A, B and C) and Weigert Hematoxylin-Victoria blue'B-Ponceau staining (D, E, F). Magnification ×400.).

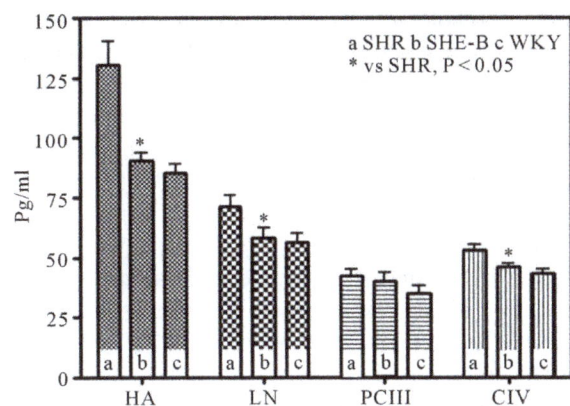

Figure 3. Serum HA, LN, PCIII and CIV levels (The recorded levels of serum HA LN, PCIII and CIV in Untreated SHR, treated SHR and WKY. There was difference in HA, LN, CIV between Untreated SHR and treated SHR ($P < 0.05$).).

3.3. Blood Plasma Ang II, ALD, NOS and iNOS Levels

Treatment with BCC caused significantly reduction in both the level of Ang II and ALD (**Figure 4(a)**), but augmentation in both the level NOS and iNOS of SHR. The untreated SHR, treated SHR and WKY showed inverse proportion for Ang II and NOS (**Figure 4(c)**). The proportion of iNOS and NOS in treated SHR were distinctive 1:2, but the iNOS level was about 90% of NOS in WKY (**Figure 4(b)**). Comparison of the three groups showed that untreated SHR had ALD of 298.3 ± 57.7 pg/ml, whereas the SHR treated with BCC demonstrated reduced ALD of 138.96 ± 25.2 pg/ml, which was near to WKY ALD of 100.18 ± 38.8 pg/ml (**Figure 4(a)**).

4. Discussion

The results of our study showed an anti-hypertensive and a reversal of the heart remodeling effect of the supercritical fluid extraction of Dahurian Angelica Root and Szechwan Lovage Rhizome on SHR. The SHR treated with a daily dose of BCC over a period of 12 weeks not only demonstrated arrest of the development of hypertension, but a significant reduction myocardial fibrosis and coherent index. Cardiac hypertrophy is a well-established major risk factor for cardiovascular disease, including sudden death. But, we also found that that LVW/BW of the untreated SHR was higher than WKY rats, and animals treated with BCC had significantly lower LVW/BW compared with untreated animals in the model group. Most antihypertensive drugs lower BP and also cause regression of LVH (Jennings *et al.*, 1997). However, the classic arterial vasodilators, hydralazine and minoxidil, cause minimal regression [12] and can increase LV mass in hypertensive rats and humans. BCC not only can protect BP, but also can cause regression of LVH. Morphological studies indicate that the increment in myocardial mass is caused by muscle hypertrophy and a disproportionate accumulation of fibrillar collagen in the interstitial space. Aldosterone emerges as important determinants of myocardial fibrosis [13,14]. This factor increases the synthesis of collagen I and III by cardiac fibroblasts [6]. The direct pro-fibrotic effect of ALD is mediated through specific corticoid receptors in cardiac fibroblast [15], and is independent of cardiac load and LVH. In addition, experimental evidence has been collected on a cross-talk between ALD and ET. ET-1 has been demonstrated to stimulate ALD secretion, both in animals and in humans, having a direct secretagogue effect on the adrenal cortex [16], equipotent to that of Ang II, and ALD infusion in experimental models of salt-loaded rats has been shown to enhance ET-1 production [17]. The possible effect of ALD on myocardial performance is not obvious. Increased collagen content

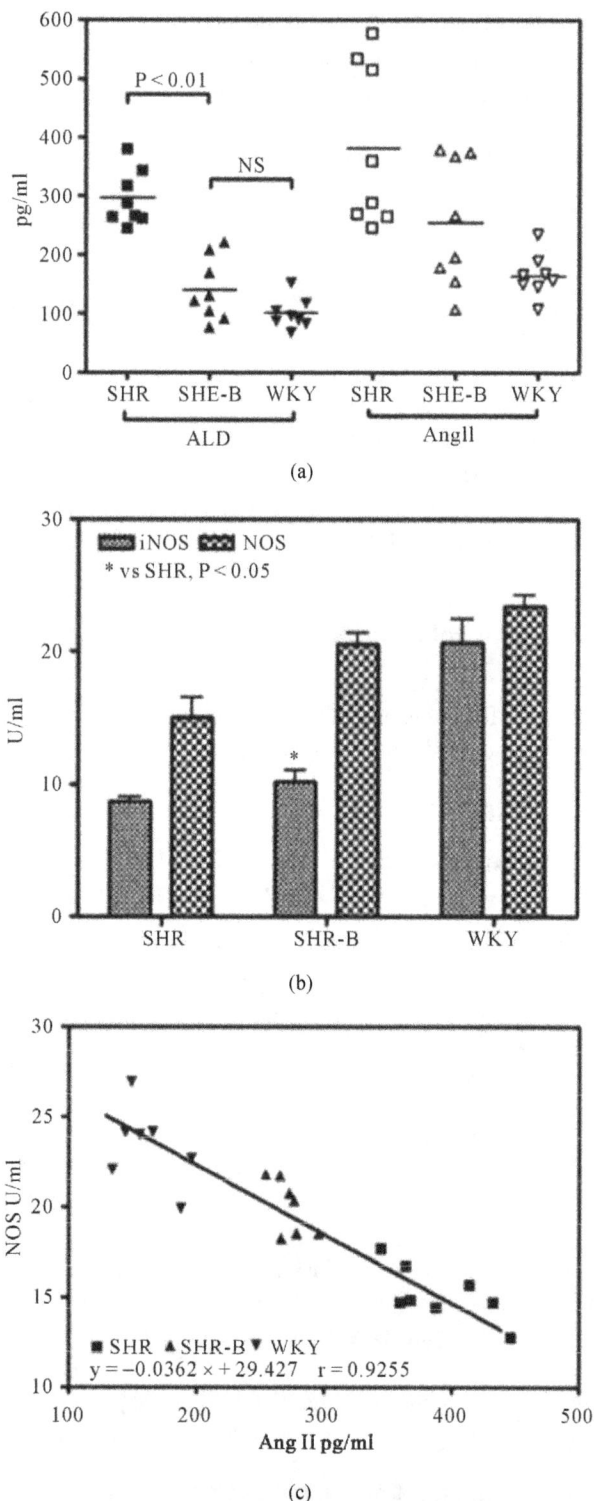

(a)

(b)

(c)

Figure 4. Blood plasma Ang II, ALD, NOS and iNOS levels (Comparison of Ang II and ALD in the three experimental groups (a). Comparison of NOS and iNOS in the three experimental groups (b). The correlation between NOS and plasma Ang II in Untreated SHR, treated SHR and WKY (c; r = 0.93; P < 0.01). Data are expressed as the mean ± S.D. (n = 8 rats/group). *P < 0.01 means significantly different from SHR group.).

within myocardial interstitium can be presumed to impair contractile behavior of myocardial fibers. Our data suggest that ALD-induced alterations in myocardial composition and geometry result in a subtle impairment of myocardial performance. These alterations can also modify myocardial stiffness and therefore LV diastolic properties. The left ventricle morphology and histology results show that collagen fibers in media were hyperplastic, elastic fibers decreased and disordered, part of which were substituted by collagen fibers.

Recently, study has demonstrated that macrophage infiltration is an early key event for reactive myocardial fibrosis, especially perivascular fibrosis in this model [18]. Also, it has been shown that Ang II supports leukocyte transmigration via AT1 receptor-dependent, but arterial pressure-independent, mechanisms [19,20]. Taken together, the present study provides in vivo evidence that Ang II might play an important role in early fibrotic changes and the resultant reactive myocardial fibrosis in hearts by activating the macrophage-mediated inflammatory process. Of course, Ang II is not the only proinflammatory mediator. Recent studies have suggested that it is a strong proinflammatory factors, because mechanical strain can induce inflammatory cytokines, growth factors, and oxidative stress, as well as tissue RAS in the vessel wall [21]. The interplay of these factors might regulate tissue Ang II production and the fibrotic process in hearts.

Our study clearly demonstrated that BCC supplementation could block the effects of high blood pressure on plasma Ang II, NOS level, Biochemical indicators of myocardial fibrosis levels, and BP in SHR. These observations indicated that BCC might influence NOS by inhibiting the Ang II production and preventing the BP elevation. The pharmacological results demonstrated that the effective component of BCC in CMC system can act on rat artery cell membrane as Verapamil, a calcium antagonist. And further studies showed that the effective component had the effects of inhibiting vasoconstriction *in vitro* on rat abdominal aorta segments. It would be our next research project.

REFERENCES

[1] K. Michaela, B. Simona, P. Carlo, B. Giampaolo, M. Angelica, F. Stefania, *et al.*, "Myocardial Ultrasonic Backscatter in Hypertension Relation to Aldosterone and Endothelin," *Hypertension*, Vol. 41, No. 2, 2003, pp. 230-236. doi:10.1161/01.HYP.0000052542.68896.2B

[2] Y. Hu and N. S. Cai, "Reconstitution of LVH in High Blood Pressure," *Chinese Journal of Internal Medicine*, Vol. 36, No. 6, 1997, pp. 424-426.

[3] L. M. De, A. Estevez, D. Bunout, C. Klenner, M. Oyonarte and S. Hirsch, "Ventricular Mass in Hypertensive and Normotensive Obese Subjects," *International Journal of Obesity and Related Metabolic Disorders*, Vol. 18, No. 4, 1994, pp. 193-197.

[4] M. S. Lauer, K. M. Anderson and D. Levy, "Separate and Joint Influences of Obesity and Mild Hypertension on Left Ventricular Mass and Geometry: The Framingham Heart Study," *Journal of the American College of Cardiology*, Vol. 19, No. 1, 1992, pp. 130-134. doi:10.1016/0735-1097(92)90063-S

[5] C. Li and F. Lu, "Change of Myocardial Interstitial Fibrosis Index in Hypertension Complicated with Left Ventricular Hypertrophy and Influence of ACET Therapy," *Chinese Journal of Cardiovascular Rehabilitation Medicine*, Vol. 12, No. 1, 2003, pp. 22-24.

[6] C. G. Brilla, G. Zhou, L. Matsubara and K. T. Weber, "Collagen Metabolism in Cultured Adult Rat Cardiac Fibroblasts: Response to Angiotensin II and Aldosterone," *Journal of Molecular and Cellular Cardiology*, Vol. 26, No. 7, 1994, pp. 809-820. doi:10.1006/jmcc.1994.1098

[7] F. J. Villarreal, N. N. Kim, G. D. Ungab, M. P. Printz and W. H. Dillmann, "Identification of Functional Angiotensin II Receptors on Rat Cardiac Fibroblasts," *Circulation*, Vol. 88, No. 6, 1993, pp. 2849-2861. doi:10.1161/01.CIR.88.6.2849

[8] W. Sibylle, R. Cornelia, W. Sandra, R. Joachim, K. Georg and S. Klaus-Dieter, "Lack of Endothelial Nitric Oxide Synthase-Derived Nitric Oxide Formation Favors Hypertrophy in Adult Ventricular Cardiomyocytes," *Hypertension*, Vol. 49, No. 1, 2007, pp. 193-200.

[9] H. C. Shih, T. H. Lee, S. C. Chen, C. Y. Li and T. Shibuya, "Antihypertension Effects of Traditional Chinese Medicine Ju-Ling-Tang on Renal Hypertensive Rats," *The American Journal of Chinese Medicine*, Vol. 33, No. 6, 2005, pp. 913-921. doi:10.1142/S0192415X05003545

[10] W. H. Zhao, Y. X. Cao, J. Liu and L. C. He, "The Influence of Bai Chuan Capsule to Awake Rats," *Journal of Xi'an Medical University*, Vol. 22, No. 4, 2001, pp. 315-336.

[11] Y. Zhang, L. C. He, H. J. Duan and Y. Z. Zhan, "Effects of Bai Chuan Capsule on Left Ventricular Hypertrophy and Correlative Indexes," *Journal of Chinese Medicinal Materials*, Vol. 33, No. 8, 2010, pp. 1290-1292.

[12] J. M. Cruickshank, J. Lewis, V. Moore and C. Dodd, "Reversibility of Left Ventricular Hypertrophy by Differing Types of Antihypertensive Therapy," *Journal of Human Hypertension*, Vol. 6, No. 2, 1992, pp. 85-90.

[13] N. Varo, M. J. Iraburu, M. Varela, B. Lùpez, J. C. Etayo and J. Dìez, "Chronic AT1 Blockade Stimulates Extracellular Collagen Type I Degradation and Reverses Myocardial Fibrosis in Spontaneously Hypertensive Rats," *Hypertension*, Vol. 35, No. 6, 2000, pp. 1197-1202. doi:10.1161/01.HYP.35.6.1197

[14] K. T. Weber and G. G. Brilla, "Pathological Hypertrophy and Cardiac Interstitium: Fibrosis and Renin-Angiotensin-Aldosterone System," *Circulation*, Vol. 83, No. 6, 1991, pp. 1849-1865. doi:10.1161/01.CIR.83.6.1849

[15] M. Lombès, N. Alfaidy, E. Eugene, A. Lessana, N. Farman and J. P. Bonvalet, "Prerequisite for Cardiac Aldosterone Action: Mineralcorticoid Receptor and 11-Hydroxysteroid Dehydrogenase in the Human Heart," *Circula-*

tion, Vol. 92, No. 2, 1995, pp. 175-182. doi:10.1161/01.CIR.92.2.175

[16] G. P. Rossi, A. Sacchetto, M. Cesari and A. C. Pessina, "Interaction between Endothelin-1 and Renin-Angiotensin-Aldosterone System," *Cardiovascular Research*, Vol. 43, No. 2, 1999, pp. 300-307. doi:10.1016/S0008-6363(99)00110-8

[17] E. L. Schiffrin, "Role of Endothelin-1 in Hypertension and Vascular Disease," *American Journal of Hypertension*, Vol. 14, No. 6, 2001, pp. 83S-89S. doi:10.1016/S0895-7061(01)02074-X

[18] F. Kuwahara, H. Kai, K. Tokuda, H. Niiyama, N. Tahara, K. Kusaba, *et al.*, "Roles of Intercellular Adhesion Molecule-1 in Hypertensive Cardiac Remodeling," *Hypertension*, Vol. 41, No. 3, 2003, pp. 819-823.

[19] W. B. Strawn, P. E. Gallagher, E. A. Tallant, D. Ganten and C. M. Ferrario, "Angiotensin II AT1-Receptor Blockade Inhibits Monocyte Activation and Adhesion in Transgenic (mRen2) 27 Rats," *Journal of Cardiovascular Pharmacology*, Vol. 33, No. 3, 1999, pp. 341-351. doi:10.1097/00005344-199903000-00001

[20] L. Pastore, A. Tessitore, S. Martinotti, E. Toniato, E. Alesse, M. C. Bravi, *et al.*, "Angiotensin II Stimulates Intracellular Adhesion Molecule-1 (ICAM-1) Expression by Human Vascular Endothelial Cells and Increases Soluble ICAM-1 Release *in Vivo*," *Circulation*, Vol. 100, No. 15, 1999, pp. 1646-1652. doi:10.1161/01.CIR.100.15.1646

[21] A. Nicoletti and J. B. Michel, "Cardiac Fibrosis and Inflammation: Interaction with Hemodynamic and Hormonal Factors," *Cardiovascular Research*, Vol. 41, No. 3, 1999, pp. 532-543. doi:10.1016/S0008-6363(98)00305-8

21

PIP, Not FiO$_2$ Regulates Expression of MMP-9 in the Newborn Rabbit VILI with Different Mechanical Ventilation Strategies

Shaodong Hua[1], Xiaoying Zhang[1], Shengli An[2], Xiuxiang Liu[3], Zhichun Feng[4*]

[1]Department of Pediatrics, BaYi Children's Hospital of the General Military Hospital of Beijing PLA, Beijing, China
[2]Department of Biostatistics, South Medical University, Guangzhou, China
[3]The Hospital Affiliated Binzhou Medicall University, Binzhou, China
[4]Department of Pediatrics, BaYi Children's Hospital of the General Military Hospital of Beijing PLA, Beijing, China
Email: *fengzhichun81@163.com

ABSTRACT

Background: Results from experimental and clinical studies have shown that mechanical ventilation or/and hyperoxia may aggravate a pre-existing lung injury or even cause lung injury in healthy lungs by affecting the expression of MMP-9, but the MMP-9 effects are controversial. How are MMP-9 regulated when multicausative factors of injury such as different FiO$_2$, PIP, and respiratory time (RT) impose simultaneously on lungs? **Methods:** Newborn New Zealand white rabbits were randomly allocated to an unventilated air control group or to one of the $2 \times 3 \times 3$ ventilation strategies by using a factorial design, with different FiO$_2$, PIP, and RT. Then, lung wet-to-dry ratio (W/D), lung histopathology scores, transmission electron microscope, and cells in BALF were analyzed in these different groups. MMP-9 levels were studied by immunohistochemistry and ELISA. **Results:** MMP-9 levels were significantly different among 3 PIP ventilation regimes (F = 7.215) and MPIP group was the highest among 3 PIP groups. The lung histopathology score in 100% oxygen was significantly higher than in 45% oxygen group (F = 9.037) and MPIP group was the lowest among 3 PIP groups (F = 57.515) and RT 6 h was more serious than RT 1 h. MMP-9 positively correlated with monocytes, but negatively correlated with neutrophils and lung injury histopathology scores. **Conclusions:** Different PIP and FiO$_2$ exert simultaneously on newborn lung in newborn rabbits ventilation, only mechanical stretch stimulation affects MMP-9 synthesis. Advisable mechanical stretch can promote MMP-9 expression and has protective role in lung in VILI. HPIP causes barotraumas and LPIP induces atelectrauma.

Keywords: Mechanical Ventilation; Lung Injury; Matrix Metalloproteinase; Newborn Rabbit; Fraction of Inspired Oxygen; Peak Inspiratory Pressure

1. Introduction

Mechanical ventilation (MV) is a life-saving therapy that can also damage the lungs. Matrix Metalloproteinase-9 (MMP-9) can degrade the complex components structure of the lungs and airway, such as extracellular matrix (ECM) and the basement membrane to participate in the lungs and airway reconstruction [1]. On the relationship between MMP-9 and lung injury, there were plenty of studies showing that expression of MMP-9 was regulated by factors of MV [2,3] and high concentrations of oxygen [4] as well as the expression of MMP-9 increases led to lung injury [5,6], but there were also some studies on

protective role in MMP-9 [7,8], absence of MMP-9 worsens mechanical ventilation-induced lung injury (VILI) [9]. These conclusions are based on single-factor condition model and different condition animal models have different experimental results [10]. However, clinically, VILI was multi-factorial, not only including oxygen concentrations, peak inspiratory pressure (PIP), but also including duration of ventilation and so on. To support gas exchange, the parameters about oxygen concentrations and PIP are usually regulated. Importantly, PIP, hyperoxia and duration of ventilation (respiratory time, RT) can induce lung injury, but it has not yet to be determined whether these 3 factors regulated individually

---

*Corresponding author.

or simultaneously the expression of MMP-9 causing lung injury when multi-factors impose simultaneously on lungs. Did these factors interact, and/or was one more dominant than the other? Assessment of lung injury was only carried out in animal experiment. We hypothesized that these causative factors of injury could not simultaneously promote MMP-9 producing, otherwise, VILI was impossible to be cured.

2. Methods

2.1. Ethics

The use of animals was approved by hospital of Beijing Institutional Animal Care and Use Committee (IACUC) and conformed to the guidelines of the National Institutes of Health for the care and use of laboratory animals.

2.2. Animals and Experimental Protocol

We employed 114 newborn New Zealand white rabbits (postnatal days, 1 - 5; 44.84 g). The rabbits were randomly allocated to either an unventilated air control group (n = 6) or to one of the $2 \times 3 \times 3$ ventilation strategies by using a factorial design FiO_2: $FiO_2 = 100\%$ and $FiO_2 = 45\%$; PIP: high PIP (HPIP) = 25 cmH_2O, mid PIP (MPIP) = 18 cmH_2O and low PIP (LPIP) = 10 cmH_2O; respiratory time (RT): 1 h, 3 h and 6 h; Each group had 6 rabbits, and there were 108 rabbits in the ventilated groups.

2.3. Mechanical Ventilation

The rabbits were anesthetized with intraperitoneal sodium pentobarbital, 25 mg/kg. Their body-temperatures were maintained at 39°C by a heating pad. A tracheostomy was performed near the thyroid eminence, and an endotracheal tube (1.3×25 mm^2 intravenous catheter needles) was inserted via tracheostomy (the depth was 1.5 - 2.0 cm), and the endotracheal tube was regulated on the basis of the symmetry of thorax fluctuation after ventilation to avoid atelectasis. Then the rabbits were ventilated (Siemens-900C, Germany) with a fixed positive end-expiratory pressure (PEEP) at 2 cmH_2O with a respiratory rate of (RR) 50 min^{-1}, and an inspiratory time of 0.33 sec at differing levels of FiO_2 and PIP depending on the RT according to a factorial design. No additional fluid support was given in any of the conducted experiments. At the end of the experiment, the rabbits from each experiment group were euthanized at 1, 3, and 6 h with a lethal dose of pentobarbital (100 mg/kg, i.p.). Immediately after sacrifice, lungs were isolated and measurements were performed as described below.

2.4. Measurements

The left lung was weighed and subsequently dried for 2 days in an oven at 70°C for estimating the wet-to-dry ratios (W/D). Bronchoalveolar lavage fluid (BALF) was obtained by instilling 1.0 ml saline 3 times by using a T catheter (Abbott, Sligo, Ireland) into the left trachea to lavage the left lung, and approximately 2.7 ml of BALF was retrieved per rabbit. Subsequently, BALF was centrifuged at 2000 g for 10 min, supernatants were snap-frozen in liquid nitrogen for later analysis, and wright-stained smears of cytospin slides of tracheal aspirates were examined for cell density (cells/ $\times$ 400 high power field) with white blood cells (WBC) and differential WBC counts (percentage) being done by an observer masked to the group identities.

2.5. Lung Histopathology

To analyze the histopathology of the lungs, the right lung lower lobe was fixed in 4% formalin and embedded in paraffin. Sections of 4 μm in thickness were stained with hematoxylin and eosin (HE) and analyzed by a pathologist who was blinded to the group identities. To score lung injury, we used a modified VILI histopathology scoring system as previously described [11,12]. An overall score of VILI was obtained on the basis of the summation of all the scores from air control or ventilated lungs (n = 6 per group).

2.6. Electron Microscopy

Electron microscopy was performed to investigate the morphological changes in different ventilation groups. Lung tissues were fixed with 2.5% glutaraldehyde in 0.1 M phosphate buffer at pH 7.4 for 18 h. Lung tissues were post-fixed for 1.5 h in 1% osmium tetroxide (OsO_4), dissolved in 0.1 M phosphate buffer at pH 7.4, dehydrated in an ascending acetone series, embedded in epon, sectioned at 70 nm, stained with uranyl-acetate and lead nitrate, and examined under an H-7500 transmission electron microscope (HITACHI, Japan).

2.7. Matrix Metalloproteinase-9 Assay

At each RT point, the right lung middle lobe was harvested and weighted 0.12 g pulmonary tissue samples and frozen at −70°C until use. The concentrations of MMP-9 in lung tissue homogenate were assayed using a commerically available kit according to the manufacture's protocol (Rabbit MMP-9 ELISA Kit, Catalog No: E0553Rb, Wuhan EIAab Science.co., Ltd., China; http://www.eiaab.com). The concentrations of MMP-9 in lung tissue homogenate were expressed ng·mL^{-1}.

2.8. Immunohistochemistry

Immunohistochemical analysis of protein expression was performed on paraffin slides with the use of SABC kits

(Boster Biological Technology, Ltd., Wuhan, China), Dako peroxidase kit (Dako, CA) and DAB reagent (DAKO, Denmark) as previously described [13], Tissue sections were incubated with primary antibodies (biotinylated anti rabbit MMP-9) and appropriate secondary antibodies (biotinylated goat anti rabbit). The sections were lightly counterstained with hematoxylin and bound antibody was visualized according to the standard avidin-biotinperoxidase complex protocol with a microscope (Nikon, Japan). The primary antibody was replaced by PBS for negative control slides and the known-positive slice was used as the positive control slides. The immunoreactivities of the lung tissue specimens were scored independently by two pathologists who were blinded to the protocol and experimental groups using the following scheme: the yellow intensity of positive immunoreactivity stained: 0 = no stain; 1 = stramineous; 2 = buffy; 3 = brown and the area of positive yellow stained (0 = 0; 1 = 0 - 1/3; 2 = 1/3 - 2/3; 3 = 2/3 - 1). MMP-9 expression was examined randomly in five HPFs (magnification ×400), and the total scores of the two parts represented the expression of MMP-9.

2.9. Statistical Analysis

All data in the results section are expressed as mean ± standard deviation. $2 \times 3 \times 3$ factorial design analysis of variance (ANOVA) was performed. Interaction significant needed to analyze simple effect with one-way ANOVA after fixed certain factor. Post Hoc Test for multiple comparisons, if equal variances assumed, LSD was perform; equal variances not assumed, Tamhane's T2 test was performed. The χ^2 test was used to compare the distribution of atelectasis. Bivariate correlation was used to determine the correlation of variable. The statistical significance level was set at $p < 0.05$.

3. Results

3.1. FiO2, PIP and RT Contribute to W/D. There Are Interactions to W/D between FiO2 and PIP

Factorial design analysis of variance results show: there were significances in different FiO2 (F = 7.164, p = 0.009) and 100% oxygen group was higher than 45% oxygen groups, or in different PIP (F = 27.563, p = 0.000) groups and 18 cmH2O was the lowest among 3 PIP groups, or in different RT groups (F = 3.233, p = 0.044) and RT6 group was higher than RT1 group (p = 0.016). Furthermore, there were interaction effect between FiO2 and PIP (F = 3.674, p = 0.029) (R squared = 0.479, Adjusted R squared = 0.381). The simple effect was analyzed. When FiO2 was 100% or 45%, One way ANOVA showed that 18 cmH2O group was the lowest in 3 PIP groups , respectively, (p = 0.000, 0.010) or (p = 0.000, 0.000). As

for PIP, there was significance in different FiO2 groups and 100% oxygen groups was higher than 45% oxygen when PIP was fixed at 25 cmH2O (F = 4.209, p = 0.048) or 18 cmH2O (F = 10.241, p = 0.003), whilst, there was no significance in different FiO2 groups when PIP was fixed at 10 cmH2O (F = 0.270, p = 0.607) (Table 1).

3.2. PIP, RT 2 Factors Contribute to WBCs in BALF. There Are Interactions to Cells between FiO2 and RT as well as PIP and RT

Factorial design ANOVA (Table 2) showed that the number of WBCs in BALF was similar in the 2 FiO2 groups (F = 0.122, p = 0.728), whereas PIP (F = 78.437, p < 0.001) and RT (F = 9.114, p < 0.001) had a significant effect on the number of WBCs. Moreover, there were interaction effects between FiO2 and RT (F = 6.206, p = 0.003) or between PIP and RT (F = 3.468, p = 0.011) (R Squared = 0.693, Adjusted R Squared = 0.636). The simple effect was analyzed. when FiO2 was 100%, ONE-WAY ANOVA showed that there were no significance in cells among RT 1 h, 3 h and 6 h groups (F = 2.386, p = 0.102), but fixed FiO2 was 45%, there were significance in cells among RT 1 h, 3 h and 6 h groups (F = 3.481, p = 0.038), multiple comparisons with Tamhane were no significance. when fixed RT was 3 h, 100% oxygen group was lower than 45% oxygen group in cells (F = 5.393, p = 0.026). But there were no significance when fixed RT was 1 h (F = 0.051, p = 0.822) and 6 h (F = 1.027, p = 0.318). When fixed PIP was 25 cmH2O, ONE-WAY ANOVA showed that there were significance in CELLS among RT 1 h, 3 h, 6 h groups (F = 3.923, p = 0.030) and RT 6 h group was the highest compared with RT 1 h and 3 h (p = 0.024, 0.019). When fixed PIP was 18 cmH2O, ONE-WAY ANOVA showed that there were significance in cells among 3 RT groups (F = 8.862, p = 0.001) and RT 3 h group was the highest compared with RT 1 h and 6 h (p = 0.000, 0.013). When fixed PIP was 10 cmH2O, ONE-WAY ANOVA showed that there were significance in cells among 3 RT groups (F = 6.611, p = 0.004) and RT 1 h group was the lowest compared with RT3 h and 6 h (p = 0.001, 0.040). As for fixed RT 1 h,3 h and 6 h, ONE-WAY ANOVA showed that there were significance in cells among 3 PIP groups, (F = 39.001, 11.188, 33.732, respectively, p = 0.000) and 25 cmH2O group was the highest compared with 18 and 10 cmH2O group in fixed RT 1 h, 3 h and 6 h.

3.3. FiO2, PIP, RT 3 Factors Contribute to Neutrophil in BALF. There Are Interactions to Neutrophil between FiO2 and PIP as well as PIP and RT

Factorial design ANOVA showed that the neutrophil levels were significantly different in these ventilation regimes (Table 2). These results show that neutrophil le-

Table 1. W/D in different ventilation groups.

RT	100% oxygen				45% oxygen			
	HPIP	MPIP	LPIP	Total	HPIP	MPIP	LPIP	Total
1 h	5.65 ± 0.16	5.54 ± 0.22	5.59 ± 0.24	5.59 ± 0.20	5.52 ± .16	5.16 ± 0.14	5.62 ± 0.29	5.43 ± 0.28
3 h	5.79 ± 0.26	5.47 ± 0.15	5.73 ± 0.23	5.66 ± 0.25	5.59 ± 0.27	5.32 ± 0.21	5.74 ± 0.22	5.55 ± 0.29
6	5.87 ± 0.09	5.43 ± 0.37	5.73 ± 0.19	5.68 ± 0.30	5.77 ± 0.19	5.25 ± 0.22	5.81 ± 0.22	5.61 ± 0.33
Total	5.77 ± 0.20	5.48 ± 0.25	5.68 ± 0.22	5.64 ± 0.25	5.62 ± 0.23	5.24 ± 0.19	5.72 ± 0.25	5.53 ± 0.30

Table 2. Cells count and cells classification in BALF in different ventilation groups.

RT	100% oxygen				45% oxygen			
	HPIP	MPIP	LPIP	Total	HPIP	MPIP	LPIP	Total
Cells in BALF								
1 h	26.08 ± 4.82	12.26 ± 3.00	9.08 ± 1.53	15.80 ± 8.23	26.59 ± 7.89	10.71 ± 2.33	12.12 ± 7.01	16.47 ± 9.43
3 h	29.63 ± 10.10	19.98 ± 3.09	16.88 ± 2.49	22.16 ± 8.11	22.36 ± 6.79	14.73 ± 3.63	12.62 ± 2.98	16.57 ± 6.22
6 h	31.57 ± 7.18	11.85 ± 3.76	16.65 ± 5.61	20.02 ± 10.16	37.34 ± 11.22	15.48 ± 1.23	18.55 ± 5.63	23.79 ± 12.07
Total	29.09 ± 7.58	14.69 ± 4.94	14.20 ± 5.07	19.33 ± 9.11	28.77 ± 10.54	13.64 ± 3.25	14.43 ± 5.95	18.94 ± 9.98
Neutrophils in BALF								
1 h	32.83 ± 10.11	8.00 ± 2.61	19.17 ± 5.34	20.00 ± 12.23	26.50 ± 5.01	8.17 ± 4.12	17.00 ± 5.14	17.22 ± 8.91
3 h	21.67 ± 13.69	10.33 ± 4.03	12.17 ± 2.32	14.72 ± 9.36	12.33 ± 2.58	9.17 ± 2.32	12.67 ± 4.23	11.39 ± 3.38
6 h	16.67 ± 3.39	8.17 ± 2.64	26.00 ± 6.03	16.94 ± 8.50	5.33 ± 1.86	9.17 ± 2.93	18.83 ± 4.79	11.11 ± 6.67
Total	23.72 ± 11.70	8.83 ± 3.17	19.11 ± 7.38	17.22 ± 10.20	14.72 ± 9.61	8.83 ± 3.05	16.17 ± 5.18	13.24 ± 7.18
Monocytes in BALF								
1 h	37.83 ± 9.15	64.17 ± 7.39	17.00 ± 4.15	39.67 ± 20.98	23.17 ± 2.99	62.00 ± 11.19	50.33 ± 5.89	45.17 ± 18.16
3	34.50 ± 13.81	49.50 ± 12.23	31.67 ± 10.56	38.56 ± 14.06	31.17 ± 5.71	64.67 ± 4.84	29.83 ± 6.37	41.89 ± 17.42
6 h	19.00 ± 9.30	47.00 ± 18.06	41.33 ± 6.56	35.78 ± 16.99	23.83 ± 11.09	65.00 ± 7.56	41.00 ± 6.32	43.28 ± 19.15
Total	30.44 ± 13.32	53.56 ± 14.72	30.00 ± 12.51	38.00 ± 17.32	26.06 ± 7.89	63.89 ± 7.90	40.39 ± 10.40	43.44 ± 17.96
Lymphocytes in BALF								
1 h	29.33 ± 10.29	27.83 ± 7.22	63.83 ± 7.11	40.33 ± 18.82	50.33 ± 4.03	29.83 ± 8.98	32.67 ± 6.83	37.61 ± 11.37
3 h	43.83 ± 12.02	40.00 ± 10.45	56.17 ± 12.02	46.67 ± 12.94	56.50 ± 5.17	26.17 ± 4.54	57.50 ± 9.59	46.72 ± 16.27
6 h	67.33 ± 5.85	44.83 ± 16.53	32.67 ± 5.39	48.28 ± 17.82	70.83 ± 10.09	25.83 ± 5.34	40.17 ± 8.04	45.61 ± 20.75
Total	46.83 ± 18.53	37.56 ± 13.49	50.89 ± 15.88	45.09 ± 16.77	59.22 ± 10.98	27.28 ± 6.45	43.44 ± 13.20	43.31 ± 16.77

vels were correlated with FiO_2, PIP, and RT (F = 14.405, 37.958, 10.665, respectively, p < 0.001). 100% oxygen group was higher than 45% oxygen group in neutrophil (F = 14.405, p = 0.000.). 18 cmH_2O group was the lowest compared with 25 and 10 cmH_2O group in neutrophil (p = 0.000, 0.000) and RT 1 h group was higher than RT 3 h group in neutrophil (p = 0.035). Furthermore, there were interaction effects between FiO_2 and PIP (F = 6.378, p = 0.003) or between PIP and RT (F = 18.228, p < 0.001) (R Squared = 0.692, Adjusted R Squared = 0.633). The simple effect was analyzed. When fixed FiO_2 was 100%, 18 cmH_2O group was the lowest compared with 25 and 10 cmH_2O group in neutrophil (p = 0.000, 0.000). When fixed FiO_2 was 45%, 18 cmH_2O group was the lower than 10 cmH_2O group in neutrophil (p = 0.000). when fixed PIP was 25 cmH_2O, 100% oxygen group was the higher than 45% oxygen group in neutrophil (p = 0.017), but there were no significance between 100% oxygen group and 45% oxygen group when fixed PIP was 10 cmH_2O or 18 cmH_2O. When fixed RT was 6 h,

RT 1 h group was the highest compared with RT 6 h and 3 h group in neutrophil (p = 0.001, 0.000).When fixed PIP was 10 cmH_2O, RT 6 h group was the highest and RT 3 h was the lowest compared with RT 1 h, 3 h and 6 h group in neutrophil (p = 0.010, 0.000, 0.045), but there were no significance among 3 RT groups when fixed PIP was 18 cmH_2O. When fixed RT was 1 h, the 25 cmH_2O group was the highest and 18 cmH_2O group was the lowest among 3 PIP groups in neutrophil (p = 0.000, 0.000, 0.000). When fixed RT was 6 h, the 10 cmH_2O group was the highest compared with 25 cmH_2O and 18 cmH_2O group in neutrophil (p = 0.001, 0.000), but there were no significance among 3 PIP groups in neutrophil When fixed RT was 3 h.

3.4. FiO_2, PIP 2 Factor Contribute to Monocytes in BALF, There Are Interactions to Monocytes between FiO_2 and PIP, PIP and RT as well as FiO_2, PIP and RT

Factorial design ANOVA showed that the monocytes

counts in 100% oxygen group were lower than that of 45% oxygen group ($F = 9.305$, $p = 0.003$). There were significance in 3 PIP groups ($F = 106.749$, $p = 0.000$) and 18 cmH_2O group was the highest than 25 and 10 cmH_2O ($p = 0.000$, 0.000), but RT were no difference ($F = 0.952$, $p = 0.390$). Furthermore, there were interaction effects between FiO_2 and PIP ($F = 7.588$, $p = 0.001$) or between PIP and RT ($F = 5.092$, $p = 0.001$) or among PIP, RT and FiO_2 (R Squared $= 0.771$, Adjusted R Squared $= 0.728$). The simple effect was analyzed. When fixed FiO_2 was 100%, 18 cmH_2O group was the highest compared with 25 and 10 cmH_2O groups in monocytes ($p = 0.000$, 0.000). When fixed FiO_2 was 45%, 18 cmH_2O group was the highest and 25 cmH_2O group was the lowest among 3 PIP groups in monocytes ($p = 0.000$, 0.000, 0.000). When fixed PIP was 18 cmH_2O or 10 cmH_2O, 45% oxygen group was higher 100% oxygen group in monocytes ($F = 6.887$ or 7.339. $p = 0.013$ or 0.010), but 25 cmH_2O group was no difference. As for interaction effects between PIP and RT, when fixed PIP was 25 cmH_2O, RT 3 h was higher than RT 6 h in monocytes ($p = 0.009$); When fixed PIP was 10 cmH_2O, RT 6 h was higher than RT 3 h in monocytes ($p = 0.007$); however, there was no difference among 3 RT group in monocytes. When fixed RT 1 h or 3 h, 18 cmH_2O group was the highest among 3 PIP groups(all of p were 0.000); When fixed RT 6 h, 18 cmH_2O group was the highest and 25 cmH_2O was the lowest among 3 PIP groups ($p = 0.000$, 0.000, 0.030) (**Table 2**).

3.5. PIP and RT Contributes to Lymphocytes. There Are Interactions to Lymphocytes between FiO₂ and PIP, PIP and RT as well as FiO₂, PIP and RT

Factorial design ANOVA showed that the lymphocytes counts in 100% and 45% oxygen group were no difference ($F = 1.081$, $p = 0.301$). There were significance in 3 PIP groups ($F = 51.462$, $p = 0.000$) and 18 cmH_2O group was the lowest among 3 PIP groups ($p = 0.000$, 0.000). RT were difference ($F = 9.366$, $p = 0.000$.), but Post Hoc Test for 3 RT groups were no difference with Tamhane ($p = 0.092$, 0.157, 1.000). Furthermore, there were interaction effects between FiO_2 and PIP ($F = 17.386$, $p = 0.001$) or between PIP and RT ($F = 20.852$, $p = 0.000$) or among FiO_2, RT and PIP ($F = 11.785$, $p = 0.000$). (R Squared $= 0.762$, Adjusted R Squared $= 0.717$) (**Table 2**).

3.6. FiO₂, RT, PIP 3 Factors Contribute to Lung Injury Histopathology Scores

Factorial design ANOVA showed that the lung histopathology scores in 100% oxygen was significantly higher than in 45% oxygen group ($F = 9.037$, $p = 0.003$) (**Table**

3) and 18 cmH_2O group lung histopathology scores was the lowest among 3 PIP groups ($F = 57.515$, $p < 0.000$). RT were significant differences ($F = 3.586$, $p = 0.032$) and RT 6 h groups was higher than RT 1 h group ($p = 0.010$). However, there were no interaction effects among FiO_2, RT and PIP.

3.7. PIP Contributes to MMP-9 Levels. There Was Interaction to MMP-9 between FiO₂ and PIP in Lung Tissue Bomogenate

Factorial design ANOVA showed that the MMP-9 levels were significantly different among 3 PIP ventilation regimes ($F = 7.215$, $p = 0.932$) and 18 cmH_2O groups was the highest than the other 2 PIP groups ($p = 0.000$, 0.008), but there were no significance between the 25 and 10 cmH_2O. FiO_2 and RT did not contribute to MMP-9 ($F = 0.007$, 0.401; $p = 0.932$, 0.671, respectively). There were interaction to MMP-9 between FiO_2 and PIP. When fixed PIP was 25 cmH_2O, there were no significance between 100% and 45% oxygen group in MMP-9 ($F = 0.583$, $p = 0.450$). When fixed PIP was 18 cmH_2O, 100% oxygen group was higher than 45% oxygen group in MMP-9 ($F = 4.403$, $p = 0.043$). When fixed PIP was 10 cmH_2O, 100% oxygen group was lower than 45% oxygen group in MMP-9 ($F = 4.392$, $p = 0.044$). when fixed FiO_2 was 100%, there were significances among 3 PIP groups ($F = 10.622$, $p = 0.000$) and the 18 cmH_2O group was the highest than the others PIP groups ($p = 0.002$, 0.003) in MMP-9, ut there was no significance between 25 and 10 cmH_2O. There were no significance among 3 PIP groups in MMP-9 ($F = 1.248$, $p = 0.296$) when fixed FiO_2 was 45% (**Table 4**).

3.8. Pathology

Ten of 108 rabbits were induced with pulmonary atelectasis (**Figure 1(c)**, **Table 5**), and PIP ($\chi^2 = 6.834$, $p < 0.05$) or RT ($\chi^2 = 8.154$, $p < 0.05$) induced atelectasis significantly, but FiO_2 did not ($\chi^2 = 0.441$, $p > 0.05$). Although the histopathological changes in the ventilation groups were greatly different from the control groups (**Figure 2(a)**), they shared the common structural changes among these ventilation group. Change in lung structure with patchy areas of parenchymal thickening and small airspaces interspersed with areas of enlarged airspaces, with inflammatory cell infiltrated. Pathological features from the exudative phase to the early proliferative phase of diffuse alveolar damage such as: epithelial destruction, capillary congestion, interstitial oedema, intra-alveolar oedema, haemorrhage, mononuclear infiltration, polymorphonuclear infiltration, interlobular septal thickening, hyaline membrane formation, uneven alveolar ventilation and microatelectasis were observed in the present experimental groups. The hemorrhage in the 100% oxygen

Table 3. Lung injury histopathology scores in different ventilation groups.

	100% oxygen				45% oxygen			
RT	HPIP	MPIP	LPIP	Total	HPIP	MPIP	LPIP	Total
1 h	7.67 ± 1.21	4.33 ± 1.03	7.50 ± 1.05	6.50 ± 1.89	7.17 ± 0.98	4.33 ± 1.03	5.67 ± 1.03	5.72 ± 1.53
3 h	8.17 ± 1.47	4.50 ± 0.84	8.00 ± 2.00	6.89 ± 2.25	7.67 ± 1.75	4.17 ± 0.41	5.83 ± 1.60	5.89 ± 1.97
6 h	8.33 ± 2.07	5.67 ± 0.8	7.67 ± 1.21	7.22 ± 1.80	8.17 ± 1.94	4.50 ± 0.55	7.33 ± 1.63	6.67 ± 2.14
Total	8.06 ± 1.55	4.83 ± 1.04	7.72 ± 1.41	6.87 ± 1.97	7.67 ± 1.57	4.33 ± 0.69	6.28 ± 1.56	6.09 ± 1.91

Table 4. MMP-9 assay in lung tissue homogenate.

	100% oxygen				45% oxygen			
RT	HPIP	MPIP	LPIP	Total	HPIP	MPIP	LPIP	Total
1 h	61.09 ± 13.68	93.46 ± 27.08	59.38 ± 10.78	71.31 ± 23.77	69.77 ± 10.02	76.72 ± 21.78	89.38 ± 26.94	78.62 ± 21.27
3 h	77.45 ± 13.14	89.78 ± 25.80	67.36 ± 12.46	78.20 ± 19.53	72.74 ± 12.36	86.93 ± 18.49	70.69 ± 12.67	76.79 ± 15.74
6 h	66.41 ± 16.99	102.39 ± 25.09	75.81 ± 30.28	81.54 ± 28.03	73.31 ± 17.31	72.89 ± 25.55	83.64 ± 12.90	76.61 ± 18.85
Total	68.32 ± 15.49	95.21 ± 25.03	67.52 ± 19.93	77.02 ± 23.96	71.94 ± 12.85	78.84 ± 21.66	81.24 ± 19.35	77.34 ± 18.42

Table 5. Pulmonary atelectasis in different ventilation groups (n/group).

	PIP			RT			FiO2	
	HPIP	MPIP	LPIP	1 h	3 h	6 h	100%	45%
Atelectasis	1	2	7	0	3	7	4	6
Normal	35	34	29	36	33	29	50	48
χ^2		6.834			8.154			0.441	
p		<0.05			<0.05			>0.05	

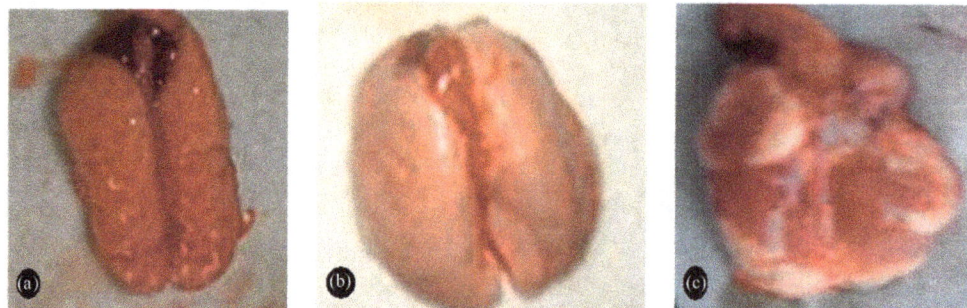

Figure 1. Gross appearance of lung tissue.

ventilation groups was more serious than that in the 45% oxygen ventilation groups (**Figures 1(a)** and **(b)**). Uneven al-veolar sizes, microatelectasis, significant hyaline membrane formation, interlobular septal thickening and interlobular septal destruction were obviously observed in LPIP ventilation groups (**Figures 1** and **2((b),(c), (h),(i)**). Pulmonary hemorrhage, significant pulmonary bullae formation and the hemorrhage were obviously observed not only within the interlobular septal and alveolar spaces but also within bronch-walls in HPIP ventilation groups, but the atelectasis were less observed (**Figures 2 (f),(g),(l),(m)**). Compared with the HPIP ventilation groups and LPIP ventilation groups, the pathological changes in the MPIP groups were better (**Figure 1(b)**; **Figures 2(d),(e),(k),(l)**): alveolar distention even, pulmonary hemorrhage, intra-alveolar oedema, atelecta-

sis, the hyaline membrane formation and pulmonary bullae were decreased significantly. To further confirm our results, we performed transmission electron microscope to illustrate the lung structural features. Lung tissue without ventilation had the continuous vascular endothelial cells and the integrity basement membrane. But with the ventilation going, disappeared and collapse cell conjunction were found in HPIP groups (**Figure 3(a)**) and microatelectasis were found in LPIP groups (**Figure 3(c)**). The lung structural or air-blood barrier of MPIP groups were normal (**Figure 3(b)**).

3.9. Immunohistochemical Detection the Express of MMP-9 in Lung Tissue (Figure 4)

Positivion MMP-9-expression was observed in alveolar

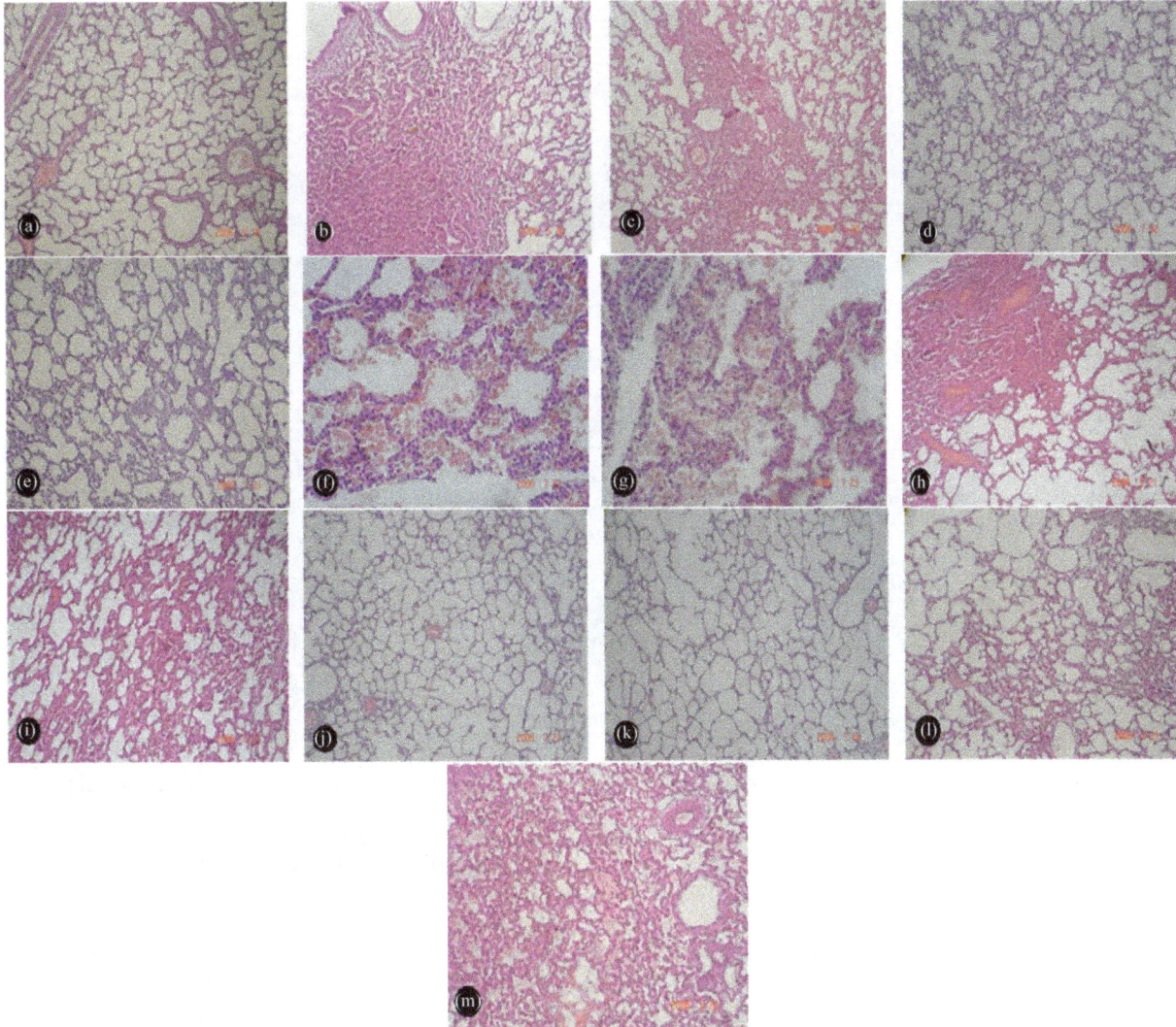

Figure 2. Microscopic changes in Hematoxylin-eosin (H&E) staining lungs tissues. No ventilation control group (a); 100% oxygen LPIP ventilation for 1 h (b) and 100% oxygen LPIP ventilation for 6 h (c); 45% oxygen LPIP ventilation for 1 h (h), 45% oxygen LPIP ventilation for 6 h (i) show the evidence of extensive lung injury with microatelectasis, hyaline membrane formation and interlobular septal thickening. 100% MPIP ventilation for 1 h (d) and 100% oxygen MPIP ventilation for 6 h (e); 45% oxygen MPIP ventilation for 1 h (j) and 45% oxygen MPIP ventilation for 6 h (k) illustrate the pathological changes in the moderate pressure groups are better: alveolar distention are even; After 1 h, 6 h 100% oxygen HPIP (f), (g) and 45% oxygen HPIP (l), (m) ventilate, severe infiltration of inflammatory cells into the interstitium, hyaline membrane formation, severe haemorrhage, and pulmonary bullae are observed.

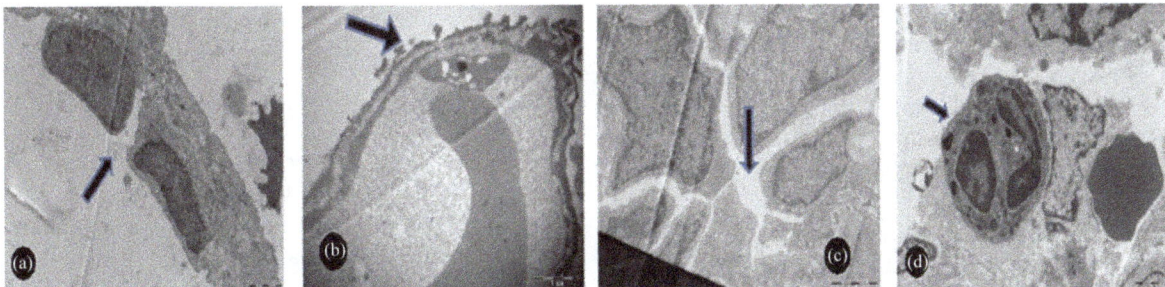

Figure 3. Transmission electron microscope changes in lungs tissues. (a) 45% oxygen and HPIP ventilation for 1 h, magnification ×10000; (b) 100% oxygn MPIP 6 h magnification ×3000; (c) 45% oxygen and LPIP ventilation for 6 h, magnification ×15000, atelectasis alveolar space. (d) 100% oxygen LPIP 6 h, alveolar neutrophilic infiltration (magnification ×3000).

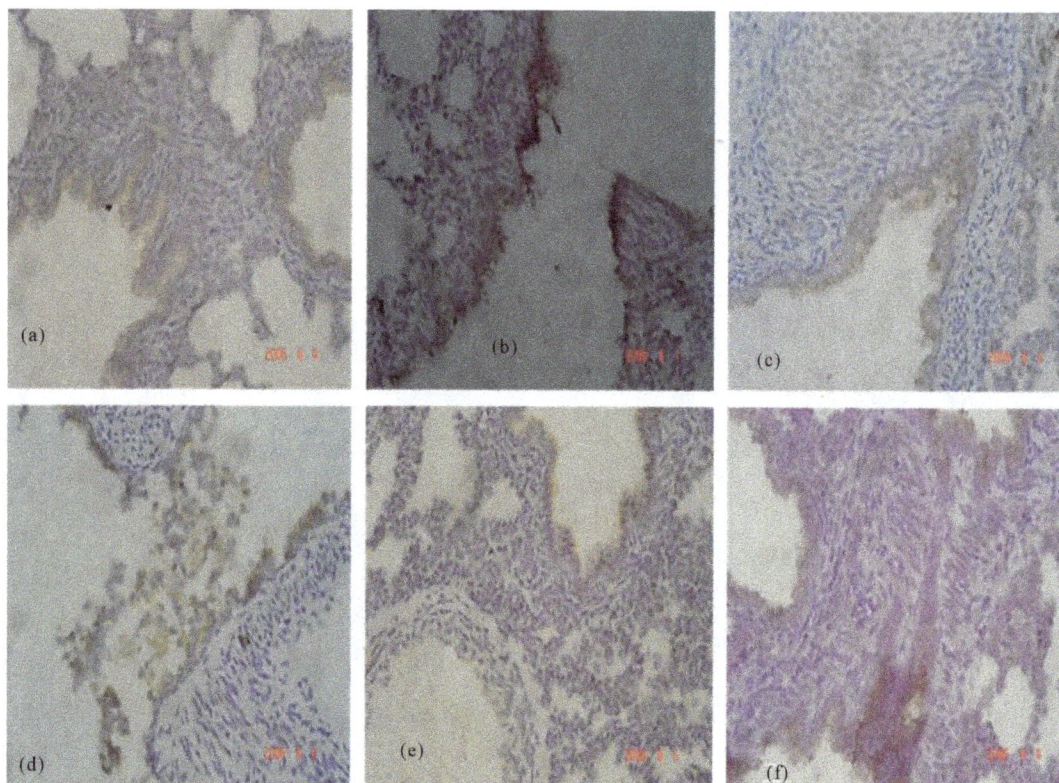

Figure 4. Immunohistochemical localization of MMP-9 in lung tissue sections. (a): Normal control lung tissue (magnification, ×200). (b): Strong expression of MMP-9 in Ventiliation 1 h with 100% oxygen and MPIP. (c): Weak expression of MMP-9 in Ventilation 3 h with 100% oxygen and HPIP. (d): MMP-9 expressed increase in ventilation 6 h with 45% oxygen and LPIP, (e): Less normal control lung tissue expression of MMP-9 in ventilation 6 h with 100% oxygen and HPIP. (f): Almost normal control lung tissue of MMP-9-expression in ventilation 1 h with 45% oxygen and HPIP.

macrophages, alveolar lining epithelium, alveolar septal interstitium, and interstitium cells in unventilated rabbits (**Figure 4(a)**). Strong expression of MMP-9 was detected in ventilation for 1 h with 100% oxygen and MPIP (**Figure 4(b)**). In newborn rabbits Ventilation for 3 h with 100% oxygen and HPIP, Weak expression of MMP-9 was detected in alveolar lining epithelium and inflammatory cells (**Figure 4(c)**). After 6 h ventilation with 45% oxygen and LPIP, MMP-9 was strong expressed in alveolar macrophages, neutrophils, and alveolar lining epithelium. Injury and defluxion airway epithelium mucosae was also observed (**Figure 4(d)**). In ventilation for 6 h with 100% oxygen and HPIP, less normal control lung tissue expression of MMP-9 was detected (**Figure 4(e)**). However, in ventilation for 1 h with 45% oxygen and HPIP, it was almost normal control lung tissue of MMP-9-expression in alveolar lining epithelium and inflammatory cells (**Figure 4(f)**).

3.10. MMP-9 Positively Correlated with Monocytes, but Negatively Correlated with Neutrophils, Lung Injury Histopathology Scores

To understand the relationship between these variables in the different ventilation regimes, pearson correlation analysis was performed. The results revealed that MMP-9 positively correlated with monocytes in BALF ($r = 0.262$, $p = 0.006$), MMP-9 negatively correlated with neutrophils in BALF ($r = -0.235$, $p = 0.014$), lung injury histopathology scores ($r = -0.280$, $p = 0.003$). However, there were no relationship between MMP-9 and W/D ($r = -0.021$, $p = 0.827$), Cells ($r = -0.067$, $p = 0.494$), lymphocytes ($r = -0.150$, $p = 0.122$) in BALF.

W/D positively correlated with lung injury histopathology scores ($r = 0.462$, $p = 0.000$). Cells ($r = 0.322$, $p = 0.001$), lymphocytes ($r = 0.409$, $p = 0.000$) in BALF, but negatively correlated with monocytes in BALF ($r = -0.460$, $p = 0.000$). $n = 108$.

4. Discussion

Our study indicated that atelectasis increases significantly in 10 cmH$_2$O PIP ventilation groups and RT 6 h groups, but different oxygen has no effect on atelectasis. These also confirmed that the lower PIP, the easier to induce uneven alveolar ventilation. W/D and the lung histopathology scores were positive relationship ($r = 0.462$, $p = 0.000$) and they were the marker of lung injury. Different FiO$_2$, PIP and RT could cause lung injury and the degree of lung injury in 100% oxygen groups was more severe than in 45% oxygen groups. Lung injury in RT 6 h groups was more severe than in RT 1 h groups. The fact that lung injury in MPIP group was the lightest among 3 PIP groups was confirmed by W/D, the lung histopathology scores and lung histopathology. There was significant pulmonary hemorrhage in pulmonary alveoli and bronch-walls in HPIP groups, so only MPIP caused uniform alveolar distention (**Figure 1(b)**), HPIP was easy to cause barotraumas (**Figure 1(a)**) [14,15] and LPIP was easy to atelectasis (**Figure 1(c)**).

MMP-9 is a metalloproteinase secreted by a wide variety of cell types. In the lung, MMP-9 is synthesized by normal resident structural and inflammatory cells such as bronchial epithelial cells [16], alveolar epithelial cells [17], and alveolar macrophages [18]. All of these cell types can greatly increase their MMP-9 secretion after stimulation [16-18]. In our experiment, the cell count and cell classification were researched in BALF and the results found that MMP-9 was not correlated with the cell count, lymphocytes and W/D. It is agreed with Gushima report that MMP-9 expression was not correlated with the number of total cells or lymphocytes [19], MMP-9 was negatively correlated with lung histopathology scores and neutrophils, but MM-9 was positively correlated with alveolar macrophages. On the basis of these findings, it has been suggested that MMP-9 may derive from alveolar macrophages. Macrophages are a type of inflammatory cell that synthesizes hundreds of bioactive substances and enzymes. Macrophages are sensitive to cyclic pressure stretching and pressure-stretching stimulus. Macrophages respond to pressure-stretching strain by secreting MMP-9 and the chemokine IL-8 [20]. All of these results (fractorial design ANOVA, lung histopathology and immunohistochemisty) confirmed that the higher alveolar macrophages, the higher the level of MMP-9, the lower alveolar neutrophilic granulocyte, the lighter lung injury. MMP-9 is the production of macrophages. Normally, protected lung cell is alveolar macrophages, but not neutrophilic granulocyte [21]. Absence of MMP-9 led to a more severe injury with neutrophil increase in the alveolar spaces in 100% oxygen LPIP 6 h (**Figure 3(d)**). It appeared that MMP-9 has advantage over VILI. Mice lacking MMP-9 developed more severe lung damage after high-pressure ventilation than their wildtype counterparts [9], and MMP-9 deficiency worsened lung injury in a model of bronchopulmonary dysplasia [8]. MMP-9 had protective role in O_3-induced lung neutrophilic inflammation and hyperpermeability. MMP-9 deficiency was associated with enhanced airway epithelial injury and neutrophil recruitment [7]. MMP-9 deficiency impairs host defense against abdominal sepsis [22]. Other authors have shown a similar protective role in MMP-9 in different models of lung injury [7-9,22-24].

It is known that proteolytic function of MMP-9 affects cytokine and chemokine levels as well as their activities. MMP-9 could cleave different cytokine and chemokines, like IL-1β [25]. MMP-9 protected against ventilator-induced lung injury by decreasing alveolar neutrophilic infiltration, probably by modulation of the cytokine response in the air spaces [9]. MMP-9 was first identified in neutrophils and could also be expressed by neutrophils [26], but neutrophils-derived MMP-9 differs from MMP-9 expressed by other cell types in two major ways. First, mature neutrophils do not synthesize MMP-9 de novo. Rather, MMP-9 is produced during the late stages of maturation of neutrophils precursors in the bone marrow [27]. These may explain why the numbers of neutrophils were negatively correlated with total MMP-9 level in our study.

There was no significant difference in MMP-9 between 100% oxygen ventilation groups and 45% oxygen ventilation groups. It indicated that FiO_2 was not the regulation factor for the express of MMP-9 in this ventilation animal model. However, the expression of MMP-9 has significant difference in different PIP, in other words, the different mechanical stretch regulated the expression of MMP-9. The application of high pressures to lungs during mechanical ventilation can induce a severe injury type, known as ventilator-induced lung injury [28,29]. Physical stimulus can lead to an inflammatory response within the respiratory system and in distal organs [30]. Several of these pathways result in the synthesis, release, and activation of MMPs [2,31]. Mechanical stretch differentially affects MMP-2/9 and their inhibitors in fetal lung cells [32]. Furthermore, advisable mechanical stretch could promote MMP-9 secretion and decrease the lung injury by our study. The mechanism may be that advisable mechanical stretch activated and enlarged the signal password of MMP-9, leading to MMP-9 synthesis and discharge increase, so the expression of MMP-9 was up-regulated. However, HPIP ventilation formed obvious pulmonary bullae and destroyed the normal pulmonary alveoli structures as well as interrupted the signal connection between cell and cell (**Figure 3(a)**). Finally, the signal password of MMP-9 was broken and the MMP-9 could not be synthesized. Over-mechanical stretch of epithelial cells decreased MMP-9 activity and the MMP-9/TIMP-1 ratio by 60% - 70% [32]. Accordingly, lung injury was inevitable. In LPIP ventilation, there were obvious uneven alveolar ventilation and microatelectasis, suggesting that the stimulation signal transmission of mechanical stretch was uneven in pulmonary alveoli and could not active the signal password of MMP-9, because MMP-9 is not produced constitutively, but needs a trigger to be expressed [33]. MMP-9 is synthesized and stored in the granules of neutrophils and eosinophils in the bone marrow, but is secreted from the cells outside of the bone marrow in an inducible manner [34,35]. Therefore, atelectasis cannot pass the signal to alveolar epithelial cell, macrophages and fibroblasts and cannot induce MMP-9 synthesis. MMP-9 expression decreased in LPIP and caused lung injury.

In conclusion, different PIP and different oxygen concentrations exert simultaneously on newborn lung in newborn rabbits ventilation; only mechanical stretch stimulation affects MMP-9 synthesis. Advisable mechanical stretch can promote MMP-9 expression and has protective role in lung in VILI. HPIP causes barotraumas and LPIP induces atelectrauma.

5. Acknowledgements

We thank Prof. Yanping Chen (Department of Biostatistics, Southern medical University) for his valuable advice in relation to this study.

REFERENCES

[1] P. L. Davies, O. B. Spiller, M. L. Beeton, *et al.*, "Relationship of Proteinases and Proteinase Inhibitors with Microbial Presence in Chronic Lung Disease of Prematurity," *Thorax*, Vol. 65, No. 3, 2010, pp. 246-251. http://dx.doi.org/10.1136/thx.2009.116061

[2] H. D. Foda, E. E. Rollo, M. Drews, *et al.*, "Ventilator-Induced Lung Injury Upregulates and Activates Gelatinases and EMMPRIN: Attenuation by the Synthetic Matrix Metalloproteinase Inhibitor, Prinomastat (AG3340)," *American Journal of Respiratory Cell and Molecular Biology*, Vol. 25, No. 6, 2001, pp. 717-724. http://dx.doi.org/10.1165/ajrcmb.25.6.4558f

[3] J. H. Kim, M. H. Suk, D. W. Yoon, *et al.*, "Inhibition of Matrix Metalloproteinase-9 Prevents Neutrophilic Inflammation in Ventilator-Induced Lung Injury," *American Journal of Physiology Lung Cellular and Molecular*, Vol. 291, No. 4, 2006, pp. L580-L587. http://dx.doi.org/10.1152/ajplung.00270.2005

[4] S. Buckley, B. Driscoll, W. Shi, *et al.*, "Migration and Gelatinases in Cultured Fetal, Adult, and Hyperoxic Alveolar Epithelial Cells," *American Journal of Physiology Lung Cellular and Molecular*, Vol. 281, No. 2, 2001, pp. L427-L434.

[5] C. Delclaux, M. P. d'Ortho, C. Delacourt, *et al.*, "Gelatinases in Epithelial Lining Fluid of Patients with Adult Respiratory Distress Syndrome," *American Journal of Physiology*, Vol. 272, No. 3, 1997, pp. L442-L451.

[6] B. Ricou, L. Nicod, S. Lacraz, *et al.*, "Matrix Metalloproteinases and TIMP in Acute Respiratory Distress Syndrome," *American Journal of Respiratory and Critical Care Medicine*, Vol. 154, No. 2, 1996, pp. 346-352. http://dx.doi.org/10.1164/ajrccm.154.2.8756805

[7] H. K. Yoon, H. Y. Cho and S. R. Kleeberger, "Protective Role of Matrix Metalloproteinase-9 in Ozone-Induced Airway Inflammation," *Environmental Health Perspectives*, Vol. 115, No. 11, 2007, pp. 1557-1563. http://dx.doi.org/10.1289/ehp.10289

[8] H. Lukkarinen, A. Hogmalm, U. Lappalainen, *et al.*, "Matrix Metalloproteinase-9 Deficiency Worsens Lung Injury in a Model of Bronchopulmonary Dysplasia," *American Journal of Respiratory Cell and Molecular Biology*, Vol. 41, No. 1, 2009, pp. 59-68. http://dx.doi.org/10.1165/rcmb.2008-0179OC

[9] G. M. Albaiceta, A. Gutierrez-Fernandez, D. Parra, *et al.*, "Lack of Matrix Metalloproteinasec9 Worsens Ventilator-Induced Lung Injury," *American Journal of Physiology Lung Cellular and Molecular*, Vol. 294, No. 3, 2008, pp. L535-L543. http://dx.doi.org/10.1152/ajplung.00334.2007

[10] V. Lagente, B. Manoury, S. Nenan, *et al.*, "Role of Matrix Metalloproteinase in the Development of Airway Inflammation and Remodeling," *Brazilian Journal of Medical and Biological Research*, Vol. 38, No. 10, 2005, pp. 1521-1530. http://dx.doi.org/10.1590/S0100-879X2005001000009

[11] E. K. Wolthuis, A. P. Vlaar, G. Choi, *et al.*, "Mechanical Ventilation Using Non-Injurious Ventilation Settings Causes Lung Injury in the Absence of Pre-Existing Lung Injury in Healthy Mice," *Critical Care*, Vol. 13, No. 1, 2009, p. R1. http://dx.doi.org/10.1186/cc7688

[12] E. K. Wolthuis, A. P. Vlaar, G. Choi, *et al.*, "Recombinant Human Soluble Tumor Necrosis Factor-Alpha Receptor Fusion Protein Partly Attenuates Ventilator-Induced Lung Injury," *Shock*, Vol. 31, No. 3, 2009, pp. 262-266. http://dx.doi.org/10.1097/SHK.0b013e31817d42dd

[13] P. Svedin, H. Hagberg, K. Sävman, *et al.*, "Matrix Metalloproteinase-9 Gene Knock-out Protects the Immature Brain after Cerebral Hypoxia-Ischemia," *The Journal of Neuroscience*, Vol. 27, No. 7, 2007, pp. 1511-1518. http://dx.doi.org/10.1523/JNEUROSCI.4391-06.2007

[14] D. Dreyfuss and G. Saumon, "Ventilator-Induced Lung Injury: Lessons from Experimental Studies," *American Journal of Respiratory and Critical Care Medicine*, Vol. 157, No. 1, 1998, pp. 294-323. http://dx.doi.org/10.1164/ajrccm.157.1.9604014

[15] D. Dreyfuss, P. Soler, G. Basset, *et al.*, "High Inflation Pressure Pulmonary Edema: Respective Effects of High Pressure, High Tidal Volume and Positive End-Expiratory Pressure," *American Review of Respiratory Disease*, Vol. 137, No. 5, 1988, pp. 1159-1164.

[16] P. M. Yao, J. M. Buhler, M. P. d'Ortho, *et al.*, "C. Expression of Matrix Metalloproteinase Gelatinases A and B by Cultured Epithelial Cells from Human Bronchial Explants," *The Journal of Biological Chemistry*, Vol. 271, No. 26, 1996, pp. 15580-15589. http://dx.doi.org/10.1074/jbc.271.26.15580

[17] A. Pardo, K. Ridge, B. Uhal, *et al.*, "Lung Alveolar Epithelial Cells Synthesize Interstitial Collagenase and Gelatinases A and B *in Vitro*," *The International Journal of Biochemistry & Cell Biology*, Vol. 29, No. 6, 1997, pp. 901-910. http://dx.doi.org/10.1016/S1357-2725(97)00030-7

[18] H. G. Welgus, E. J. Campbell, J. D. Cury, *et al.*, "Neutral Metalloproteinases Produced by Human Mononuclear Phagocytes. Enzyme Profile, Regulation, and Expression

during Cellular Development," *Journal of Clinical Investigation*, Vol. 86, No. 5, 1990, pp. 1496-1502. http://dx.doi.org/10.1172/JCI114867

[19] Y. Gushima, K. Ichikado, M. Suga, *et al.*, "Expression of Matrix Metalloproteinases in Pigs with Hyperoxia-Induced Acute Lung Injury," *European Respiratory Journal*, Vol. 18, No. 5, 2001, pp. 827-837. http://dx.doi.org/10.1183/09031936.01.00049201

[20] J. Pugin, I. Dunn, P. Jolliet, *et al.* "Activation of Human Macrophages by Mechanical Ventilation *in Vitro*," *American Journal of Physiology*, Vol. 275, No. 6, 1998, pp. L1040-L1050.

[21] D. F. Gibbs, R. L. Warner, S. J. Weiss, *et al.*, "Characterization of Matrixmetallop Roteinases Produced by Rat Alveolar Macrophages," *American Journal of Respiratory Cell and Molecular Biology*, Vol. 20, No. 6, 1999, pp. 1136-1144. http://dx.doi.org/10.1165/ajrcmb.20.6.3483

[22] R. Renckens, J. J. Roelofs, S. Florquin, *et al.*, "Matrix Metalloproteinase-9 Deficiency Impairs Host Defense against Abdominal Sepsis," *The Journal of Immunology*, Vol. 176, No. 6, 2006, pp. 3735-3741.

[23] K. Bry, A. Hogmalm and E. Bäckström, "Mechanisms of Inflammatory Lung Injury in the Neonate: Lessons from a Transgenic Mouse Model of Bronchopulmonary Dysplasia," *Seminars in Perinatology*, Vol. 34, No. 3, 2010, pp. 211-221. http://dx.doi.org/10.1053/j.semperi.2010.02.006

[24] S. Cabrera, M. Gaxiola, J. L. Arreola, *et al.*, "Overexpression of MMP9 in Macrophages Attenuates Pulmonary Fibrosis Induced by Bleomycin," *The International Journal of Biochemistry & Cell Biology*, Vol. 39, No. 12, 2007, pp. 2324-2338. http://dx.doi.org/10.1016/j.biocel.2007.06.022

[25] A. Ito, A. Mukaiyama, Y. Itoh, *et al.*, "Degradation of Interleukin 1beta by Matrix Metalloproteinases," *The Journal of Biological Chemistry*, Vol. 271, No. 25, 1996, pp. 14657-14660. http://dx.doi.org/10.1074/jbc.271.25.14657

[26] W. C. Parks and R. P. Mecham, "Gelatinase B: Structure, Regulation, and Function," In: *Matrix Metalloproteinases*, Academic Press, San Diego, 1998, pp. 115-148.

[27] C. A. Owen, Z. Hu, B. Barrick, *et al.*, "Inducible Expression of Tissue Inhibitor of Metalloproteinases-Resistant Matrix Metalloproteinase-9 on the Cell Surface of Neutrophils," *American Journal of Respiratory Cell and Molecular Biology*, Vol. 29, No. 3, 2003, pp. 283-294. http://dx.doi.org/10.1165/rcmb.2003-0034OC

[28] A. S. Slutsky, "Ventilator-Induced Lung Injury: From Barotrauma to Biotrauma," *Respiratory Care*, Vol. 50, No. 5, 2005, pp. 646-659.

[29] C. C. dos Santos and A. S. Slutsky, "The Contribution of Biophysical Lung Injury to the Development of Biotrauma," *Annual Review of Physiology*, Vol. 68, 2006, pp. 585-618. http://dx.doi.org/10.1146/annurev.physiol.68.072304.113443

[30] L. Gattinoni, E. Carlesso, P. Cadringher, *et al.*, "Physical and Biological Triggers of Ventilator-Induced Lung Injury and Its Prevention," *European Respiratory Journal*, Vol. 47, 2003, pp. 15s-25s. http://dx.doi.org/10.1183/09031936.03.00021303

[31] F. Kheradmand, E. Werner, P. Tremble, *et al.*, "Role of Rac1 and Oxygen Radicals in Collagenase-1 Expression Induced by Cell Shape Change," *Science*, Vol. 280, No. 5365, 1998, pp. 898-902. http://dx.doi.org/10.1126/science.280.5365.898

[32] R. L. Hawwa, M. A. Hokenson, Y. Wang, *et al.*, "Differential Expression of MMP-2 and -9 and Their Inhibitors in Fetal Lung Cells Exposed to Mechanical Stretch: Regulation by IL-10," *Lung*, Vol. 189, No. 4, 2011, pp. 341-349. http://dx.doi.org/10.1007/s00408-011-9310-7

[33] G. Opdenakker, P. E. Van den Steen, J. Van Damme, "Gelatinase B: A Tuner and Amplifier of Immune Functions," *Trends in Immunology*, Vol. 22, No. 10, 2001, pp. 571-579. http://dx.doi.org/10.1016/S1471-4906(01)02023-3

[34] J. J. Atkinson and R. M. Senior, "Matrix Metalloproteinase-9 in Lung Remodeling," *American Journal of Respiratory Cell and Molecular Biology*, Vol. 28, No. 1, 2003, pp. 12-24. http://dx.doi.org/10.1165/rcmb.2002-0166TR

[35] S. Chakrabarti and K. D. Patel, "Matrix Metalloproteinase-2 (MMP-2) and MMP-9 in Pulmonary Pathology," *Experimental Lung Research*, Vol. 31, No. 6, 2005, pp. 599-621. http://dx.doi.org/10.1080/019021490944232

22

Houttuynia cordata Thunb: A Review of Phytochemistry and Pharmacology and Quality Control

Jiangang Fu, Ling Dai, Zhang Lin, Hongmei Lu[*]

College of Chemistry and Chemical Engineering, Central South University, Changsha, China

Email: [*]hongmeilu@csu.edu.cn

ABSTRACT

Houttuynia cordata Thunb is an important medicinal plant widely distributed in East Asia. The collected information is an attempt to cover recent developments in the pharmacology, phytochemistry and quality control of this species. During the past several decades, the medicinally important phyto-constituents have been identified including essential oil, flavonoids and other polyphenols, fatty acids and alkaloids. A survey of the literatures shows *H. cordata* possesses a variety of pharmacological activities including antiviral, antitumor, antimicrobial, anti-inflammatory, and antioxidative effects. Little attempt has been done to review the techniques used for its quality control. Future efforts should concentrate more on *in vitro*, *in vivo* studies and clinical trials in order to confirm traditional wisdom in the light of a rational phytotherapy. The information summarized here is intended to serve as a reference tool to practitioners in the fields of ethnopharmacology and natural products chemistry.

Keywords: *Houttuynia cordata* Thunb; Phytochemical Constituents; Pharmacological Activity; Quality Control

1. Introduction

There is a long history of herbal medicine in far Eastern countries; in particular, Chinese people have utilized herbs and plants to treat various diseases for more than 8000 years [1]. With the advance of modern medicine and drug research, chemical synthesis has replaced plants as the primary source of medicinal agents in industrialized countries. However, in 1985, the World Health Organization estimated that about 80% of the world's population relied on traditional medicines including herb medicines for their primary health care needs [2]. Several aspects: 1) the high cost of chemical synthesis drug discovery, 2) the efficiency of herb medicine on complex illnesses such as cancer and cardiovascular disease, 3) the unique activities of herbal medicine aiming at the system level via interactions with a multitude of targets in the human body, make people return to the herbal medicine, a potential reservoir for new drugs [3].

Houttuynia cordata Thunb, the sole species in the genus *Houttuynia* that belongs to the *Saururaceae* family, is a flowering and perennial herb native to China, Japan, Korea and Southeast Asia. In China, this plant is distributed widely, eastwards to Taiwan, southwest to Yunnan

and Tibet, and north to Shaanxi and Gansu. It grows optimally on moist, shady hillside, wayside and ridge of field with an altitude of 300 - 2600 m.

H. cordata is a well known traditionally used medicinal material in the indigenous medicine systems of Southeast Asia. It is commonly called *Yu-Xing-Cao, Ji-Cai*, historically called *Cen-Cao (Wuyue Chunqiu), Ji (Mingyi Bielu), Zi-Bei-Yu-Xing-Cao (Lü Chan Yan Ben Cao), Zi-Ji (Jiuji Yifang), Zu-Zi (Bencao Gangmu), Zu-Cao (Xinxiu Bencao), Chou-Zhu-Cao (Yilin zuan-yao‧yaoxing), Ce-Er-Gen (Zunyifu Zhi), Zhu-Bi-Kong (Tianbao Bencao), Jiu-Jie-Lian (Lingnan Caiyao Lu), Zhe-Er-Gen* or *Fei-Xing-Cao (Guizhou Mingjian Fangyao Ji)*, and *Chou-Xing-Cao (Quanzhou Bencao)* in China; *dokudame* in Japan; *E-Sung-Cho* in Korea; *Khaotong* or *Plu-khao* in Thailand; *giấp cá* or *diếp cá* in Vietnam. It has the functions of relieving fever, resolving toxin, reducing swelling, draining pus and promoting urination [4]. During the period of the Severe Acute Respiratory Syndrome (SARS) outbreak, it was one of the ingredients in the SARS prevention formulas recognized by the Health Ministry of China. Recently, several studies also provided scientific data to support and unveil its anti-SARS [5], anti-inflammatory [6,7], anti-allergic [8,9], virucidal [10,11], antileukemic [12], anti-oxidative

---

[*]Corresponding author.

[13,14] and anti-cancer [15] activities. It was reported that *H. cordata* contains groups of such chemical components as flavones, essential oil and alkaloids [16].

Over the last few years, there has been a rapid increase in the information available on the structures and pharmacological activities of *H. cordata* (**Figure 1**). In this review, we present recent *H. cordata* plant research in three sections: phytochemistry, pharmacological activities and quality control. The information was mainly collected from databases (Scifinder, ISIWeb of Knowledge) and several books.

2. Morphological Description

H. cordata is herbaceous perennial plant growing to 20 - 80 cm, the flowers are greenish-yellow, borne on a terminal spike 2 - 3 cm long with 4 - 6 large white basal bracts; spike terminal yellowish-brown. The odour is fishy on rubbing and the taste is slightly adstringent (**Figure 2**).

3. Traditional Uses of *H. cordata*

The uses differ from one country to another. In China, *H. cordata* has been used to treat anisolobis sores. The documented folk uses and indications in China were listed in detail in **Table 1**. In Korea, it has been used for the treatment of cough, pneumonia, bronchitis, dysentery, dropsy, leukorrhea, uteritis, eczema, herpes simplex, acne, chronic sinusitis and nasal polyps [11,17]. In Thailand, it has been used for immune stimulization and as anticancer agent [18]. In Japan, it has been mainly used as diuretics [19] and also used for the treatment of stomach ulcers [20], the control of the infection [21], and as antimicrobial [22,23], antitumor [24], promoting agents for the production of an antibiotic substance by a strain of gram-positive, spore-bearing bacilli [25]. In India, the shoot has been used for the freshness, good sleep, heart disorders by Apatani who have traditionally settled in seven villages in the Ziro valley of Lower Subansiri district of Arunachal Pradesh in the Eastern Himalayan region of India [26]. Besides general medicinal uses, *H. cordata* is employed as food (**Table 2**) and cosmetic formulations. In Korea and Japan, *H. cordata* is frequently used in combination with other herbal medicines as cosmetic. Its extraction are used as cosmetic composition for preventing or treating wrinkle [27], preventing chapped skin [28], antiaging [29,30], improving the skin conditions [31], removing freckles and skin-whitening [30]. The fermented extract with other herbal medicine are used for alleviating atopic dermatitis [32] and other skin troubles [33], owing to the anti-inflammatory and skin-calming effect, pruritus-alleviating effect, and humidifying effect of this composition. The extraction is also used for protecting or nourishing hair and preventing dandruff

[34,35]. In addition, *H. cordata* is used to prepare the massage pack which is able to treat acne, chloasma, atopy, and freckle without leaving any scar [36].

4. Phytochemistry

To date, the majority of phytochemical studies on *H. cordata* have focused on three types, namely: essential oil, flavonoid and alkaloids components [16]. Recent pharmacological studies indicated the essential oil components in *H. cordata* possess anti-inflammatory, antibacterial and antiviral activities [6,10]. The flavonoid components revealed antineoplastic, antioxidant, antimutagenic and free radical scavenging capacity [14, 37,38]. Similarly, the alkaloid components demonstrated significant potent antiplatelet and cytotoxic activities [15].

4.1. Essential Oil

Most of previous studies were mainly focused on the chemistry of essential oil. The volatile oils of *H. cordata* were extracted by various methods, supercritical CO_2 extraction [39,40], steam distillation [41-43], petroleum ether extraction [39,42], solid-phase microextraction [43], flash evaporation and simultaneous distillation-extraction [44,45], isolated by preparative HPLC [45,46], and analyzed qualitatively and quantitatively by GC , GC-MS, GC-MS with on-column derivatization procedure [41] TLC [47,48], flash GC [49], combined gas-liquid chromatography and mass spectroscopy [48]. The considerable differences may depend on the extraction procedure, the season, the part, the dry process, the stage of development and the distinct habitat in which the plant has been collected [47,50-54]. A total of 346 volatile components were reported. They were composed mainly of terpenoids (27.0%), hydrocarbons (16.8%), esters (11.9%), alcohols (11.6%), ketones (7.2%), aldehydes (4.9%), acids (3.8%), phenols (1.7%), aethers (0.9%) and mixed compounds (14.2%). Among these, which were found with higher frequency are: methyl *n*-nonyl ketone, *β*-myrcene, houttuynin, decanal, trans-caryophyllene, decanoic acid, camphene, *β*-pinene, lauraldehyde, bornyl acetate, *α*-pinene, limonene, 4-terpineol, caryophyllene oxide, nonanol and linalool so on.

4.2. Flavonoids and Other Polyphenols

As would be expected in biologically active plants, a number of flavonoids and other polyphenols have been isolated and identified from *H. cordata* (**Table 3**). The quercitrin is the first flavonoids extracted from the leaves and stems of *H. cordata* [55]. Quercetin-3-*O*-*β*-D-galactoside-7-*O*-*β*-D-glucoside, kaempferol 3-O-[*α*-L-rhamnopyranosyl-(1→6)-*β*-D-glucopyranoside], quercetin

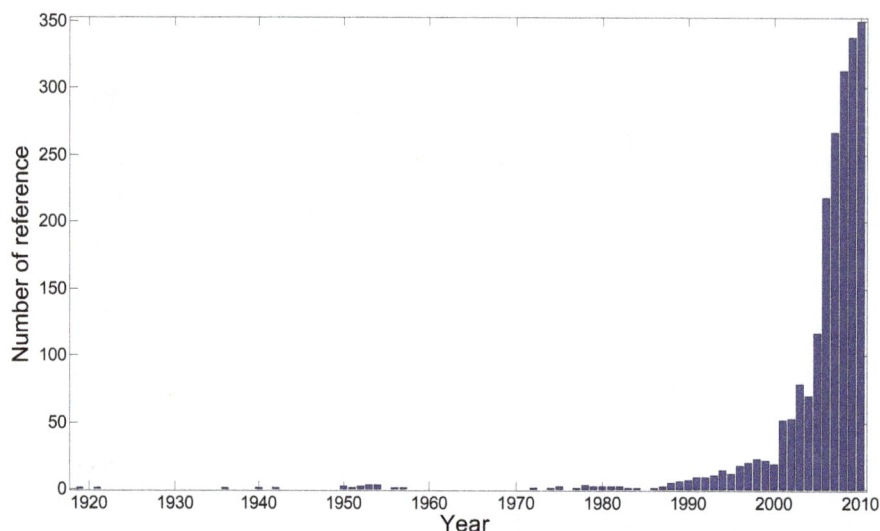

Figure 1. The increasing trend of the research work about *H. cordata* (The data was collected from Scifinder database).

Table 1. Ethnomedical uses of *H. cordata* in China.

Traditional uses	Document	Historial period
Anisolobis sores	*Mingyi Bielu* (*Appendant Records of Famous Physicians*)	220-450 AD
Sores, tinea capitis	*Rihuazi Bencao* (*The Herbal Medicine of Rihuazi*)	935-965 AD
Heatstroke	*Lü Chan Yan Ben Cao*	1220 AD
Lung carbuncles and refractory hemoptysis, large intestine heat-toxin, hemorrhoids	*Diannan Bencao*	1436 AD
Heat-toxin, carbuncle, hemorrhoids and rectocele, malaria, salammoniac poison	*Bencao Gangmu* (*Compendium of CMM*)	1592-1596 AD
Lung carbuncles and cough with pyoid blood	*Shennong Bencao Jingshu*	1625
Tonsillitis, chronic phlegm	*Bencao Fengyuan*	1695 AD
Diuresis, resolving mass and swelling, miasma, heatstroke, toxin from the viper and insect, dermatophytosis, sores and carbuncles with pyogenesis, gore	*Yilin zuanyao··yaoxing*	1758 AD
Swelling, malaria	*Yaoxing Kao*	1772 AD
Scrotal abscess, whitlow	*Bencao Qiu Yuan*	1848 AD
Deobstruant, febrifuge	*Caomu Bianfang*	1870 AD
Hydropsy, weakness, wooden belly	*Fenlei Caoyaoxing*	1906
skin ulcer, diarrhoea, dysentery	*Lingnan Caiyao Lu*	1936
Sores and tinea, eczema, lumbago, coronary heart disease angina	*Xiandai Shiyong Zhongyao*	1956
Syphilis, urethritis, tummy, purulent disease, cellulitis, tympanitis, mastitis, lung abscess, tuberculosis, hysteritis, first-aid emetic for taking poison	*Zhongguo… Yaoyong Zhiwu Tujian*	1960
Stenocardia	*Shaanxi Zhongyao Zhi*	1962
clearing heat and detoxifying, mastitis, cellulitis, tympanitis, enteritis	*Changyong Zhongcaoyao Shouce*	1969
Lung abscess, lobar pneumonia, malaria, chincough, diarrhoea, dysentery, appendicitis, urethritis, infantile diarrhea, heatstroke, cold, tonsillitis, cholecystitis, stubborn dermatitis, boils, wound by the viper	*Fujian Yaowu Zhi*	1979

3-*O*-α-*L*-rhamnopyranosyl-7-*O*-β-*D*-glucopyranoside three flavonoid glycosides [56], chlorogenic acid methyl ester, 4-[(2E)-3-(β-D-glucopyranosyloxy)-2-buten-1-yl]-4-hydroxy-3,5,5-trimethyl-2-cyclohexen-1-one, 2-(4-hydroxyphenyl)ethyl-β-D-glucopyranoside, 2-(3,4-dihydro-xyphenyl) ethyl-β-D-glucopyranoside, 4-(β-D-glucopy-rano-syloxy)-3-hydroxybenzoic acid five polyphenols [57], catechin, procyanidin B, houttuynamide A, houttuynoside A [18,58] (**Figure 3**), were isolated from *H. cordata*. The structures of new compounds are listed in

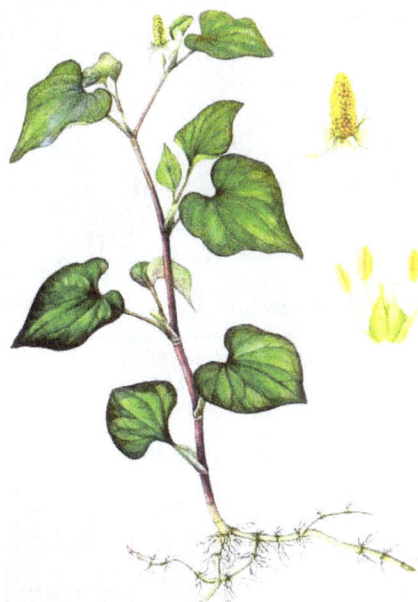

Figure 2. *Houttuynia cordata* **Thunb.**

Figure 3.

The flavonoids and other polyphenols of *H. cordata* were extracted by various methods, hot soaking extraction [59,60], EtOAc extraction [61], ethanol/methanol refluent extraction [56], Soxhlet extraction [59], ultrasonic extraction [62], microwave-assisted extraction [63, 64] and pressurized liquid extraction [60], isolated and purified by macroreticular resin [65], various column chromatography [57] and bioactivity-guided fractionation and isolation [66], and identified and analyzed by physiochemical properties analysis [67], capillary electrophoresis with wall-jet amperometric detection [68], TLC [67,69], GC [69], HPLC [69-72], HPLC-MS [73], HPLC-DAD-ESI-MS [66,74] and spectral analysis including UV-VIS [59,67], NMR and MS [56,75]. Among the above-mentioned extraction methods, microwave-assisted extraction and pressurized liquid extraction are favorable to the other methods. The microwave-assisted extraction not only has higher extraction efficiency but also the advantages of being fast and energy saving.

The amounts of five flavonoid glycosides contained in *H. cordata*, quercitrin, hyperin, rutin, isoquercitrin and afzelin, were determined by HPLC [70,76]. The order of the flavonoids content in the different parts was as: flower > leaf > fruit > stem. No flavonoid was found in rhizome.

A correlation between flavonoid glycoside contents of *H. cordata* and light intensity has been reported. The flavonoid glycoside content was the highest when the plant was cultivated without shade and decreased as the shading rate increased [77].

The contents of flavonoids in freeze-dried *H. cordata* from different habitats were measured by HPLC-MS. It was found that flavonoids in Hongkong were higher than those in Sichuan and Guangdong Province. The relationship between the content of flavonoids in *H. cordata* and their biological characteristics such as morphologic and growth traits or a geographic origin were analyzed. The result revealed that the levels of three major flavonoids, hyperin, quercitrin, and quercetin, varied remarkably in the plants from different provinces, and variation in quercitrin was significantly correlated to the biological characteristics of the plant but not correlated to the geographic region where the plant grows [72].

4.3. Alkaloids

During the past 20 years, many kinds of alkaloid have been isolated from *H. cordata*, including aporphine, pyridine and the others. The structures of these compounds are shown in **Table 4**. *cis-N-*(4-Hydroxystyryl) benzamide and *trans-N-*(4-Hydroxystyryl) benzamide were isolated from the CHCl$_3$ extraction of this herb by a combination of HPLC and other techniques [78]. Probstle and co-workers isolated aristolactam A, aristolactam B, piperolactam A and norcepharacdione B from *H. cordata*. Jong and Wang isolated 7-chloro-6-demethyl-cepharadione, long chain substituted pyridine alkaloids 3,5-didecanoyl-pyridine,2-nonyl-5-decanoylpyridine which are rare in nature and *N*-methyl-5-methoxy-pyr-rolidin-2-one from this plant [79,80], respectively.

4.4. Organic Acid and Fatty Acid

Palmitic acid, stearic acid, heptanoic acid, nonanoic acid, undecanoic acid, octanoic acid, hexanoic acid, lauric acid, capric acid, heptadecanoic acid, tetradecanoic acid, tridecanoic acid, pentadecanoic acid, octadecenoic acid, hexadecenoic acid, octadecadienoic acid, aspartic acid, glutamic acid capric acid, lauric acid and palmitic acid in this plant were identified using gas chromatograph [81]. In addition, chlorogenic acid, crypto-chlorogenic acid, neo-chlorogenic acid, quinic acid and caffeic acid were identified using mass spectra and fragmentation patterns [18]. Takagi and coworkers extracted chlorogenic acid, detected palmitic acid, linoleic acid, oleic acid, and stearic acid in the benzene fraction [82]. Wu and co-workers seperated and purified the chemical components by solvent extraction, thin-layer chromatograph and silica gel column chromatograph, and identified the structures by IR, EI-MS, 1H-NMR and ^{13}C-NMR [83]. Bauer and colleagues identified linolenic, linoleic, oleic, palmitic and stearic acid by phytochemical examination [16]. Wang and colleagues isolated and purified succinic acid from dried rhizome of this plant by solvent extraction, silica gel and Sephadex LH-20 column chromatographs [80].

Table 2. Food applications of *H. cordata*.

Countries	Used part	Traditional uses	References
China, Vietnam	Root, leaves	Vegetable	[145,146]
Japan	Leaves, entire plant	Beverage, deodorant	[147,148]
Korea	Entire plant	Kimchi, soy sauce, knife-cut noodles, syrup, carbonated drinks	[149-151]
Thailand	Young leaves	vegetable	[18]

Table 3. Flavonoids and other polyphenols from *H. cordata*.

Number	Compounds	Classes	Parts	References
1	Quercetin	Flavonoids	E, A	[61,75,150]
2	Rutin	Flavonoids	A, L, SP, S	[68-70,76,82,150]
3	Hyperin	Flavonoids	A, SP, L, S	[69,70,75,76,82,85,149,150]
4	Afzelin	Flavonoids	E, A, L, SP, S	[61,70,75,76,82,85,150]
5	Quercitrin	Flavonoids	A, E, L, SP, S	[24,55,56,61,69,70,75,76,84,85,103,150]
6	Isoquercitrin	Flavonoids	A, L, SP, S	[69,70,76,88,149,150]
7	Apigenin	Flavonoids	A	[75]
8	Quercetin-3-*O*-*β*-*D*-galactoside-7-*O*-*β*-*D*-glucoside	Flavonoids*	E, L, R, S	[56]
9	Kaempferol 3-O-[*α*-L-rhamnopyranosyl-(1→6)-*β*-D-glucopyranoside]	Flavonoids*	E, L, R, S	[56,71]
10	Quercetin 3-*O*-*α*-*L*-rhamnopyranosyl-7-*O*-*β*-*D*-glucopyranoside	Flavonoids*	E, R, S	[56]
11	Quercetin hexoside	Flavonoids	L	[18]
12	Kaempferol	Flavonoids	E	[71]
13	Isorhamnetin	Flavonoids	E	[71]
14	Phloridzin	Flavonoids	L	[152]
15	Avicularin	Flavonoids	L	[152]
16	Protocatechuic acid	Polyphenols	E, A	[61,75,85,150]
17	Chlorogenic acid	Polyphenols	A, E, L, R, S	[18,82,150]
18	Vanillic acid	Polyphenols	NR	[85,153]
19	*p*-Hydroxy-benzoic acid methyl ester	Polyphenols	NR	[84,153]
20	Chlorogenic acid methyl ester	Polyphenols*	E	[57]

Continued

21	4-[(2E)-3-(β-D-glucopyranosyloxy) -2-buten-1-yl]-4-hydroxy-3,5, 5-trimethyl-2-Cyclohexen-1-one	Polyphenols*	E	[57]	
22	2-(4-Hydroxyphenyl)ethyl-β- D-Glucopyranoside	Polyphenols*	E	[57]	
23	2-(3,4-Dihydroxyphenyl)ethyl- β-D-Glucopyranoside	Polyphenols*	E	[57]	
24	4-(β-D-glucopyranosyloxy)-3 -hydroxybenzoic acid	Polyphenols*	E	[57]	
25	Cryptochlorogenic acid	Polyphenols	L	[18]	
26	Neochlorogenic acid	Polyphenols	L	[18]	
27	Procyanidin B	Polyphenols*	L	[18]	
28	Catechin	Polyphenols*	L	[18]	
29	Quinic acid	Polyphenols	L	[18]	
30	Caffeic acid	Polyphenols	L	[18]	
31	cis-Methyl ferulate	Polyphenols	E	[85]	
32	trans-Methyl ferulate	Polyphenols	E	[85]	
33	Methyl vanillate	Polyphenols	E	[85]	
34	Vanillin	Polyphenols	E	[85]	
35	Houttuynamide A	Polyphenols*	E	[85]	
36	Houuttuynoside A	Polyphenols*	E	[85]	

*Novel compound; E, entire plants; A, aerial parts; R, roots; S, stems; SP, spikes; B, barks; L, leaves; NR, not reported.

4.5. Sterols

A number of common sterols have been isolated from *H. cordata*. Stigmast-4-en-3-one, 3β-hydroxystigmast-5-en-7-one, 5α-stigmastane-3,6-dione and stigmast-4-ene-3,6-dione were isolated from this plant [84]. Stigmast-3,6-dione, sitoindoside I and daucosterol were isolated and purified from dried rhizome of *H. cordata* by solvent extraction, silica gel and Sephadex LH-20 column chromatographs [80]. β-Sitosterol [4,82,85], β-sitosterol glucoside [85], brassicasterol [4], stigmasterol [4], spinasterol [4], and stigmast-4-ene-3,6-dione [16] were also found in this plant.

4.6. Amino Acid and Microelements

H. cordata contains more than 20 amino acids, including alanine, valine, glutamic acid, aspartic acid, isoleucine, proline, leucine, glycine, serine, lysine, cystine, tyrosine, methionine, phenylalanine, histidine, threonine, tryptophane, arginine, hydroxyproline and citrulline [81,86]. The major components were alanine, valine, glutamic acid, aspartic acid, isoleucine, proline leucine [81]. Among all amino acids, the glutamic acid content was the highest followed by leucine and aspartic acid [86]. Many microelements including iron, magnesium, manganese, potassium, copper, zinc and calcium, etc., can be in *H. cordata* [86,87]. The involucre of *H. cordata* contains high levels of zinc, copper, and Zn/Cu ratios at the stages of fructification [86].

4.7. Other Compounds

N-phenethyl-benzamide, glyceryl linoleate and *n*-butyl-α-D-fructopyranoside were isolated and purified from dried rhizome of *H. cordata* by solvent extraction, silica gel and Sephadex LH-20 column chromatographs [80]. Vomifoliol, sesamin and 1,3,5-tridecanoylbenzene were isolated from the aerial parts of *H. cordata*. 1,3,5-tridecanoylbenzene was also isolated [84]. Chou characterized N-(1-hydroxymethyl-2-phenylethyl) benzamide, N-(4-hydroxyphenylthyl) benzamide, 4-hydroxybenzamide, 4-hydroxy-3-methoxybenzamide, 6,7-dimethyl-1-ribitol-1-yl-1,4-dihydroquinoxaline-2,3-dione, (1H)-quinolinone, indole-3-carboxylic acid, dihydrovomifoliol, reseoside, 7-(3,5,6-trihydroxy-2,6,6-trimethylcyclohexyl)but-3-en-2-one, 6-(9-hydroxy-but-7-enyl)-1,1,5-trimethylcyclhexane-3,5,6-triol, 4-hydroxybenzoic acid, methylpara-ben, *p*-hydroxybenzaldehyde, benzyl-β-D-glucopyranoside and cycloart-25-ene-3β,24-diol from *H. cordata using* 1D and 2D NMR and mass spectra [85]. The carotenoids were observed in *H. cordata*. The content of β-carotene and violaxanthin are relatively high in the cotyledonous stage and decreased in fructification, while the content of lutein is low in the cotyledonous stage and progressively increased with the growth [86].

5. Pharmacological Activities

5.1. Diuretic Effects

The components quercitrin extracted from the leaves and

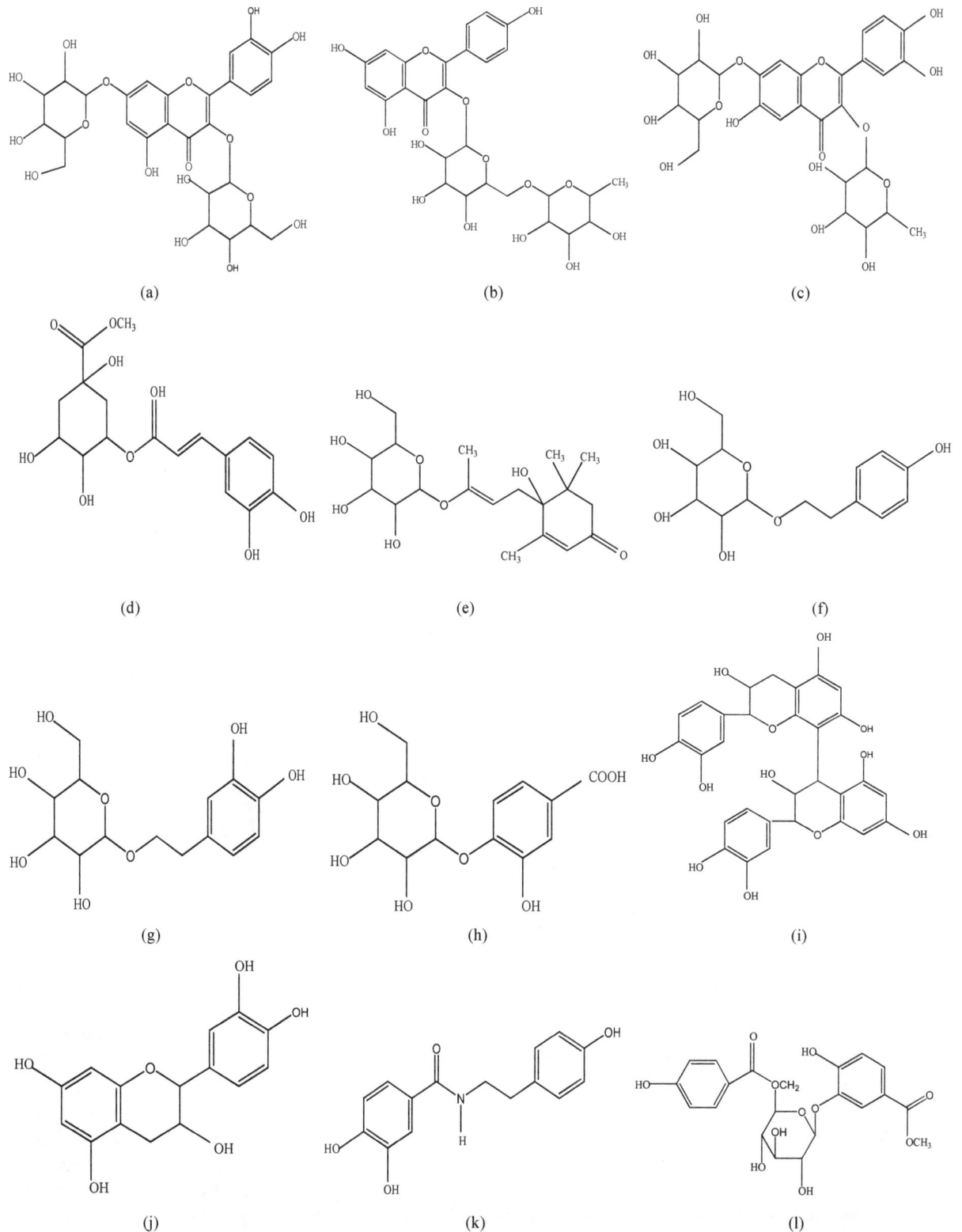

Figure 3. Flavonoids and other polyphenols were isolated or detected from *H. cordata* for the first time. (a) Quercetin 3-*O*-α-*L*-rhamnopyranosyl-7-*O*-β-*D*-glucopyranoside; (b) Kaempferol 3-O-[α-L-rhamnopyranosyl-(1→6)-β-D-glucopyrano-side]; (c) Quercetin 3-*O*-α-*L*-rhamnopyranosyl-7-*O*-β-*D*-glucopyranoside; (d) Chlorogenic acid methyl ester; (e) 4-[(2E)-3-(β-D-glucopyranosyloxy)-2-buten-1-yl]-4-hydroxy-3,5,5-trimethyl-2-cyclohexen-1-one; (f) 2-(4-Hydroxyphenyl)ethyl-β-D-glucopyranoside; (g) 2-(3,4-Dihydroxyphenyl)ethyl-β-D-glucopyranoside; (h) 4-(β-D-glucopyranosyloxy)-3-hydroxybenzoic-acid; (i) Procyanidin B; (j) Catechin; (k) Houttuynamide A; (l) Houttuynoside A.

Table 4. Alkaloids from *H. cordata*.

Number	Compounds	Structures	References
1	Aristolactam A		[15,85,120,153]
2	Aristolactam B		[15,16,74,79,85,120,153]
3	Piperolactam A		[15,16,74,85,120,153]
4	3,4-Dimethoxy-N-methyl aristolactam		[85]
5	Lysicamine		[85]
6	Noraritolodione		[85]
7	Norcepharadione B		[15,85,120,153]

Contimued

8	Cepharadione B		[15,61,79,85,153]
9	Splendidine		[15,85]
10	3,5-Didecanoylpyridine		[16,79,154]
11	2-Nonyl-5-decanoylpyridine		[16,79,131,154]
12	3,5-Didecanoyl-4-nonyl-1,4-dihydropyridine		[16,154]
13	3-Decanoyl-4-nonyl-5-dodecanoyl-1,4-dihydropyridine		[16,154]
14	3,5-Didodecanoyl-4-nonyl-1,4-dihydropyridine		[16,154]

Contimued

15	7-chloro-6-demethylcepharadione B		[79,153]
16	3-Nonylpyrazole		[96]
17	N-methyl-5-methoxy-pyrrolidin-2-one		[80]
18	*cis-N*-(4-Hydroxystyryl) benzamide		[78]
19	*trans-N*-(4-Hydroxystyryl) benzamide		[78]

stems, isoquercitrin from the floral spikes and fruit spikes of this herb show diuretic action [55,88]. The diuretic action is attributed to quercitrin, KCl and K_2SO_4 [89]. The extract of *H. cordata* showed similar diuretic action of acetylcholine, lactic acid and aspartic acid [19].

5.2. Antimicrobial Effects

Zhang [90] found that oil extract had inhibitory effect on β-Hemolytic streptococcus, *Streptococcus aureus*, Pseudomonas aeruginosa and *Escherichia coli*. Kwon [44] noticed that the volatile flavor components showed strong antibacterial activities against Bacillus cereus, Bacillus subtilis, Vibrio cholerae and Vibrio parahaemolyticus. Meng [91] found that water and ethanol extracts of fresh and dry *H. cordata* showed antimicrobial activity against *Staphylococcus aureus* and *Escherichia coli*. The

minimal inhibitory concentrations (MICs) against *Staphylococcus aureus* of water extracts of fresh and dry *H. cordata* were 12.5 and 100 mg/mL, and those of ethanol extracts were 25 and 100 mg/mL respectively. The fresh extract had better pharma-cological activity than dry one, and water extract had better pharmacological activity than ethanol extract. Lu *et al* reported that oils obtained by hydrodistillation from the above and the below ground parts shows antimicrobial activity with MIC values of 0.0625×10^{-3} to 4.0×10^{-3} mL/mL against Staphylococcus aureus and Sarcina ureae [53]. Zhang *et al.* found that the MICs of the essential oil against Staphylococcus aureus and Sarcina increased with the storage time [92]. Moderate antibacterial activities are observed against Escherichia coli and Staphyloccocus aureus by [93,94], but not by [95].

The volatile essential oil isolated from H. cordata was seperated into 11 fractions by preparative HPLC. In a test of the antibacterial activity of 11 fractions, the growth of nine Gram-negative bacteria was inhibited when treated with Fraction 6 including methyl n-nonyl ketone, β-myrcene, β-ocimene, 1-decanol and houttuynin, and fraction 5 including decanal, bornyl acetate, fenchene and decanoic acid, respectively [46]. Houttuynin isolated from the rhizome of H. cordata suppressed the growth of yeasts and molds [22] and 3-nonylpyrazole inhibited the growth of Staphylococcus aureus, Bacillus subtilis, Trichophytons, Zygosaccharomyces salsus, and Aspergillus niger [96]. Kim et al. observeed that the antibacterial activity of H. cordata water extract (HCWE) against Salmonella typhimurium increased in a dose-dependent manner at concentrations from 25 to 100 mg/ml during 8-h incubation in vitro, without showing cytotoxicity in RAW 264.7 cells. Furthermore, HCWE showed virulence reduction effects in S. typhimurium-infected BALB/c mice in vivo [97].

5.3. Antiviral Effects

Over the past decade, substantial progress has been made in research on the natural products for the treatment of AIDS. Several plants and their products including H. cordata have shown anti-HIV activity [98]. The distillate and three major compounds from fresh plants of H. cordata showed dose-dependent virucidal acitivity against HIV-1 without showing cytotoxicity in vitro. At 2-fold dilution, approximately 20% and 40% of HIV-1 were inactivated by the pretreatment with the distillate for 2 h and 6 h, respectively. While no significant activity was observed at the concentrations less than 0.0017% (w/v), each of three components exerted virucial activity against HIV-1 at 0.0083% (w/v). Lauryl aldehyde was found to be the most potent constituent of the three components [10]. Vpr, an accessory gene product of HIV-1 induced abnormality in cell cycle leading to the increased HIV replication, was supposed to be a possible target for anti-AIDS drugs. Quercetin, a compound from this crude drug, efficiently inhibited Vpr function without affecting its expression. Furthermore, the data suggested that Vpr-induced transcription from HIV-LTR was considerably abrogated by quercetin. These in vitro data indicated that quercetin, a flavonoid previously reported inhibited HIV replication, also targeted Vpr [99].

An in vitro study evaluated the anti-HSV (herpes simplex virus) activity of H. cordata, using XTT-based colorimetric assay. BCC-1/KMC cells were infected with HSV and were cultured in HCWE. The results showed that HCWE significantly inhibited the replication of HSV at a concentration of 250 µg/mL, 10.2% for HSV type 1 (HSV-1) ($p < 0.05$) and 32.9% for HSV type 2 (HSV-2) ($p < 0.005$). The ED_{50} of HSV-1 and HSV-2 were 822.4

µg/mL and 362.5 µg/mL respectively. H. cordata had better effect against HSV-2 than HSV-1, and had a low ED_{50} against HSV-2 [11]. The distillates extracted from fresh plants of H. cordata and three components, methyl n-nonyl ketone, lauryl aldehyde, and capryl aldehyde are also assayed for anti-HSV activity. The distillates, lauryl aldehyde and capryl aldehyde exhibited moderate antiviral activity against HSV-1 (ED_{50} = 0.0013%, ED_{50} = 0.0008%, ED_{50} = 0.00038%, w/v). Methyl n-nonyl ketone was not so effective against it (ED_{50} = 0.0091%, w/v) [10]. In another in vitro study, norcepharadione B isolated from the whole plant of H. cordata significantly suppresses HSV-1 replication by 46.38% at the concentration of 100 µM [58].

Severe acute respiratory syndrome (SARS) is a life-threatening form of pneumonia caused by SARS coronavirus (SARS-CoV). From late 2002 to mid 2003, it infected more than 8000 people worldwide, of which over 7000 cases were found in China (http://www.who.int/en/). Owing to the high infectious rate and the absence of definitive therapeutic Western medicines, State Administration of Traditional Chinese Medicine of the People's Republic of China proposed six traditional Chinese medicine formulae to general public as preventive measures on 24 April 2003 (http://www.satcm.gov.cn/zhuanti/jbfz/20060901/100052.shtml). H. cordata was one of the component herbs in a heatremoving and detoxifying formula. Recently, immunomodulatory effect H. cordata was investigated in mouse splenic lymphocytes, inhibitory activity on SARS coronaviral 3C-like protease (3CLpro) and RNA-dependent RNA polymerase (RdRp). The results showed that HCWE stimulated the proliferation of mouse splenic lymphocytes significantly and dose-dependently. By flow cytometry, it revealed that H. cordata increased the proportion of CD4(+) and CD8(+) T cells. H. cordata exhibited significant dose-dependent inhibitory effects on SARS-CoV 3C-like protease (3CL (pro)) and RdRp activity. At concentration of 200 µg/ml or above, significantly inhibited the activity of 3CLpro ($p < 0.05$). At the highest testing dose (1000 µg/ml), the 3CLpro activity was decreased by 50%. The essential oil could inhibit the growth of influenza virus in cultures with ED_{50} = 41% (v/v) [100], and a complete inhibition at 250 mg/mL [90]. The antiviral assays demonstrated that quercetin 3-rhamnoside (Q3R) possessed strong antiviral activity of about 86% against influenza A/WS/33 virus at concentration of 100 µg/ml and antiviral activity of about 66% at the same virus at concentration of 10 µg/ml. The research on antivirus activities was carried out using amantadine, ribavirin and H. cordata injection (HCI) in vitro and in vivo. The abilities of treating pneumonia of mice when three kinds of drugs were used cooperatively were far higher than those alone in BALB/c mice [101]. Therefore, these findings provided important information for the utilization of *H. cordata* for influenza treatment.

Another one flavonoid compound, quercetin 7-rhamnoside (Q7R), showed antiviral activity against rotavirus and rhinovirus [102]. Q7R was used to inhibit porcine epidemic diarrhea virus (PEDV), was the predominant cause of severe entero-pathogenic diarrhea in swine. It inhibited PEDV replication by 50% using 0.014 μg/mL. Several structural analogues of Q7R, quercetin, apigenin, luteolin and catechin, also showed moderate anti-PEDV activity. Q7R did not directly interact with or inactivate PEDV particles and affect the initial stage of PEDV infection by interfering of PEDV replication. The effectiveness of Q7R against transmissible gastroenteritis virus (TGEV) and porcine respiratory coronavirus (PRCV), was lower compared to PEDV. Q7R could be considered as a lead compound for development of anti-PEDV drugs [103].

The inhibitory effect of *H. cordata* on epidemic hemorrhagic fever virus (EHFV) infection was also reported [104]. *H. cordata* extract (HCE) could neutralize EV71-induced cytopathic effects in Vero cells. The IC_{50} of HCE for EV71 was 125.92 ± 27.84 μg/mL. Antiviral screening of herb extracts was also conducted on 3 genotypes of EV71, coxsackievirus A16 and echovirus 9. HCE had the highest activity against genotype A of EV71. A plaque reduction assay showed that HCE significantly reduced plaque formation. Viral protein expression, viral RNA synthesis and virus-induced caspase 3 activation were inhibited in the presence of HCE, suggesting that it affected apoptotic processes in EV71-infected Vero cells by inhibiting viral replication. The antiviral activity of HCE was greater in cells pretreated with extract than those treated after infection. Therefore, it was concluded that HCE had antiviral activity, and it offered a potential to develop a new anti-EV71 agent [105].

5.4. Anticancer/Antitumour Effects

Some extracts and compounds from *H. cordata* and some traditional Chinese medicine formulae containing *H. cordata* were reported to have anticancer effect. A traditional Chinese medicine formulae containing *H. cordata* was used for treating lung cancer and improving human immunity. It had the advantages of good curative effect, no obvious toxic or side effect, simple manufacturing process, and low cost [106,107].

HCE treatment caused lowering of cell viability in various human cancer cell lines [108], and administered on the acupuncture point prevented the increase of mass weight of melanoma BBL16 tumor cells inoculated into mice [109]. The cellular effects of HCE and the signal pathways of HCE-induced apoptosis in HL-60 human promyelocytic leukemia cell line were investigated. HCE

treatment caused apoptosis of cells as evidenced by discontinuous fragmentation of DNA, the loss of mitochondrial membrane potential, release of mitochondrial cytochrome c into the cytosol, activation of procaspase-9 and caspase-3, and proteolytic cleavage of poly(ADP-ribose) polymerase (PARP). Pretreatment of Ac-DEVD-CHO, caspase-3 specific inhibitor, or cyclosporin A, a mitochondrial permeability transition inhibitor, completely abolished HCE-induced DNA fragmentation. Together, these results suggested that HCE possibly caused mitochondrial damage leading to cytochrome c release into cytosol and activation of caspases resulting in PARP cleavage and execution of apoptotic cell death in HL-60 cells [110]. The 100 μg/mL of methanolic extract of *H. cordata* root showed significant protective effects (p < 0.01) against hydrogen peroxide-induced DNA damage in HepG2 cells and increased cell viability against hydrogen peroxide. The study indicated that *H. cordata* root methanol extract acted as a potential antioxidant, and exhibited potential anticancer properties [111]. The investigation examined the anticancer activity of the methanol extract from *H. cordata* on ICR mouse with induced abdominal cancer and L1210 cancer cells. To get an insight into the reaction mechanism undelying the anticancer activity, O_2^- ion quantity and antioxidant enzyme activities such as superoxide dismiutase (SOD) and glutathione peroxidase (GPx) of L1210 cells in the presence of HCE were measured. The increased values of SOD and GPx enzyme activities in addition to the augmented generation of O_2^- ion in L1210 cells implied that the reactive oxygen species including O_2^- ion which were presumably induced by HCE might have participated in the process of L1210 cells cytotoxicity [112,113]. In another study, HCWE inhibited five leukemic cell lines, namely L1210, U937, K562, Raji and P3HR1, with IC50s between 478 μg/mL and 662 μg/mL. It was proved to be a potential medicinal plant for treating leukemia [12].

In a study, forty-eight Sprague-Dawley rats were fed with a diet containing 0%, 2% or 5% *H. cordata* powder and 15% fresh soybean oil or 24-h oxidized frying oil (OFO) for 28 days. The level of microsomal protein, total cytochrome 450 content (CYP450) and enzyme activities including NADPH reductase, ethoxyresorufin O-deethylase (EROD), pentoxyresorufin O-dealkylase (PROD), aniline hydroxylase (ANH), aminopyrine demethylase (AMD), and quinone reductase (QR) were determined. The oxidized frying oil feeding produced a significant increase in the content of CYP450, microsomal protein, activities of NADPH reductase, EROD, PROD, ANH, AMD and QR in rats (P < 0.05). In addition, the activities of EROD, ANH and AMD decreased and QR increased after feeding with *H. cordata* in OFO-fed group (P < 0.05). The feeding with 2% *H. cordata* diet showed the most significant effect. The findings suggested that polyphenol in *H. cordata* could be an important and necessary factor in the defense against CYP450-mediated cancers and other chronic diseases [114].

The anticancer activity of flavonoid extracts from *H. cordata* was studied on Sarcoma-180. They exhibited cytotoxic activity on S-180. The total flavonoid extract of *H. cordata* gave highest rate of death and showed good inhibitory effect on the growth of ascites tumor by S-180 in mice [37]. The inhibiting rate of flavonoids was detected by MTT assay. The apoptosis of HL60 and B16-BL6 was detected by FCM. Flavonoid from *H. cordata* also inhibited HL60 and B16BL6 and induced cell apoptosis. The IC50 in HL60 and B16BL6 was 0.410 and 0.122 g/L respectively [115].

Furthermore, six alkaloids exhibited cytotoxicity against five human tumor cell lines (A-549, SK-OV-3, SK-MEL-2, XF-498 and HCT-15) *in vitro*, including aristolactam B, piperolactam A, aristolactam A, norcepharadione B, cepharadione B and splendidine isolated by bioactivity-guided fractionation of a methanolic extract. Among them, splendidine exhibited the strongest cytotoxicity and aristolactam B selectively suppressed XF-498 (ED$_{50}$ = 0.84 µg/ml) [15].

5.5. Anti-Inflammatory Effects

Many kinds of extracts from *H. cordata* showed anti-inflammatory activity. The inflammation induced by xylene in the mice ear edema model was adopted to study the anti-inflammatory activity of chloroform extract, water extract, ethanol extract and *n*-butanol extract. All forms showed good anti-inflammatory activity, and the water extract had better pharmacological activity than ethanol extract, while the extract of fresh *H. cordata* had better pharmacological activity than that of dry one [91,116].

Shuang-Qing-Cao (SQC), a folk Chinese medicinal formula composed of *Lonicera japonica* Thunb (Caprifoliaceae), *Isatis indigotica* Fort (Cruciferae) and *H. cordata*, was used for treating diseases related with inflammation in the folk of China. The results indicated that SQC extract in β-cyclodextrin was greatly effective on an experimental model of acute lung inflammation induced by the intratracheal instillation of lipopolysaccharide (LPS) *in vivo* [117]. 40 - 400 mg·kg^{-1} of fresh HCE reduced the increase of LPS-induced leucocytes in brochoalveolar lavage fluid (BALF) in ICR mice, and alleviated the infiltration of inflammatory cells in pathological lung tissue, which showed that fresh HCE inhibited the LPS-induced lung inflammation [118].

A study investigated the effect of HCE on the migration of the human mast cell line, HMC-1, in response to stem cell factor (SCF). Treatment with HCE at a concentration of 10 µg/mL for 24 h showed no significant de-

crease in the survival rate of the HMC-1 cells. SCF showed the typical bell-shape curve for the HMC-1 cell chemoattraction with the peak of the curve at the SCF concentration of 100 ng/mL. HC-1, which was the whole plant extracted with 80% EtOH, and HC-3, which was the residue successively partitioned with EtOAc, both had inhibitory effects on HMC-1 cell movement. After the treatment with 10 µg/mL HC-1 extract for 6 and 24 h, the chemotactic index (CI) of HMC-1 cells decreased to 74% and 63%, respectively. HC-3 extract treatment for 6 and 24 h lowered the CI to 72% and 44%, respectively. The HC-1 and HC-3 extracts had no inhibitory effect on the mRNA and surface protein expressions of c-kit, SCF receptor. SCF mediated the chemotaxis signaling via nuclear factor κB (NF-κB) activation, and both extracts inhibited the activation. Therefore, the results indicated that HC-1 and HC-3 extracts decreased the chemotactic ability of HMC-1 cells in response to SCF by inhibiting NF-κB activation, and these substances may be useful for treating mast cell-induced inflammatory diseases [8]. Ethanol fraction was obtained from dried and powdered whole plants of *H. cordata*. The residue was diluted with water and was successively partitioned with *n*-hexane, EtOAc and BuOH. *H. cordata* fractions (HcFs) inhibited the expression of IL-4 and IL-5 in response to phorbol 12-myristate 13-acetate (PMA) and calcium ionophore (CaI) in Jurkat T cells and the human mast cell line, HMC-1. IL-4 and tumor necrosis factor-alpha (TNF-α)-induced thymus and activationregulated chemokine (TARC) production was blocked by HcFs in skin fibroblast CCD-986sk cells, particularly by the ethanol extract of Hc. Stimulants included in PMA, phytohemagglutinin (PHA) and CaI, increase the mRNA level of CC chemokine receptor 4 (CCR4), a receptor of TARC, in Jurkat T cells, and the ethanol extract of HcF weakly blocks the increased mRNA level. The ethanol extract inhibited TARC-induced migration, as well as basal migration of Jurkat T cells. Recent studies showed the usefulness of HcFs in the ethnopharmacological treatment of Th2-mediated or allergic inflammation, through the down-regulation of the production of Th2 cytokines, TARCand cell migration [119].

The effects of aqueous extract of *H. cordata* on the production of the pro-inflammatory mediators, nitric oxide (NO) and TNF-α were examined in an activated macrophage-cell line; RAW 264.7. The aqueous extract from *H. cordata* inhibited NO production in a dose-dependent manner, but minimally (~30%) TNF-α secretion at 0.0625 and 0.125 mg/mL [7]. Another study investigated the effects of aqueous extract on passive cutaneous anaphylaxis (PCA) in mice and on IgE-mediated allergic response in rat mast RBL-2H3 cells. Oral administration of aqueous extract inhibited IgE-mediated systemic PCA in mice. It also reduced antigen (DNP-BSA)-induced release of β-hexosaminidase, histamine, and reactive oxygen species in IgE-sensitized RBL-2H3 cells. In addition, it inhibited antigen-induced IL-4 and TNF-α production and expression in IgE-sensitized RBL-2H3 cells. It inhibited antigen-induced activation of NF-κB and degradation of IKB-α, and suppressed antigen-induced phosphorylation of Syk, Lyn, LAT, Gab2, and PLCγ2 and phosphorylation of Akt and MAP kinases (ERK1/2 and JNK1/2 but not p38 MAP kinase).

HCE showed remarkable COX inhibitory activity. Phytochemical investigation of HCE has led to the isolation of three aristolactams, two 4,5-dioxoaporphine derivatives, and several pyridine and dihydropyridine derived alkaloids. Finally it was found that unsaturaed fatty acids, like oleic and linoleic acid, were responsible for the high acitivity of the extract (IC$_{50}$: 13, 4 and 0, 25 μM respectively; indomethacin: 1, 15 μM) [120]. The anti-inflammatory activities of quercitrin isolated from *H. cordata* were evaluated in mice, rats, and guinea pigs. Quercitrin (50, 100, and 200 mg/kg orally) inhibited the rat hind paw edema induced by carrageenin, dextran, histamine, serotonin, and bradykinin in a dose-dependent manner; at 200 mg/kg this compound also inhibited the scald edema induced by 54°C hot water. Quercitrin did not show any inhibition of the UV light-induced erythema in guinea-pigs and of the increase of vascular permeability induced by acetic acid in mice. Quercitrin did not affect the granuloma formation in a cotton pellet implant and the development of adjuvant arthritis in rats. Quercitrin had an inhibitory effect on acute inflammation [121].

HCI, an aqueous solution of the steam distillate from plants of *H. cordata*, was used to treat ulcerative colitis (UC). Forty-two first episode type UC patients were randomly divided into HCI treatment group (n = 21) and Sulfasalazine group (n = 21). Clinical effects were observed in the 2 groups while ultrastructure of colonic mucosa, ICAM-1 and the pressure of distant colon were studied in HCI group. The clinical effect of HCI group (complete remission in 20, 95.2%; improvement in 1, 4.8%) was better than that of Sulfasalazine group (complete remission in 15, 72.4%, improvement in 5, 23.8%; inefficiency in 1, 3.8%, P < 0.01). The time of stool frequency recovering to normal (5.6 ± 3.3 d), and blood stool disappearance (6.7 ± 3.8 d) and abdominal pain disappearance (6.1 ± 3.5 d) in HCI group compared with Sulfasalazine group (9.5 ± 4.9 d, 11.7 ± 6.1 d, 10.6 ± 5.3 d, P < 0.01). HCI inhibited the epithelial cell apoptosis of colonic mucous membrane and the expression of ICAM-1 (45.8 ± 5.7% vs 30.7 ± 4.1%, P < 0.05). Compared with normal, the mean promotive speed of contraction wave steped up (4.6 ± 1.6 cm/min vs 3.2 ± 1.8 cm/min, P < 0.05) and the mean amplitude of the wave decreased (14.2 ± 9.3 kPa vs 18.4 ± 8.0 kPa, P < 0.05) in active UC

patients. After treatment with HCI, these 2 indexes improved significantly (17.3 ± 8.3 kPa, 3.7 ± 1.7 cm/min, P < 0.05). In normal persons, the postprandial pressure of sigmoid (2.9 ± 0.9 kPa) was higher than that of descending colon (2.0 ± 0.7 kPa) and splenic flexure (1.7 ± 0.6 kPa), while the colonic pressure (1.5 ± 0.5 kPa, 1.4 ± 0.6 kPa, 1.3 ± 0.6 kPa) decreased significantly (P<0.05) in active UC patients. The pain threshold of distant colon (67.3 ± 18.9 mL) in active UC patients decreased significantly compared with normal persons (216.2 ± 40.8 mL, P < 0.05) and recovered to normal after treatment with HCI (187.4 ± 27.2 mL, P < 0.05) [122]. Injection of carrageenan into the pleural cavity elicited an acute inflammatory response characterized by protein rich fluid accumulation and leukocyte infiltration in the pleural cavity. The inflammatory responses including fluid volume, protein concentration, C-reactive protein and cell infiltration reached peak after 24 h. The results showed that these parameters were attenuated by HCI and touched bottom at dose of 0.54 mL/100g. The results clearly indicated that HCI had anti-inflammatory activity [6]. The subsequent GC-MS analysis result indicated that main effect compounds in HCIs were methyl *n*-nonyl ketone, houttuynin, lauryl aldehyde, capryl aldehyde, β-pinene, β-linalool, 1-nonanol, 4-terpineol, α-terpineol, bornyl acetate, *n*-decanoic acid and acetic acid, geraniol ester etc [123,124].

5.6. Antioxidative Effects

Chen [14] showed that both aqueous and methanolic extracts of *H. cordata* had antioxidant properties under OFO feeding-induced oxidative stress on Sprague-Dawley rats. The rats were fed diets containing 0%, 2%, or 5% *H. cordata* and 15% fresh or OFO for 28 days. The levels of polyphenols in feces, blood plasma, and liver were determined. The low-density lipoprotein (LDL) oxidation lag time, plasma total antioxidant status (TAS), and levels of thiobarbituric acid-reactive substances (TBARS) were used as antioxidant indexes and the protein carbonyl groups were used as oxidative index. The polyphenol levels decreased in blood plasma and increased in feces when feeding OFO; the apparent absorption of polyphenols also decreased. The polyphenol levels in plasma increased when feeding *H. cordata*. The OFO-fed rats had higher plasma TBARS and hepatic protein carbonyl group concentrations and shorter LDL lag times than controls. The total TAS was elevated and the LDL lag time was prolonged with *H. cordata* feeding.

Ng [13] examined the antioxidant properties of *H. cordata* and its protective effect on bleomycin-induced pulmonary fibrosis in rats. Results showed that aqueous extract of *H. cordata* exhibited a different magnitude of antioxidant activities in all model systems tested. Although *H. cordata* showed weaker free radical scavenging and xanthine oxidase inhibitory activity than vitamin E, its anti-lipid peroxidation activity in rat liver homogenate was close to that of vitamin E. In animal studies, *H. cordata* significantly decreased the levels of superoxide dismutase, malondialdehyde, hydroxyproline, interferon-γ, and TNF-α. However, an increase in the concentration of catalase was noted in the bronchoalveolar lavage fluid. *H. cordata* also remarkably improved the morphological appearance of the lung of bleomycin-treated rats. This protective effect was more pronounced than that of vitamin E. In Korea, the reactive oxygen radical species (ROS) scavenging effects of 50 kinds of Korean medicinal plant leaves were examined. *H. cordata* exhibited over a 95% scavenging effect of superoxide anion in 1 ppm concentration of test solution. The correlation coefficient of total phenolic content with superoxide anion, hydrogen peroxide, hydroxyl radical and DPPH radical scavenging effects were 0.8111, 0.8057, 0.8809 and 0.9810, respectively [125]. Furthermore, the polyphenols isolated from *H. cordata*, quercetin, quercetin-3-O-*β*-D-galactoside, quercetin-3-O-*α*-L-rhamnoside and kaempferol-3-O-*α*-L-rhamnoside, exerted strong DPPH radical-scavenging activity [126]. In addition, the antioxidative activities of those medicinal plants and the compounds were investigated using the thiocyanate method to evaluate inhibitory effects on lipid peroxidation in the linoleic acid system. The peroxide levels gradually increased during incubation in the presence of linoleic acid over 3 days, and most of the plants inhibited lipid peroxidation. The aerial part *of H. cordata* reduced lipid peroxidation more effectively as lipid peroxidation progressed, resulting in inhibition of about 80% relative to the control value by the 3rd day of incubation. The polyphenols isolated from *H. cordata*, quercetin, quercetin-3-O-*β*-D-galactoside and quercetin-3-O-*α*-L-rhamnoside, also showed marked and dose-dependent inhibitory effects on lipid peroxidation. Moreover, quercetin glycosides showed stronger activity than quercetin, suggesting that glycosylation increased the antioxidative activity of quercetin [127]. The antioxidative and anti-lipid peroxidative efficacies of the fractions (H_2O, 20% MeOH, 40% MeOH, 60% MeOH, 100% MeOH) from *H. cordata* were measured by DPPH method and TBARS assay on rat liver homogenate. It was revealed that 60% MeOH fractions had potential antioxidative activity and inhibited lipid peroxidation significantly. The DNA damage was analyzed by tail moment (TM) and tail length (TL), which used markers of DNA strand breaks in SCGE. The 100 μg/mL of methanolic extract of *H. cordata* root showed significant protective effects ($P < 0.01$) against H_2O_2-induced DNA damage in HepG2 cells and increased cell viability against H_2O_2. The results of this study indicated that *H. cordata* root methanol extract acted as a potential

antioxidant, and exhibited potential anticancer properties, which might provide a clue to find applications in new pharmaceuticals for oxidative stability. The free radical scavenging capacities and antioxidant activities of *H. cordata* were evaluated using commonly accepted assays, including xanthine-xanthine oxidase assay, linoleic acid peroxidation and DPPH spectrophotometric assays, rapid screening of antioxidant by dot-blot and DPPH staining, TLC analysis with DPPH staining and DNA strand scission by hydroxyl radicals. *H. cordata* was extracted with dichloromethane, methanol or ethanol, respectively and selected for the best antioxidant results. Each sample under assay condition showed a dose-dependent free radical scavenging effect of DPPH and a dose-dependent inhibitory effect of xanthine oxidase and lipid peroxidation. They also showed a protective effect on DNA damage caused by hydroxyl radicals generated from UV-induced photolysis of hydrogen peroxide. A rapid evaluation for antioxidants using TLC screening and DPPH staining methods demonstrated each extract having various free radical scavenging capacity. Stained silica layer revealed a purple background with yellow spots at the location of drops, which showed radical scavenging capacity [138].

5.7. Antidiabetic Effects

The essential oils from *H. cordata* has been shown to have an effect on improving fat metabolism, the urinary albumin and insulin resistance of diabetes mellitus rats [128,129]. The rat model of diabetes mellitus was induced with streptozotocin (STZ) and high glucose-lipoids animal feeds, treated with *H. cordata* for 8 weeks. After treatment, fasting insulin level was lower in *H. cordata* group than in control, rosiglitazone and losartan group ($P < 0.05$). Insulin sensitivity index increased in *H. cordata* group and rosiglitazone group ($P < 0.05$ compared with the losartan group). The urinary albumin and 24 h urine volume were the lowest in *H. cordata* group ($P < 0.05$). The concentration of triglyceride in serum was lower in *H. cordata* and rosiglitazone group than that in control group ($P < 0.05$). *H. cordata* had a protective effect on the renal tissues in diabetic rats, which was probably correlated with the decrease of the expression of transforming growth factor-*β*1 and collagen I and with the increase of the expression of bone morphogenetic protein-7 in the renal tissues [130,131].

5.8. Anti-Allergic Effects

Human basophilic KU812F cells express a high-affinity immunoglobulin (Ig) E receptor, FcεRI, which plays an important role in IgE-mediated allergic reactions. Flow cytometric analysis showed that the FcεRI expression and the IgE binding activity were suppressed when the cells were cultured with HCE. Reverse transcription-polymerase chain reaction analysis showed that levels of the mRNAs for $Fc\varepsilon RI\alpha$- and γ-chains were decreased by the treatment of HCE. Addition of HCE to culture medium also resulted in a reduction in the release of histamine from the cells. These results suggested that HCE may exert its anti-allergic activity through down-regulation of $Fc\varepsilon RI$ expression and a subsequent decrease in histamine release [17]. Oral administration of HCWE inhibited compound 48/80-induced systemic anaphylaxis in mice. HCWE also inhibited the local allergic reaction, PCA, activated by anti-dinitrophenyl (DNP) IgE antibody in rats. HCWE reduced the compound 48/80-induced mast cell degranulation and colchicine-induced deformation of rat peritoneal mast cells (RPMC). Moreover, HCWE dose-dependently inhibited histamine release and calcium uptake of RPMC induced by compound 48/80 or anti-DNP IgE. Another study investigated the effects of HCWE on PCA in mice and on IgE-mediated allergic response in rat mast RBL-2H3 cells. Oral administration of HCWE inhibited IgE-mediated systemic PCA in mice, and reduced antigen (DNP-BSA)-induced release of β-hexosaminidase, histamine, and reactive oxygen species in IgE-sensitized RBL-2H3 cells. In addition, HCWE inhibited antigen-induced IL-4 and TNF-α production and expression in IgE-sensitized RBL-2H3 cells. HCWE inhibited antigen-induced activation of NF-κB and degradation of IκB-α. To investigate the inhibitory mechanism of HCWE on degranulation and cytokine production, the activation of intracellular $Fc\varepsilon RI$ signaling molecules were examined. HCWE suppressed antigen-induced phosphorylation of Syk, Lyn, LAT, Gab2, and PLC $\gamma 2$, further downstream, inhibited antigen-induced phosphorylation of Akt and MAP kinases (ERK1/2 and JNK1/2 but not p38 MAP kinase).

5.9. Antimutagenic Effects

The antimutagenic effects of both aqueous and methanolic extracts of *H. cordata* were examined using the Ames test. They had dose-dependent antimutagenic effects on benzo(a)pyrene, aflatoxin B1, and OFO, and the antimutagenic ability of aqueous extracts was higher than of methanolic extracts [14]. The inhibitory actions of chloroform extracts from *H. cardata* on the mutagenicity of Trp-P-2 and 1-NP was examined [132]. Inhibitory action was clarified on the following three points: 1) extract had the repressive effect on the two kinds of mutagenic substances which were composed of the indirect mutagen (Trp-P-2) requiring metabolic activation with S-9mix and of the direct mutagen (1-NP), 2) extract had the repressive effect on Trp-P-2 (NHOH), an activated form of Trp-P-2, and 3) extract had the repressive effect on metabolic process of Trp-P-2 with S-9mix. These results suggested that the antimutagens in chloroform extracts

had wide mechanism of repression.

5.10. Others

Two compounds, *cis*- and *trans*-N-(4-hydroxystyryl) benzamide, were isolated from the CHCl$_3$ extract of *H. cordata*, and proved to be potent inhibitors of platelet aggregation [78]. The injection and aqueous extract of *H. cordata* were illustrated to enhance immune function by modulating *ex vivo* pro-inflammatory cytokine and NO production as well as the expression of iNOS and COX-2 [133,134]. Effects of *H. cordata* extracts on the level of lipid peroxide and the enzyme activities of the liver were investigated in bromobenzene-induced rats. Lipid peroxide content in liver was increased by bromobenzene. It was decreased when the methanol extract of *H. cordata* was given to the rat. The methanol extract reduced the activities of aminopyrine N-demethylase and aniline hydroxylase that increased by bromobenzene, however did not affect glutathione S-transferase activity. The methanol extract recovered the activity of epoxide hydrolase activity that decreased significantly by bromobenzene. It was suggest that the extract might play an important play in the prevention of hepatotoxicity by reduction of aminopyrine N-demethylase and aniline hydroxylase activities as well as enhancement of epoxide hydrolase activity [75].

6. Quality Control

During our market surveillance, *H. cordata* has been sold in medicinal materials, tablet, injection, formula, grain, capsule and oral liquid, either presenting as single herb or as collections of herbs. However, like most of tradional herbal medicines and their preparations, despite its existence and continued use over many centuries, and its popularity and extensive use during the last decade, the quantity and quality of the safety and efficacy data are far from sufficient to meet the criteria needed to support its use world-wide. During the past several decades, with the extensive herbal treatment, adverse drug reactions accompany. HCI, the extract of sterile volatile oils from distillation of fresh *H. cordata* with a milliliter equivalent to 2 g of herbal materials, was reported a substantial incidence of life threatening anaphylaxis. The Chinese National Adverse Reaction Monitoring Center reports over 5000 adverse reactions to HCI from January 1988 to April 2006 including 222 serious cases [135]. The State Food and Drug Administration of China (SFDA) halted the use of HCI in hospitals in June 2006. Later, Lei and co-worker found that polysorbate-80, one of supplementary material in the injection caused serious adverse reactions in dogs with intravenous drip of HCI, when the concentration of polysorbate-80 was greater than 0.01 mg/ml. The distillate without polysorbate-80 showed no adverse reaction. This revealed that the adverse reactions of this injection may cause by supplementary material, not by the raw material herb [136,137]. Then, after re-examining HCI manufacturing conditions and quality control, the SFDA gave permission to few manufacturers to recommence HCI production. An allergen-warning label was requested to be added to the product.

As metioned above, *H. cordata* herb contains dozens of components. However, only one or two markers or pharmacologically active components is currently employed for evaluating the quality and authenticity, identifying the single herb or herb medicine preparations. The quality of HCI is assured based on the content of methyl *n*-nonyl ketone, whose content is set to the least 1.0 µg/ml injection. The quality of "*fufang yuxingcao*" tablet is assured based on the content of baicalin, whose content is set to the least 2.7 mg per tablet [138]. This standard is neither sufficient to determine the identity of an extracted plant material nor to ensure the quality of products. The chemical constituents in *H. cordata* vary depending on harvest seasons, plant origins, drying processes and other factors. Thus, it is necessary to develop accepted guideline for evaluating traditional medicine [139] and for determining most of the phytochemical constituents of herbal products in order to ensure the reliability and repeatability of pharmacological and clinical research, to understand their bioactivities and possible side effects of active compounds and to enhance product quality control [140].

The concept of phytoequivalence is developed in Germany in order to ensure consistency of herbal products [141]. According to this concept, a chemical profile concept, such as a fingerprint, is developed and proposed for standardizing medicinal products manufactured from herb medicines and their raw materials. In 2004, the Chinese State Food and Drug Administration (SFDA) regulated the compositions of liquid injection with herb medicine ingredients, using stringent quality procedures such as chemical assay and standardization. Fingerprints of herb medicine liquid injections are compulsorily carried out for this purpose. Comparing with conventional method focusing mainly on the determination of a certain active compound, fingerprinting can offer integral characterization of a complex system with a quantitative degree of reliability. The method for authentication and quality assessment of herb medicine has recently been accepted by the World Health Organization (WHO) as a strategy for the assessment of herbal medicines [142].

Under such circumstances, China Pharmacopoeia Committee organizes several scientific research institutions including our group, Research center for modernization of Chinese herbal medicine, college of chemistry and chemical engineering, Central south university, to establish the fingerprint of 70 traditional Chinese medicine injections and the technology platforms.

7. Conclusions

Throughout our literature review, many modern chemical, physical and biological methods are applied for the investigation of *H. cordata*. Despite the great progress, there are still some key tasks to do:

1) Find actual bioactive components. As mentioned above, the chemical composition of this herb is complex and diverse. Essential oil, alkaloids, flavonoids and other polyphenols are studied frequently in this species. The remaining chemical compounds are not well studied. Most of the mentioned studies focus on crude preparations of *H. cordata*, and the chemical profiles are not well detailed or standardized. There is a scarcity of detailed isolation studies works published. We believe that the isolation of new active principles for drug discovery from individual perspective, and establishment of detail chemical profiles for standardized extracts from holistic perspective would be of great scientific merit.

2) Understand the mechanism. Despite the extensive past and present traditional uses, and recent progress in pharmacological studies, biological data to correlate the ethnobotany to the chemistry are still lacking. In addition to recognized antibacterial ingredients such as decanoyl acetaldehyde and undecanone, some non-volatile components such as flavonoids, alkaloids and water-soluble polysaccharide have been found to have strong pharmacological activities gradually. Many studies on the pharmacological effects of *H. cordata* are reported, but the anti-inflammatory effects and immune mechanism are not clear, which are more important. The quantification of individual phytoconstituents and pharmacological profile of extracts based on *in vitro*, *in vivo* studies and on clinical trials are urgently needed in order to confirm traditional wisdom in the light of rational phytotherapy.

3) Find new ways. It is very difficult to find how the mixtures of ingredients act in concert, partly due to the complexity of *H. cordata* but also due to the lack of appropriate approaches within research of complex herbal mixtures. Recent arisen technologies, such as proteomics and metabolomics, offer additional complementary approaches and provide a deeper and holistic insight in systems biology. They are addressed as promising tools to investigate herb medicines [143].

4) Establish effective quality control methods. Allergic compounds in the product HCI are not entirely clear. And the current Chinese Pharmacopoeia only provides TLC distinction of undecanone for this herb [144]. The comprehensive and effective quality control methods for complex active ingredients of this herb are lack.

Although HCI has been halted, there is no doubt about the efficacy of this herb. This herb, particularly its oral formulations, has high value and broad application prospects. Therefore, in order to better development and utilization of this herb, it is urgent to use modern technology to clarify the material basis of its efficacy and mechanism, improve the quality control standards, and expand the clinical use for traditional efficacy and pharmacological effect. The collected information reviewed here provides a resource for future ethnopharmacological and phytochemical studies of the genus. The scientific validation for the popular use of *H. cordata* deserves more investigations.

8. Acknowledgements

The authors would like to thank National Natural Science Foundation of China for support of the projects (No. 20975115, 21175157 and 21375151), China Hunan Provincial science and technology department for support of the project (No. 2012FJ4139), Central South University for special support of the basic scientific research project (No. 2010QZZD007), China Postdoctoral Science Foundation for support of the project (No. 201104511).

REFERENCES

[1] P. Drasar and J. Moravcova, "Recent Advances in Analysis of Chinese Medical Plants and Traditional Medicines," *Journal of Chromatography B*, Vol. 812, No. 1-2, 2004, pp. 3-21.

[2] N. R. Farnsworth, O. Akerele, A. S. Bingel, D. D. Soejarto and Z. Guo, "Medicinal Plants in Therapy," *Bulletin of the World Health Organization*, Vol. 63, No. 6, 1985, pp. 965-981.

[3] S. Frantz, "Drug Discovery: Playing Dirty," *Nature*, Vol. 437, No. 7061, 2005, pp. 942-943. doi:10.1038/437942a

[4] H. Zheng, Z. Dong and J. She, "Modern Study of Traditional Chinese Medicine," Xue Yuan Press, Beijing, 1998.

[5] K.-M. Lau, K.-M. Lee, C.-M. Koon, C. S.-F. Cheung, C.-P. Lau, H.-M. Ho, M. Y.-H. Lee, S. W.-N. Au, C. H.-K. Cheng, C. B.-S Lau, *et al.*, "Immunomodulatory and Anti-SARS Activities of Houttuynia Cordata," *Journal of Ethnopharmacology*, Vol. 118, No. 1, 2008, pp. 79-85. doi:10.1016/j.jep.2008.03.018

[6] H. Lu, Y. Liang, L. Yi and X. Wu, "Anti-Inflammatory Effect of *Houttuynia cordata* Injection," *Journal of Ethnopharmacology*, Vol. 104, No. 1-2, 2006, pp. 245-249. doi:10.1016/j.jep.2005.09.012

[7] E. Park, S. Kum, C. Wang, S. Y. Park, B. S. Kim and G. Schuller-Levis, "Anti-Inflammatory Activity of Herbal Medicines: Inhibition of Nitric Oxide Production and Tumor Necrosis Factor-Alpha Secretion in an Activated Macrophage-Like Cell Line," *American Journal of Chinese Medicine*, Vol. 33, No. 3, 2005, pp. 415-424. doi:10.1142/S0192415X05003028

[8] I. S. Kim, J.-H. Kim, J. S. Kim, C.-Y. Yun, D.-H. Kim and J.-S. Lee, "The Inhibitory Effect of *Houttuynia cor-*

data Extract on Stem Cell Factor-Induced HMC-1 Cell Migration," *Journal of Ethnopharmacology*, Vol. 112, No. 1, 2007, pp. 90-95. doi:10.1016/j.jep.2007.02.010

[9] G. Z. Li, O. H. Chai, M. S. Lee, E.-H. Han, H. T. Kim and C. H. Song, "Inhibitory Effects of *Houttuynia cordata* Water Extracts on Anaphylactic Reaction and Mast Cell Activation," *Biological & Pharmaceutical Bulletin*, Vol. 28, No. 10, 2005, pp. 1864-1868. doi:10.1248/bpb.28.1864

[10] K. Hayashi, M. Kamiya and T. Hayashi, "Virucidal Effects of the Steam Distillate from *Houttuynia cordata* and Its Components on HSV-1, Influenza Virus, and HIV," *Planta Medica*, Vol. 61, No. 3, 1995, pp. 237-241. doi:10.1055/s-2006-958063

[11] L.-C. Chiang, J.-S. Chang, C.-C. Chen, L.-T. Ng and C.-C. Lin, "Anti-Herpes Simplex Virus Activity of *Bidens pilosa* and *Houttuynia cordata*," *American Journal of Chinese Medicine*, Vol. 31, No. 3, 2003, pp. 355-362. doi:10.1142/S0192415X03001090

[12] J.-S. Chang, L.-C. Chiang, C.-C. Chen, L.-T. Liu, K.-C. Wang and C.-C. Lin, "Antileukemic Activity of *Bidens pilosa* L. var. *minor* (Blume) Sherff and *Houttuynia cordata* Thunb," *American Journal of Chinese Medicine*, Vol. 29, No. 2, 2001, pp. 303-312. doi:10.1142/S0192415X01000320

[13] L.-T. Ng, F.-L. Yen, C.-W. Liao and C.-C. Lin, "Protective Effect of *Houttuynia cordata* Extract on Bleomycin-Induced Pulmonary Fibrosis in Rats," *American Journal of Chinese Medicine*, Vol. 35, No. 3, 2007, pp. 465-475. doi:10.1142/S0192415X07004989

[14] Y.-Y. Chen, J.-F. Liu, C.-M. Chen, P.-Y. Chao and T.-J. Chang, "A Study of the Antioxidative and Antimutagenic Effects of *Houttuynia cordata* Thunb. Using an Oxidized Frying Oil-Fed Model," *Journal of Nutritional Science and Vitaminology*, Vol. 49, No. 5, 2003, pp. 327-333. doi:10.3177/jnsv.49.327

[15] S.-K. Kim, S. Y. Ryu, J. No, S. U. Choi and Y. S. Kim, Cytotoxic Alkaloids from *Houttuynia cordata*," *Archives of Pharmacal Research*, Vol. 24, No. 6, 2001, pp. 518-521. doi:10.1007/BF02975156

[16] R. Bauer, A. Proebstle and H. Lotter, "Cyclooxygenase Inhibitory Constituents from *Houttuynia cordata*," *Phytomedicine*, Vol. 2, No. 4, 1996, pp. 305-308. doi:10.1016/S0944-7113(96)80073-0

[17] S.-Y. Shim, Y.-K. Seo and J.-R. Park, "Down-Regulation of Fc.vepsiln.RI Expression by *Houttuynia cordata* Thunb Extract in Human Basophilic KU812F Cells," *Journal of Medicinal Food*, Vol. 12, No. 2, 2009, pp. 383-388. doi:10.1089/jmf.2007.0684

[18] N. Nuengchamnong, K. Krittasilp and K. Ingkaninan, "Rapid Screening and Identification of Antioxidants in Aqueous Extracts of *Houttuynia cordata* Using LC-ESI-MS Coupled with DPPH Assay," *Food Chemistry*, Vol. 117, No. 4, 2009, pp. 750-756. doi:10.1016/j.foodchem.2009.04.071

[19] H. Masuzawa, "The Diuretic Action of the Extract of Phytolacca Root (*Phytolacca esculenta*) and of Extracts of Some Plants and Drugs. II. The Diuretic Action of Some Plants and Drugs," *Journal of Okayama Medical*

Association, Vol. 52, No. 1, 1940, pp. 1813-1821.

[20] S. Oyama, "Extraction of an Active Principle from *Houttuynia cordata*," JP Patent No. 25000880, 1950.

[21] G. Inagak, "*Houttuynia cordata* Extracts for Treatment of Athlete's Foot," JP Patent No. 53050313, 1978.

[22] Y. Isogai, "An Antimicrobial Substance Isolated from the Rhizome of *Houttuynia cordata*," Scientific Papers of the College of General Education, University of Tokyo, Tokyo, 1952.

[23] H. Chikane, S. Yuka and Y. Takao, "Antibacterial Activity of Extracts from *Houttuynia cordata* and It's Components," *Bulletin of Saitama Medical School Junior College*, Vol. 14, No. 2, 2003, pp. 1-6.

[24] C. Lee and S.-J. Lin, "Constituents of *Houttuynia cordata*," *Beiyi Xuebao*, Vol. 6, No. 1, 1974, pp. 75-78.

[25] K.-I. Hoshishima and H. Okabe, "Promoting Agents Obtained from *Houttuynia cordata* for the Production of an Antibiotic Substance by a Strain of Gram-Positive, Spore-Bearing Bacilli," *Tohoku Journal of Experimental Medicine*, Vol. 52, No. 3, 1950, pp. 265-271.

[26] C. P. Kala, "Ethnomedicinal Botany of the Apatani in the Eastern Himalayan Region of India," *Journal of Ethnobiology and Ethnomedicine*, Vol. 1, No. 11, 2005, pp. 11-18. doi:10.1186/1746-4269-1-11

[27] J. W. Kim, H. J. Ji, J. H. Ahn and M. S. Kim, "Cosmetic Composition Containing Herbal Medicine Extracts for Preventing Wrinkle," KR Patent No. 2009002678, 2009.

[28] M. Ida, "Cosmetics," JP Patent No. 54145226, 1979.

[29] T. Tehara, "Antiaging Cosmetics Containing Natural Products," JP Patent No. 2006241036, 2006.

[30] Y. S. You, "*Houttuynia cordata* Face Lotion," KR Patent No. 2001016594, 2001.

[31] M. Araki, "Additives for Cosmetics to Improve the Skin Conditions," JP Patent No. 2007246516, 2007.

[32] S. H. So and Y. O. Kim, "Cosmetic Composition for Alleviating Skin Inflammation," KR Patent No. 2009-049401, 2009.

[33] H. M. Kim, H. J. Kim, S. G. Park, J. J. Kim and J. H. Choi, "Cosmetic Composition for Alleviating Skin Trouble," KR Patent No. 2009002678, 2009.

[34] N. Takagi, M. Kamiya and K. Yoshida, "Cosmetics Containing *Rhinacanthus nasuta* Extracts, *Ganoderma lucidum* Extracts and/or *Houttuynia cordana* Extracts for Skin Aging Control and Hair Protection," JP Patent No. 09143025, 1997.

[35] J. S. Choi, "Hair Care Product for Nourishing Hair and Preventing Dandruff and Method for Manufacturing the Same," KR Patent No. 2004037057, 2004.

[36] Y. S. You, "Method of Preparing Functional Massage Pack Useful for Treating Acne from Rice Powder, Houttuynia Cordata Thunb. And Green Tea Leaves," KR Patent No. 2006059930, 2006.

[37] T. H. Hoang, V. B. Ha, Q. H. Tran and V. H, Ha, "Antineoplastic Activity of Flavonoid Components Extracted from Leaves of *Houttuynia cordata* Thunb. in Vietnam," *Tap Chi Duoc Hoc*, Vol. 51, No. 10, 2003, pp. 9-10.

[38] C. W. Choi, S. C. Kim, S. S. Hwang, B. K. Choi, H. J. Ahn, M. Y. Lee, S. H. Park and S. K. Kim, "Antioxidant Activity and Free Radical Scavenging Capacity between Korean Medicinal Plants and Flavonoids by Assay-Guided Comparison," *Plant Science*, Vol. 163, No. 6, 2002, pp. 1161-1168. doi:10.1016/S0168-9452(02)00332-1

[39] H. Zeng, L. Jiang and Y. Zhang, "Chemical Constituents of Volatile Oil from *Houttuynia cordata* Thunb," *Journal of Plant Resources and Environment*, Vol. 12, No. 3, 2003, pp. 50-52.

[40] J. Meng, X. Dong, Y. Zhou, Z. Jiang, S. Liang and Z. Zhao, "Orthogonal Experiment Using SFE-CO2 in Extraction of Essential Oil from Fresh *Houttuynia cordata* and Analysis of Essential Oil by GC-MS," *China Journal of Chinese Materia Medica*, Vol. 32, No. 3, 2007, 215-217.

[41] M. I. Ch, Y. F. Wen and Y. Cheng, "Gas Chromatographic/Mass Spectrometric Analysis of the Essential Oil of *Houttuynia cordata* Thunb by Using On-Column Methylation with Tetramethylammonium Acetate," *Journal of AOAC International*, Vol. 90, No. 1, 2007, pp. 60-67.

[42] X. Hao, L. Li, Z. Ding and Y. Yi, "Analysis of Essential Oil from *Houttuynia cordata* in Guizhou," *Acta Botanica Yunnanica*, Vol. 17, No. 3, 1995, pp. 350-352.

[43] Z. Zeng, Y. Liang and C. Xu, "Comparing Chemical Fingerprints of Herbal Medicines Using Modified Window Target-Testing Factor Analysis," *Analyical And Bioanalytical Chemistry*, Vol. 381, No. 4, 2005, pp. 913-924

[44] H.-D. Kwon, I.-H. Cha, W.-K. Lee, J.-H. Song and I.-H. Park, "Antibacterial Activity of Volatile Flavor Components from *Houttuynia cordata* Thunb," *Journal of Food Science and Nutrition*, Vol. 1, No. 2, 1996, pp. 208-213.

[45] J.-M. Kang, I.-H. Cha, Y.-K. Lee and H.-S. Ryu, "Identification of Volatile Essential Oil, and Flavor Characterization and Antibacterial Effect of Fractions from *Houttuynia cordata* Thunb. I. Identification of Volatile Essential Oil Compounds from *Houttuynia cordata* Thunb," *Han'guk Sikp'um Yongyang Kwahak Hoechi*, Vol. 26, No. 2, 1997, pp. 209-213.

[46] J.-M. Kang, I.-H. Cha, Y.-K. Lee and H.-S. Ryu, "Identification of Volatile Essential Oil, and Flavor Characterization and Antibacterial Effect of Fractions from *Houttuynia cordata* Thunb. II. Flavor Characterization and Antibacterial Effect of Fraction from *Houttuynia cordata* Thunb Obtained by Preparative HPLC," *Han'guk Sikp'um Yongyang Kwahak Hoechi*, Vol. 26, No. 2, 1997, pp. 214-221.

[47] L. Chen, W. Wu and Y. Zheng, "TLC Analysis on Essential Oil in *Houttuynia cordata* with Different Chromosome Numbers," *Chinese Traditional and Herbal Drugs*, Vol. 35, No. 12, 2004, pp. 1399-1402.

[48] Y.-L. Liu and Z.-F. Deng, "Study on the Chemical Constituents of the Essential Oil from *Houttuynia cordata* Thunb," *Chinese Bulletin of Botany*, Vol. 21, No. 3, 1979, pp. 244-249.

[49] M. Qi, X. Ge, M. Liang and R. Fu, "Flash Gas Chromatography for Analysis of Volatile Compounds from *Hout-*

tuynia cordata Thunb," *Analytica Chimica Acta*, Vol. 527, No. 1, 2004, pp. 69-72. doi:10.1016/j.aca.2004.08.073

[50] H. Lu, "Fingerprint and Fingerprint-Efficacy Study of *Houttuynia cordata* Thunb. and Injection, a Traditional Chinese Medicine (TCM)," Central South University, Chemistry & Chemical Engineering College, Changsha, 2006.

[51] C. Huang, W. Wu and Y. Zheng, "Analysis on the Chemical Constituents of Essential Oil from Different Parts of *Houttuynia cordata* Thunb," *Chinese Journal of Pharmaceutical Analysis*, Vol. 27, No. 1, 2007, pp. 40-44.

[52] W.-F. Yang, Y. Chen and Y.-Y. Cheng, "Essential Oils from Various Parts of *Houttuynia cordata* Thunb," *Chinese Traditional and Herbal Drugs*, Vol. 37, No. 8, 2006, pp. 1149-1151.

[53] H. Lu, X. Wu, Y. Liang and J. Zhang, "Variation in Chemical Composition and Antibacterial Activities of Essential Oils from Two Species of *Houttuynia cordata* Thunb," *Chemical & Pharmaceutical Bulletin*, Vol. 54, No. 7, 2006, pp. 936-940. doi:10.1248/cpb.54.936

[54] H. Lu, Y. Liang, X. Wu, L. Yi and S. Chen, "Comparative Study of Fingerprints of *Houttuynia cordata* Injection Made of Fresh and Dry Raw Material," *Chinese Journal of Analytical Chemistry*, Vol. 34, No. 6, 2006, pp. 813-816.

[55] H. Nakamura, T. Ota and G. Fukuchi, "The Constituents of Diuretic Drugs. II. The Flavonol Glucoside of *Houttuynia cordata* Thunb," *Journal of the Pharmaceutical Society of Japan*, Vol. 56, No. 3, 1936, p. 68.

[56] J. Meng, X. Dong, Z. Jiang, S. Leung and Z. Zhao, "Study on Chemical Constituents of Flavonoids in Fresh Herb of *Houttuynia cordata*," *China Journal of Chinese Materia Medica*, Vol. 31, No. 16, 2006, pp. 1335-1337.

[57] J. Meng, X. P. Dong, Y. S. Zhou, Z. H. Jiang, S.-Y. K. Leung and Z. Z. Zhen, "Studies on Chemical Constituents of Phenols in Fresh *Houttuynia cordata*," *China Journal of Chinese Materia Medica*, Vol. 32, No. 10, 2007, pp. 929-931.

[58] S.-C. Chou, C.-R. Su, Y.-C. Ku and T.-S. Wu, "The Constituents and Their Bioactivities of *Houttuynia cordata*," *Chemical & pharmaceutical Bulletin*, Vol. 57, No. 11, 2009, pp. 1227-1230. doi:10.1248/cpb.57.1227

[59] S. H. Li and X. J. Wu, "Studies on Flavonoids Extracting Methods in Different Parts of *Houttunia cordata* Thunb," *Journal of Jishou University*, Vol. 28, No. 3, 2007, pp. 117-118.

[60] Y. Zhang, S. Li and X. Wu, "Pressurized Liquid Extraction of Flavonoids from *Houttuynia cordata* Thunb," *Separation and Purification Technology*, Vol. 58, No. 3, 2008, pp. 305-310. doi:10.1016/j.seppur.2007.04.010

[61] D. S. Jang, J. M. Kim, Y. M. Lee, J. L. Yoo, Y. S. Kim, J.-H. Kim and J. S. Kim, "Flavonols from *Houttuynia cordata* with Protein Glycation and Aldose Reductase Inhibitory Activity," *Natural Product Sciences*, Vol. 12, No. 4, 2006, pp. 210-213.

[62] S. Huang, C. Wan, Y. Zou and R. Li, "Extraction and Identification of Flavones from *Houttuynia cordata*

Thunb. by Ultrasonic Wave," *Li Shizhen Medicine And Materia Medica Research*, Vol. 17, No. 11, 2006, pp. 2261-2262.

[63] C. Ye, J. Kan, S. Tan, J. Fan and G. Yang, "Microwave Assisted Extraction of Total Flavonoids from *Houttuynia cordata* Thunb. Leaves," *China Brewing*, No. 1, 2009, pp. 134-137.

[64] C. Ye, J. Kan, S. Tan, Q. Zhu, L. Xu and G. Yang, "Extraction and Separation of Flavonoids from *Houttuynia cordata* Thunb. Leaves," *Transactions of the Chinese Society of Agricultural Engineering*, Vol. 24, No. 10, 2008, pp. 227-232.

[65] S. Y. Xu, J. X. Hong, G. M. Yan, Y. F. Lin and J. Y. Sun, "Study on Purification Process of Extract of the Fresh *Houttuynia cordata*," *Research and Practice on Chinese Medicines*, Vol. 22, No. 2, 2008, pp. 55-58.

[66] T. Zhang and D. Chen, "Anticomplementary Principles of a Chinese Multiherb Remedy for the Treatment and Prevention of SARS," *Journal of Ethnopharmacology*, Vol. 117, No. 2, 2008, pp. 351-361. doi:10.1016/j.jep.2008.02.012

[67] Y. Guo and J. Xu, "Extraction and Purification of *Houttuyniae cordata* Flavonoids and Identification of Flavonoids Type," *Food Science*, Vol. 28, No. 9, 2007, pp. 287-291.

[68] X. Xu, H. Ye, W. Wang, L. Yu and G. Chen, "Determination of Flavonoids in *Houttuynia cordata* Thunb. and *Saururus chinensis* (Lour.) Bail. by Capillary Electrophoresis with Electrochemical Detection," *Talanta*, Vol. 68, No. 3, 2006, pp. 759-764. doi:10.1016/j.talanta.2005.05.027

[69] K. H. Choe, S. J. Kwon and D. S. Jung, "A Study on Chemical Composition of Saururaceae Growing in Korea. 4. On Flavonoid Constituents of *Houttuynia cordata*," *Analytical Science & Technology*, Vol. 4, No. 3, 1991, pp. 285-288.

[70] J.-I. Fuse, H. Kanamori, I. Sakamoto and S. Yahara, "Flavonol Glycosides in *Houttuynia cordata*," *Natural Medicines*, Vol. 48, No. 4, 1994, pp. 307-311.

[71] Q. C. Eng, Z. N. Yang, J. W. Hu, W. S. Cheng and C. X. Li, "Determination of Contents of Seven Flavonoids in *Houttuynia cordata* Thunb by HPLC," *Journal of Jiangxi Normal University*, Vol. 32, No. 6, 2008, pp. 645-648, 661.

[72] L.-S. Wu, J.-P. Si and X.-Q. Yuan, "Quantitive Variation of Flavonoids in *Houttuynia cordata* from Different Geographic Origins in China," *Chinese Journal of Natural Medicines*, Vol. 7, No. 1, 2009, pp. 40-45.

[73] J. Meng, H. Liao, X. Dong and Z. Zhao, "Quantitative Analysis of Flavonoids in Freeze-Dried *Houttuynia cordata* from Different Habitats by HPLC-MS," *Journal of Guangdong College of Pharmacy*, Vol. 24, No. 2, 2008, pp. 114-117.

[74] J. Meng, K. S.-Y. Leung, Z. Jiang, X. Dong, Z. Zhao and L.-J. Xu, "Establishment of HPLC-DAD-MS Fingerprint of Fresh *Houttuynia cordata*," *Chemical & Pharmaceutical Bulletin*, Vol. 53, No. 12, 2005, pp. 1604-1609. doi:10.1248/cpb.53.1604

[75] J.-C. Park, J.-M. Hur, J.-G. Park, S.-J. Park, J.-H. Lee, N.-J. Sung, M.-R. Choi, S.-H. Song, M.-S. Kim and J.-W. Choi, "The Effects of *Houttuynia cordata* on the Hepatic Bromobenzene Metabolizing Enzyme System in Rats and Isolation of Phenolic Compounds," *Korean Journal of Pharmacognosy*, Vol. 31, No. 2, 2000, pp. 228-234.

[76] T. Kawamura, Y. Hisata, K. Okuda, Y. Noro, T. Tanaka, M. Yoshida and E. Sakai, "Pharmacognostical Studies of Houttuyniae Herba. (1) Flavonoid Glycosides Contents of *Houttuynia cordata* Thunb," *Natural Medicines*, Vol. 48, No. 3, 1994, pp. 208-212.

[77] E. Sakai, T. Shibata, T. Kawamura, Y. Hisata, Y. Noro, M. Yoshida and T. Tanaka, "Pharmacognostical Studies of Houttuyniae Herba: 2. Growth and Flavonoid Glycoside Contents of *Houttuynia cordata* Thunb. Cultivated under Shade Condition," *Natural Medicines*, Vol. 50, No. 1, 1996, pp. 45-48.

[78] H. Nishiya, K. Ishiwata, K. Komatsu, O. Nakata, K. Kitamura and S. Fujii, "Platelet Aggregation Inhibitors from Jyu-Yaku (Houttuyniae Herb)," *Chemical & Pharmaceutical Bulletin*, Vol. 36, No. 5, 1988, pp. 1902-1904. doi:10.1248/cpb.36.1902

[79] T. T. Jong and M. Y. Jean, "Alkaloids from *Houttuynia cordata*," *Journal of the Chinese Chemical Society*, Vol. 40, No. 3, 1993, pp. 301-303.

[80] L. Wang, Y. Zhao, L. Zhou and J. Zhou, "Chemical Constituents of *Houttuynia cordata*," *Chinese Traditional and Herbal Drugs*, Vol. 38, No. 12, 2007, pp. 1788-1790.

[81] K. H. Choe, S. J. Kwon and K. C. Lee, "Chemical Composition of Saururaceae Growing in Korea. (3). On Fatty Acids and Amino Acids of *Houttuynia cordata* and *Saururus chinensis*," *Punsok Kwahak*, Vol. 2, No. 2, 1989, pp. 285-292.

[82] S. Takagi, M. Yamaki, K. Masuda and M. Kubota, "On the Constituents of the Terrestrial Part of *Houttuynia cordata* Thunb," *Shoyakugaku Zasshi*, Vol. 32, No. 2, 1978, pp. 123-125.

[83] X. Wu, S. Li, A. Li and J. Zhang, "Chemical Components from Herba of *Houttuynia cordata* Thunb," *Journal of Chinese Medicinal Materials*, Vol. 31, No. 8, 2008, pp. 1168-1170.

[84] T. T. Jong and M. Y. Jean, "Constituents of *Houttuyniae cordata* and the Crystal Structure of Vomifoliol," *Journal of the Chinese Chemical Society*, Vol. 40, No. 4, 1993, pp. 399-402.

[85] S.-C. Chou, "The Constituents of the *Houttuynia cordata* Thumb," National Cheng Kung University, Tainan, 2005.

[86] M. Mori, K. Suzuki, Y. Tsukahara and M. Nada, "Changes in the Components of *Houttuynia cordata* during Growth," *Sagami Joshi Daigaku Kiyo, Shizenkei*, Vol. 59B, No. 3, 1995, pp. 89-95.

[87] X. Gong and M. Cheng, "Analysis and Appraisal of Nutrients of *Houttuynia cordata* Thunb," *Food and Fermentation Industries*, Vol. 30, No. 11, 2004, pp. 102-105.

[88] Y. Kimura and Y. Nishikawa, "Standardization of Crude Drugs. III. 2. Component of *Houttuynia cordata*," *Journal of the Pharmaceutical Society of Japan*, Vol. 73, No. 47, 1953, pp. 196-198.

[89] T. Ohta, "The Diuretic Components of *Houttuynia cordata*," *Journal of the Pharmaceutical Society of Japan*, Vol. 62, No. 2, 1942, pp. 105-106.

[90] W. Zhang, F. Lu, S. Pan and S. Li, "Extraction of Volatile Oil from *Houttuynia cordata* and Its Anti-Biotic and Anti-Virus Activities," *Practical Preventive Medicine*, Vol. 15, No. 2, 2008, pp. 312-316.

[91] J. Meng, X. Zong and X. Dong, "Study on Pharmacological Effects of Fresh and Dry *Houttuynia cordata* Thunb," *Li Shizhen Medicine and Materia Medica Research*, Vol. 19, No. 6, 2008, pp. 1315-1316.

[92] J. Zhang, X. Wu, Z. Luo and X. Zhong, "Determination of Chemical Components and Antibacterial Activities of *Houttuynia cordata* Thunb. during Desiccation and Storage," *Food Science*, Vol. 28, No. 11, 2007, pp. 565-569.

[93] M. Fu, X. Wu, D. Liu, J. Zhang, L. Wei and X. Jiang, "Research on Antibacterial Activity *in Vitro* of the *Houttuynia cordata* Thunb Injection," *Journal of Anhui Agricultural Science*, Vol. 35, No. 8, 2007, pp. 2264-2265.

[94] P. Qian, Y. Liang and H. Lu, "The Study of Antibacterial Activity in Quality Control of *Houttuynia cordata* Injection," *Journal of Xiangtan Normal University*, Vol. 29, No. 3, 2007, pp. 12-14.

[95] Y. Hou and X. Zhang, "Antiphlogistic Action of *Houttuynia cordata* Injection *in Vitro* and in Mice," *China Journal of Chinese Materia Medica*, Vol. 15, No. 4, 1990, pp. 221-222, 255.

[96] T. Kosuge and H. Okeda, "Nonylpyrazole, a New Antimicrobial Substance," *Journal of Biochemistry*, Vol. 41, No. 2, 1954, pp. 183-186.

[97] G. Kim, D. Kim and J. Lim, "Biological and Antibacterial Activities of the Natural Herb *Houttuynia cordata* Water Extract against the Intracellular Bacterial Pathogen Salmonella within the RAW 264.7 Macrophage," *Biological & Pharmaceutical Bulletin*, Vol. 31, No. 11, 2008, pp. 2012-2017. doi:10.1248/bpb.31.2012

[98] S. B. Bharate, "Medicinal Plants with Anti-HIV Potential," *Journal of Medicinal and Aromatic Plant Sciences*, Vol. 25, No. 2, 2003, pp. 427-440.

[99] M. Shimura, Y. Zhou, Y. Asada, T. Yoshikawa, K. Hatake, F. Takaku and Y. Ishizaka, "Inhibition of Vpr-Induced Cell Cycle Abnormality by Quercetin: A Novel Strategy for Searching Compounds Targeting Vpr," *Biochemical and Biophysical Research Communications*, Vol. 261, No. 2, 1999, pp. 308-316. doi:10.1006/bbrc.1999.0994

[100] N. Morita, K. Hayashi, A. Fujita and H. Matsui, "Extraction of Antiviral Substances from *Houttuynia cordata* Thunb," JP Patent No. 07118160, 1995.

[101] Y. Yan, X. Chen, X. Yang, S. Wu, D. Fang and C. Dong, "Cooperative Anti-Influenza Virus Activities of Amantadine, Ribavirin and Herb Houttuynia," *Virologica Sinica*, Vol. 17, No. 2, 2002, pp. 192-194.

[102] D. H. Kwon, W. J. Choi, C. H. Lee, J. H. Kim and M. B. Kim, "Flavonoid Compound Having an Antiviral Activity," WO Patent No. 2007069823, 2007.

[103] H.-J. Choi, J.-H. Kim, C.-H. Lee, Y.-J. Ahn, J.-H. Song, S.-H. Baek and D.-H. Kwon, "Antiviral Activity of

Quercetin 7-Rhamnoside against Porcine Epidemic Diarrhea Virus," *Antiviral Research*, Vol. 81, No. 1, 2009, pp. 77-81.

[104] X. Zheng, X. Tang and X. Su, "Experimental Study of Inhibitory Effect of the Four Traditional Chinese Herb Medicines on Epidemic Hemorrhagic Fever Virus," *Bulletin of Hunan Medical University*, Vol. 18, No. 2, 1993, pp. 165-167.

[105] T.-Y. Lin, Y.-C. Liu, J.-R. Jheng, H.-P. Tsai, J.-T. Jan, W.-R. Wong and J.-T. Horng, "Anti-Enterovirus 71 Activity Screening of Chinese Herbs with Anti-Infection and Inflammation Activities," *American Journal of Chinese Medicine*, Vol. 37, No. 1, 2009, pp. 143-158.

[106] X. Kou, "Traditional Chinese Medicine Composition Containing Taraxacum and Glycyrrhiza and Others for Treating Lung Cancer," CN Patent No. 101406657, 2009.

[107] Q. Li, "Chinese Medical Honeyed Pill for Treating Lung Carcinoma," CN Patent No. 101391036, 2009.

[108] H. Jung, J. Choi and C. Jin, "Effects of Flos Lonicerae and Herba Houttuyniae on Human Cancer Cell-Lines," *Korean Journal of Oriental Physiology & Pathology*, Vol. 10, No. 3, 1996, pp. 126-132.

[109] W. Bae, H. Go and C. Kim, "Experimental Study on the Effect of Houttuyniae Herbal Accupuncture on the Growth of Melanoma B16 in Mice," *The Korean Acupuncture and Moxibustion Journal*, Vol. 18, No. 2, 2001, pp. 186-201.

[110] K.-B. Kwon, E.-K. Kim, B.-C. Shin, E.-A. Seo, J.-Y. Yang and D.-G. Ryu, "Herba Houttuyniae Extract Induces Apoptotic Death of Human Promyelocytic Leukemia Cells via Caspase Activation Accompanied by Dissipation of Mitochondrial Membrane Potential and Cytochrome c Release," *Experimental and Molecular Medicine*, Vol. 35, No. 2, 2003, pp. 91-97.

[111] D. S. Hah, C. H. Kim, J.-D. Ryu, E. K. Kim and J. S. Kim, "Evaluation of Protective Effects of *Houttuynia cordata* on H_2O_2-Induced Oxidative DNA Damage Using an Alkaline Comet Assay in Human HepG2 Cells," *Journal of Toxicology and Public Health*, Vol. 23, No. 1, 2007, pp. 25-31.

[112] H. Ha, D. Y. Jung and S. W. Park, "Anticancer Effect of *Houttuynia cordata* Extract on Cancered ICR Mouse and L1210 Cells with Changes of SOD and GPx Activities," *Yakhak Hoechi*, Vol. 48, No. 4, 2004, pp. 219-225.

[113] A. Murakami, S. Jiwajinda and K. Koshimizu, "Screening for *in Vitro* Anti-Tumor Promoting Activities of Edible Plants from Thailand," *Cancer Letters*, Vol. 95, No. 1-2, 1995, pp. 139-146.

[114] Y.-Y. Chen, C.-M. Chen, P.-Y. Chao, T.-J. Chang and J.-F. Liu, "Effects of Frying Oil and *Houttuynia cordata* Thunb on Xenobiotic-Metabolizing Enzyme System of Rodents," *World Journal of Gastroenterology*, Vol. 11, No. 3, 2005, pp. 389-392.

[115] H. Fan, W. Qu, Y. Li and M. Sun, "Experimental Investigation for Anti-Tumor Activity of Flavonoid from the *Houttuynia cordata* Thunb. *in Vitro*," *Chinese Journal of Hospital Pharmacy*, Vol. 28, No. 7, 2008, pp. 528-531.

[116] J. Meng, D. He, Y. Zhou and X. Dong, "Comparison on the Pharmacological Effects of Different Extract Parts from *Houttuynia cordata* Thunb," *Li Shizhen Medicine And Materia Medica Research*, Vol. 19, No. 5, 2008, pp. 1050-1051.

[117] Q. Feng, Y. Ren, Y. Wang, H. Ma, J. Xu, C. Zhou, Z. Yin and L. Luo, "Anti-Inflammatory Effect of SQC-Beta-CD on Lipopolysaccharide-Induced Acute Lung Injury," *Journal of Ethnopharmacology*, Vol. 118, No. 1, 2008, pp. 51-58.

[118] J. Hong, B. Wang, Y. Gao, B. Feng, J. Mo, Y. Wang, H. Yao, X. Xu, W. Zhao and F. Tang, "Effect of Fresh Herba Houttuyniae Extract on Lipopolysaccharide-Induced Inflammation in Mice," *The Chinese Journal of Modern Applied Pharmacy*, Vol. 25, No. 5, 2008, 376-378.

[119] J. Lee, I. Kim, J. Kim, J. Kim, D. Kim and C. Yun, "Suppressive Effects of *Houttuynia cordata* Thunb (Saururaceae) Extract on Th2 Immune Response," *Journal of Ethnopharmacology*, Vol. 117, No. 1, 2008, pp. 34-40.

[120] A. Probstle and R. Bauer, "Aristolactams and a 4,5-Dioxoaporphine Derivative from *Houttuynia cordata*," *Planta Medica*, Vol. 58, No. 6, 1992, pp. 568-569.

[121] K. Taguchi, Y. Hagiwara, K. Kajiyama and Y. Suzuki, "Pharmcological Studies of Houttuyniae Herba: The Antiinflammatory Effect of Quercitrin," *Journal of the Pharmaceutical Society of Japan*, Vol. 113, No. 4, 1993, pp. 327-333.

[122] X.-L. Jiang and H.-F. Cui, "Different Therapy for Different Types of Ulcerative Colitis in China," *World Journal of Gastroenterology*, Vol. 10, No. 10, 2004, pp. 1513-1520.

[123] H.-M. Lu, Y.-Z. Liang and P. Qian, "Profile-Effect on Quality Control of *Houttuynia cordata* Injection," *Acta pharmaceutica Sinica*, Vol. 40, No. 12, 2005, pp. 1147-1150.

[124] H.-M. Lu, Y.-Z. Liang, X.-J. Wu and P. Qiu, "Tentative Fingerprint-Efficacy Study of *Houttuynia cordata* Injection in Quality Control of Traditional Chinese Medicine," *Chemical & Pharmaceutical Bulletin*, Vol. 54, No. 5, 2006, pp. 725-730.

[125] Y.-C. Kim and S.-K. Chung, "Reactive Oxygen Radical Species Scavenging Effects of Korean Medicinal Plant Leaves," *Food Science and Biotechnology*, Vol. 11, No. 4, 2002, pp. 407-411.

[126] E. Cho, T. Yokozawa, D. Rhyu, S. Kim, N. Shibahara and J. Park, "Study on the Inhibitory Effects of Korean Medicinal Plants and Their Main Compounds on the 1,1-diphenyl-2-picrylhydrazyl Radical," *Phytomedicine*, Vol. 10, No. 6-7, 2003, pp. 544-551.

[127] E. J. Cho, T. Yokozawa, D. Y. Rhyu, H. Y. Kim, N. Shibahara and J. C. Park, "The Inhibitory Effects of 12 Medicinal Plants and Their Component Compounds on Lipid Peroxidation," *American Journal of Chinese Medicine*, Vol. 31, No. 6, 2003, pp. 907-917.

[128] H. Wang and Y. Xiu, "Effect of *Houttuynia cordata* on Urinary Albumin and Insulin Resistance of Diabetes Mellitus Rats," *Traditional Chinese Drug & Clinical Pharmacology*, Vol. 19, No. 1, 2008, pp. 12-14.

[129] H. Wang, Y. Xiu and K. Sun, "Effect of *Houttuynia cordata* on Fat Metabolism in Plasma and Insulin Resistance

of Diabetes Mellitus Rats," *Chinese Journal of Basic Medicine in Traditional Chinese Medicine*, Vol. 15, No. 1, 2009, pp. 72-73, 78.

[130] F. Wang, F. Lu, G. Chen and L. Xu, "Influence of *Houttuynia cordata* Thumb on Expression of TGF-β1 and HGF in Kidney Tissue of Streptozotocin Induced Diabetic Rats," *The 3rd World Integrative Medicine Congress Abstracts*, Guangzhou, 21-24 September 2007, p. 722.

[131] F. Wang, F. Lu and L. Xu, "Effects of *Houttuynia cordata* Thumb on Expression of BMP-7 and TGF-β1 in the Renal Tissues of Diabetic Rats," *Journal of Traditional Chinese Medicine*, Vol. 27, No. 3, 2007, pp. 220-225.

[132] Y. Kimata, Y. Eto, M. Asanoma, Y. Sakabe and H. Horitsu, "Inhibitory Actions of Chloroform Extracts from Natural Medicines on the Mutagenicity of Trp-P-2 and 1-NP," *Chukyo Joshi Daigaku Kenkyu Kiyo*, Vol. 31, No. 2, 1997, pp. 123-130.

[133] Z. Song, C. Wang, J. Cheng, F. Li, Z. Zhu, Y. Ning and M. Zhang, "Effect of Injection of *Houttuynia cordata* Thunb, *Hyperiaum japonlcum* Thunb and *Erycibe obtusifolia* Benth on Immune Function of Rats," *Chinese Traditional and Herbal Drugs*, Vol. 24, No. 12, 1993, pp. 643-644, 438.

[134] J. Kim, C.-S. Park, Y. Lim and H.-S. Kim, "*Paeonia japonica, Houttuynia cordata*, and *Aster scaber* Water Extracts Induce Nitric Oxide and Cytokine Production by Lipopolysaccharide-Activated Macrophages," *Journal of Medicinal Food*, Vol. 12, No. 2, 2009, pp. 365-373.

[135] K.-M. Ji, M. Li, J.-J. Chen, Z.-K. Zhan and Z.-G. Liu, "Anaphylactic Shock and Lethal Anaphylaxis Caused by *Houttuynia cordata* Injection, a Herbal Treatment in China," *Allergy*, Vol. 64, No. 5, 2009, pp. 816-817.

[136] L. Lei, X. Pu, K. Yang, H. Wang, Y. Liu, D. Zhang and L. Zhang, "Adverse Response Caused by Intravenous Drip of *Houttuynia cordata* Injection I," *Pharmacology and Clinics of Chinese Materia Medica*, Vol. 23, No. 5, 2007, pp. 131-133.

[137] Y. Liu, X. Pu and L. Lei, "Adverse Response Caused by Intravenous Drip of *Houttuynia cordata* Injection II," *Pharmacology and Clinics of Chinese Materia Medica*, Vol. 24, No. 2, 2008, pp. 61-63.

[138] China TPCo (Ed.), "The Chinese Pharmacopoeia," China Medical Science Press, Beijing, 2010.

[139] WHO "General Guidelines for Methodologies on Research and Evaluation of Traditional Medicines," 2000, p.

1.

[140] Y.-Z. Liang, P. Xie and K. Chan, "Quality Control of Herbal Medicines," *Journal of Chromatography B*, Vol. 812, No. 1-2, 2004, pp. 53-70.

[141] V. E. Tyler, "Phytomedicines: Back to the Future," *Journal of Natural Products*, Vol. 62, No. 11, 1999, pp. 1589-1592.

[142] WHO "Guidelines for the Assessment of Herbal Medicines," 1991.

[143] J. Wang, R. van der Heijden, S. Spruit, T. Hankermeier, K. Chan, J. van der Greef, G. Xu and M. Wang, "Quality and Safety of Chinese Herbal Medicines Guided by a Systems Biology Perspective," *Journal of Ethnopharmacology*, Vol. 126, No. 1, 2009, pp. 31-41.

[144] C. P. Commission (Ed.), "The Pharmacopoeia of the People's Republic of China," China Medical Science Press, Beijing, 2010.

[145] China Mohotpsro, "Farther Standardization of Raw Materials Administrators for Health Foods," 2002.

[146] http://en.wikipedia.org/wiki/Houttuynia

[147] Y. Wata, "Therapeutic Drinks from *Houttuynia cordata*," JP Patent No.56097234, 1981.

[148] K. Mori, "Deodorizing Fish Oil," JP Patent No. 35240, 1919.

[149] J. S. Choi, "Knife-Cut Noodles Using Houttuyniae Herba and Method for Preparing the Same," KR Patent No. 2004063884, 2004.

[150] S. H. Kwon and M. S. Kim, "Method for Manufacturing Soy Sauce by Using Houttuynia Cordata and Saururus Chinensis," KR Patent No. 2009076250, 2009.

[151] Y. S. You, "Method for Manufacturing Carbonic Drink of Houttuynia Cordata," KR Patent No. 2002028976, 2002.

[152] T. H. Hoang, Q. H. Tran, V. B. Ha and D. T. Nguyen, "Study on the Flavonoid Component Extracted from Leaves of *Houttuynia cordata* Thunb in Vietnam," *Tap Chi Duoc Hoc*, No. 9, 2002, pp. 13-15.

[153] H. Wagner, R. Bauer, P. Xiao, J. Chen and A. Probstle, "Herba *Houttuyniae cordatae*," *Chinese Drug Monographs and Analysis*, Vol. 1, No. 6, 1997, pp. 1-11.

[154] A. Proebstle, A. Neszmelyi, G. Jerkovich, H. Wagner and R. Bauer, "Novel Pyridine and 1,4-Dihydropyridine Alkaloids from *Houttuynia cordata*," *Natural Product Letters*, Vol. 4, No. 3, 1994, pp. 235-240.

23

Attention Points of Research and Education in TCMP across Taiwan Strait and Recommendations for Future Research and Development of TCM in China Mainland Especially Fujian and Taiwan

Shengyan Xi[1], Yanhui Wang[1*], Yaochen Chuang[2], Linchao Qian[1],
Xiaoyan Qian[1], Pengcheng Li[1], Dawei Lu[1]

[1]Department of Traditional Chinese Medicine of Medical College, Xiamen University, Xiamen, China
[2]Center of General Education, Central Taiwan University of Science and Technology, Taichung, Taiwan
Email: *2076110@126.com

ABSTRACT

Objective: China mainland and Taiwan are separated by the Taiwan Strait, but their land edges are close to each other, blood relationship is very compact, and the origin is profound, the communication of Traditional Chinese Medicine (TCM) between China mainland especially Fujian and Taiwan district is more and more frequent. From the actuality and situation of traditional Chinese medicine and pharmacy (TCMP), the objective of this study was to briefly expound the points to which attention should be attached urgently in education, research and development of TCM between China mainland especially between Fujian and Taiwan, and be provide with several resolving threads and recommend-dations to aim directly at the attention points, and wish it can offer some assistance to the development and generalization of the cross-Strait TCMP. **Methods:** The *China Statistical Yearbook of Chinese Medicine* (1987-2010), the *Yearbook of Public Health of Taiwan* (2009), the full-text data base of China National Knowledge Infrastructure (CNKI) (1993-2009), provides information on research and education in TCMP across Taiwan Strait in the last 10 years. The methods of analysis and comparison are applied in this study to show the TCMP situation between Taiwan and China mainland. **Result:** Due to the differences in history, district, policy and legislation, the TCMP's industry and trade, education, research and exploitation, standard and so on, have lots of differences between Taiwan and China mainland, and many barriers are produced in the communication and cooperation of cross-Strait TCM and pharmacy. **Conclusion:** China mainland especially Fujian and Taiwan have the fierce intention to carry out thorough investigation in many territories of TCMP. The prospects and development space of communication and cooperation of cross-Strait TCMP are quite broad.

Keywords: Traditional Chinese Medicine and Pharmacy (TCMP); Traditional Chinese Drug; Traditional Chinese Medicine (TCM); Chinese Herbal Medicine; Research and Development (R&D); China Mainland; Fujian and Taiwan District; Recommendation

1. Introduction

Traditional Chinese medicine (TCM) is the splendid cultural treasure of the Chinese nation, and with long history and several thousand years of medication experience, it has accumulated a great deal of valuable materia medica data, which has an important guiding role on new medicine research and development (R&D). Although with thousands of years of practice, Chinese herbal medicine

has formed its own unique and complete pharmacological system, due to the traditional route of administration and dosage form is more backward, effect shows slowly, and is difficult to standardize and normalize, especially the complicated ingredients in Chinese herbal medicine, the substantial basis of effect is not wholly clear, pharmacodynamic mechanism of action is not well known, and the content determination method is relatively rough. This greatly limits the industry development of Chinese medicine in China. In recent years, because of many de-

*Corresponding author.

ficiencies in the basic research of Chinese herbs, and unreasonable application, parts of the traditional Chinese drugs have shown some serious adverse drug reactions in clinic. The problem is highlighted particularly in the injections made by decoction pieces of traditional Chinese medicine in mainland, which is badly in need of new breakthrough [1]. Across the Taiwan Strait, the authority of Taiwan has constantly thought highly of the scientization of Chinese herbal drugs and the exploitation of Chinese Herbals [2], and the obvious developing advantages of Chinese herbal drugs of Taiwan, which comes from the good quality and the fine international image of the Chinese patent medicines produced in Taiwan [3]. Recently, the development of Chinese herbal industry in Taiwan district has been emphasized, and the research on traditional Chinese drug has been motivated to become the most activated branch in the domain of Taiwan present scientific research. Its research center is the new traditional Chinese drugs' exploitation. To surround this center, scientific researchers have carried out the items on exploiting for dried medicinal herbs, controlling on the quality of Chinese crude drugs, and studying their pharmacology [4]. We should thoroughly utilize this opportunity to positively strengthen the cooperation and communication on traditional Chinese medicine and pharmacy between China mainland and Taiwan district and to make up for each other's deficiencies, overcome the existing problems and share the benefits.

2. Application and Trade of Chinese Herbal Medicine across Taiwan Strait

Traditional Chinese medicine in Taiwan and Fujian has come from the same continuous Chinese culture, with distinct regional characteristics of Fujian province and Taiwan; traditional Chinese drugs have been widely used. About 66% Taiwan populace usually apply traditional Chinese drugs. According to the investigation of Taiwan Pharmaceutical Manufacture's Association (TPMA), the most commonly used ten great Chinese crude drugs by Taiwan are Danggui (*Radix Angelicae Sinensis*), Shudihuang (*Radix Rehmanniae preparata*), Gancao (*Radix Glycyrrhizae*), Chuanxiong (*Rhizoma Chanxiong*), Fuling (*Poria*), Baishao (*Radix Paeoniae Alba*), Huangqi (*Radix Astragali Mongolici*), Baizhu (*Rhizoma Atractylodis Macrocephalae*), Renshen (*Radix Ginseng*), and Banxia (*Rhizoma Pinelliae*) respectively [5]. At present, more than 600 kinds of Chinese herbal medicines in Taiwan are dependent on imports, and of which 90% come from the district of China mainland, and to some kinds of which, China mainland is the single source to import. In 2009, the export amount of mainland's Chinese crude drugs & decoction pieces and extracts to Taiwan amounts to 98% of the total amount of exports of

traditional Chinese drugs to Taiwan [3] (**Figure 1**). In 2010, Taiwan imported about 5000 batches of traditional Chinese medicinal materials, the gross weight of which was more than 13,000 tons, the market value of which was 5.5 hundred million *Yuan*, among which Hongzao (*Fructus Jujubae*), Huangqi (*Radix Astragali Mongolici*), Danggui (*Radix Angelicae Sinensis*) and Gancao (*Radix Glycyrrhizae*) count for nearly 4.0 hundred million *Yuan*. Throughout Taiwan, Chinese herbal medicine is also often used as health food material. Now more than 170 health food products in Taiwan have obtained their conformity certifications, among which 61 products has used Chinese herbal medicine as raw materials, the tea, g*inseng*, fungi and Hongqu (*Ultivarietas Oryzae Sativae et Monasci*) are the most, which occupied by 35.88% [6]. It is thus evident that the dependency of Taiwan on China mainland's traditional Chinese drugs is high.

3. Research of Chinese Herbal Medicine and Compound Recipe in Taiwan District

About the study of traditional Chinese medicine and pharmacy, since the 1970s, Taiwan authorities began opening up to the scientific research on Chinese herbal drugs. And the basic and clinical research on the disease that had a significant effect by TCM and the prescription that commonly used was carried out, which under the efficacy assessment of Chinese medicine. For example, Prof. Shih TB had researched the immunoregulation effects of Four-Ingredient Decoction (*Siwu Tang*), Tonifying the Middle and Replenishing Qi Decoction (*Buzhong Yiqi Tang*) and Pulse-Generating Powder (*Shengmai San*), who found that the three compound recipes had the different stimulating effects on many kinds of founder cells of hematopoietic community, and the protecting actions to the decrease of leucocytes caused by 5-Fluorouracil (5-FU) and could repair the hematopoiesis function [7]. The processing methods, quantitative analysis and safety testing to herbal medicines, have been in depth study. Prof. Wun WC has found that unprocessed Pinellia tuber or Ban Xia (*Rhizoma Pinelliae*) processed for seven days follow the incunabula had no toxicity in cell experiments or no acute lethal dose (LD) in rat experiments [8]. Prof.

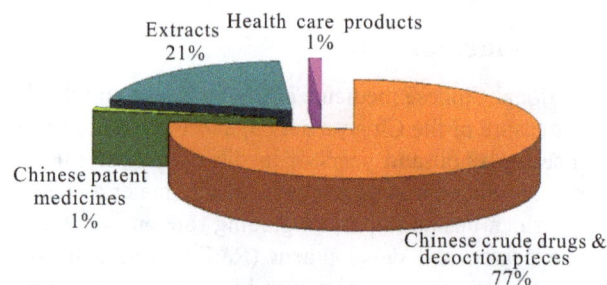

Figure 1. Product structure statistics of mainland's export amount of traditional Chinese drugs to Taiwan in 2009.

Attention Points of Research and Education in TCMP across Taiwan Strait...

187

Liou SS's research has shown that the content of Magnolol and Honokiol in Houpu (*Cortex Magnoliae Officinalis*) parched by ginger pop were respectively increased 5.6 and 4.1 times [9]. And it had been also continuously mixed with the modern scientific and technological achievements, and to explore the combination between Chinese medicine research and genomics research, and planning a "correlated research between TCM and genome" to develop the study of sthenic *zheng* of TCM [10]. In the modernization of traditional Chinese medicine research, the extraction, analysis and purification of Chinese herbal medicine are mainly in application. For example, the plant Jia Ci Shu (*Casearia membranacea Hance*) in Taiwan, Prof. Guh JH [11] has purified ten kinds clerodane diterpenoids from which have anticancer active, which all could effectively promote the apoptosis of tumor cells. It is worth mentioning that Taiwan has established the high-end platform of development and verification of Traditional Chinese Medicine, and by means of "Drug-similar" concept to find the drugs that are similar to the profiles of gene expression of Chinese herbal medicine to further understand the mechanism or effect of Chinese herbal medicine, may accelerate the opportunity that the effective Chinese herbal medicine or other drugs can enter the clinical trial [12]. And the obvious modern progress has been made in TCMP research of Taiwan.

4. Higher Education of TCMP in Taiwan

At present, the normal higher educational institutions of TCMP in Taiwan are mainly the two private universities, China Medical University (CMU) and Chang Gung University (CGU). The former has set up the college of TCM, school of Chinese medicine for eight years and school of post baccalaureate Chinese medicine for five years, and Master's and doctor degree programs of Graduate Institute of Chinese Medical Science, Master's degree program of Graduate Institute of Integrated Medicine (GIIM), and Master's degree program of Graduate Institute of Acupuncture Science. The latter only has the school of Chinese medicine for eight years and Master's degree program of Graduate Institute of Traditional Chinese Medicine [13] (**Table 1**). Except the CMU, the

other schools are all relatively less scale of TCMP education. Concretely speaking, the education courses of Chinese medicine in Taiwan's higher schools are mainly as follows: The Graduate Institute of Natural Products of Chang Gung University, which has set up the "Pharmacology of TCM", "Information Research of Chinese Medicine", etc.; China Medical University has the school of Chinese Pharmaceutical Sciences and Chinese Medicine Resources, and has cultivated the professional persons who mastered the resources of herbs, research and development of herbs by biotechnology, and management of herb resources. The master curriculums of CMU have "Monography of Herbalism", "Special Discussion of Chinese Materia Medica", "Industry Technology of Chinese Herbal Medicine", etc. The doctor curriculums have "Special Topics of Herbalism", "Special Topics of Chinese Pharmacy", "Special Topics of Research Methods of Chinese Pharmacy", etc. The Department of Pharmacy and Graduate Institute of Pharmaceutical Technology of Tajen University has set up the "Special Topics of Pharmacology of Traditional Chinese Drug", "Special Topics of Pharmacological Identification", "Pharmaco preparing Process of Traditional Chinese Drug", "Special Topics of Materia Medica Formulas", etc. The Biological Resources Department of Taipei Medical University has set up the "General Discussion of Traditional Medicine", "Herbalogy", "Medicated Diet and Food Therapy" and other courses [14]. We know that every hierarchical education of TCMP from the under graduate course to doctor curriculum has been opened in Taiwan now. But compared with China mainland's TCM courses that are complete in ranges, curriculum taxons of Taiwan TCM are not enough, and the contents' profundity and scope are also more inferior.

5. Attention Points of Cross-Strait TCMP Research and Education Needed Urgently

With the development of the economy, the society and culture exchanges between the mainland and Taiwan are more and more close. TCM that carries the history characteristics of the Chinese nation has taken the lead on cooperative research for standardization, normalization, and modernization of cross-Strait traditional Chinese

Table 1. Overview of Taiwan bachelor education of TCM.

School Name	Department Name	Study Time Limit	Established Time	Annual Enrollment	Number of Graduate
China Medical University	School of Chinese Medicine	Seven years	1966-1995	120	2180
		Eight years	1996-up to now	120	404
Chang Gung University	School of Chinese Medicine	Eight years	1998-up to now	50	81
China Medical University	School of Post Baccalaureate Chinese Medicine	Five years	1984-up to now	100	1449

Notes: Data from *Public Health Reports* (2005) and *Chinese Medicine Administration Indicators* (2007).

drug with a series of positive and effective exploration. Through the constant exchange and joint research, it has made significant progress and formed a good development momentum. But there also both exist considerable problems that inheriting traditional characteristics of TCM and carrying forward to TCM or generalizing TCM are not enough, post marketing of traditional Chinese drug and quality requirements of Materia Medica are not strict, the groundbreaking of new traditional Chinese drug is insufficient, and the key technology breakthrough is difficult, and so on, especially in the development and research of Chinese crude drugs and decoction pieces.

5.1. Analysis in Industry and Trade of TCMP

In China mainland, the Chinese medicine agriculture has started for many years. Prof. Huang SL pointed out that the sustainable development and rational utilization of traditional Chinese drug resources, and related ecological or environmental problems were not resolved effectively; some Chinese drug industrial arts and engineering technologies in some industries were relatively backward; the production efficiency and utilization capacity were relatively low; some industries lack standardized and tailor-made pharmaceutical industry equipments [15]. From the above-mentioned application of Chinese herbal drugs of Taiwan and the cross-Strait import or export amount of Chinese crude drugs, we know that the Taiwan industry of Chinese medicine has faced many problems, such as few natural resources of Chinese medicinal materials, Materia Medica depending on China Mainland extremely, small scale of Chinese patent medicine industry, difficult exploitation of fire new patent medicine, and so on. To obtain Chinese medicine Taiwan needs to import it. As for the Chinese crude drugs, they are quite abundant in Mainland, but the ratio of Taiwan importing the health care products and Chinese patent medicines from China Mainland is tiny [16]. And in order to enhance the competitiveness, since 2009, "the Executive Yuan" of Taiwan has listed Chinese herbal medicine industry as one of the Taiwan's major development projects, strengthened infrastructure and improved the industrial environment to impulse the market development [17]. In China Mainland, the situation about the exports of Chinese medicine mainly depends on the bulk drugs and the old species has no significant change [15]. Therefore, there exist strong complementarities of cross-Strait Chinese medicine industry and trade, and there will be more co-operation items.

5.2. Analysis in Education and Elite Cultivating in TCMP

Today's main international medicine is the modern western medicine, the economy income and social status of

traditional profession doctor is not better than western medicine doctor's, especially in Taiwan. The phenomenon of westernizing tendency in TCMP is the best annotation for this embarrassing reality. Prof. Su XY [14] pointed out that all the mode of education and training of traditional Chinese medicine and pharmacy in Taiwan trends to westernizing for its high proportion western medical courses, and higher education of traditional Chinese drug usually ignore the "patient-oriented pharmaceutical care education". For instance, the purpose of running China Medical University is to "unify the Chinese and western medicine to establish new medical science", and to emphasize the important position of western medicine in TCMP education. Currently, except the westernizing tendency, there are still lots of problems in the education of TCMP in Taiwan that need to be resolved urgently, such as that the teaching faculty of TCMP is quite insufficient, the teachers who have abundant clinical experience but less teaching experience, the deficient teaching materials of TCMP that unitively compiled by Taiwan natives, and few clinical teaching hospitals of TCM [13]. The supply of teachers in School of Chinese Medicine of Chang Gung University is mostly the visiting professors who are invited from TCM colleges or universities in China mainland, their TCM teaching materials are the fifth edition teaching materials of the mainland high medicine schools; but CMU mostly uses the self-compiled teaching materials [18]. Prof. Shen JZ points out that the teaching materials applied by school of Chinese medicine and post baccalaureate Chinese medicine are out of date to cause some learning perplexity to students, that mainly because the materials had no unity and no systematicness, and been compiled too early [19]. Except this problem, there are few magazines about TCMP in Taiwan, just several kinds like "Journal of Chinese Medicine", "Taiwan Clinical Journal of Traditional Chinese Medicine". Nowadays, there are no departments of Chinese traditional medicine set up in Taiwan's public hospitals, and its medical service laws restrict the traditional Chinese physicians to use western medicines, so the self-sustaining traditional Chinese hospitals provide little TCM service to in-patients for the deficiency in emergency treatment assisting to patients by western medicine, and furthermore, no health insurance has been internalized to the in-patients of TCM hospitals, and the clinic beds of TCM are less [20]. The Quantity of Traditional Chinese Medical Hospital in China Mainland are increasing steadily from 2141 hospitals in 1990 to 3232 hospitals in 2010 [21]; but the Quantity of TCM Hospital in Taiwan was in decrease year by year from 109 hospitals in 1994 to 22 hospitals in 2008 [22], see **Figure 2**. And as a result, the clinical education and development of TCMP needs urgent focus by the Taiwan authority. To touch upon the medical

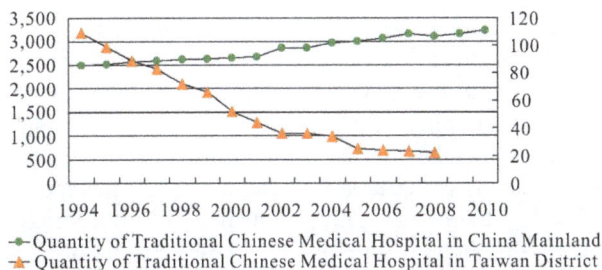

Figure 2. Comparison of quantity of Traditional Chinese Medical Hospital between China mainland and Taiwan District.

education pattern in Taiwan from the annual enrollment, discipline setup, curriculum or study time limit, it is certainly the Alma education. Generally speaking, the atmosphere and cultural heritage of TCMP education in Taiwan is not profound, and inferior to China mainland. But it is advisable to develop the TCM and Western medicine simultaneously, to thin the course offering, and emphasize the practice skills cultivation in Taiwan. By special examinations, people can obtain the qualifications of physicians and practitioners in Taiwan. Although the educational background of personnel participated in this special examination is increasing to some extent, most has low culture degree, high proportion personnel who passed the examination has no systemic and normal clinical skills training [18]. Furthermore, there is no examination system of licensed TCM pharmacists in Taiwan. The in-service education to Taiwan professional person in traditional Chinese drug, actually, is a remedied method to redeem the deficiency of pure TCM pharmacists in Taiwan, which aims at improving diathesis to pharmacists and practitioners of Chinese medicine, and belongs to irregular education of academic career. Just as a scholar pointed out that the cultivation of pure pharmacists of Chinese medicine in Taiwan needs to be achieved through subject differentiation and curriculum reform urgently [23]. In a word, in Taiwan District, the professional personnel for work or research engaged in traditional Chinese drug, the systematical studying about the basic theory of traditional Chinese drug, or professional training institutions are less, but the westernized phenomenon is quite serious. Taiwan TCM education has not yet formed the scale, and not still been brought into the formal trajectory. Lots of graduates possess the western medicine license and deal with western medicine or change to do something else. Therefore, the number of practitioners in TCMP is limited, elite mastered traditional Chinese medicine is lost.

5.3. Analysis in Characteristics Maintaining to TCMP

In China mainland, people in some developed coastal districts in economy such as Fujian, Guangdong usually

trust the TCM relatively, but the supporting diagnostic facilities in Chinese medical institutions in part of mountain area of China mainland are in need of development. The characteristics and culture building of TCMP still need to be further strengthened by Chinese medical authorities. In these districts, taking advantages of characteristics and clinic techniques of TCMP to diagnose and treat, compared with the developed areas of TCMP, is not enough. In Taiwan, the phenomena also exist extensively. As the above-mentioned, the TCMP education and research is westernizing, the traditional Chinese medical hospitals are few. Especially in the effect study on Chinese crude drugs, compared with China mainland, more attention should be paid to purify the monomers to test their actions, not to the compatibility of traditional Chinese medicine prescriptions and the basic theory like drug-nature of Chinese medicine. Unfortunately, with the amount increasing of TCM hospitals in China mainland, the great problem is the westernizing in diagnosis and treatment [24]. Keeping the characteristics and culture of TCM becomes more and more difficult.

5.4. Analysis in Research and Exploitation of Chinese Herbal Medicine or New Chinese Materia Medica Preparation

Due to the historical reasons between Taiwan and China mainland, even if depending on their own advantages and painstaking research respectively, Chinese Herbal Medicine research in both Taiwan and China mainland still exist some insufficiency like the problems of the material basis clarification of perplexing mechanisms of action and of how to bring Chinese Herbal Medicine in line with modern science. The new drugs of TCM that have real curative effects in clinic and good economic benefits are seldom [25]. The reasons are multifold, such as emphasizing inadequately on prophase screening to effective prescriptions, pursuing the high and new preparation level and ignoring the potency of formula itself, falling short of standardization and normalization in clinical trials of Chinese Herbal Medicines, rare clinical revaluation to postmarketing new drugs, the shortage of basic research on drugs that only several hundred CHMs have been lucubrated in more than ten thousand kinds, having restricted the preparation development, not undertaking researches to aim directly at the market since the scientific research institutions and universities have the powerful strength on drug exploitation, and not closing up on the connection of the resources between the scientific research institutions, universities, and enterprises [25,26]. At present, Taiwan's Chinese materia medica preparations authorized by the Taiwan TCM Committee are all recorded in traditional ancient books and records, and the therapeutical indications all belong to the conceptual category of TCM. The new drug of TCM research in Taiwan is mainly involved in the anticancer, lowering blood pressure or blood fat, anti-osteoporosis, anti-gastrelcoma, relieving cough and antiasthma, treating stroke and melancholia, drug abstinence and so on [27]. Compared with the numerous scientific research institutions and multitude researchers, and strong support from Ministry of Public Health, Ministry of Science and Technology and State Administration of Traditional Chinese Medicine in China mainland, the research scope of Taiwan Chinese Herbal Medicine is narrower, and the number of Taiwan CHM research items is also less. Though the research of material basis and effect mechanism of some Taiwan idiomatical Chinese herbal medicines or minority ethnic drugs such as Niu Zhang Zhi (Antrodia Camphorata) [28,29] has been gradually carried out in China mainland, the cooperation and research in natural resources investigation, introduction and cultivation, and exploitation of cross-Strait idiomatical Chinese herbal medicines are not enough. The Chinese medicinal products with fine quality and high efficiency are still the chasing target of the TCM industry both in Taiwan District and China mainland. The capabilities in independent research, development, innovation and generalization of Chinese drugs in both sides across the Taiwan Strait are required to expand and accelerate. To develop the Chinese medicine products with cross-Strait common intellectual property rights is required urgently. Therefore, the cross-Strait thorough joint to research traditional Chinese drugs is imperative, meanwhile, has quite broad prospects and development space. Just as the researcher Huang Y [4] has pointed out that the future direction and priorities of traditional Chinese medicine research in Taiwan was still around the development of new Chinese drugs, and to undertake a series research of scientization, modernization and internationalization of traditional Chinese drugs.

5.5. Analysis in Standard, Policy and Management in TCMP

Taiwan and China mainland have been cut off from each other for more than 40 years, and development of TCMP between them has formed some differences. For example, some Chinese herbal medicines are not unified in species, such as Ji Xue Teng in China mainland is referred to the Spatholobus suberectus, but in Taiwan is referred to Millettia dielsiana, Mucuna birdwoodiana, or Mucuna sempervireus; and Fang Ji, Niu Xi, Shayuan Zi, Fang Feng, Xi Xin, Baijiang Cao, Kun Bu, also exist this phenomena [30]. These differences may be resulting in some obstacles for cooperation each other. The standards of preparation and application of traditional Chinese drugs are also not uniform. Both sides have such problems, so

there are efforts should be made to develop appropriate legislation to reform and update. But the evaluation methods and standards system that are suitable for research of traditional Chinese medicine with its own characteristics has not been established [15]. The problems such as the criteria for determining the therapeutic effect of traditional Chinese medicines still restricted them to the international market; the exchanges and cooperation of TCM between China mainland and Taiwan are still restrained by the historical and geographical multifactor, cross-Strait policies and regulations, and so on. For example, Taiwan's traditional Chinese medicine research and application follows the "Taiwan Traditional Pharmacopoeia (TWTP)", but in China mainland it follows the "Pharmacopoeia of the People's Republic of China (PPRC)", which some standards of CHM origin and pharmaceutics have the distinctions. Furthermore, there are many differences in the quality testing standards of cross-Strait traditional Chinese drugs [31]. The research and control to the active ingredient in China mainland is higher than in Taiwan, but Taiwan pays more attention to the control of the security index. To the Chinese crude drugs purchased from China mainland before the use, the test items such as the heavy metal contamination and pesticide residues are more, and the limited requirements are higher. Just as the chairman of TCM Committee of Department of Health of the Executive Yuan in Taiwan Huang LH [3] pointed out that "the current import of Chinese crude drugs was short of the all round borderland checkout mechanism, and between China mainland and Taiwan, the pharmacopoeia norm, test standard and management also had great differences. Meanwhile, the channel of the correlated experience and technical exchange was deficient, and there were no report windows for intercommunication and coordinating mechanism to be established for the disqualified Chinese crude drugs by the sampling inspection".

5.6. Analysis in Safety and Quality of Traditional Chinese Drugs

Currently, to the Chinese herbal medicines, the Taiwan populaces mostly worry about that the heavy metals, pesticide residue, too many microorganisms and flavacin contained inside [3,16]. In China mainland, these problems also exist. Furthermore, the safety issues of traditional Chinese drug injections, especially the anaphylactic responses, are paid more and more close attention to [1]. In our opinions, the safety problems on the clinical application of some toxic Chinese herbal medicines or Chinese patent medicines especially containing the poisonous herbs or ingredients also need to be thought highly of. The processing or preparation quality of traditional Chinese drug should be put on the first place to some extent.

Attention Points of Research and Education in TCMP across Taiwan Strait...

191

6. Recommendations for R&D of TCMP between China Mainland Especially Fujian and Taiwan

Fujian and Taiwan District, although facing each other across the Taiwan Strait, having the common ancestry and the same Fukienese, the similar customs and climate, but were isolated by the historical anthropogenic factors for a long time. Along with the alleviation of Cross-Strait Relations step by step, for the recent years, communication between China mainland especially the Fujian province and Taiwan District is increasing. It is quite frequent and direct more than the other provinces. The technology and culture exchange become active. Cross-Strait Relations get into a new period. And further understanding of the current situation between each other in science technology development, creating conditions to enhance the two districts' communication in medical science, has the far-reaching history and reality meaning with regard to promoting development of cross-Strait Medical treatment and health service, improving the health level of bilaterial compatriots, and multiplying and thriving of the whole Chinese nation [32]. These attention points, contained so many differences of cross-Strait, which need to be improved and overcome or resolved by the substantial investment of human, material and financial resources and time, may provide a good way for China mainland and Taiwan to get in touch with each other. It is the major subjects in cross-Strait TCM field to organize first-class researchers and educators jointly by both sides, and to use the advanced R&D and education platform, to adopt the advanced, reasonable methods and education cooperation for the development of traditional Chinese medicine and pharmacy.

6.1. Strengthen the Cooperation of Industry and Trade of Traditional Chinese Drugs

In order to resolve the obstacles in the cooperation of industry and trade of Chinese medicine, we think that the industrial platforms of cross-Strait traditional Chinese drug especially the one of the specific ethnic drugs in Fujian and Taiwan must be established first to exploit several Chinese medicine products with cross-Strait common intellectual property rights through utilizing each other's advanced experience. The pharmaceutical enterprises in both sides should consummate the pharmacectic flow sheet in common, penetrate each other deeply to be familiar with the respective custody laws and regulations of drugs and market demands, and avoid blindness in investment and market risk. Both sides should try their best to reduce the differences in legislation to improve the confidence in investment and cooperation. With regard to the trade of TCMP, due to the demand for body health care and diagnosis and treatment

to disease, Taiwan District should enhance the import proportion of Chinese patent medicines and TCM health care products from China mainland. The cooperation of industry and trade of cross-Strait traditional Chinese drug is the future objective requirement, and also the necessity of history development.

6.2. Strengthen the Education and Elite Cultivating in TCMP

In view of the current situation of cross-Strait TCMP, we think that strengthening the education cooperation of cross-Strait traditional Chinese medicine and the cultivation of specialized elite who can master the related information of cross-Strait traditional Chinese medicine and pharmacy is quite necessary. Firstly, Taiwan District should organize experts to compile the unified teaching materials that are fit for the district characteristic and establish the complete supply system of teachers, and increase the TCMP curriculums in TCM discipline to change the tendency of over-emphasizing western medicine education, and expand the space and level of knowledge and academic exchange of cross-Strait Chinese herbal medicine, expand collection and sorting of the documents of traditional Chinese drugs in both sides, especially in Taiwan; and carry out the deep learning of ancient and modern Chinese medicine literature of Fukien and Taiwan with multi-disciplinary theoretical approaches and technologies of philosophy, social sciences, history, information science, computer technology and so on [33]. Secondly, Taiwan District should set up the regular examination system of traditional Chinese physicians and traditional Chinese pharmacists by drawing assistance from China mainland, and establish a joint cultivation system to cultivate the traditional Chinese pharmacist who can master the cross-Strait Chinese medicine, and allow the genuine pharmacists who know the clinical application and research of Chinese drugs to give full play the guiding role in these areas. Thirdly, Taiwan District should increase the number of TCM hospital and set up the department of TCM in public hospitals to give the TCM students more practice opportunities. Finally, Taiwan District may increase the kinds of magazines in TCMP to expand people's understanding of TCMP and strengthen the influence of TCM.

6.3. Outstanding the Characteristics of TCMP

How to keep the characteristics of traditional Chinese medicine in clinical practice and research is an important topic to the authority and TCMP workers both in Taiwan District and China mainland. We think that the urgent priority is to stop the westernizing of cultivation plan of TCM student in university or college, and take the cultivation model of the "disciple-following-teacher" convention that imparted and inherited since ancient times according to the growth regularity of famous veteran teran doctors of TCM to cultivate TCM student. During the clinic process, the traditional Chinese physicians should try their best to make use of four diagnostic methods (inspection, listening and smelling, inquiry, palpation and pulse taking) to diagnose disease and CHMs, compound recipes or acupuncture to treat, especially in the TCM department of general hospitals. And in the R&D of TCM, researchers must insist on the instruction of basic theory of TCM.

6.4. Strengthen the Research and Exploitation of Chinese Herbal Medicine or New Compound Recipe

Firstly, we think that it is urgent to strengthen the investigation of resources of the famous-region drugs in Taiwan and their introduction, breeding and developing in China mainland especially in Fujian province, including identifying the biogenesis of local Chinese herbal medicines that commonly used in Fujian and Taiwan, and summing up the nature and flavor, efficacy, usage, information about medicinal and edible dual purpose of the herbs. Relying on the advantages of wildlife resources, patterns implantation and medicinal industrial park of Fujian and Taiwan region, both sides should take the natural resources investigation, monitoring and regional planning to special local famous-region drugs, and establish gene banks of wild herbs and banks of germplasm resources, especially focus on carrying out the standardized planting of Chinese herbal medicines, the mutual introduction of cross-Strait herbs, and research and development of medicinal resources, and establish the introduction viewing area, the interzonal region test area, and demonstration area of good agriculture practice (GAP) stock breeding of cross-Strait famous-region drugs and endangered or bare drugs, and cultivate the modern raw material depot of traditional Chinese drugs to begin to take shape. Secondly, we think that both sides should aim directly at the Chinese herbal drugs that have cross-Strait national or local characteristics, and enlarge the pharmacy research. The focal point is to strengthen the research on therapeutic effect and mechanism of active components of idiomatical Chinese herbal medicines in China mainland especially Fujian and Taiwan. For example, the thorough research for drug-nature and channel entry, efficacy, and active constituents of Niu Zhang Zhi (*Antrodia Camphorata*), Xiao Ye Shan Pu Tao (*Vitis Thunbergi*), Jian Qu (*Massa Medicata Fermentata*), Feng Ju Dou Cao (*Sarcopyramis Nepalensis Wall.*), Ba Ji Tian (*Morindae Officinalis How.*), Tai Wan San Jian Shan (*Cephalotaxus Wilsoniana Hayata.*) [34] and so on, is very worthy to carry out. The research on the material basis, mechanism of action, clinical thera-

peutic effect evaluation, and clinical safety evaluation of the cross-Strait new specific Chinese drugs or new compound preparations being used for the treatment to some common momentous diseases such as multiple tumor, diabetes, cardiovascular disease, neurogenic disease, hepatopathy and nephropathy in Fujian and Taiwan, also should be impelled actively. But the most important centric position of "therapeutic effect" should be established in the drug manufacturing. Thirdly, we think that both sides should choose the potential species to take the secondary thorough research and development from the existing idiomatical compound preparations in Fujian and Taiwan. China mainland especially Fujian and Taiwan may aim directly at the cross-Strait idiomatical traditional Chinese patent medicines and simple preparations, and use a variety of combinatorial chemical or biological methods to explain their scientific connotation, and exploit their upgrade and update Chinese herbal products. The Research Priorities are the differences in components, effects and toxicity between Taiwan's "Scientific Chinese medicine granule" and China mainland's "Traditional Chinese medicine preparation", and promote the Taiwan's "Scientific Chinese medicine granule" to get into China mainland through Fujian province's R&D platform. According to the standard of new drug approval of China mainland, Fujian pharmaceutical enterprises should combine with Taiwan's enterprises and scientific research units to proceed the clinical pharmaco-research of cross-Strait idiomatical new drugs, which is the Clinical Trials and Clinical Verification of new drug, and hasten the West Bank of Taiwan Strait to become the China mainland industrialization hatching station of Taiwan's traditional Chinese medicine products. Fourthly, both sides should actively carry out the method research of the quality control of cross-Strait Chinese crude drugs and decoction pieces, and the famous-region genuineness of cross-Strait CHMs, and the content analysis of active ingredients, and improve the value of application. Finally, China mainland especially Fujian and Taiwan should optimize and integrate the resources in new drug exploitation and marketing sufficiently, increase the R&D investment to Chinese herbal drugs, make the technological research findings transform into the productivity quickly and create proper economic effectiveness and social benefit.

6.5. Try to Unify the Standard, Management and Policy in TCMP

Firstly, the different comprehension of the concept of "disease", "syndrome", "sign", "disease entity", "disease type", "name of TCM syndrome" between Taiwan and China mainland, always causes some disturbance in the communication and cooperation of cross-Strait TCMP. The terminology of cross-Strait TCMP should be unified as early as possibly and also should be in line with international medicine educational circles. Secondly, the CHM species that have inconsistent origins also should be unified for the common standard, especially the species included in both Taiwan's and China mainland's pharmacopoeia. So the standard of pharmacopoeia should be unified too. Thirdly, China mainland and Taiwan District should establish the common overall borderland checkout mechanism to manage the export and import of Chinese crude drugs, and set up the report windows for intercommunication and coordinating mechanism to disqualified Chinese crude drug. Finally, the cross-Strait drug custody departments and industry associations should work together to explore the mutual recognition of cross-Strait standards and the co-operation of related testing technology. Aiming directly at the unconformity of quality standards for cross-Strait Chinese medicines, in accordance with the limited requirements of *"Green Industry Standards for the Export and Import of Medicinal Plants and Preparation"* to lead, cadmium, mercury, arsenic and other heavy metals, and the requirements of the 2010 edition *"Pharmacopoeia of the People's Republic of China"* to pesticide residues of organophosphates and pyrethroids, both sides should understand the quality control methods of cross-Strait Chinese herbal medicines and try to find a common method to unify the standard. The main focus is investigating the cross-Strait standards for Fujian bulk famous-region drugs, and comparing the standard differences, providing the technical support for the West Bank of Taiwan Strait to form the Taiwan export depot to Chinese herbal medicines. Ultimately through combining to enact the TCM pharmaceutical standards and the export of pharmaceutical certification, it will be as soon as possible to narrow the differences of cross-Strait TCM management laws and regulations and quality standards to achieve mutual recognition.

6.6. Strengthen the Safety Detection of Traditional Chinese Drugs

Both sides should focus on the safety assessment of Chinese herbs. Before the export of Chinese crude drugs or traditional Chinese patent medicines and simple preparations in China mainland, we should strength the detection of toxic substances, harmful substances and heavy metals, moreover, take the same detected methods with Taiwan. To Taiwan's import, the detection also should be done like this.

7. Conclusion

To face the development and opportunities in the new history period, the cross-Strait medical academia and industry both generate the resonance from the academic to the industrial cooperation, give full play to their re-

spective preponderance to jointly study and resolve the key issues that constraining the development of traditional Chinese medicine, and establish the long-term mechanism of cross-Strait TCMP cooperation. In order to make traditional Chinese drug modernize, the two sides of Taiwan Strait must be sharing the resources, have the mutual benefit and win-win to obtain collaborative progress, and make it widely to the international market. TCMP, passed down as one of the excellent treasures of the Chinese nation for safeguarding public health, its notable efficacy is extensively recognized by the people of China mainland and Taiwan District. Traditional Chinese medicine and pharmacy is the common wealth of the compatriots on both sides of the Taiwan Strait, and is also the important link to maintain the feelings of cross-Strait compatriots. To promote the prosperity and development of cross-Strait TCMP is the same aspiration of the Chinese people. The pharmaceutical industries in the both sides are willing to establish the combined research and development platform of Chinese medicine, so as to establish unified TCMP standards to improve the quality of varieties of cross-Strait Chinese medicine products and speed up their replacement, and improve the competitiveness and rapid, healthy development of cross-Strait TCMP industry.

8. Acknowledgements

The authors thank the Research Grant of Xiamen City Key Science and Technology Plan (No. 3502Z20100006) "Strait Science and Technology Platform (Xiamen, China) of Traditional Chinese Medicine and Pharmacy" to support this article.

REFERENCES

[1] X. C. Li, "Correlation between Quality Standard of Traditional Chinese Medicine Injections and Medication Safety," *Chinese Journal of Pharmacoepidemiology*, Vol. 21, No. 11, 2012, pp. 38-40.

[2] S. X. Wang, "The Scientization of Chinese Herbal Drugs and the New Drug Exploitation of Chinese Herbals Have Been Emphasized by Taiwan," *Hebei Journal of Traditional Chinese Medicine*, Vol. 25, No. 2, 2003, p. 113.

[3] Z. B. Yu, "From the Forum of Traditional Chinese Medicine and Pharmacy across Taiwan Strait to View the Trade Prospect of Traditional Chinese Drugs between Taiwan and Mainland China," *Modern Chinese Medicine*, Vol. 12, No. 7, 2010, pp. 42-43.

[4] Y. Huang, "The Progress and Tendency of Research of Traditional Chinese Medicine in Taiwan District," *World Journal of Integrated Traditional and Western Medicine*, Vol. 4, No. 6, 2009, pp. 452-454.

[5] "Six Cooperating Protocols Forming Complementation to Push about the Development of Traditional Chinese Medicine and Pharmacy in Taiwan District and China

Mainland,"
http://www.chemdrug.com/databases/detail/3-13214.html
2010-07-08

[6]   X. J. Gao, "10 Kinds of Chinese Crude Drugs Getting into Taiwan Will Be Put into Source Management and Needs to Provide the Inspection Unit Testimonial by China State Administration of Quality Supervision and Be Confirmed by Taiwan," *Journal of Traditional Chinese Medicine Management*, Vol. 19, No. 9, 2011, p. 859.

[7]   T. B. Shih, "Research of System Analysis of Tonifying Chinese Herbal Medicines and Their Prescriptions Used on Human Stem Cells," *Yearbook of Chinese Medicine and Pharmacy*, Vol. 24, No. 1, 2006, pp. 29-51.

[8]   W. C. Wun. "Research on Processing Technique of Rhizoma Pinelliae (2-1)," *Yearbook of Chinese Medicine and Pharmacy*, Vol. 24, No. 3, 2006, pp. 1-39.

[9]   S. S. Liou, "To Establish the Processing Standard and Processing Factory Norm of Chinese Crude Drug and Decoction Pieces of Cortex Magnoliae Officinalis," *Yearbook of Chinese Medicine and Pharmacy*, Vol. 25, No. 4, 2007, pp. 89-146.

[10] L. R. Xiao, "The History Origin and Modern Development of Traditional Chinese Medicine in Fujian and Taiwan," *Journal of Fujian University of Traditional Chinese Medicine*, Vol. 16, No. 1, 2006, pp. 58-59.

[11] J. H. Guh, "Effect Research of Chinese Herbals' Ingredients on Antagonizing Cancer and Neovascularization and the Identification the Origin of Active Components (3 - 2)," *Yearbook of Chinese Medicine and Pharmacy*, Vol. 24, No. 2, 2006, pp. 75-94.

[12] M. D. Lin, "Taiwan Establishes the High-End Platform of Development and Verification of Traditional Chinese Medicine," *China Medicine and Pharmacy*, Vol. 1, No. 5, 2011, pp. 4-5.

[13] J. Z. Fu, "The New Change and Tendency of Traditional Chinese Medicine Education in Taiwan Recent Years," *Journal of Traditional Chinese Medicine Management*, Vol. 17, No. 8, 2009, pp. 686-688.

[14] X. Y. Su, "Current Situation of Higher Education of traditional Chinese Drug in Taiwan," *Chinese Journal of Information on Traditional Chinese Medicine*, Vol. 14, No. 9, 2007, pp. 107-108.

[15] S. L. Huang, X. Y. Chen and C. M. Yang, "Play Area Advantage, Promote the Exchange and Development of Cross-Strait Traditional Chinese Medicine," *Strait Pharmaceutical Journal*, Vol. 20, No. 10, 2008, pp. 142-145.

[16] N. Liao, "To Analyze the Cooperation and Development of Cross-Strait Industry of Chinese Medicine," *Journal of Traditional Chinese Medicine Management*, Vol. 19, No. 6, 2011, pp. 497-500.

[17] X. F. Lin and D. Y. Lin, "General Situation of Administration of Traditional Chinese Medicine in Taiwan Area in 2009," *Journal of Fujian University of Traditional Chinese Medicine*, Vol. 21, No. 1, 2011, pp. 70-72.

[18] D. C. Tang, "Pre-Test on Education of under Graduate Course of Traditional Chinese Medicine in Taiwan," *Lishizhen Medicine and Materia Medica Research*, Vol. 17, No. 10, 2006, pp. 2096-2097.

[19] J. J. Shen, Y. L. Zhang and W. Q. Xu, "Present Situation and Suggestions of the Education of Chinese Medicine in Taiwan," *Education of Chinese Medicine*, Vol. 21, No. 1, 2002, pp. 41-43.

[20] W. H. Bao, X. M. Liu, S. L. Ren and L. Li, "Compare the Setting Standards of TCM Hospitals in China Mainland with that in Taiwan District," *World Chinese Medicine*, Vol. 5, No. 6, 2010, pp. 436-439.

[21] Department of Planning and Finance of State Administration of Traditional Chinese Medicine, "China Statistical Yearbook of Chinese Medicine (1987-2010)," http://www.satcm.gov.cn/1987-2010/start.htm

[22] Department of Health, the Executive Yuan of Taiwan, "The Statistical Annual Report of Medical Institutions Status and Hospital's Utilization," Yearbook of Public Health of Taiwan, 2009, p. 23.

[23] B. W. Cheng, "Overview of Education of Professional Talented Person of Traditional Chinese Drug in Taiwan," *Pharmaceutical Education*, Vol. 11, No. 1, 1995, pp. 60-61.

[24] L. Liu, "Many Points of View on Westernizing of Traditional Chinese Medical Hospitals," *Hospital Management Forum*, Vol. 22, No. 11, 2005, pp. 36-40.

[25] X. H. Xiao, L. Q. Huang and X. J. Ma, "Discussion on the New Connotation and Significance of Traditional Chinese Drug and Its Modernization," *China Journal of Chinese Materia Medica*, Vol. 28, No. 3, 2003, pp. 282-286.

[26] L. Jin, "Current Situation of Research and Development of Traditional Chinese Drugs and Thinking about the Future Development," *China Medicine and Pharmacy*, Vol. 1, No. 18, 2011, pp. 32-33.

[27] L. R. Xiao, "Characteristics, Research and Development of New Drugs of Traditional Chinese Medicine in Taiwan District for Recent Ten Years," *Journal of Fujian University of Traditional Chinese Medicine*, Vol. 20, No. 2, 2010, pp. 64-65.

[28] G. Wang, J. Wang and W. Xu, "Study on the Extracting Condition of Antrodia Camphorata Polysaccharide," *Fujian Journal of Traditional Chinese Medicine*, Vol. 42, No. 1, 2011, pp. 52-53.

[29] W. Xu, J. Wang and G. Wang, "Study on Toxicity Test for Antrodia Camphorata Capsule," *Strait Pharmaceutical Journal*, Vol. 23, No. 5, 2011, pp. 41-43.

[30] L. H. Pan and W. Lu, "Analysis of Easy Confusion Species of Cross-Strait Traditional Chinese Drugs," *Journal of Fujian College of Traditional Chinese Medicine*, Vol. 7, No. 1, 1997, pp. 33-34.

[31] D. Huang and L. L. Li, "Preliminary Discussion about Differences of TCM Quality Standards between Taiwan and Mainland China," *Chinese Pharmaceutical Affairs*, Vol. 24, No. 11, 2010, pp. 1088-1090.

[32] D. S. Zhuang, P. Lin, Y. L. Zhang and L. Ye, "Strengthen the Technology Communication of Medical Science between Fujian and Taiwan to Promote the Development of Cross-Strait Health Service," *Fujian Medical Journal*, Vol. 17, No. 3, 1995, pp. 102-103.

[33] N. Liao, "Play Area Advantage and Carry forward Tradi-

tional Culture: Fujian University of Traditional Chinese Medicine Paves the Way for the Bypass for the Exchange of Traditional Chinese Medicine between Fujian and Taiwan," *Relations across Taiwan Straits*, Vol. 13, No. 3, 2009, pp. 52-53.

[34] M. Z. Lin, Z. B. Chen, "The Situation of Pharmaceutical Plant Resources in Southern Fujian," *Journal of Zhangzhou Normal University*, Vol. 22, No. 4, 2009, pp. 99-103.

24

Clinical Practice Examples of Dachaihu Decoction

Hongmei Zhu

Department of Chinese Medicine, Medical School, Xiamen University, Xiamen, China

Email: z5913778@126.com

ABSTRACT

This paper mainly describes the experiences of clinical application of Dachaihu Decoction in treating chronic pelvic infection, coronary heart disease, insomnia, and hepatolithiasis.

Keywords: Dachaihu Decoction; Coronary Heart Disease; Insomnia; Chronic Pelvic Infection; Hepatolithiasis

1. Introduction

Dachaihu Decoction, originating from Treatise on Febrile Diseases, is a commonly used formula in clinic. Modifying from Xiaochaihu Decoction by excluding Radix et Rhizoma Glycyrrhizae, Radix et Rhizoma Ginseng and including Radix et Rhizoma Rhei, Fructus Aurantii Immaturus, and Radix Paeoniae Alba, it aims at harmonizing Shaoyang and relieving excess Fu syndrome by promoting defecation. It is used to treat syndrome of pathogenic evils in Shaoyang combining interior excess in Yangming by Zhang Zhongjing. In clinical practice, the formula has been flexibly modified to treat varied miscellaneous diseases with significant effects by focusing on its pathogenesis, namely, Shaoyang disorder with Fu qi obstruction. Now the writer would like to give four detailed examples as follows.

2. Coronary Heart Disease

Mr. Bai, male, 61 yr, who has coronary heart disease for over five years with chest distress in anterior thoracic region at intervals, initially came to my clinic for treatment on July 8th, 2010. He used to take Compound Danshen Tablet and Diao Xinxuekang Capsule to relieve symptoms. With the months getting hotter, Bai noticed the aggravated symptoms such as frequent occurrence of chest pain, together with shortness in breath, fatigue, dry mouth and bitter taste. The patient added that he has abdominal distension in the afternoon in recent two to three years, especially after the nap, with difficulty in defecation. Last year, he had three severe abdominal distensions with no defection and was diagnosed as intestinal obstruction. The condition got relieved then after appropriate treatment, but still occurred sometimes. At that time,

the patient showed dark red tongue, with thin yellow coating and dark sublingual venae, thready and taut pulse for left hand, taut, slippery and rapid for right hand. He was diagnosed as chest obstruction with stagnated heat obstructing chest, combining Yangming excess syndrome. The method of regulating Shaoyang, removing blood stasis to unblock the channels, eliminating excess fu syndrome was selected and the combined Dachaihu Decoction with Guizhi Fuling Tablet was modified as follows: Radix Bupleuri 12 g, Radix Scutellariae 10 g, Rhizoma Pinelliae Praeparata 10 g, Radix Codonopsis 10 g, Fructus Aurantii Immaturus 10 g, Rhizoma Zingiberis Recens 3 slices, Fructus Jujubae 10 g, Radix Paeoniae Rubra 10 g, Radix Paeoniae Alba 10 g, Radix et Rhizoma Rhei 6 g, Ramulus Cinnamomi 6 g, Poria 15 g, Cortex Moutan 10 g, Radix et Rhizoma Salviae Miltiorrhizae 15 g, Semen Persicae 10 g, Semen Armeniacae Amarum 10 g, and Fructus Trichosanthis 20 g. One week later, his chest pain disappeared, chest distress relieved greatly, abdominal distention occurred only occasionally, and bowel movement better regulated. Then, the patient was suggested to take the decoction for another one week, with Radix et Rhizoma Rhei 6 g in the previous formula increased to 9 g, and Fructus Cannabis 18 g included. Later, the patient telephoned to inform us that everything was good.

Comment: Coronary heart disease pertains to Chest obstruction in Chinese medicine, in which the approach of invigorating qi, accelerating blood movement and removing phlegm is frequently used. In this case, the patient only showed deficiency syndrome manifested by symptoms such as shortness in breath and fatigue, and excess syndrome in pulses, just as Synopsis of Golden Chamber-Chest obstruction, heart pain and shortness in breath states: For patient with no obvious aversion to cold or hot, if he shows shortness in breath, he has an excess syndrome [1]. This chest obstruction is an excess syndrome caused by phlegm-heat obstructing chest, where Shaoyang meridian covers. For patient with problems in Shaoyang meridian, he usually has symptoms such as bitter taste, dry throat and taut pulse [2]. It is beyond doubt that in this case, the disease was resulted from Shayang meridian, combining symptoms such as abdominal distention and constipation. Thus, Dachaihu Decoction was used to clear away stagnated heat in Shaoyang, regulating Shaoyang meridian, and eliminating excess Fu syndrome in Yangming. Together with Guizhi Fuling Tablet, which specializes in accelerating blood circulation and removing stasis and phlegm, the formula meets the syndrome and focuses on regulating both qi and blood, phlegm and blood stasis with significant effects.

3. Insomnia

Ms Lin, female, 46yrs, first turned to me for help on May 11th, 2010. Since diagnosed as insomnia ten years ago, she has tried varied Western and Chinese medicine, only to find herself severely disappointed. According to Lin, she always have chest suppression, and feel upset, palpitation, sense of frightening and difficulty in falling sleep every night, which commonly lead to sleepless all night. Meanwhile, Lin has dry mouth and bitter taste, discomfort in stomach, constipation, dark red tongue with yellow greasy coating, deep, thready and slippery pulse. She was diagnosed as insomnia with heart qi deficiency, phlegm-heat disturbance internally combining heart and gallbladder inquietude in Chinese medicine. Thereby the approach of tonifying heart qi, clearing heat in heart and gallbladder, removing phlegm-heat and calming down the spirit was prescribed and Chaihu Jia Longgu Muli Decoction was modified as follows: Radix Bupleuri 12 g, Radix Scutellariae 10 g, Rhizoma Pinelliae Praeparata 10 g, Radix Codonopsis 10 g, Ramulus Cinnamomi 6 g, Radix et Rhizoma Rhei Praeparata 5 g, Fossilia Ossis Mastodi 30 g, Concha Ostreae 30 g, Sclerotium Poriae Pararadicis 20 g, Rhizoma Zingiberis 3 slices, Fructus Jujubae 10 g, Cortex Albiziae 20 g, Caulis Polygoni Multiflori 20 g, Radix et Rhizoma Salviae Miltiorrhizae 20 g, Radix Curcumae 10 g, and Semen Ziziphi Spinosae 20 g. Five days later, the patient told us that she can now sleep for 4 hours every night with her chest suppression reduced, upset and palpitation relieved. In consideration of her stubborn constipation, Radix Codonopsis 10 g and Ramulus Cinnamomi 5 g in the previous formula were excluded, Radix et Rhizoma Rhei Praeparata 5 g replaced by Radix et Rhizoma Rhei 9 g, but Fructus Aurantii Immaturus 10 g and Radix Paeoniae Alba 15 g were included. Two days later, her bowel movement was promoted a little, chest suppression eradicated with more

than five hours' sleep every night. Later, the decoction was suspended due to the hysteromyoma surgery, which brought back the chest suppression. At present, the patient shows red tongue with yellow coating at the root, thready and slippery pulse, no dry mouth or bitter taste regular movement by taking more fruits and vegetable. She is suggested to take the formula ten more days to consolidate effects.

Comment: In this case, the insomnia started after delivery ten years ago, it is not only long in course but also leads to intermingled deficiency and excess syndrome. Heart qi deficiency, together with phlegm-heat disturbing heart and gallbladder, brought about all the symptoms mentioned above. At the beginning, its syndrome fit into Chaihu Jia Longgu Muli Decoction, which resulted in obvious effects. Since heart qi was promoted and phlegm-heat was eliminated, symptoms such as palpitation and upset were relieved gradually, yet constipation existed as before. Hence, in her second visit, Dachaihu Decoction was applied mainly, combining drugs for calming down spirit, so as to promote bowel movement, clear away the internal phlegm-heat and clam down heart and gallbladder, thus freeing the patient from her stub-born insomnia.

4. Chronic Pelvic Infection

Ms Lin, female, 31 yr who initially called on my clinic on April 17th, 2008, has already had pain and sagging distention in the lower abdomen for over three years with increased pain before or after the menstruation. Her menstruation was described as profuse but dark with blood clots. The patient had chronic pelvic infection and left oviduct obstruction in accordance with Western medicine. Other symptoms were stated as follows: dry mouth, bitter taste, sore waist, breast distending pain before menstruation, disturbance of frequent dreams, irritable feeling, constipation (once a week), dark and purple tongue with slight yellow but thick greasy coating, taut, thready but rapid pulse. Lin was diagnosed as abdominal pain with stagnant heat in Chong and Ren Channels, combining excess Fu syndrome in Yangming by Chinese medicine. In consequence, the approach of clearing away the heat located in Shaoyang, dissipating blood stasis and unblocking channels, relieving excess Fu syndrome though promoting defecation was determined and the combined Dachaihu Decoction with Guizhi Fuling Tablet was modified as follows: Radix Bupleuri 15 g, Radix Paeoniae Rubra 12 g, Radix Paeoniae Alba 12 g, Rhizoma Pinelliae Praeparata 10 g, Radix et Rhizoma Rhei Praeparata 9 g, Ramulus Cinnamomi 9 g, Cortex Moutan 10 g, Radix et Rhizoma Salviae Miltiorrhizae 20 g, Poria 15 g, Semen Persicae 10 g, Fructus Aurantii Immaturus 10 g, Radix Scutellariae 10 g, Radix et Rhizoma Glycyrrhizae Praeparata cum Melle 6 g, Caulis Sargentodoxae 20 g, Radix Dipsaci 15 g, Fructus Toosendan 10 g, Rhizoma Corydalis 10 g, Concha Ostreae 30 g, and Semen Ziziphi Spinosae 15 g and prescribed to the patient. Five days later, the abdominal pain was greatly relieved with smoothing bowel movement and after another one month, the abdominal pain was eliminated completely with regular bowel movement and menstruation. Later, with combined Guizhi Fuling Tablet and Dan Zhi Xiaoyang Tablet as consolidation therapy for two more months, the patient obtained a negative result at left oviduct B-ultrasonic examination.

Comment: the Liver Meridian of Foot-Jueyi travels around the reproductive organs and reaches to lower abdomen [3]. Abdominal pain in gynaecology usually occurs at lower abdomen, therefore, it can be treated from the liver meridian: for deficiency syndrome, one can use Danggui Shaoyao Decoction to nourish blood and regulate liver, Dachaihui Decoction for excess syndrome to promote qi movement, expel heat and eliminate the excess. Moreover, since gynecological diseases often go deep to the blood phrase and Dachaihu Decoction mainly focuses on regulating qi, one should add Guizhi Fuling Tablet, which specializes in accelerating blood movement, removing stasis and promoting urination in order to strengthen its effects. In this case, with typical Shangyang syndrome, Yangming syndrome as well as qi stagnation and blood stasis syndrome, it is very effective to use combined Dachaihu Decoction with Guizhi Fuling Tablet.

5. Hepatolithiasis

Ms Zhang, female, 69 yrs, a retired doctor who has suffered from recurrent epigastric pain over ten years with more frequent occurrence in recent two years, paid her first visit here on May 10th, 2008. She used to take gastric motor drugs, spasm relaxants, or antibiotics to relieve pain; however, during the last three months recurrence, all the medicine did not help a little. Barium meal indicated chronic superficial gastritis and B-ultrasonic examination results showed negative results (She had cholecystectomy twenty years ago due to cholelithiasis). The patient described her symptoms as follows: continuous distension or pain in the stomach, reluctance to eat, slight nausea, bitterness in the mouth, annoyed and perplexed feeling, scanty, soft and impeded bowel movement. Meanwhile, she was yellow in complexion, thin in figure and exhausted in spirit with redness at tongue tip and white coating from inspection, deep and thready in pulse diagnosis. The patient was initially administrated with Xiaochaihu Decoction for three days, which resulted smoothing in the stomach and growing appetite as she described. Next, Zhang was given the same formula for three days more with no significant effects. When I tried to figure out the reason, I was told that she felt quite annoyed and restless, with tendency to

sweat after taking the decoction this time. All of a sudden, I recalled one article from Treatise on Febrile Diseases, which states: For patients with persistent vomiting, discomfort in the stomach, low but slightly annoyed in spirit, one should use Dachaihu Decoction [4]. In spite of persistent vomiting, the rest symptoms all fit in the article. Hence, Dachaihu Decoction was applied and modified as follows: Radix Bupleuri 15 g, Radix Scutellariae 10 g, Rhizoma Pinelliae Praeparata 12 g, Pericarpium Citri Reticulatae 10 g, Radix Paeoniae Alba 15 g, Radix et Rhizoma Rhei Praeparata 9 g, Radix Codonopsis 12 g, Rhizoma Zingiberis Recens 15 g, Radix et Rhizoma Glycyrrhizae 6 g, Fructus Setariae Germinatus 10 g, Fructus Hordei Germinatus 10 g, and Endothelium Corneum Gigeriae Galli 10 g. In the formula, Rhizoma Zingiberis Recens was applied in large dosage not for the vomiting as usual but for her low in spirit by helping Radix Bupleuri and Radix Scutellariae to clear away stagnated heat in Shaoyang with its spicy and warm nature, Rhizoma Pinelliae Praeparata for harmonizing stomach, relieving oppression and preventing vomiting, Radix Paeoniae Alba for relaxing spasm and releving pain, and Radix et Rhizoma Rhei Praeparata for removing excess Fu syndrome. Meanwhile, in consideration of her age, Radix et Rhizoma Glycyrrhizae and Radix Codonopsis were applied to invigorate spleen and strengthen the body resistance. All the symptoms were relieved after taking the latest formula for three days. Since her hepatolithiasis was highly indicated, the patient was suggested to maintain light diet with less oily food and regular administration of Yidan Tablet. No occurrence was reported in the one-year follow-up.

Comment: Dachaihu Decoction has significant antibacterial and anti-inflammatory, cholagogue and calculus removing effects [5], which is frequently used in the treatment of cholecystitis and cholelithiasis in clinic. The case mentioned above is not very typical on account of its imperfection in Western diagnosis and atypical symptoms. Thus, it is suggested that the clinical application of Dachaihu Decoction should not be confined to Western diagnosis, and more emphasis should be given to the comprehension of articles from Treatise on Febrile Diseases, for instance: in this case, discomfort in the stomach, low but slightly annoyed in spirit, scanty but inhibited diarrhea all indicate obstruction of Fu qi in Yangming.

REFERENCES

[1] Z. J. Zhang, "Theory of Synopsis of Golden Chamber," Publishing House of Chinese Medicine, Beijing, 2006.

[2] Z. J. Zhang, "Treatise on Febrile Diseases," Shanghai People'S Publishing House, Shanghai, 1976.

[3] P. J. Yang, "Spiritual Axis," Xueyuan Publishing House, Beijing, 2008.

[4] Z. J. Zhang, "Treatise on Febrile Diseases," Shanghai People's Publishing House, Shanghai, 1976.

[5] W. L. Deng, "Pharmacology of TCM Formula and Its Application," Chongqing Publishing House, Chongqing, 1990.

25

Antioxidant Activity of 50 Traditional Chinese Medicinal Materials Varies with Total Phenolics

Zhengyou He[1,2*], Minbo Lan[1], Dongying Lu[1], Hongli Zhao[1], Huihui Yuan[1]

[1]Research Center of Analysis & Test and Institute of Advanced Materials, East China University of Science & Technology, Shanghai, China

[2]Sichuan Industrial Institute of Antibiotics, Chengdu University, Chengdu, China

Email: *Hezhengyou@aliyun.com

ABSTRACT

This study was designed to determine the total phenolic content of 50 herbs and to examine their antioxidant potential. In the sample preparation, 60% ethanol was chosen as the extraction solvent for the subsequent experiments. Folin-Cicolteau phenol reagent and a colorimetric method were used to determine the total phenolic content of the selected herbs. The result showed that total phenolic content of those herbs ranged from 2 to 185 mg/g. In antioxidant assay, the ferric reducing/antioxidant power (FRAP) values ranged from 2 to 134 mg GAE/g; the IC_{50} values of DPPH•, •OH and O_2^- scavenging were in the range of 0.06 - 5.50 mg/mL, 0.017 - 0.636 mg/mL and 0.050 - 0.681 mg/mL respectively.

Flos caryophylli was the exceptant in the O_2^- scavenging assay because there was no linear relation between the concentration and the scavenging percentage. Compared to gallic acid, ascorbic acid and butylated hydroxytoluene (BHT) in antioxidant assay as positive control, the most potential antioxidant herbs were *Cacumen platycladi*, *Radix et Rhizoma rhei*, *Rhizoma rhodiolae crenulatae*, and *Rhizoma sanguisorbae* with considerable content of phenolics. Especially, a positive and significant correlation was found between the total phenolic content and FRAP value or DPPH• scavenging percentage.

Keywords: Traditional Chinese Medicinal Material; Total Phenolics; Antioxidant Activity; Ferric Reducing/Antioxidant Power; Free Radical Scavenging Activity

1. Introduction

Roles of the reactive oxygen species (ROS) and reactive nitrogen species (RNS) are increasingly recognized in physiological processes, pathogenesis of many diseases, and molecular mechanisms in many drug-therapies [1]. ROS are generated by all aerobic organisms and their production seems to be essential for signal-transduction pathways that regulate multiple physiological processes. Excessive amount of ROS, however, can initiate toxic and lethal chain reactions, which disable the biological structures that are required for cellular integrity and survival. Recently, there is a growing interest in substances exhibiting antioxidant properties that are supplied to human and animal organisms as food components or as specific redox-therapy drugs [1]. Substantive experiments have already testified that many phytochemicals and extracts from plants possess antioxidant effects.

Many synthetic antioxidants, such as butylated hydroxyanisole (BHA), butylated hydroxytoluene (BHT) and tert-butylhydro-quinone (TBHQ), are widely used in food and pharmaceutical industries against oxidative damage. However, animal tests have demonstrated that those synthesized compounds would accumulate in rats and result in liver-damage and carcinogenesis [2]. Interestingly, some important antioxidants, including ascorbic acid and the tocopherols, cannot be synthesized by humans and must be taken in diet [3]. It has long been recognized that some naturally occurring substances in plants process antioxidant activity. Therefore, the development and utilization of more effective and non-toxic antioxidants from natural products are desired, not only for the food and drug storage, but also for the nutritional and clinical applications.

It is well known that the traditional Chinese herbs have been used in food and medicine over two thousand years. There are more than 11,000 officinal plants, 1500 offici-

*Corresponding author.

nal animals and 80 officinal minerals used as the traditional Chinese medicine [4]. For the reason of biodiversity, the chemical composition and bioactivity of the medicinal materials are also varied. Epidemiological studies have shown that many natural antioxidant compounds possess anti-inflammatory, antiatherosclerotic, antitumor, antimutagenic, anticarcinogenic, antibacterial, or antiviral activities to a greater or lesser extent [5,6]. Apparently, the Chinese medicinal plants may contain a wide variety of chemical composition, including phenolic compounds (e.g. phenolic acids, flavonoids, quinones, coumarins, lignans, stilbenes, tannins), nitrogen compounds (alkaloids, amines, betalains), vitamins, terpenoids (including carotenoids), with potential antioxidant activities [7]. In free radical biology, the balance between antioxidation and oxidation is believed to be a critical concept to maintain a healthy biological system, which is similar to the concept of the balance between "Yin" and "Yang" in the Traditional Chinese Medicine (TCM). The effective compositions in the yin-tonic herbs were mainly flavonoids with strong antioxidant activities six times higher than that of the yang-tonic herbs [8]. Contrarily, Szeto and Benzie indicated that the yin nature of herbs may not be necessarily associated with superior antioxidative effect to yang-tonic herbs, at least in terms of DNA protection against oxidant challenge [9]. The synergetic antioxidant effects of the traditional Chinese herbs should be considered in the view of systems biology [10], but the literature partially revealed the inner correlation between the antioxidant capacity and the traditional usages. Consequently, it is necessary to evaluate the antioxidant activity of traditional Chinese herbs systematically using different types of free radical.

50 Traditional Chinese herbs, grown and processed under the standard operating procedures, were selected and prepared for the initial investigation. According to the classification of their traditional usages [4], 18 of those herbs, including 11 stanchers, are used as the haematic. The next is the heat-clearing drug, and 10 medicinal materials are ranged to this class. The third is the tonic, including one yin-tonic, eight yang-tonics, and four weaktonics. Other medicinal materials are sorted into diaphoretic, damp-resolving, cathartic, and antitussive respectively. The main objectives of this paper were a) to determine the content of total phenolics in above medicinal materials; b) to evaluate their *in vitro* antioxidant activity of ferric reducing and antioxidant power (FRAP), and free radicals (DPPH•, •OH and $O_2^{•-}$) scavenging capacities.

2. Materials and Methods

2.1. Materials from the Traditional Chinese Medicine

50 Chinese medicinal materials were purchased from a local pharmacy (Jiamei medicine chain Co., Ltd., Shanghai, China). The planting, harvesting, drying, processing, and storage of the medicinal materials were conducted according to strict traditional procedures, namely the standard operating procedures implemented in China. Names of those Chinese medicinal materials are listed in **Table 1**, all of them have been identified according to the literature [4]. All the voucher specimens have been deposited at the Specimen-room of the Research Center of Analysis & Test, East China University of Science and Technology, Shanghai, China.

2.2. Preparation of Extracts

Dried and pulverized sample (1 g) was extracted using 20 ml of 60% (v/v) ethanol. It was mixed continuously with magnetic stirrer under refluxing at 60°C for 1 h. Then, the extracts were filtered over Xinhua filter paper. The residue was re-extracted under the same conditions. The obtained extracts were conflated and concentrated *in vacuo* under 40°C using a rotary evaporator (ZX98-1 Rotavapor, Shanghai Organic Chemistry Institute, Shanghai, China) to yield dry extracts, which were stored at 4°C for further analysis.

2.3. Total Phenolic Contents (TPCs) Analysis

The TPCs of those extracts were analyzed using Folin-Ciocalteu's phenol reagent [11]. The extracts were dissolved in 60% (v/v) ethanol at the concentrations to fit the TPC analysis. The solutions (0.5 mL) of different concentrations were put in a 10 mL volumetric flask, 4.5 mL of distilled water and 1.0 mL of Folin-Ciocalteu reagent were added, and the flask was shaken thoroughly. After 3 min, 4 mL of 2% Na_2CO_3 was added, and the mixture was allowed to stand for 2 h with intermittent shaking. The absorbance was measured at 770 nm (UV-2102, Unico Instruments Co., Ltd., Shanghai, China). Experiments were carried out in triplicate. The results were expressed as gallic acid equivalent per gram raw material (mg GAE/g). The same procedure was repeated

Table 1. Extraction efficiencies of various dilutions of ethanol in water on *Folium artemistae argyi*, *Rhizoma rhodiolae crenulatae*, and *Cortex eucommiae*.

Species	TPC [a] (mg GAE/g dried sample)			
	95% ethanol	60% ethanol	30% ethanol	10% ethanol
Folium artemistae argyi	18.49 ± 0.46	34.72 ± 0.72	28.33 ± 0.70	24.13 ± 0.56
Rhizoma rhodiolae crenulatae	93.61 ± 1.72	184.56 ± 3.78	169.02 ± 3.95	151.70 ± 1.87
Cortex eucommiae	22.07 ± 0.61	40.04 ± 0.80	34.15 ± 0.66	31.28 ± 0.59

[a]Results are means ± SD (n = 3).

for all of the standard gallic acid solutions (0 - 10,000 μg/mL), and the standard curve was determined using the equation:

$$\text{Absorbance} = 0.0011 \times \text{gallic acid} \,(\mu g) + 0.0027.$$

2.4. Antioxidant Screening

2.4.1. Ferric Reducing and Antioxidant Power (FRAP) Assay

The total antioxidant potential of those herbs was determined using ferric reducing and antioxidant power (FRAP) assay [12]. FRAP reagent was freshly prepared and mixed in the proportion of 10:1:1 (v:v:v) for A:B:C solutions, where A = 300 mmol/L sodium acetate trihydrate in glacial acetic acid buffer (pH = 3.6); B = 10 mmol/L TPTZ in 40 mmol/L HCl; and C = 20 mmol/L $FeCl_3$. Gallic acid was used for a standard curve with all solutions, including samples dissolved in 60% ethanol. The assay was carried out at 37°C (pH = 3.6) using 0.4 mL sample or standard solution plus 4.0 mL FRAP reagent shown above. After 10 min incubation at room temperature, the absorbance was read at 593 nm. Results were expressed in mg gallic acid equivalent per gram dried herb weight (mg GAE/g). Experiments were carried out in triplicate.

2.4.2. DPPH Radical Scavenging Activity Assay

This spectrophotometric assay used the stable DPPH radical as the reagent to determine the DPPH• scavenging activity [13]. The extracts and standards were dissolved in 60% (v/v) ethanol at the concentrations to fit the DPPH assay. Ethanolic extracts or standards of 0.1 mL at various concentrations was added to 4.0 mL 0.004% DPPH• methanol solution in a 10 mL test tube respectively. After 30 min incubation at room temperature, the absorbance was read against a contrast only containing all solvents at 517 nm. Inhibition of the free radical of DPPH in percent (I%) was calculated as follow:

$$\text{Inhibition}\% = \left[\left(A_{blank} - A_{sample}\right) / A_{blank}\right] \times 100\%$$

where A_{blank} is the absorbance of the control reaction (containing all of the reagents except the test compound) and A_{sample} is the absorbance of the test samples. Exact concentration providing 50% inhibition (IC_{50}) was calculated from the graph plotted from the regression analysis as inhibition percentage against concentration of the medicinal materials. Gallic acid, ascorbic acid, and BHT were measured at the same procedure. Tests were carried out in triplicate. Results were expressed in milligram medicinal materials per milliliter (mg/mL).

2.4.3. •OH Scavenging Activity Assay

The scavenging ability of different extracts on hydroxide radical was measured in the $CuSO_4$-Phen-Vc-H_2O_2 che-miluminescence (CL) system. The CL of hydroxyl radical formation was monitored under the described method [14] using a BPCL Ultra-weak luminescence analyzer (Institute of Biophysics, Academia Sinica, China). The extracts were dispersed in 1% Tween 20 and standards were dissolved in redistilled water, those solutions were diluted to fit the •OH scavenging assay. The volume of the reaction was composed of 50 μL of the sample solution, 50 μL of 1.0 mmol/L $CuSO_4$ solution, 50 μL of 1 mmol/L 1,10-phenanthroline solution, 700 μL of 0.05 mol/L borate buffer (pH 9.0), 100 μL of 1 mmol/L ascorbic acid solution, and 50 μL of 1% H_2O_2 solution. The reaction was initiated immediately after the injection of H_2O_2 solution, and kinetic curves were obtained at 2 s intervals over a period of 400 s. Varying degrees of sudden drops of CL counts observed represent the different degrees of •OH scavenging abilities. As the inhibiting percentage of CL counts had been calculated, comparison of the correlativity between the •OH scavenging efficacy and the concentration of each sample is possible. The integrated area of the curve expressed the relative luminescent intensity. The scavenging activity was represented by the following formula:

$$\text{Inhibition}\% = \frac{\left[\left(CL_{control} - CL_0\right) - \left(CL_{sample} - CL_0\right)\right]}{\left(CL_{control} - CL_0\right)} \times 100\%$$

where $CL_{control}$ is the relative luminescent intensity of the control group, CL_0 is the relative luminescent intensity of the background group, and CL_{sample} is the relative luminescent intensity of the experimental group. Exact concentration providing 50% inhibition (IC_{50}) was calculated from the graph plotted as scavenging percentage against concentration of medicinal materials. Gallic acid was also measured at the same procedure. Tests were carried out in triplicate. IC_{50} values were expressed in milligram medicinal materials per milliliter (mg/mL).

2.4.4. $O_2^{\cdot-}$ Scavenging Activity Assay

The $O_2^{\cdot-}$ scavenging activity of the selected herbs was determined by the nitrite reduction method [15]. The tested solutions were prepared in the •OH scavenging assay and diluted to fit the $O_2^{\cdot-}$ scavenging assay. The reaction mixture contained 0.6 mL 1 mmol/L hypoxanthine, 0.3 mL 220 μmol/L hydroxylammonium-chloride, 1mL buffer solution (pH 8.2, the solution containing 15.6 mmol/L $Na_2B_4O_7$ and 20.8 mmol/L KH_2PO_4), and 40 μL 0.7 U/mL xanthine oxidase. The diluted solution of 1.0 mL was added to the reaction mixture and incubated for 30 min at 37°C. Then 2.0 mL 1.73 mmol/L sulfanilic acid, which was dissolved in 1.36 mmol/L acetic acid, and 2.0mL of 19.29 μmol/L N-1-naphthylethylenediamine were injected to the solution and shook. After standing at room temperature in the dark for 20 min, the absorbance was measured at 550 nm. A control solution was measured, in which sample was replaced by redistilled water. The scavenging rate was obtained according to the formula:

$$\text{Scavenging rate}(\%) = \frac{A_c - A_s}{A_c - A_b} \times 100\%$$

where A_c is the absorbance of the control solution, A_s is the absorbance of the test sample, and A_b represents the absorbance of the blank, in which xanthine oxidase was replaced by the buffer. Exact concentration providing 50 % inhibition (IC_{50}) was calculated from the graph plotted from the regression analysis as inhibition percentage against the concentration. The results were expressed in milligram raw materials per milliliter (mg/mL). Gallic acid and ascorbic acid were measured at the same procedure. Experiments were carried out in triplicate.

2.5. Data Analysis

Data were processed using origin 6.1 software (Microcal Software, Inc., Northampton, MA, USA). The regression equations and correlation coefficients were fitted by the least-squares method. All experiments were repeated at least three times. The results were expressed as means ± SD. Standard differences were considered significant at $P < 0.05$.

3. Results and Discussions

3.1. Selection of Extraction Solvents

In order to select the best solvent for extraction of those medicinal materials, four different percentages of ethanol (10%, 3 %, 60% and 95% v/v) were used in the extraction of *Folium artemistae argyi*, *Rhizoma rhodiolae crenulatae*, and *Cortex eucommiae* respectively. The extraction solvent of 60% ethanol, indicated by the TPC values (**Table 2**), was found to give the highest extraction efficiency for the selected three herbs, while 95% ethanol had the lowest extraction efficiency. Consequently, 60% ethanol was chosen as the extraction solvent for the subsequent antioxidant assays. The average extraction efficiency of 60% ethanol was determined by multiple extraction experiments and was found in range from 95% to 97% after the first and the second extraction depending on the selected medicinal materials (**Table 3**). Therefore, the selected medicinal materials were extracted twice using 60% ethanol under refluxing for further investigations respectively.

3.2. Total Phenolic Contents of 50 Medicinal Materials

There was a wide range of the total phenolic contents among the selected medicinal materials. As shown in **Ta-**

ble 1, the TPC values, determined by the Folin-Ciocalteau method, varied from 2 to 185 mg GAE/g (average 39.9 mg GAE/g) depending on the biological origin of the plant. It is well known that plant polyphenols are widely distributed in the plant kingdom and sometimes in surprisingly high concentrations [16,17]. According to the results, there are 7 medicinal materials with the lowest total phenolics concentration (<10 mg GAE/g), including *Semen nelumbinis* < *Rhizoma atractylodis macrocephalae* < *Flos magnolia officinalis* < *Herba portulacae* < *Semen ginkgo* < *Folium mori* < *Radix dipsaci*. Five herbs had total phenolics concentrations > 90 mg GAE/g: *Rhizoma rhodiolae crenulatae* > *Herba cirsii japonici* > *Rhizoma sanguisorbae* > *Radix rubiae* > *Radix et rhizoma rhei*. The highest total phenolics content (> 150 mg GAE/g) was found in *Rhizoma rhodiolae crenulatae*, the roots collected from *Rhodiola crenulata* (Hook. f. et. Thoms.) H. Ohba. According to the literature [11], various phenolic compounds have different responses in TPC assay. The molar response of this method is roughly proportional to the number of phenolic hydroxyl groups in a given substrate, whereas the reducing capacity is enhanced when two phenolic hydroxyl groups are oriented ortho or para [18]. Since these structural features of phenolic compounds are also responsible for antioxidant activity, measurements of phenols in food or medicinal materials may be related to their antioxidant properties.

3.3. Antioxidant Capacity

3.3.1. FRAP of 50 Medicinal Materials

As shown in **Table 1**, the total antioxidant capacities (FRAP) are different from each other between the selected 50 medicinal materials. The FRAP values varied from 2 to 134 (the mean was calculated as 25.6) mg GAE/g of the dried material weight. In FRAP assay, the

Table 2. Extraction efficiencies of *Folium artemistae argyi*, *Rhizoma rhodiolae crenulatae*, and *Cortex eucommiae*.

Species	Extraction	Average TPC[a] (mg GAE/g dried sample)	Average extraction efficiencies (%)
Folium artemistae argyi	1st	30.09 ± 0.67	85.38 ± 1.83
	2nd	3.61 ± 0.16	10.24 ± 0.46
	3rd	1.54 ± 0.09	4.37 ± 0.28
Rhizoma rhodiolae crenulatae	1st	139.24 ± 3.45	74.83 ± 1.76
	2nd	33.04 ± 1.52	17.76 ± 0.83
	3rd	13.80 ± 0.94	7.42 ± 0.45
Cortex eucommiae	1st	35.34 ± 0.87	87.82 ± 2.03
	2nd	3.61 ± 0.18	8.97 ± 0.44
	3rd	1.29 ± 0.08	3.20 ± 0.21

[a]The average of TPC and extraction efficiencies were based on triplicates from a single batch; the results are means ± SD (n = 3).

Table 3. The total phenolic content (TPC) values and the *in vitro* antioxidant activities of fifty traditional Chinese medicines[a].

Plant materials (medicinal name)	Total phenolic contents[b] (mg GAE/g)	FRAP[b] (mg GAE/g)	IC$_{50}$ of DPPH scavenging activity[c] (mg/mL)	IC$_{50}$ of OH scavenging activity[c] (mg/mL)	IC$_{50}$ of O$_2^-$ scavenging activity[c] (mg/mL)
Cacumen platycladi	74.59 ± 1.49	47.99 ± 0.96	0.140 ± 0.004	0.045 ± 0.001	0.076 ± 0.001
Cortex eucommiae	40.04 ± 0.80	26.59 ± 0.55	0.262 ± 0.005	0.270 ± 0.004	0.220 ± 0.006
Cortex magnoliae officinalis	24.34 ± 0.44	16.59 ± 0.31	0.504 ± 0.010	0.057 ± 0.001	0.069 ± 0.002
Cortex moutan	80.09 ± 1.50	53.48 ± 1.00	0.127 ± 0.002	0.089 ± 0.001	0.093 ± 0.003
Flos caryophylli	53.99 ± 1.10	36.64 ± 0.78	0.198 ± 0.006	0.021 ± 0.001	nd[d]
Flos chrysanthemi	11.08 ± 0.20	8.43 ± 0.21	1.037 ± 0.019	0.099 ± 0.001	0.083 ± 0.001
Flos chrysanthemi indici	10.76 ± 0.22	7.15 ± 0.14	0.994 ± 0.022	0.208 ± 0.006	0.143 ± 0.005
Flos magnolia officinalis	5.44 ± 0.09	3.68 ± 0.08	2.066 ± 0.046	0.047 ± 0.001	0.050 ± 0.002
Folium artemistae argyi	34.72 ± 0.72	21.71 ± 0.41	0.297 ± 0.008	0.132 ± 0.004	0.094 ± 0.002
Folium eucommiae ulmoides	23.54 ± 0.41	11.25 ± 0.23	0.505 ± 0.010	0.282 ± 0.005	0.108 ± 0.002
Folium ginkgo	36.64 ± 0.73	21.32 ± 0.46	0.281 ± 0.008	0.087 ± 0.002	0.084 ± 0.001
Folium mori	8.94 ± 0.20	6.30 ± 0.11	1.213 ± 0.025	0.227 ± 0.003	0.127 ± 0.002
Folium nelumbinis	14.17 ± 0.25	9.30 ± 0.20	0.725 ± 0.014	0.088 ± 0.001	0.064 ± 0.001
Folium phyllostachydis henonis	40.32 ± 0.77	25.84 ± 0.54	0.253 ± 0.006	0.450 ± 0.012	0.477 ± 0.010
Fructus arctii	17.07 ± 0.30	9.19 ± 0.15	0.704 ± 0.017	0.234 ± 0.005	0.158 ± 0.003
Fructus crataegi	44.97 ± 0.82	26.95 ± 0.59	0.232 ± 0.006	0.098 ± 0.002	0.093 ± 0.001
Fructus lycii	27.16 ± 0.54	17.98 ± 0.37	0.411 ± 0.010	0.089 ± 0.002	0.152 ± 0.003
Fructus psoraleae	36.86 ± 0.71	23.84 ± 0.52	0.297 ± 0.003	0.135 ± 0.003	0.364 ± 0.012
Herba asari	18.65 ± 0.32	10.57 ± 0.23	0.610 ± 0.014	0.533 ± 0.011	0.431 ± 0.008
Herba cirsii	82.06 ± 1.51	51.90 ± 1.02	0.128 ± 0.004	0.094 ± 0.002	0.101 ± 0.002
Herba cirsii japonici	147.64 ± 2.99	90.36 ± 1.83	0.085 ± 0.002	0.102 ± 0.002	0.076 ± 0.001
Herba epimedii	28.38 ± 0.57	14.24 ± 0.28	0.365 ± 0.007	0.296 ± 0.007	0.075 ± 0.001
Herba erodii	10.06 ± 0.20	5.64 ± 0.12	1.085 ± 0.026	0.131 ± 0.003	0.086 ± 0.002
Herba moslae	16.03 ± 0.30	11.02 ± 0.21	0.645 ± 0.015	0.636 ± 0.012	0.478 ± 0.010
Herba portulacae	6.06 ± 0.11	6.94 ± 0.15	1.686 ± 0.034	0.150 ± 0.005	0.142 ± 0.004
Herba senecionis scandentis	17.27 ± 0.38	13.09 ± 0.27	0.607 ± 0.011	0.094 ± 0.002	0.100 ± 0.002
Radix angelicae sinensis	19.92 ± 0.42	13.50 ± 0.28	0.519 ± 0.009	0.148 ± 0.004	0.076 ± 0.001
Radix astragali	27.75 ± 0.56	19.11 ± 0.36	0.380 ± 0.007	0.216 ± 0.002	0.108 ± 0.002
Radix dipsaci	9.50 ± 0.20	6.76 ± 0.15	1.168 ± 0.022	0.102 ± 0.003	0.058 ± 0.001
Radix et rhizoma rhei	90.21 ± 1.90	57.83 ± 1.21	0.126 ± 0.002	0.085 ± 0.001	0.078 ± 0.002
Radix glycyrrhizae	26.71 ± 0.55	16.67 ± 0.32	0.379 ± 0.007	0.092 ± 0.001	0.060 ± 0.001
Radix notoginseng	27.81 ± 0.59	12.84 ± 0.26	0.362 ± 0.006	0.174 ± 0.003	0.111 ± 0.002
Radix paeoniae alba	31.31 ± 0.63	21.20 ± 0.47	0.338 ± 0.008	0.152 ± 0.005	0.106 ± 0.003
Radix paeoniae rubra	46.21 ± 0.92	30.30 ± 0.69	0.232 ± 0.005	0.101 ± 0.002	0.089 ± 0.002
Radix pulsatillae	16.51 ± 0.34	11.72 ± 0.24	0.685 ± 0.014	0.187 ± 0.003	0.225 ± 0.005
Radix rubiae	93.56 ± 1.87	56.45 ± 1.12	0.109 ± 0.002	0.099 ± 0.002	0.222 ± 0.006
Radix scutellartae	80.24 ± 1.62	52.14 ± 1.01	0.146 ± 0.005	0.056 ± 0.001	0.093 ± 0.002
Ramulus uncariae cum uncis	31.53 ± 0.65	20.40 ± 0.30	0.340 ± 0.009	0.091 ± 0.002	0.153 ± 0.002
Rhizoma atractylodis macrocephalae	2.88 ± 0.06	4.73 ± 0.05	4.175 ± 0.081	0.074 ± 0.002	0.086 ± 0.002
Rhizoma belamcandae	23.89 ± 0.53	14.71 ± 0.31	0.488 ± 0.013	0.073 ± 0.001	0.163 ± 0.004
Rhizoma chuanxiong	27.62 ± 0.56	16.97 ± 0.33	0.406 ± 0.007	0.244 ± 0.008	0.249 ± 0.007
Rhizoma cimicifugae	22.27 ± 0.45	12.67 ± 0.25	0.511 ± 0.018	0.313 ± 0.010	0.412 ± 0.008
Rhizoma polygont cuspidati	60.96 ± 1.25	41.38 ± 0.53	0.190 ± 0.006	0.097 ± 0.003	0.064 ± 0.002
Rhizoma rhodiolae crenulatae	184.56 ± 3.78	133.98 ± 2.73	0.062 ± 0.002	0.017 ± 0.001	0.109 ± 0.002
Rhizoma sanguisorbae	128.93 ± 2.56	72.38 ± 1.55	0.084 ± 0.002	0.035 ± 0.001	0.059 ± 0.001
Semen euryales	48.42 ± 0.99	30.98 ± 0.66	0.213 ± 0.003	0.225 ± 0.007	0.153 ± 0.005

Continued

Semen ginkgo	7.81 ± 0.20	4.96 ± 0.07	1.569 ± 0.031	0.217 ± 0.003	0.681 ± 0.009
Semen nelumbinis	2.20 ± 0.05	2.34 ± 0.05	5.477 ± 0.111	0.303 ± 0.009	0.125 ± 0.003
Spica prunellae	13.86 ± 0.24	9.17 ± 0.16	0.828 ± 0.018	0.216 ± 0.006	0.516 ± 0.015
Thallus eckloniae	59.97 ± 1.22	38.75 ± 0.79	0.175 ± 0.005	0.175 ± 0.004	0.151 ± 0.006
Gallic acid	[f]	-	0.0153 ± 0.0004	0.0123 ± 0.0004	0.101 ± 0.003
Ascorbic acid	-	510 ± 7	0.0042 ± 0.0001	-	0.0248 ± 0.0006
BHT[e]	-	-	0.0191 ± 0.0003	-	-

[a]Results were means ± SD (n = 3); [b]Total phenolic contents were expressed in gallic acid equivalent of the dried medicinal materials; [c]IC_{50} was defined as the concentration sufficient to obtain 50% scavenging activity; [d]The linear relation could not be constructed; [e]BHT represents butylated hydroxytoluene; [f]Not detected.

antioxidant activity was based on the ability of the antioxidant components in the samples to reduce Fe^{3+} to Fe^{2+} in a redox-linked colourimetric reaction that involves single electron transfer [12]. According to their reducing ability/antioxidant power (FRAP) values, 50 medicinal plants can be divided into five groups: a) very low FRAP (<5 mg GAE/g), n = 4; b) low FRAP (5 - 30 mg GAE/g), n = 32; c) good FRAP (30 - 50 mg GAE/g), n = 6; d) high FRAP (50 - 100 mg GAE/g), n = 7; and e) very high FRAP (>100 mg GAE/g) n = 1. On the basis of the FRAP values of the selected chemicals, the ratio of the slope of the linear curve of ascorbic acid to that of $FeSO_4 \cdot 7H_2O$ was 1.96, and the ratio of gallic acid to $FeSO_4 \cdot 7H_2O$ was 4.02. Gallic acid, bearing a pyrogallol moiety, exhibited more potent activity than ascorbic acid (gallic acid vs asorbic acid = 2.05:1). The significant linear correlation (coefficient "r" = 0.9918, and two-tailed "P"-value < 0.0001) was confirmed between TPC values and their related FRAP values of the selected medicinal materials (**Figure 1**).

There are many methods to determine the total antioxidant capacity [19]. These *in vitro* and *in vivo* methods differ in terms of their assay principles and experimental conditions. Consequently, antioxidant components may individually have varying contributions to the total antioxidant capability in different methods. Because FRAP assay is quick and simple to perform, and the reaction is reproducible and linearly related to the molar concentration of the antioxidant(s) [20], the FRAP assay was applied in the determination of the total antioxidant capacity of those herbs. This method was initially developed to assay plasma antioxidant capacity, and popularly used to measure the antioxidant capacity from a wide range of biological samples in recent years, including teas, vegetables, fruits, wines, plants, and animal tissues [21,22]. In sharp contrast to the medicinal plants with high or very high FRAP values, the positive properties of the medicinal plants with very low FRAP are unlikely related to their antioxidant capacity. As a result, eight medicinal materials, namely *Rhizoma rhodiolae crenulatae, Herba cirsii japonici, Rhizoma sanguisorbae, Radix et rhizoma rhei, Radix rubiae, Cortex moutan, Radix scutellartae,*

and *Herba cirsii*, have the highest FRAP values among those selected herbs.

3.3.2. DPPH Radical Scavenging Activity

DPPH assay was applied to test the ability of the antioxidative compounds as well as different plant extracts functioning as proton radical scavengers or hydrogen donors [23]. IC_{50} values of DPPH radicals scavenging activity were in the range of 0.06 - 5.50 mg/mL according to the results listed in **Table 1**. A negative correlation was found between the TPCs and IC_{50} values, indicating that the materials or the extracts at high TPC levels would have low IC_{50} values but strong potency to scavenge DPPH radicals. Among 50 selected materials, 12 medicinal materials with lowest IC_{50} values (<0.2 mg/mL) were *Rhizoma rhodiolae crenulatae < Rhizoma sanguisorbae < Herba cirsii japonici < Radix rubiae < Radix et rhizoma rhei < Cortex moutan < Herba cirsii < Cacumen platycladi < Radix scutellartae < Thallus eckloniae < Rhizoma polygont cuspidati < Flos caryophylli.* Gallic acid and BHT, determined with the IC_{50} values of 15.3 µg/mL and 19.6 µg/mL respectively, were used as the positive control in DPPH assay. The correlation was investigated between the concentration and the antioxidant capacity at different concentrations of individual medicinal materials. The results indicated that the selected herbs have liner relation between the DPPH radicals scavenging percentages and the TPC concentrations. It could be concluded that the DPPH radicals scavenging nature of those materials might depend on their total phenolics tentatively. As a result, a parabola regressive model could be built from those data. In other words, the reciprocals of the TPCs values were linear to the IC_{50} values (coefficient "r" = 0.9985, and two-tailed "P"-value <0.0001) (**Figure 2**).

3.3.3. •OH and O_2^- Scavenging Activities

To evaluate the ROS scavenging properties of those medicinal materials, we have used two different reactive oxygen species (ROS): the hydroxyl radical and superoxide anion radical. •OH was produced and monitored by the $CuSO_4$-Phen-Vc-H_2O_2 chemiluminescence system,

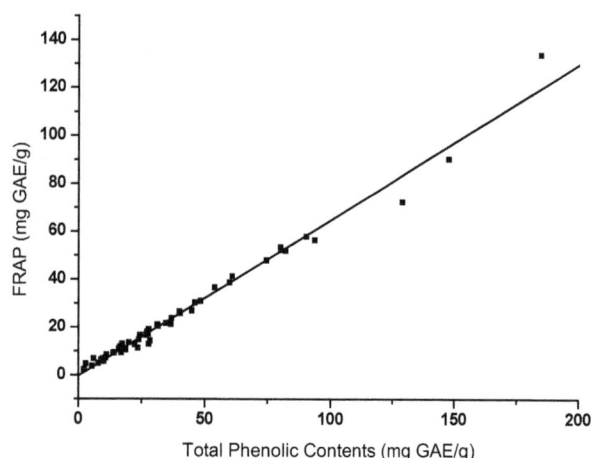

Figure 1. Linear correlation between the amount of total phenolics and the total antioxidant capacity (FRAP), y = 0.6509x − 0.3783. Correlation coefficient "r" = 0.9918. The two-tailed P value is <0.0001, considered extremely significant.

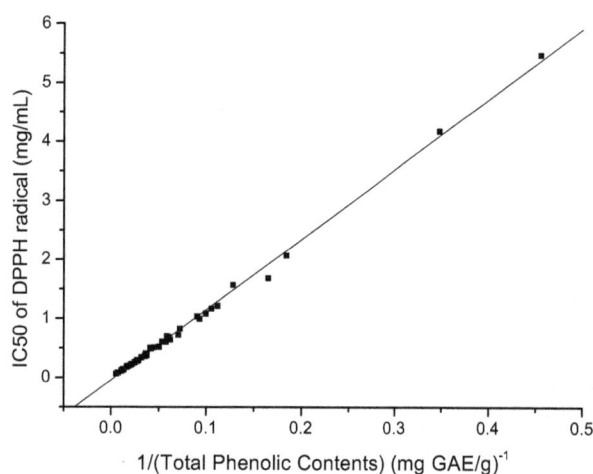

Figure 2. Linear correlation between the reciprocals of the total phenolic content and IC$_{50}$ values of DPPH scavenging activity, y = 11.9209x − 0.0406. Correlation coefficient "r" = 0.9985. The two-tailed P value is < 0.0001, considered extremely significant.

whereas O_2^- was generated by the hypoxanthinexanthine oxidase system and detected by UV-Vis spectrophotometry. The results of the ROS scavenging capacities, in the form of IC$_{50}$ values of those herbs, were presented in **Table 1**. The IC$_{50}$ values of •OH and O_2^- varied in the ranges of 0.017 - 0.636 mg/mL and 0.050 - 0.681 mg/mL respectively. In the superoxide anion radical assay, only *Flos caryophylli* did not exhibit correlation between the free radicals scavenging percentage and the concentration. Comparison of the ROS scavenging characteristics of those medicinal materials, *Herba moslae* has the highest potency to scavenge the hydroxyl radicals, whereas *Semen ginkgo* is the highest in the superoxide anion radical assay. According to the results,

there was a weak linear relation between IC$_{50}$ values of the hydroxyl radical and the superoxide anion radical scavenging activities (coefficient "r" = 0.6442, and two-tailed "P"-value <0.0001). The individual extracts, which could scavenge the hydroxyl radicals, can not necessarily eliminate the superoxide anion radicals. As a result, traditional Chinese herbs have specific ROS scavenging properties respectively, which can be applied in the explanation of the rules of compatibility of medicines in the traditional Chinese medicine.

In the ROS scavenging experiments, there was no linear response between the total phenolic contents and the free radicals scavenging activities, other factors should be considered in the evaluation of the ROS scavenging capacities. There were several methods to screen the ROS scavengers, different methods could give varied results for the unstable characteristics of the ROS in chemical or biochemical systems. The total phenolics content in the extracts could be correlated linearly with the oxygen depletion, but not with the ROS scavenging effect by different methods using ESR spin trapping and electrochemical measurement [24]. Other scientists also have not found linear response between the total phenolics and the ROS scavenging capacities [8]. The difference between the sterical structures of antioxidants or the free radicals played a more important role in the abilities to scavenge different types of free radicals [25], which could be applied in the explanation of the antioxidant variations between the DPPH•, •OH, and O_2^- scavenging activities. In DPPH assay, the 60 % ethanol extracts showed higher scavenging activity than the 95 % ethanol extracts. The similar conclusion could be drawn from the results of the extracts by different polar solvents in •OH and O_2^- assays. It suggests that more-polar components presented in extracts have contributed towards the increased ROS scavenging activities. Although there was no direct evidence in this study, the antioxidant activities of 60% ethanol extracts could be related to the presence of phenolic compounds, peptides, saccharides, and other polar compounds because they contain hydroxyl moiety [26,27].

3.3.4. Comparison of Antioxidant Activities of 50 Medicinal Materials

Influenced by several biofactors, such as the ROS and other free radicals occurrence, the redox status in human body, and the bioavailability of the phytochemicals, the traditional Chinese herbs would act as more complicated roles in the life processes than the chemical or biochemical systems *in vitro*. According to the classification of their medicinal usages in the traditional Chinese medicine, 18 of those herbs, including 11 stanchers, were traditionally used as the haematic. Those haematic drugs, especially the stanchers, have highest TPC values and strongest antioxidant capacities in comparison with other herbs. The next is the heat-clearing drugs, totally 10 herbs are ranged to this class. According to the results, those heat-clearing drugs owned higher total phenolic contents and moderate antioxidant activities. The other medicinal materials, traditionally defined as the tonic, the diaphoretic and damp-resolving, have quite low TPC values and low antioxidant activities. On the other hand, the diseases are usually treated by complex prescriptions using the drug matching principles in traditional Chinese medicine. So, it would be of great importance to investigate the antioxidant characteristics of the traditional Chinese medicinal materials using the different antioxidant screening systems.

The total antioxidant (FRAP) and DPPH•, •OH and $O_2^{\cdot-}$ scavenging activities have different mechanisms in the antioxidant effects, so the herbs with the highest capacities were chose as the potential antioxidants. Four traditional Chinese herbs, namely *Cacumen platycladi*, *Radix et rhizoma rhei*, *Rhizoma rhodiolae crenulatae* and *Rhizoma sanguisorbae*, have antioxidant potency in comparison with some well known natural and synthetic antioxidants. Contrarily, *Folium mori*, *Fructus arctii*, *Semen ginkgo*, *Semen nelumbinis* and *Spica prunellae* were the weak antioxidants correspondingly. It has been revealed that various phenolic antioxidants, such as flavonoids, tannins, coumarins, xanthones, and procyanidins, can scavenge free radicals dose-dependently [28], thus they are viewed as promising therapeutic drugs for the free radical related disorders or illnesses. There are more than 4000 naturally occurring flavonoids described in the literature [29], including chalcones, flavonones, flavones, biflavonoids, dihydroflavonols, anthrocyanidins, and flavonols. Other polar natural products, such as proteins, saccharides, etc., also have the antioxidant capacities, but as a rule, phenolic compounds were applied in the evaluation of the correlation between the results of the antioxidant capacities and the botanic materials [26,27]. Therefore, the antioxidant activities of plant original medicinal materials are dependent on the chemical type of antioxidant compounds, the polarity of the extracting solvent, and the test systems or the substrates to be protected.

Interestingly, many complex prescriptions can be assembled from the selected 50 herbs according to the traditional Chinese medicine. Among those prescriptions, the herbs from at least two types are discriminated as monarch, minister, assistant and guide by the roles of their actions in the diseases treatment. The composition of abundant substances in the complex prescription will provide more complicated and synergistic antioxidant effects in the human body than the individual herbs.

4. Conclusion

In conclusion, our results further support the point of view that some medicinal materials are promising sources of natural antioxidants. Among 50 selected traditional Chinese herbs, the total phenolic content and the antioxidant capacity differed significantly. There were significant linear correlations between the total phenolic concentration and the values of FRAP or DPPH radicals scavenging percentage. We also have found that three stanchers, namely *Cacumen platycladi*, *Rhizoma Rhodiolae crenulatae*, *Rhizoma sanguisorbae*, and one cathartic, that is *Radix et rhizoma rhei*, have significant ferric reducing power and free radicals scavenging activities. Those traditional Chinese medicines have been certified with low profile of side effects and toxicities for thousands of years. Several herbs, popularly used in the traditional Chinese medicine, have already been on schedule to be investigated for their phytochemistry and their medicinal applications.

5. Acknowledgements

We gratefully acknowledge Shanghai Nanotechnology Promotion Center (Grant No. 0552nm018) for the financial support.

REFERENCES

[1] B. Halliwell and M. C. G. John, "Free Radicals in Biology and Medicine," 2 Edition, Oxford University Press, Oxford, 1989, pp. 299-508.

[2] N. Ito, S. Fukushima and H. Tsuda, "Carcinogenicity and Modification of the Carcinogenic Response by BHA, BHT, and Other Antioxidants," *Critical Reviews in Toxicology*, Vol. 15, No. 2, 1985, pp. 109-150. http://dx.doi.org/10.3109/10408448509029322

[3] R. G. Cutler, "Antioxidants and Aging," *The American Journal of Clinical Nutrition*, Vol. 53, No. 1, 1991, pp. 373S-379S.

[4] X. M. Hu, "Chinese Materia Medica (in Chinese)," Vol. 1, Shanghai Science and Technology Press, Shanghai, 1999, pp. 1-252.

[5] Y. Cai, *et al.*, "Antioxidant Activity and Phenolic Compounds of 112 Traditional Chinese Medicinal Plants Associated with Anticancer," *Life Sciences*, Vol. 74, No. 17, 2004, pp. 2157-2184. http://dx.doi.org/10.1016/j.lfs.2003.09.047

[6] P. Scartezzini and E. Speroni, "Review on Some Plants of Indian Traditional Medicine with Antioxidant Activity," *Journal of Ethnopharmacology*, Vol. 71, No. 1-2, 2000, pp. 23-43. http://dx.doi.org/10.1016/S0378-8741(00)00213-0

[7] Y. Z. Cai, *et al.*, "Structure-Radical Scavenging Activity Relationships of Phenolic Compounds from Traditional Chinese Medicinal Plants," *Life Sciences*, Vol. 78, No. 25, 2006, pp. 2872-2888. http://dx.doi.org/10.1016/j.lfs.2005.11.004

[8] B. Ou, *et al.*, "When the East Meets West: The Relationship between Yin-Yang and Antioxidation-Oxidation,"

The FASEB Journal: Official Publication of the Federation of American Societies for Experimental Biology, Vol. 17, No. 2, 2003, pp. 127-129.

[9]   Y. T. Szeto and I. F. Benzie, "Is the Yin-Yang Nature of Chinese Herbal Medicine Equivalent to Antioxidation-Oxidation?" *Journal of Ethnopharmacology*, Vol. 108, No. 3, 2006, pp. 361-366. http://dx.doi.org/10.1016/j.jep.2006.05.033

[10] D. Wormuth, *et al.*, "Redox Regulation and Antioxidative Defence in Arabidopsis Leaves Viewed from a Systems Biology Perspective," *Journal of Biotechnology*, Vol. 129, No. 2, 2007, pp. 229-248. http://dx.doi.org/10.1016/j.jbiotec.2006.12.006

[11] V. L. Singleton and J. A. Rossi, "Colorimetry of Total Phenolics with Phosphomolybdic-Phosphotungstic Acid Reagents," *American Journal of Enology and Viticulture*, Vol. 16, No. 3, 1965, pp. 144-158.

[12] I. F. F. Benzie and J. J. Strain, "The Ferric Reducing Ability of Plasma (FRAP) as a Measure of 'Antioxidant Power': The FRAP Assay," *Analytical Biochemistry*, Vol. 239, No. 1, 1996, pp. 70-76. http://dx.doi.org/10.1006/abio.1996.0292

[13] T. Katsube, *et al.*, "Screening for Antioxidant Activity in Edible Plant Products: Comparison of Low-Density Lipoprotein Oxidation Assay, DPPH Radical Scavenging Assay, and Folin-Ciocalteu Assay," *Journal of Agricultural and Food Chemistry*, Vol. 52, No. 8, 2004, pp. 2391-6. http://dx.doi.org/10.1021/jf035372g

[14] C. H. Tsai, *et al.*, "Rapid and Specific Detection of Hydroxyl Radical Using an Ultraweak Chemiluminescence Analyzer and a Low-Level Chemiluminescence Emitter: Application to Hydroxyl Radical-Scavenging Ability of Aqueous Extracts of Food Constituents," *Journal of Agricultural and Food Chemistry*, Vol. 49, No. 5, 2001, pp. 2137-2141. http://dx.doi.org/10.1021/jf001071k

[15] Y. Oyangui, "Reealuative of Assay Methods and Establishment of Kit for Superoxide Dismutase Activity," *Analytical Biochemistry*, Vol. 142, No. 2, 1984, pp. 290-296. http://dx.doi.org/10.1016/0003-2697, No. 84)90467-6

[16] J. B. Harborne and C. A. Williams, "Anthocyanins and Other Flavonoids," *Natural Product Reports*, Vol. 18, No. 3, 2001, pp. 310-333. http://dx.doi.org/10.1039/b006257j

[17] J. B. Harborne and C. A. Williams, "Advances in Flavonoid Research Since 1992," *Phytochemistry*, Vol. 55, No. 6, 2000, pp. 481-504. http://dx.doi.org/10.1016/S0031-9422(00)00235-1

[18] E. N. Frankel, A. L. Waterhouse and P. L. Teissedre, "Principal Phytochemicals in Selected California Wines and Their Antioxidant Activity in Inhibiting Oxidation of Human Low-Density Lipoproteins," *Journal of Agricul-*

tural and Food Chemistry, Vol. 43, No. 4, 1995, pp. 890-894. http://dx.doi.org/10.1021/jf00052a008

[19] G. Bartosz, "Total Antioxidant Capacity," In: H. E. Spiegel, Ed., *Advances in Clinical Chemistry*, Vol. 37, 2003, Academic Press, New York, pp. 219-292.

[20] I. F. F. Benzie, W. Y. Chung and J. J. Strain, "Antioxidant (Reducing) Efficiency of Ascorbate in Plasma Is Not Affected by Concentration," *The Journal of Nutritional Biochemistry*, Vol. 10, No. 3, 1999, pp. 146-150. http://dx.doi.org/10.1016/S0955-2863(98)00084-9

[21] D. Modun, *et al.*, "The Increase in Human Plasma Antioxidant Capacity after Red Wine Consumption Is Due to Both Plasma Urate and Wine Polyphenols," *Atherosclerosis*, 2007.

[22] V. Katalinic, *et al.*, "Screening of 70 Medicinal Plant Extracts for Antioxidant Capacity and Total Phenols," *Food Chemistry*, Vol. 94, No. 4, 2006, pp. 550-557. http://dx.doi.org/10.1016/j.foodchem.2004.12.004

[23] T. Nomura, *et al.*, "Proton-Donative Antioxidant Activity of Fucoxanthin with 1,1-Diphenyl-2-picrylhydrazyl (DPPH)," *Biochemistry and Molecular Biology International*, Vol. 42, No. 2, 1997, pp. 361-370.

[24] H. L. Madsen, *et al.*, "Screening of Antioxidantive Activity of Spices. A Comparison between Assays Based on ESR Spin Trapping and Electrochemical Measurement of Oxygen Consumption," *Food Chemistry*, Vol. 57, No. 2, 1996, pp. 331-337. http://dx.doi.org/10.1016/0308-8146(95)00248-0

[25] Q. Guo, *et al.*, "ESR and Cell Culture Studies on Free Radical-Scavenging and Antioxidant Activities of Isoflavonoids," *Toxicology*, Vol. 179, No. 1-2, 2002, pp. 171-180. http://dx.doi.org/10.1016/S0300-483X(02)00241-X

[26] L. E. Netto, *et al.*, "Reactive Cysteine in Proteins: Protein Folding, Antioxidant Defense, Redox Signaling and More. Comparative Biochemistry and Physiology," *Toxicology & Pharmacology: CBP*, Vol. 146, No. 1-2, 2007, pp. 180-193.

[27] A. Kardosová and E. Machová, "Antioxidant Activity of medicinal Plant Polysaccharides," *Fitoterapia*, Vol. 77, No. 5, 2006, pp. 367-373. http://dx.doi.org/10.1016/j.fitote.2006.05.001

[28] Y. C. Zhou and R. L. Zheng, "Phenolic Compounds and an Analog as Superoxide Anion Scavengers and Antioxidants," *Biochemical Pharmacology*, Vol. 42, No. 6, 1991, pp. 1177-1179. http://dx.doi.org/10.1016/0006-2952(91)90251-Y

[29] E. Grotewold, "The Science of Flavonoids," Springer Science & Business Media, Inc., New York, 2006, pp. 1-47.

Abbreviations

FRAP: ferric reducing/antioxidant power
GAE: gallic acid equivalent
IC$_{50}$: exact concentration providing 50% inhibition
BHT: butylated hydroxytoluene
DPPH•: the free radical of di(phenyl)-(2,4,6-trinitro-

phenyl)iminoazanium
ROS: reactive oxygen species
RNS: reactive nitrogen species
TPC: total phenolic content
CL: chemiluminescence

26

The Prospect of Application of Extractive Reference Substance of Chinese Herbal Medicines

Peishan Xie[1,2*], Shuangcheng Ma[3*], Pengfei Tu[4], Zhengtao Wang[5], Erich Stoeger[6], Daniel Bensky[7]

[1]Macau University of Science and Technology, Macau, China
[2]Guangdong UNION Biochemical Development Co. Ltd., Guangzhou, China
[3]National Institute for Food and Drug Control, Beijing, China
[4]Peking University Modern Research Center for Traditional Chinese Medicine, Beijing, China
[5]Shanghai University of Traditional Chinese Medicine, Shanghai, China
[6]Plantasia GmbH, Oberndorf, Austria
[7]Independent Scholar, Seattle, USA
Email: *psxie163@163.com, xps340112@gmail.com.com, *masc@nicpgbp.org.cn

ABSTRACT

The emerging development of Extractive Reference Substance (ERS) is a methodology that meets the needs for quality control for Chinese Herbal Medicines (CHM) and respects the holistic viewpoint of Traditional Chinese Medicine (TCM) and its clinical use of multiple ingredients with synergistic effects. The convention of using just a selected few Chemical Reference Substances (CRS) cannot adequately assess the quality of intact CHM. A validated chemical spectrum of an ERS provides the global characteristics in order to more specifically identify and assess targeted CHM. This paper describes the fundamental concepts, potential significance, and basic criteria of ERS, along with methods of preparation and calibration. Given the diversity of CHM, the various problems that will occur in establishing the proper process of ERS will need to be solved in a step by step manner. The ERSs of *Ziziphi spinosae* semen and ERS of *Fritillaria thunbergii* bulbus are given as examples of the development of ERS and demonstrate why we are optimistic about the utility of this approach.

Keywords: Extractive Reference Substance (ERS); Chinese Herbal Medicine (CHM); ERS R & D Strategy; Holistic Quality Control

1. Introduction

The "reference substances" are indispensable substances for assessing the quality of Chinese herbal medicines (CHM) and their products. Currently, there are two kinds of available reference substances applied to Pharmacopoeia of People's Republic of China (ChP)—Herbal Reference Substance (HRS) and Chemical Reference Substance (CRS). HRS is used for microscopic and thin-layer chromatographic identification, while CRS is used for chromatographic identification and quantitative determination. Decades of practical experience have demonstrated the positive roles of HRS and CRS in routine CHM quality control; however some drawbacks have also become clear. While HRS is unequivocally necessary for microscopic identification, it is unsatisfactory for chemical identification (e.g., TLC identification) because

of the fluctuation of the chemical composition between different individual substances. As for CRS, in addition to its merits for the attribution of the corresponding chemical compounds distributed in the herbal drugs, it acts as an external standard for assay of the target component [1]. The primary issues are limited varieties, less specificity for holistic identification of the complex composition of CHM, and expense and waste of natural resources. Furthermore, as widely argued, any arbitrarily selected CRS (chemical marker) is almost irrelevant to the synergic efficacy of an individual herbal drug, much less complex formulated herbal products [2-5]. The high cost and enormous waste of resources for obtaining a single pure CRS cannot be ignored. To make one gram of the pure chemical extract often requires dozens of kilograms of the herbal drug and an enormous amount of organic solvents. The final products of CRS are so costly that it is prohibitively expensive for testing some low-cost herbal

*Corresponding authors.

drugs. The higher purity is needed, the lower yield will be obtained, and the more expensive it will be for obtaining a single pure CRS. Moreover, the real signifycance of a few arbitrarily selected CRS for quality control of a multi-ingredient CHM is questionable at best. There is a consensus at present that the conventional QC approach must be changed. Recently, simultaneous determination of multiple components by HPLC has made rapid progress due to the increasingly sophisticated chromatography and MS^n detection technologies, and much more information relevant to the quality has been found [6-9]. However, the aforementioned principle problems on routine quality control still remain. On the other hand, the growing QC requirement of herbal drugs is challenging the drawbacks of CRS. So the adoption of the limited extractive reference substances (ERS) ("powdered extract" in USP) by the United States Pharmacopoeia (USP) aims to coordinate expediently with the QC requirement of the corresponding Dietary supplements in the USP. The ChP has now initiated the ERS program as a candidate of reference substances in the upcoming edition. Some researchers call the ERS as "Substitute reference substance" [10]. From the perspective of researchers, the use of ERS is not just an alternative reference substance, but an advanced approach for meaningful and comprehensive quality control to match the synergistic traits of CHM. As the secondary metabolites in the herbals, the bioactive ingredients compose the chemical pattern playing the role of fingerprint for identifying each taxonomic plant species; hence regardless of what isolated chemical markers are chosen as the targets for analysis, they will likely not be relevant to the synergistic mechanisms involved in the holistic approaches of TCM [11,12]. A full-view of a chemical profile of an ERS of the given CHM through chromatographic separation may sufficiently provide the evidence to assess the samples qualitatively and semi-quantitatively (see below). Therefore, ERS can be developed as a methodology for comprehensively oriented QC reference substances. To have the ERS of CHM mature into a fully formed method of quality control and identification, the criteria for developing the ERS of CHM need to be developed in a methodical manner. This paper presents the proposal and methodologies for how this can come to fruition.

2. Prerequisites for Establishment of ERS of CHM

Since the 1960s, the concept and the practice of quality control of Chinese herbal medicines (CHM) in the Chinese Pharmacopoeia (ChP) has followed the model of European herbal drugs in western pharmacopoeias like the British Pharmacopoeia (BP). In the 1960's, there were no other examples on how to formulate a reasonable quality standard for herbal medicines that could

serve as a precedent. While at that time the only feasible way was to emulate the quality standard monograph of chemical medicines, this concept and strategy for quality control was doomed as it was rooted in the reductionist mindset of a single-compound-oriented analysis. Common sense tells us no one chemical ingredient can be responsible for the synergic efficacy of a herbal drug. One of the traits of CHM is of diverse curative effects in the context of the composition of the various formulas. This makes it impossible to pinpoint a single specific bioactive molecule as being responsible for the efficacy of a given CHM. In recent years, along with the rapid development of multivariable analytical technologies, facilities and algorithms, the publication on simultaneous determination of multiple ingredients in CHM has exploded. The new techniques remain very expensive and will tend to exhaust the expensive and scarce chemical references substances without any more ability to truly appreciate and control the inherent quality of CHM, particularly if theses approach come into effect in routine QC. Such a prospect leads to anxiety in the herbal medicine industries although such kind of research would be welcomed in academic circles. Other open-minded herbal analysts have considered how to develop appropriate strategies that utilize multivariable analysis pragmatically in a holistic manner. It is well known that specific chemical patterns in a plant can be revealed by chromatographic analysis. The acquired chromatographic profile represents the unique character for the given species which is called "chromatographic fingerprint". The chromatographic fingerprint generated from authentic species sample can be recognized as the criterion for identification of the target species. Once the criterion is established, the chromatographic fingerprint of a standardized Extractive of the given species is being able to act as the Extractive Reference Substance (ERS). To keep the full-view of the fingerprint (peak numbers, peak-peak ratio, integrated peaks area of the column chromatography (HPLC, GC etc.) or the total color image of the Planar chromatography (HPTLC) as a whole is very effective for chemical identification and assessment of the inherent quality, particularly at the stage we are at present with a lack of sufficient knowledge about the chemical bioactivity of CHM. We cannot assume at present which peaks in the fingerprint are indispensable, which are complementary and which are inessential and can be ignored in most cases when they only exist in trace amounts. Moreover, as the understanding of how to use CHM is the result of experience accumulated over thousands of years, the holistic approach of traditional Chinese Medicine (TCM) must be respected. Given this, it is impossible to pinpoint any single molecule for being responsible for the diverse effects of a complex CHM formula, the principle way in which CHM is used TCM practitioners. Understanding the fundamental characteristics of CHM is the cornerstone of development of ERS of CHM.

3. ERS—The Brand—New Reference Substance in Holism Manner for Assessing the Quality of CHM

Unlike HRS and CRS, the ERS of CHM has not yet achieved the status of a standard in spite of such limited adoption by the USP and ChP. In part, this is due to the suspicion that it is not yet truly feasible to be widely implemented. This is a normal concern at the early stages of development of any technique. There will be a process of trial and error until the method has been validated and shown to be reproducible. It will not become the panacea protocol for QA/QC of CHM. But we should take an optimistic attitude toward its research and development potential, as it will bring a new approach to the field of CHM's QC/QA: a chromatographic fingerprint as a reference that makes comprehensive quality control possible. The majority of the TCM manufacturers have always manufactured Chinese proprietary products using crude drugs as the starting materials. Given this, inconsistencies of the quality of the final products can be predicted. Over the last decade, some new emerging Chinese medicine industries have adopted new technologies and are instead using the herbal drug extracts as the starting materials. That is certainly a good beginning to improve QC/QA. Meeting the need for effective quality control of new products, ERS is also a powerful reference substance for the in-process QC. ChP get ready to launch the program of ERS of herbal medicines for upcoming edition of the Pharmacopoeia, which will undoubtedly rapidly drive forward the development of ERS.

The advantages of the ERS of CHM include:
- It can reflect the total detectable chemical characteristics of the herbal drug from a holistic view.
- It can accordingly ensure the consistent distribution of chemical ingredients batch-to-batch of the CHM products.
- The chemically attributed components in the ERS can easily be used as an available alternative for some known CRS for identification, while the intact chemical profile can provide a much more detailed quality evaluation.
- The integration value of the ERS can be used as a simple semi-quantitative analysis for quick reference.
- It is a cost/effective reference substances in quality control of CHM

4. Basic Requirements of ERS

Any kind of reference substance must meet the four basic universal requirements: Authenticity, Specificity, Consistency and Stability (ASCS). Focusing on the ERS, the primary requirements would be defined as follows: 1) The chromatographic fingerprint could reflect that of the original herbal drug, for example, the TLC image (fingerprint) of ERS basically conforms to that of the original drug. This fullfils the requirements for authenticity and specificity; 2) The physical appearance of the ERS must be robust, because most herbal drugs contain various hygroscopic components that are prone to soften and become sticky, so that the dry-powdered ERS deform. Therefore, keeping the ERS's appearance consistent is very important. The proper extraction technology should be carried out carefully to balance the diverse ingredients and principle components and be comparable with the chromatographic profiles of the original crude drugs, as well as maintaining a consistent appearance for the final ERS products. In order to fulfill the real needs, the ERS for identification and for full functionality (qualitative and quantitative) needs to take into account all four aspects of "ASCS", dealing with each aspect in turn to ensure that this project develops steadily.

Authenticity (A): Logically, the most basic source of the authenticated species of an herbal drug is from its original natural habitat. In reality, some of the so-called exemplary habitats (daodi in Chinese) have been migrating over time. For example, the exemplary habitat of the famous species of Di-Huang (Rehmannia radix) was originally in the Shanxi province of the north-west zone of China in ancient times, but it had migrated to Henan province in the Central plains zone of China by the early Ming Dynasty (1368-1644 AC). So nowadays, people know Henan province (Huaiqing county) as the exemplary habitat of Di-Huang. In the wake of increasing demand in recent decades, the area where Di-Huang is cultivated has been extended to a rather wide region. Furthermore, some Good Agriculture Practice (GAP) bases have been established beyond the original region. On the other hand, some of the original exemplary habitats of some Chinese herbal drugs have suffered environmental contamination resulting is a significant loss of quality. Additionally, as farmers have migrated to the cities, some areas that used to grow herbal drugs have been left uncultivated. Some examples of commonly-used Chinese herbal drugs that are still cultivated in the traditional exemplary habitats like Dang-Gui (Angelicae sinensis radix), Chuan-Xiong (Chuanxiong rhizoma), Bai-Zhi (Angelicae dahuricae radix), Gan-Cao (Glycyrrhizae radix et rhizoma) and Fu-Zi (Aconiti lateralis radix praeparata).

Wild-crafted Chinese herbal drugs have gradually declined due to overharvesting along with a decrease in their habitats, to the point where some have become endangered species. Therefore, we need to let go of any dogma regarding exemplary habitats given the reality of the situation today. While it is still preferable to collect samples of a given species from its traditional exemplary habitat if possible, often this is no longer practical and the next best approach is to obtain sufficient samples from the wholesale herbal drug markets in the main cities to ensure that they represent the main stream of the herbal distribution.

Ensuring authenticity is the first priority when dealing with the samples collected from outside the exemplary habitats. The basic testing should be carried out according to the standard in Chinese Pharmacopoeia including subjective observation of the appearance, the taste and smell, as well as chemical identification, testing and assay if necessary. Only the qualified samples can be involved in the list of candidates. It is worth noting that different samples from different habitat may have quite different chemical compositions. Sometimes, we may look at an unexpected astonishing picture in individual cases [13] (**Figure 1**).

Specificity (S): The ERS produced from the candidates of the given species must present a chemical ingredient pattern similar to the original crude drug in order to be considered of adequate quality. It has been well known that the most practical approach to this is to conduct chromatographic fingerprint analysis. Thin-layer chromatography method is preferred, as instant comparison is possible via the picture-like TLC image. A rough estimate can be done rapidly of the similarity among the sample images on the same plate via comparative observation of the bands numbers, band positions (Rf values), color and intensity (**Figure 2**); scanning profiles of the HPTLC images via corresponding digital software can be further comparative observation in detail and make more convincing assessment by similarity analysis [14] (**Figures 3** and **4**). HPLC fingerprint can be also applied for identification if necessary. Generally the validated chemical fingerprint of the ERS is sufficient to meet this basic requirement of an authentic herbal drug.

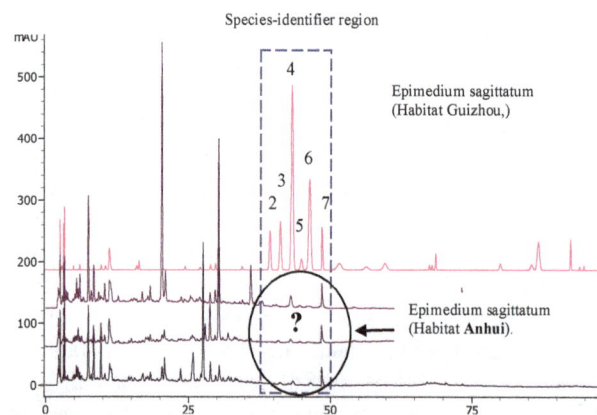

Figure 1. HPLC fingerprint of Epimedii herba (*Yin-Yang-Huo*) grown in different habitats. (2) epimedin A, (3) epimedin B, (4) epimedin C, (6) icariin. The three samples from the Anhui province showed none of the main bioactive flavonoids detected in "species Identifier region" of its HPLC fingerprint.

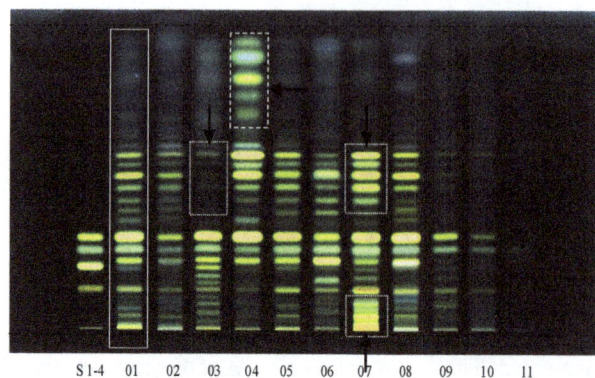

Figure 2. HPTLC fluorescence image of Bupleuri Radix (*Chai-Hu*). (S1): saikosaponin f; (S2) saikosaponin b2; (S3) saikosaponin a; (S4) saikosaponin d; (01) *Bupleurum chinense* DC.; (02) *B. scorzonerifolium* Willd; (03) *B. longiradiatum* Turcz; (04) *B. bicaule* Helm; (05) *B. polyclonum* Y. Li et S. L. Pan; (06) *B. wenchuanense* Shan et Y. Li (07) *B. marginatum* Wall. ex DC. var. *stenophyllum* (Wolff) Shan et Y. Li; (08) *B. falcatum* L; (09) *B. yinchowense* Shan et Y. Li; (10) *B. simithii* Wolff. var. *parvifolia* Shan et Y. Li; (11) *B. tenue* Huch. -Ham. ex D. Don. *Samples (01)-(09) roots; (10) (11) aerial parts.

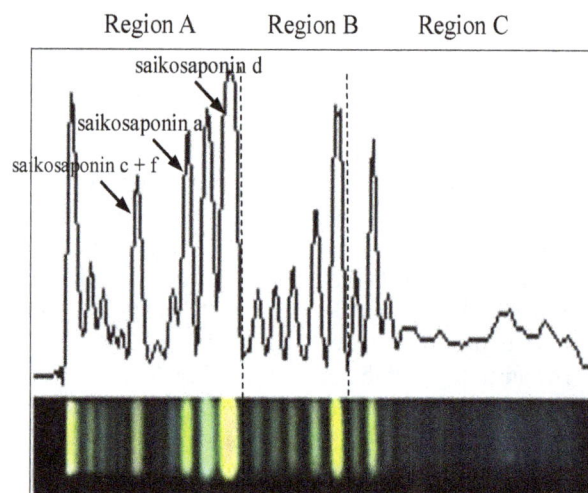

Figure 3. The digital scanning profile of the HPTLC fluorescence image of Bupleuri radix (Chai-Hu). (A): main saikosaponins region; (B): inter-species identifier region; (C) low-polarity region.

Consistency (C): A worrisome problem for ERS is inconsistencies between the chemical profiles of different batches. Therefore it is often a necessity to blend different batches of the ERS for adjustment of the ratio to reach a relatively consistent composition of the chemical ingredients based on the established common pattern of the chromatographic fingerprint and the semi-quantifiable data of the ERS.

Stability (S): The ERS must be sufficiently stable during the storage period. The tests for stability should therefore be conducted rigorously. Particularly, the phy-

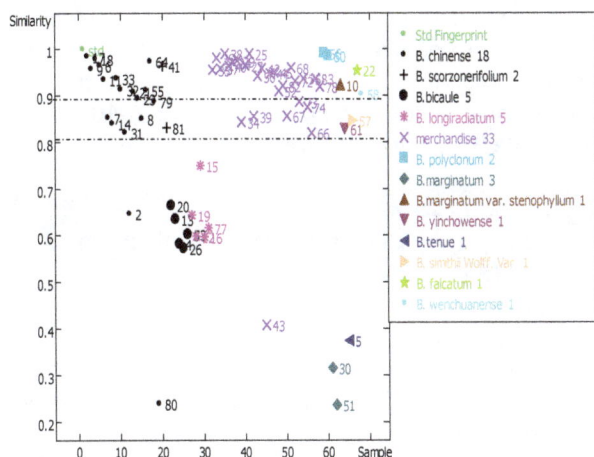

Figure 4. Similarity analysis of HPTLC fingerprint of Chai-Hu.

sical appearance of the ERS must be well preserved. Generally, stickiness or softening of the appearance of ERS that occurs during storage are common problems. The solution to such problems will rely on proper extractive technologies, packaging, and storage environments. Generally, some clean-up procedures have to be done in most cases during the preparation process, so we should as far as possible balance what needs to be removed and what needs to be retained. For example, proteins, sugars, some tannins might generally be removed during the process.

In brief, the acceptable ERS should conform to the following requirements:

- A qualified ERS must be produced from authenticated samples of the reliable habitat and include sufficient samples from various sites. Consistent raw material is necessary.
- The detected chemical composition in the ERS must be as similar as possible to that in the original herbal drug. It means that the appearance of the HPTLC image or the major composition of the HPLC profile should be fairly similar to that of original herbal drugs.
- The chemical ingredients inter-batches must be generally consistent (it works when comparing between the HPLC fingerprint or the HPTLC image). If large amount of samples need to be compared concomitantly, the similarity analysis might be conducted, then the similarity between the batches of ERS should be assumed of >0.9 (calculated by cosine or correlated coefficient) among batches.
- The physical state of the ERS must be stable during storage. The extractives of most CHM are quite hygroscopic. This is the major problem during storage to which particular attention must be paid during the production stage. The volatile oils in the herbal drugs

will be very unstable once it is extracted by e.g., steam-distillation. Special approach for its stability need to be developed.

- A fully functional ERS requires calibration of the contents of the specified markers (cf. Section 8).

5. Preparation of ERS of CHM

In principle, aqueous extraction is the closest simulation of aqueous decoction practiced in TCM. However, the traditional aqueous TCM decoction contains not only water-soluble components but also some insoluble substances in suspension as the decoction is ingested without prior fine filtration. A clear aqueous solution of the herbal drugs made in the laboratory, therefore, is not equivalent to the TCM decoction. Using 60% - 70% methanol or ethanol extraction is the reasonable protocol to approximate the real-world decoctions. The alternative option, if necessary, is to prepare two kinds of extracts; lipophilic and hydrophilic fractions depending on the need. Some special cases with special extraction procedure should be done according to those methods that have been developed previously.

The preparation procedure of ERS includes extraction, concentration and the final formation of the ERS. In addition to the conventional extraction methods, the eco-friendly extraction methods including ultrasonic, pressurized-solvent speed extraction, smashing tissue extraction, and High-performance, High-pressure, differentially Low-temperature Successive Extraction (HHLS). This last can could be selected if the method can bear the scale of the bulk products. Some clean-up steps need to be conducted with careful and reasonable measures. No matter which method is adopted, in-process quality control must be conducted. Which method of extraction is to be selected for use will depend on the properties of the particular herb to tailor-make the ERS of targeted herbal drug which is also a matter of trial and error. One final step is the stability test. Needless to say, the storage location should have a low temperature, low humidity, and be dark. In brief, no matter which preparation method was selected, the ultimate concern would focus on whether can the final ERS products guarantee the four essential principles—Authenticity, Specificity Consistency, and Stability (ASCS).

6. Establishing the Specification of the ERS Finished Product

The ERS of CHM must be certified. The typical characteristics should be validated with TLC, HPLC or GC fingerprint. The standard procedure and methodology should also be validated. The characteristics of the ERS and the chromatographic fingerprint are presented together with the certification of its equivalence with the crude drug of the original species (raw material). The specification of ERS includes the name of the entity, the equivalent ratio of ERS/raw material, description, identification, test, assay (for full-functional ERS) and storage.

Referring to the volatile ingredients (essential oils) of the herbal drug, particularly the monoterpenes or sesquiterpenes, the chemical pattern of which are unstable, the chemical pattern would seriously fluctuate and the end product will be hard to finalize, so it is almost impossible to provide usable ERS of volatile ingredients of herbal drugs. A tentative fresh-prepared the extractive as reference by using a small sealed pouch pack of the powdered authentic raw material in reserve might be an option (Solvent extraction should be feasible).

7. Examples of the Process and Application of ERS

The ERS of *Suan-Zao-Ren* (*Ziziphi spinosae* semen) and *Zhe-Bei-Mu* (*Fritillariae thunbergi* bulbus) are used here as examples to demonstrate a basis for the establishment of the ERS of CHM.

7.1. ERS of *Ziziphi spinosae* Semen) (ERS Suan-Zao-Ren)

Monograph of Chinese herbs "Extractive Reference Substances" (ERS).

ERS of *Ziziphi spinosae* semen (defatted).
ERS of *Suan-Zao-Ren* (defatted)—(SZR-ERS).
Code number: SZR-RSE 2012-02 (ERS 3).

7.1.1. Definition

Defatted extract of *Ziziphi spinosae* semen for use as the Extractive Reference Substance (ERS) of Ziziphi spinosae semen. The ERS of *Ziziphi spinosae* semen (Chinese name: *Suan-Zao-Ren)* is a light grayish brown dry powder, which is 70% ethanol extraction of defatted seeds of *Ziziphus jujuba* Mill. var. *spinosa* (Bunge) Hu ex H.F. Chou (Rhamnaceae). The amount of the final product is

converted to the equivalent amount of the raw material as per the extraction ratio. The ratio of the ERS to the raw material is approximately 1:14 (g, ERS/g, crude drug).

It contains spinosin 14 mg/g; jujuboside A 10.5 mg/g; jujuboside B 5.5 mg/g (**Figure 5**).

7.1.2. Identification

1) Thin-layer chromatography identification (ChP 2010 Ed) (**Figure 6**).
2) Criteria:

The test is not valid unless the visible color TLC image of the ERS sample shows high similarity (>0.9, correlation coefficient). light grayish brown to bluish green bands of jujuboside A (Rf ca. 0.16) and jujuboside B (Rf ca. 3.3) to that of the crude drug sample solution; in addition, several other weak saponin bands as well as the residual seed oil band on the front of the image also appear. Under UV 366 nm light, a light yellowish blue fluorescence band corresponds to spinosin CRS (Rf ca. 0.44), accompanied by one just above the spinosin band and three weak fluorescence bands lower than the spinosin band as those appeared in the crude drug sample solution.

7.1.3. Consistency

More than ten batches of ERS of *Ziziphi spinosae* semen have been checked qualitatively and quantitatively.

Carry out the method for HPLC fingerprint (optional) (**Figure 7**).

Assay Chromatographic Conditions: According to the method in ChP 2010 ed [6].

7.2. ERS of *Fritillariae thunbergi* Bulbus) (ZBM-ERS) (ERS Zhe-Bei-Mu)

Monograph of Chinese herbs "Extractive Reference Substances" (ERS).

ERS of *Fritillariae thunbergii* bulbus.
ERS of *Zhe-Bei-Mu*—(ZBM-ERS).
Code number: ZBM-ERS 2012-04.

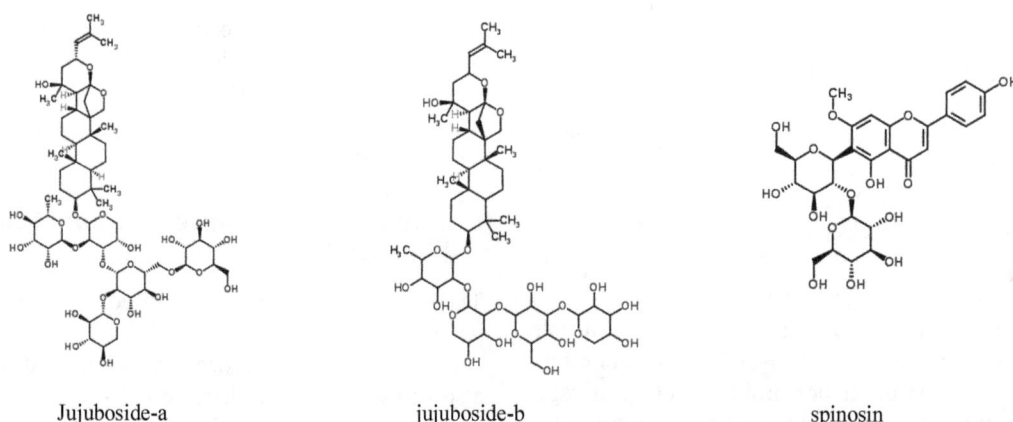

| Jujuboside-a | jujuboside-b | spinosin |

Figure 5. The chemical structures of main saponins and flavonoid in *Ziziphi spinosae* semen (Suan-Zao-Ren).

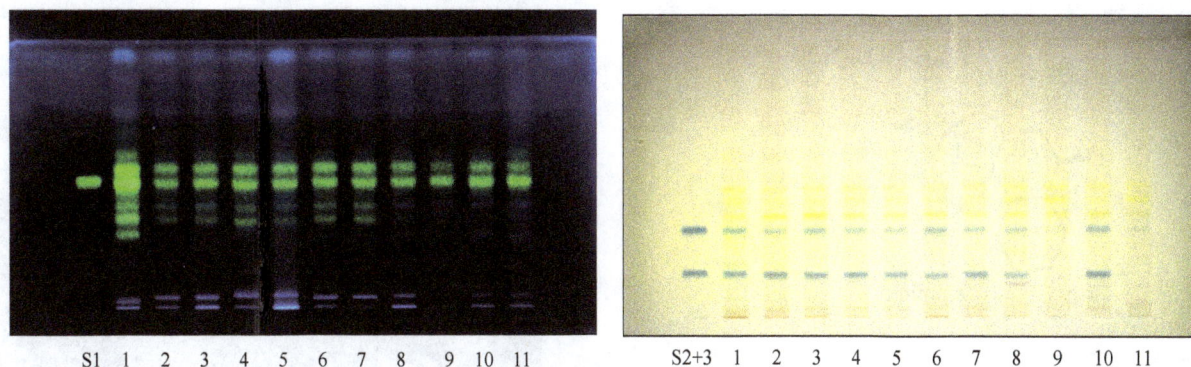

Figure 6. HPTLC images of *Ziziphi spinosae* semen (Suan-Zao-Ren). Above: fluorescence image of the flavonoids; Lower: visible color image of the saponin: (S1) spinosin; (S2) jujuboside A; (S3) jujuboside B; (1) ERS of defatted *Ziziphi spinosae* semen; (2)-(8) (10) commercial samples of *Ziziphi spinosae* semen; (9) (11): Adulterant (Ziziphi mauritianae semen). The HPTLC fluorescence (flavonoids) and visible color (saponin) images of the ERS of *Ziziphi spinosae* semen show that the authenticity and specificity of the ERS of *Ziziphi spinosae* semen are acceptable for a reference substance.

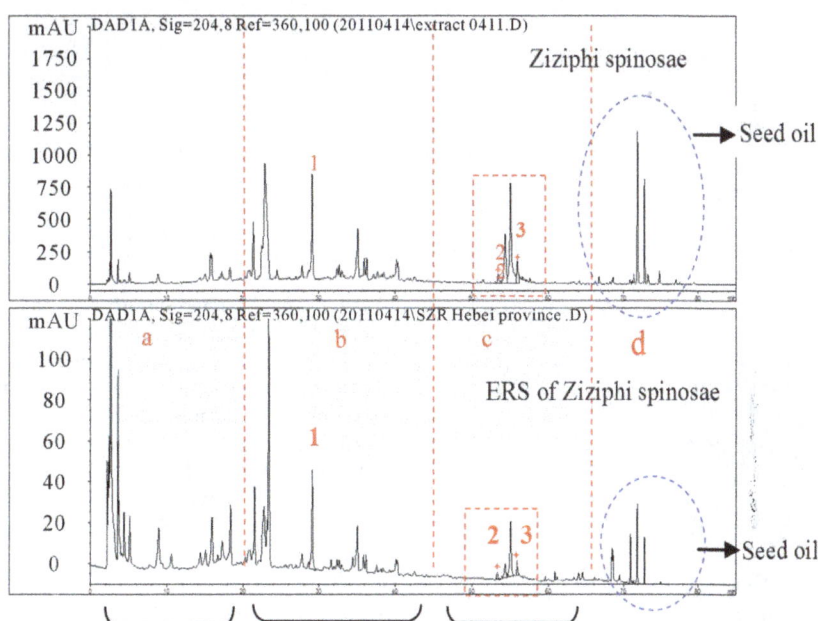

Figure 7. HPLC-DAD fingerprint of *Ziziphi spinosae* semen (above) and the ERS sample (lower). Peak (1): spinosin; (2): jujuboside (a); (3) jujuboside (b). The fingerprint can be divided into four sections for easy reorganization of the fingerprint's intact features. (a) alkaloids section; (b) flavonoids section; (c) saponin section; (d) seed oil section.

7.2.1. Definition

Extract of *Fritillariae thunbergii bulbus* (EFTB) for use as Extractive Reference Substance (ERS of *Fritillariae thunbergii* Bulbus). The EFTB is light yellowish gray dry powder, which is 70% ethanol extraction of the bulb of *Fritillaria thunbergii* Miq. The amount of the final product is converted to the equivalent amount of the bulb raw material as per the extraction ratio. The ratio of the ERS to the raw material is approximately 1: 10 (g/g).

It contains peimine 5.7 mg/g; peiminine 5.0 mg/g (**Figure 8**).

7.2.2. Identification

Carry out the method for thin-layer chromatography

(ChP 2010 Ed.) (**Figures 9** and **10**).

Criteria: should demonstrate the same TLC pattern to the HRS's HPTLC image in which peimine (S1) and peiminine (S2) dominate with another light brownish orange band just above the band of peimine when sprayed with Dragendorff reagent and viewed under white light. The fluorescence image of EFTB generated by spraying 10% sulfuric acid ethanol solution observed under UV 366 nm is also very similar to that of the crude drug which consisted of about 10 fluorescence bands. That means the EFTB can be used as a reference substance for identification.

Confirmation: For testing the feasibility of this process, 11 batches of *Fritillariae thunbergii* bulbus (**FTB**) were

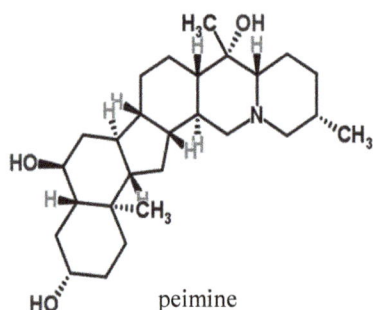

peimine

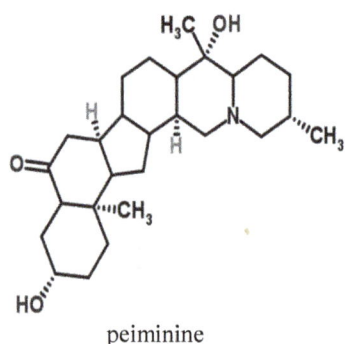

peiminine

Figure 8. Chemical structure of alkaloids—peimine and pei-minine.

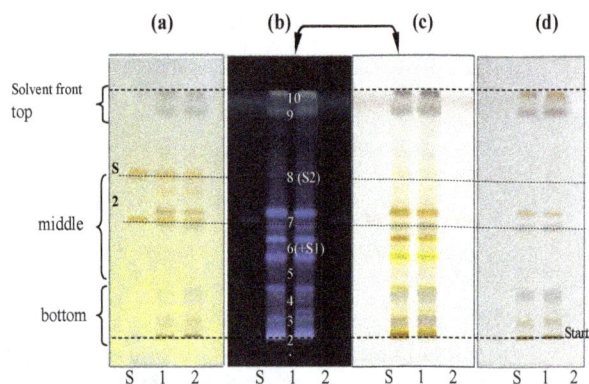

Figure 9 HPTLC images of ERS of *Fritillarae thunbergii* bulbus (Zhe-Bei-Mu) (1) and crude drug of *Fritillarae thunbergii* bulbus (2). (a): visualized by spraying Dragendorff reagent, (b): fluorescence under UV 365 nm after spraying sulfuric acid reagent, (c): the invert color image of (b); (d): visible image generated by spraying sulfuric acid reagent under white light. The main alkaloids—peimine (S1 ≈ band 6*, Rf ca. 0.46; and peiminine (S2 = band 8, Rf ca.0.65) stained brown bands with Dragendorff reagent. *The location of Peimine is very near to band 6 or they even overlap. The intact Fluorescence image consisted of mainly 10 blue or grayish blue fluorescence bands combined with the visible alkaloids image (a) constructed the characteristic fingerprint of FTB, the ERS of FTB (EFTB) provided very similar image with the crude drug. The legible invert color image (c) transformed from the fluorescence image (b) aided for more distinct observation.

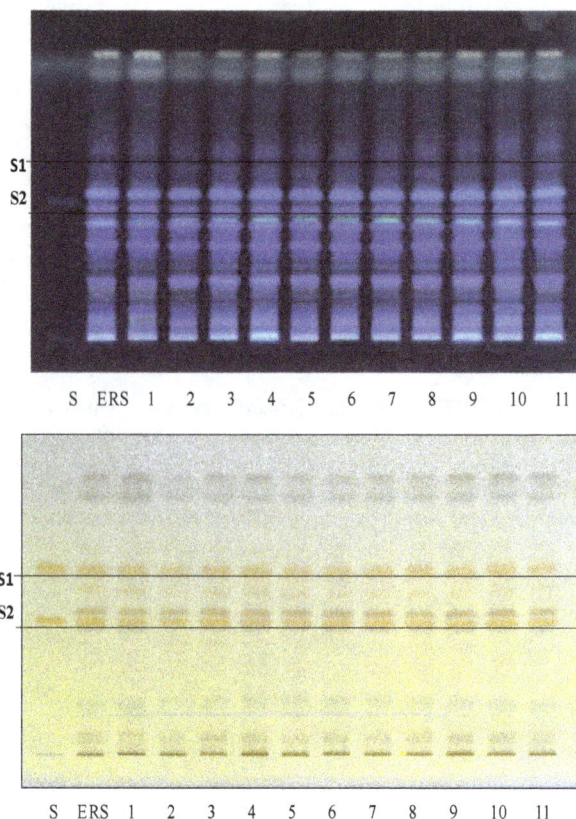

Figure 10. Application of ERS of Fritillariae thunbergii bulbus to 10 batches of Chinese herbal medicine—crude drug of Fritillariae thunbergii bulbus (FTB) T: 21℃ RH: 50%. (a)Fluorescence image after spraying 10% sulfuric acid/ethanol solution; (b) Visible color image of plate after spraying Dragendorff's reagent. (S1) = peimine; (S2) = pei-minine; Track (1) ERS of FTB; (2)-(11) commercial crude drug—FTB The images show that the authenticity and spe-cificity of the ERS of FTB are acceptable for a reference substance.

analyzed with the **EFTB** on the same plate, sample preparation and application was carried out quantita-tively; the result showed the pattern of **EFTB**'s image was basically as same as that of the crude drug **FTB**.

HPLC fingerprint of ERS of FTB provided a rather simple profile. As the main alkaloids, peimine and pei-minine were clearly separated. It can be quantitafied by external standard method for determining their contents (**Figure 11**).

8. Quantification Issue of ERS

The use of herbal reference extractive (=ERS) instead of pure reference substance for quantitative analysis is con-troversial. The issue in question is the nonequivalence between the herbal extractive reference and the corre-sponding pure substance due to the uncertain assigned value of the analyte, chromatographic resolution and stability [15]. Most analysts have also taken for granted

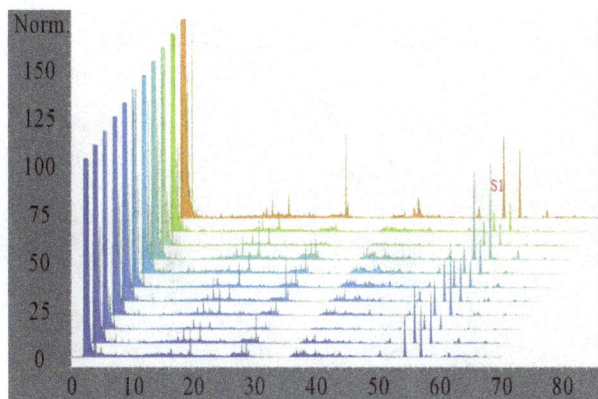

Figure 11. HPLC fingerprint of 11 batches of FTB express high similarity (cosine > 0.9) compared with ERS of FTB (S1: peimine, S2: peiminine).

that one should determine a single chemical marker precisely and accurately in a herbal drug as one does the chemical pharmaceuticals. This would be true if ERS for herbal quality control was synonymous with the CRS for QC of pure chemical medicine or natural single component product. However, the situation of CHM is completely different. Determining a chemical marker for the purpose of use in TCM has to take into consideration the fact that any chemical marker is just a few parts per thousand or even a few parts per ten thousand, when the intake dose of a prescribed herbal medicine is generally 10 - 30 g, even bigger, per potion as part of a compound formula that commonly uses 6 - 12 ingredients. This situation is obviously completely different than those that inolve pure chemical pharmaceuticals. In other words, it makes no sense to treat the herbal drug exactly the same as a chemical medicine [16]. This brings us to a fundamental question: what is the real important of determining accurately and precisely such a minute amount of one or few chemical marker(s) in a herbal medicine (except for toxic ingredients)?

We suggest that it is necessary to work out the appropriate and meaningful quantitative measurements in regards to Chinese herbal medicines. In fact, all accepted external standard quantitative determinations rely on the chromatographic integrated raw data (peak area). Why not use the integrated peak area under quantitative operation conditions to rapidly estimate the semi-quantity of the contents of the all peaks or appointed peaks at the same time as performing the chromatographic fingerprint? This would be an easy, rapid, and economical approach. The raw data is rough but practically reliable and useful. One example of its utility is demonstrated by the possibility of semi-quantitative estimation of the bioactive flavonoids in Epimedium leaves through chromatographic integrated data. It is well known that the C-8-prenylated flavonoids are special bioactive contents in *Epimedium*

spp. with the main ones being epimedin A, epimedin B, epimedin C and Icariin, (ABCI). A set of integrative peaks area of ABCI acquired from HPLC fingerprint demonstrated the ratio of ABCI peaks being concordant with the precisely determined content by external standard assay [13] (**Figure 12**). Other examples—Coptidis Rhizoma and Ginseng Radix are shown herewith the same expected results (**Figures 13** and **14**). The only issue with this is how to set the measurement unit to make it generally acceptable. Furthermore, it would be possible for the quantitative determination of some appointed peaks by means of calibrated ERS, in which some known chemical components were determined by external standards [10]. Of course, a good resolution of the target peak and good reproducibility is the prerequisite for this method's utility. There is an example for comparison of the quantitative determinations between using CRS and ERS to determine the contents of spinosin, jujuboside A and jujuboside B in *Ziziphi spinosae* semen (*Suan-Zao-Ren*). The primary results seem acceptable in terms of herbal medicines (**Table 1**).

On the quantitative analysis, Helliwell practically suggested that the key consideration on the quantification by using Herbal Drug Preparation Reference Standard (≈RES), the content of specified constituent(s) is not an absolute value, but an assigned value determined by a specified method [17]. Our testing results by using the aforementioned method exemplified the feasibility of such a suggestion.

Our argument is that application of ERS is a more meaningful strategy for identification and semi-quantification for herbal drug quality assessment. It is true that there is still work to be done to improve the preparation and application of ERS to QA/QC for chromatographic identification and rapid quantifiable estimation and see how it can be performed in a cost-effective way. There are of course other problems that will need to be solved through trial and error, so that it is necessary to go forward one step at a time. As the saying goes that "the perfect can be the enemy of the good enough".

9. Discussion

The ERS of CHM is a new methodology as well as a subject of much debate. The first issue might be what the criterion is for pragmatic useful ERS. The essential feature of the qualified ERS for identification is that it should be able to represent consistently the detected intact characteristics of the original crude drug expressed by the chromatographic fingerprint. The chemical attribution of the elements in the profile can be pinpointed by advanced technologies combined with available CRS. Considering the variety and complexity of CHM, it would be unwarranted hurdle at the early stage if over-

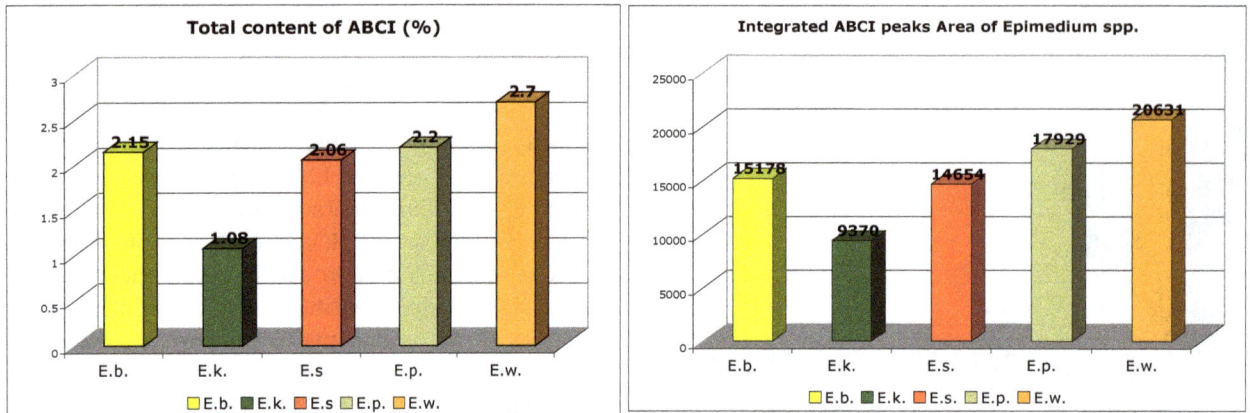

Figure 12. The comparative results of the contents of the total four C-8-prenylated flavonoids (ABCI) in epimedi herba. Light: External standard method; Right: the HPLC integrated peaks area.

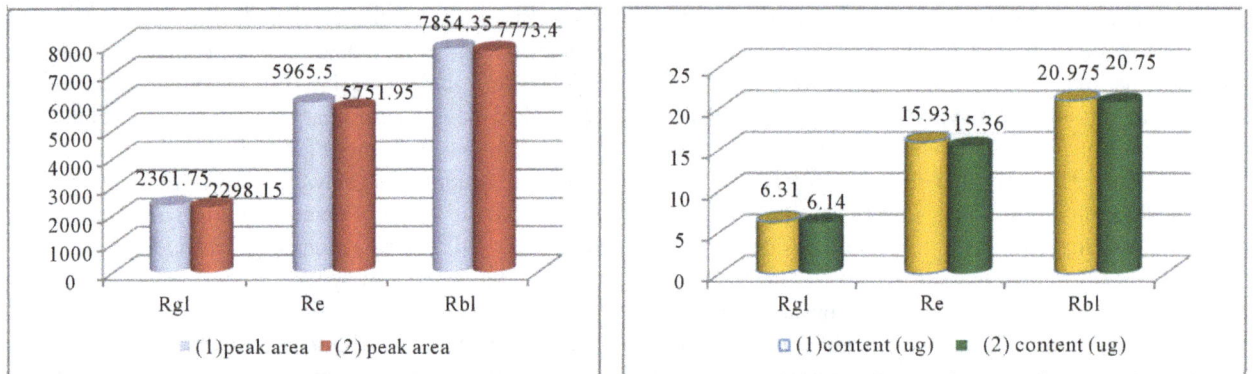

Figure 13. Comparison between integrated raw data (peak area) and external standard determination for assessing the quality of main ginsenosids in Extractive Ginseng.

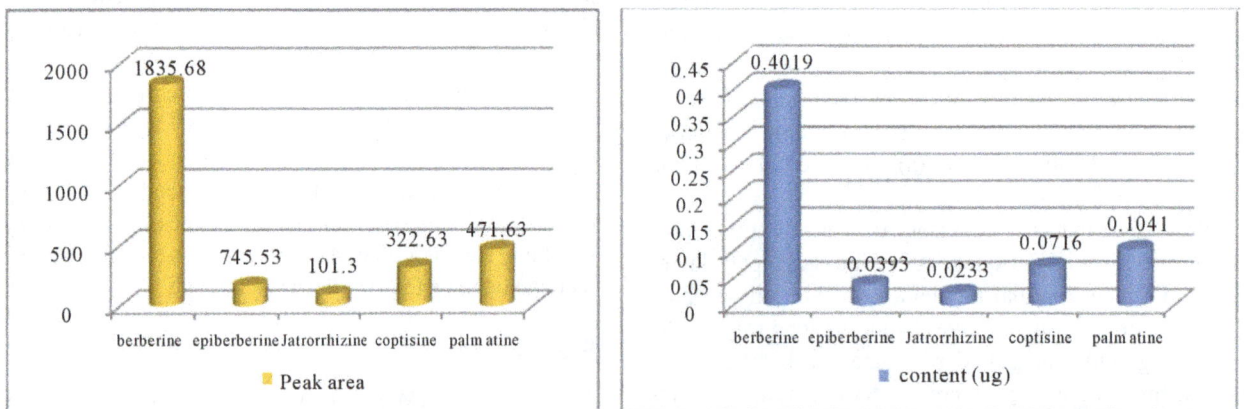

Figure 14. Comparison of the quantitative assessing between integrated raw data (peak area) and external standard method of five alkaloids in Extract of Coptidis. A rapid estimation of the contents of the five alkaloids, reading HPLC peak area value is comparable with the conventional external standard determination.

emphasizing the desire of chemical attribution in an ERS; successive exploration requires sustainable research. To be useful ERS will need to be done in a flexible manner so that it can be tailored to different situations for various types of samples. A "one-size fits all" would be impractical. The practical, economical, and relatively easily

accomplished nature of ERS is a factor pushing this approach forward, particularly for the commercial and industrial field of CHM. We need to keep in mind that the conceptual integrity of the medicine and the fuzziness of many problems will direct the research and application of ERS works in concert with effective quality control of

Table 1. Table type styles (Table caption is indispensable).

	the content (% crude drug) a		
	By CRS	By ERS	RSD
spinosin	0.0632	0.0634	0.16
Jujuboside A	0.0523	0.0531	0.76
Jujuboside B	0.0268	0.0287	3.47

[a]Using the routine external standard determination method.

CHM. Preparing a qualified practical and economical ERS of CHM requires a certain amount of expertise and diligence. Referring to the full-functional ERS, a rapid quantifiable estimation of the bioactive fraction of the whole using acquired integration data from the chromatographic fingerprint is a practical issue. Calibrating the appointed target peaks in the ERS to serve as CRS to determine the sample tested is worth investigating.

10. Conclusion

There is a fundamental difference in outlook between the antagonistic-oriented approach of single chemical pharmaceuticals and the orientation of TCM towards balancing the human body's function. Strategies of meaningful quality control need to take into account the complexity of CHM. No work into the safety and efficacy can afford to ignore the synergic action exerted by multi-ingredients in the herbals according to TCM constructs. Research and application of ERS, a standardized extractive with its detectable chemical pattern for a given species, are becoming a new trend for reference substances used for herbal medicine quality control. The criteria on the ERS of CHM should pursue the Authenticity, Specificity, Consistency and Stability (ASCS) in a holistic manner. Overcoming the inertia generated by dogma needs to be done as soon as possible to achieve real meaningful quality control of Chinese herbal medicines.

11. Acknowledgements

We appreciate our team members, Shuai Sun, Li Shao, He Li, Ruiyin Wang, Longgang Guo, Tao Kang and Xiaofeng Li, for their participation in the experiments on preparation and quality analysis of ERS cited in this paper. We also thank David Glyn Pinder for his editing assistance.

REFERENCES

[1] S. L. Li, Q. B. Han, C. F. Qiao, J. Z. Song, C. L. Cheng and H. X. Xu, "Chemical Markers for the Quality Control of Herbal Medicines: An Overview," *Chinese Medicine*, Vol. 3, No. 7, 2008, pp. 1-16.

[2] A. Y. Leung, "Tradition- and Science-Based Quality Control of Chinese Medicines—Introducing the Phyto-True System," *Journal of AOAC International*, Vol. 93,

No. 5, 2010, pp. 1355-1366.

[3] P.-S. Xie and A. Y. Leung, "Understanding the Traditional Aspect of Chinese Medicine in Order to Achieve Meaningful Quality Control of Chinese Materia Medica," *Journal of Chromatography A*, Vol. 1216, No. 11, 2009, pp. 1933-1940.
http://dx.doi.org/10.1016/j.chroma.2008.08.045

[4] P. S. Xie, "The Basic Requirement for Modernization of Chinese Herbal Medicine, Ping-Chung Leung , Annals of Traditional Chinese Medicine, Current Review of Chinese Medicine—Quality Control of Herbs and Herbal Material, 2," Chapter 1, 2006, pp. 1-10.

[5] S. S. Chitlange, "Chromatographic Fingerprint Analysis for Herbal Medicines: A Quality Control Tool," Pharmainfo.net, 2008. http://www.pharmainfo.net/

[6] S. L. Li, Y. X. Wang, L. H. Sheng and L. Yi, "Quality Evaluation of Radix Astragali through a Simultaneous Determination of Six Major Active Isoflavonoids and Four Main Saponins by High-Performance Liquid Chromatography Coupled with Diode Array and Evaporative Light Scattering Detectors," *JCA*, Vol. 1134, No. 1-2, 2006, pp. 162-169.
http://dx.doi.org/10.1016/j.chroma.2006.08.085

[7] X. J. Chen, H. Ji, Q. W. Zhang, P. F. Tu, Y. T. Wang, B. L. Guo and S. P. Li, "A Rapid Method for Simultaneous Determination of 15 Flavonoids in Epimedium Using Pressurized Liquid Extraction and Ultra-Performance Liquid Chromatography," *JPBA*, Vol. 46, No. 2, 2008, pp. 226-235.

[8] C. L. Fan, J. W. Deng, Y. Y. Yang, J. S. Liu, Y. Wang, X. Q. Zhang, K. C. Fai, Q. W. Zhang and W. C. Ye, "Multi-Ingredients Determination and Fingerprint Analysis of Leaves From Ilex Latifolia Using Ultra-Performance Liquid Chromatography Coupled with Quadrapole Time-of-Flight Mass Sepctrometry," *JPBA*, Vol. 84, 2013, pp. 20-29.

[9] S. P. Li, C. M. Lai, Y. X. Gong, K. K. W. Kan, T. T. X. Dong, K. W. K. Tsim and Y. T. Wang, "Simultaneous Determination of Ergosterol, Nucleosides and Their Bases from Natural and Cultured Cordyceps by Pressurised Liquid Extraction and High-Performance Liquid Chromatography," *JCA*, Vol. 1036, No. 2, 2004, pp. 239-243.

[10] P. Yu, S. Lei, H. Y. Jing and S. C. Ma, "Discussion on Application and Technical Requirements of Substitute Refeemce Substance Method for Simultaneous Determination of Multi-Components in Traditional Chinese Medicine," *Chin. J. Pharm. Anal*, Vol. 33, No. 1, 2013, pp. 169-177.

[11] J. S. Zhang and C. H. Lu, "Philisophical Origins of Source of Traditional Medicine's Holism and Western Medicine's Reductionism," *Journal of Anhui Traditioanal Chinese Medicine College* (in Chinese), Vol. 18, No. 1, 1999, pp. 1-3.

[12] X. D. Tang and W. W. Wang, "TCM Research: Cultural Collision and System Biology," *World Science and Technology/Modernization of Traditionl Chinese Medicine and Materia Medica* (in Chinese), Vol. 9, No. 1, 2007, pp. 119-122.

[13] P. S. Xie, Y.-Z. Yan, B.-L. Guo, C. W. K. Lam, S. H.

Chui and Q.-X. Yu, "Chemical Pattern-Aided Classification to Simplify the Intricacy of Morphological Taxonomy of Epimedium Species Using Chromatographic Fingerprinting," *Journal of Pharmaceutical and Biomedical Analysis*, Vol. 52, No. 4, 2010, pp. 452-460. http://dx.doi.org/10.1016/j.jpba.2010.01.025

[14] R.-T. Tian, P.-S. Xie and H.-P. Liu, "Evaluation of Traditional Chinese Herbal Medicine: Chaihu (*Bupleuri radix*) by Both High-Performance Liquid Chromatographic and High-Performance Thinlayer Chromatographic Fingerprint and Chemometic Analysis," *Journal of Chromatography A*, Vol. 1216, No. 11, 2009, pp. 2150-2155.

http://dx.doi.org/10.1016/j.chroma.2008.10.127

[15] P. S. Xie and S. P. Li, "Chapter 2: Back to the Future in Quality Control of Chinese Herbal Medicines/Quality Control: Developments, Methods and Applications," Nova Science Publishing Co. Ltd., 2013, pp. 47-68.

[16] M. Schwarz, B. Klier and H. Sievers, "Herbal Reference Standards," Planta Medica, No. 75, 2009, pp. 689-703.

[17] K. Helliwell, "Herbal reference Standards (Reader's Tribute)," *Pharmeuropa*, Vol. 18, No. 2, 2006, pp. 235-238.

Abbreviations

ChP = Pharmacopoeia of the Peoples Republic of China
CHM = Chinese Herbal Medicine
TCM = Traditional Chinese Medicine
CRS = Chemical Reference Substance
HRS = Herbal Reference Substance
ERS = Extractive Reference Substance
USP = The United States Pharmacopoeia
EuP = The European Pharmacopoeia

27

Effects of Single Administered Bofutsushosan-Composed Crude Drugs on Diabetic Serum Parameters in Streptozotocin-Induced Diabetic Mice

Qing Yu[1], Tatsuo Takahashi[1], Masaaki Nomura[2], Mai Yasuda[1], Kyoko Obatake-Ikeda[3], Shinjiro Kobayashi[1*]

[1]Department of Clinical Pharmacy, Faculty of Pharmaceutical Sciences, Hokuriku University, Kanazawa, Japan

[2]Department of Education Center of Clinical Pharmacy, Faculty of Pharmaceutical Sciences, Hokuriku University, Kanazawa, Japan

[3]Department of Biochemistry, Faculty of Pharmaceutical Sciences, Hokuriku University, Kanazawa, Japan

Email: *s-kobayashi@hokuriku-u.ac.jp

ABSTRACT

The 18 crude drugs in Bofutsushosan (BOF: *Pulvis ledebouriellae compositae*: 防風通聖散) are separated into 6 groups such as diaphoretic, cathartic, antidote, antipyretic, neutralizer and diuretic groups. The effects of single administered BOF and composed crude drugs in 6 groups were investigated on the levels of diabetic parameters (serum glucose, insulin, triglyceride and cholesterol) in streptozotocin-induced diabetic mice. The anti-hyperglycemic action of BOF was depended on Ephedrae Herba, Saposhnikoviae Radix and Schizonepetae Spica in diaphoretic group, Forsythiae Fructus, Saposhnikoviae Radix, Schizonepetae Spica and Cnidii Rhizoma in antidote group, Scutellariae Radix, Gardeniae Fructus and Gypsum Fibrosum in antipyretic group and Paeoniae Radix in neutralizer group. In these crude drugs, Ephedrae Herba, Saposhnikoviae Radix, Schizonepetae Spica, Forsythiae Fructus, Scutellariae Radix, Gypsum Fibrosum and Paeoniae Radix increased serum insulin level, but Cnidii Rhizoma and Gardeniae Fructus did not affect serum insulin level. From these results, it suggested that anti-hyperglycemic action of BOF was through insulin-dependent and insulin independent manners. The lowering effect of BOF on serum triglyceride level was dependent on actions of Platycodi Radix in antidote and diuretic groups and Gardeniae Fructus in antipyretic group. The lowering effect of Gardeniae Fructus was parallel with its anti-hyperglycemic action. The lowering effect of BOF on high serum triglyceride level also included both direct action and indirect action. The reducing effect of BOF on serum cholesterol level was observed together with the actions of Ephedrae Herba and Zingiberis Rhizoma in diaphoretic group, Schizonepetae Spica in diaphoretic and antidote groups and Paeoniae Radix in neutralizer group. The lowering effects of Ephedrae Herba, Schizonepetae Spica and Paeoniae Radix on serum cholesterol level were parallel with their anti-hyperglycemic actions. Zingiberis Rhizoma in diaphoretic group might be direct reducing effect on serum cholesterol level but no serum glucose level. The Ephedrae Herba in diaphoretic group, Schizonepetae Spica in diaphoretic and antidote groups and Paeoniae Radix in neutralizer group might have reduced serum cholesterol level by reducing blood glucose level. From these results, composed crude drugs in 6 groups show various mechanisms in the action of BOF.

Keywords: Bofutsushosan (BOF); 6 Groups in BOF (Diaphoretic, Cathartic, Antidote, Antipyretic, Neutralizer and Diuretic Groups); Streptozotocin (STZ); Diabetic Serum Parameters; Anti-Hyperglycemia; Anti-Hyperlipidemia

1. Introduction

Chinese medicine is used increasingly worldwide to treat chronic diseases, such as obesity, diabetes, hyperlipidemia and hypertension [1]. Metabolic syndrome is a direct consequence of diet specifically, intake of large amounts of refined carbohydrates and sugars. Chinese medicine is an excellent system in complementary and alternative medicine. It holds great and unique potential in the management of metabolic syndrome, especially in the control of glucose and lipid metabolism [2].

Bofutsushosan (BOF), typical Chinese medicine, has been reported to improve atherosclerosis [3], obesity

---

*Corresponding author.

[4-6], hypertension, hyperglycemia [6], fatty liver [7,8] visceral fat and insulin resistance [9] in both clinical practice and animal examinations [5]. BOF has the potential to prevent adipogenesis in rat white adipocytes via modulation of gene expression levels [10]. Given by oral administered, BOF lowers fatty acid accumulation in the liver and reduces the levels of several plasma parameters correlated to obesity as well as body weight in mice fed a high-fat diet [8]. BOF produces a significant decrease in fat mass and weight compared with non-treated mice, without affecting the amount of food ingested in a study of obese mice [4]. In addition we have proved that BOF improved abnormal levels of serum glucose, insulin, triglyceride and cholesterol in STZ-diabetic mice [11]. BOF is promising for developing therapeutic medicine for metabolic diseases.

Streptozotocin (STZ) has been commonly used to induce a model of insulin-dependent diabetes mellitus (IDDM, type 1). STZ-induced diabetic mice have the features such as polydipsia, polyphagia, polyuria, dyslipidemia and hyperglycemia [12]. STZ also constructs a model of non-insulin-dependent diabetes mellitus (NIDDM, type 2) by its single administration. It has been reported that oral anti-hyperglycemic agents [13,14] and Chinese medicines improved the hyperglycemia in STZ-diabetic model [15,16]. In the previous study [11], serum insulin level was increased by oral administration of BOF as well as glybenclamide in our STZ-diabetic mice. It suggested that our STZ-diabetic mice showed the feature of NIDDM.

BOF is consisted of Ephedrae Herba (麻黄), Saposhnikoviae Radix (防風), Zingiberis Rhizoma (生姜), Schizonepetae Spica (荊芥), Rhei Rhizoma (大黄), Natrium Sulfricum (芒硝), Glycyrrhizae Radix (甘草), Forsythiae Fructus (連翹), Platycodi Radix (桔梗), Cnidii Rhizoma (川芎), Scutellariae Radix (黄芩), Gardeniae Fructus (山梔子), Gypsum Fibrosum (石膏), Talcum (滑石), Angelicae Radix (当帰), Paeoniae Radix (芍薬), Atractyloidis Lanceae Rhizoma (蒼朮), and Menthae Herba (薄荷) as shown in **Table 1**. These 18 composed crude drugs are separated into 6 groups such as diaphoretic, cathartic, antidote, antipyretic, neutralizer and diuretic groups. Diaphoretic group is consisted of Ephedrae Herba, Saposhnikoviae Radix, Zingiberis Rhizoma and Schizonepetae Spica to remove the diseases through perspiration from body surface. Cathartic group

Table 1. Dosaged of drugs composed in Bofutsushosan.

	Recovery rate of extracted crude drugs % (w/w)	Dry weight of crude drugs in BOF (g)	Amount of extracted drugs in prescription (g)	Proportion of Gardeniae Fructus	Dosage of extracted crude drugs (mg/kg)
1) Ephedrae Herba	9.72	1.2	0.12	0.14	10
2) Saposhnikoviae Radix	9	1.2	0.11	0.13	10
3) Zingiberis Rhizoma	8.5	0.3	0.03	0.04	3
4) Schizonepetae Spica	7.02	1.2	0.08	0.10	10
5) Rhei Rhizoma	6.94	1.5	0.10	0.13	10
6) Natrium Sulfricum	96.7	0.7	0.68	0.71	100
7) Glycyrrhizae Radix	14.32	2.0	0.29	0.35	30
8) Forsythiae Fructus	31.76	1.2	0.38	0.47	30
9) Platycodi Radix	53	2.0	1.06	1.30	100
10) Cnidii Rhizoma	26.9	1.2	0.32	0.40	100
11) Scutellariae Radix	42.26	2.0	0.85	1.04	100
12) Gardeniae Fructus	67.7	1.2	0.81	1.00	100
13) Gypsum Fibrosum	2.12	2.0	0.04	0.05	3
14) Talcum	1.66	3.0	0.05	0.06	3
15) Angelicae Radix	32.6	1.2	0.39	0.48	30
16) Paeoniae Radix	30.6	1.2	0.37	0.45	30
17) Atractyloidis Lanceae Rhizoma	28.4	2.0	0.57	0.70	100
18) Menthae Herba	19.35	1.2	0.23	0.29	30

is consisted of Rhei Rhizoma, Natrium Sulfricum and Glycyrrhizae Radix to soft intestinal contents, regulate intestinal movements and promote defecation. Antidote group is consisted of Forsythiae Fructus, Schizonepetae Spica, Saposhnikoviae Radix, Platycodi Radix and Cnidii Rhizoma to diminish toxins. Antipyretic group is consisted of Scutellariae Radix, Gardeniae Fructus, Gypsum Fibrosum and Talcum to eliminate internal thermal or inflammation. Neutralizer group is consisted of Angelicae Radix, Paeoniae Radix, Cnidii Rhizoma, Atractyloidis Lanceae Rhizoma and Menthae Herba to palliate and reduce the stimulation from the other drugs. Diuretic group is consisted of Paeoniae Radix, Atractyloidis Lanceae Rhizoma and Talcum to promote urination and remove of waste of body.

A lot of studies have demonstrated the effects of BOF on metabolic syndrome. However, there is no publication to investigate the effects of BOF on the diabetic parameters from the aspect of composed crude drugs in 6 groups. In this study, through using STZ-diabetic mice, we compared the effects of BOF and composed crude drugs on the levels of the diabetic parameters such as glucose, insulin, triglyceride and cholesterol in serum to deeply study the mechanisms of anti-hyperglycemia and anti-hyperlipidemia in BOF.

2. Materials and Methods

2.1. Preparation of Streptozotocin-Diabetic Mice

Fed male mice (ddY strain; 4 weeks of age; 16 - 20 g; Japan SLC, Shizuoka, Japan) were injected with a single dose (150 mg/kg) of STZ (Sigma, St. Louis, MO, USA) in saline into the tail vein. STZ-induced diabetic mice (7 - 8 weeks of age; blood glucose over 600 mg/dl) were used for further experiments in 3 - 4 weeks after the injection of STZ. These mice were given by CRF-1 (Oriental Yeast Co., Tokyo, Japan) and water ad libitum and kept at 25°C - 26°C with lights on from 7 a.m. to 7 p.m. BOF, each 18 composed crude drug and water were administered intraperitoneally to 3 hours fasting STZ diabetic mice. The Ethics Review Committee for Animal Experimentation of Hokuriku University approved the experimental protocol.

2.2. Preparation and Administration of Drugs

BOF, Ephedrae Herba, Saposhnikoviae Radix, Zingiberis Rhizoma, Schizonepetae Spica, Rhei Rhizoma, Natrium Sulfricum, Glycyrrhizae Radix, Forsythiae Fructus, Platycodi Radix, Cnidii Rhizoma, Scutellariae Radix, Gardeniae Fructus, Gypsum Fibrosum, Talcum, Angelicae Radix, Paeoniae Radix, Atractyloidis Lanceae Rhizoma and Menthae Herba were purchased from Tsumura Co. (Tokyo) and extracted in 10 volumes of distilled water with an automatic extractor "Torobi" (Tochimoto, Osaka, Japan) for 1 hour. A water extract of the drug was filtered through a mesh (No. 42, Sanpo, Tokyo), lyophilized with a freeze-drier (DF-03G, ULVAC, Tokyo), and stored at 4°C [15,16]. BOF, each composed crude drug extract and water were single administered intraperitoneally (0.1 ml/10 g body weight) into 3 hours fasting STZ-diabetic mice. Drug dosages were estimated on the basis of their recovery rates of crude drugs, dry weight of crude drugs in BOF, amount drug extracts. **Table 1** showed recovery rate of extracted crude drugs, dry weight of crude drugs in BOF, amount of extracted drugs in prescription and proportion of Gardeniae Fructus. Dosages of extracted crude drugs were estimated by standardizing the dosage of Gardeniae Fructus (100 mg/kg). In our previous study, 100 mg/kg was the effective dosage [11].

2.3. Measurement of Glucose, Insulin, Triglyceride and Cholesterol Levels in Serum

Blood was collected from the neck vein plexus of STZ-diabetic mice before and 6 hours after single administration of drugs and water following 3 hours fasting. Blood samples were centrifuged at 8000 rpm at 25°C for 5 min. Serum glucose level of the supernatant was measured by the glucose oxidase method with a serum glucose monitor set (MEDISAFE MINI, Terumo, Tokyo). The fall % of serum glucose (SG) was calculated as [SG (before drug treatment) − SG (after drug treatment)]/[SG (before drug treatment) − 85] × 100. The average SG of 3 hours fasting normal mice is 85 mg/dl [17,18]. Serum insulin level was measured with a mouse ELISA kit for insulin (Morinaga, Yokohama, Japan), serum triglyceride and cholesterol levels were measured with ELISA kits (Wako, Osaka, Japan) at 6 hours after the single administration of drugs or water, respectively.

2.4. Statistical Analyses

All values were expressed as means ± S.E.M. Differences between group data were evaluated by unpaired t-test at $p = 0.05$ or 0.01. A value of $p < 0.05$ was considered statistically significant.

3. Results

3.1. Effects of Composed Crude Drugs in 6 Groups of BOF on Serum Glucose Level in STZ-Diabetic Mice

BOF (300 mg/kg) significantly lowered the high serum glucose level in STZ-diabetic mice. Effects of composed crude drugs in 6 groups of BOF, diaphoretic, cathartic, antidote, antipyretic, neutralizer and diuretic groups, were examined on the serum glucose level (**Figure 1**).

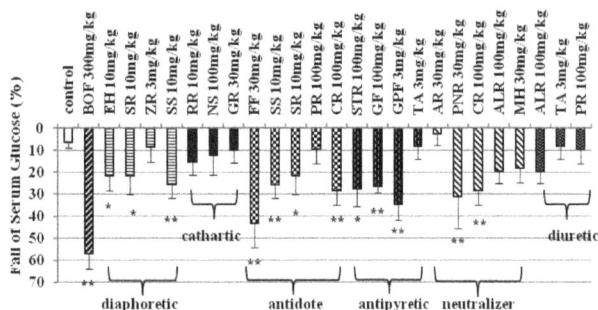

Figure 1. Effects of composed crude drugs in 6 groups of BOF on serum glucose level in STZ-diabetic mice. Serum glucose levels were measured before and 6 hours after *i.p.* administration of BOF and each composed crude drugs into 3 hours fasting STZ-diabetic mice. The values were expressed as means ± S.E.M. of 5 - 15 data. $^*p < 0.05$, $^{**}p < 0.01$: Significantly different from control water group. EH (Ephedrae Herba), SR (Saposhnikoviae Radix), ZR (Zingiberis Rhizoma), SS (Schizonepetae Spica), RR (Rhei Rhizoma), NS (Natrium Sulfricum), GR (Glycyrrhizae Radix), FF (Forsythiae Fructus), PR (Platycodi Radix), CR (Cnidii Rhizoma), STR (Scutellariae Radix), GF (Gardeniae Fructus), GPF (Gypsum Fibrosum), TA (Talcum), AR (Angelicae Radix), PNR (Paeoniae Radix), ALR (Atractyloidis Lanceae Rhizoma) and MH (Menthae Herba).

Ephedrae Herba (10 mg/kg), Saposhnikoviae Radix (10 mg/kg) and Schizonepetae Spica (10 mg/kg) in diaphoretic group significantly decreased 21.5%, 21.8% and 25.7% of serum glucose level respectively. However, Zingiberis Rhizoma (3 mg/kg) in diaphoretic group did not affect the high serum glucose level. Saposhnikoviae Radix and Schizonepetae Spica are not only in diaphoretic group but also in antidote group. In antidote group, Forsythiae Fructus (30 mg/kg) and Cnidii Rhizoma (100 mg/kg) also showed 43.4% and 28.3% fall of serum glucose level. But Platycodi Radix (100 mg/kg) in antidote group did not affect the high serum glucose level. In antipyretic group, Scutellariae Radix (100 mg/kg), Gardeniae Fructus (100 mg/kg) and Gypsum Fibrosum (3 mg/kg) showed 27.7%, 26.6% and 34.6% fall of serum glucose level. Cnidii Rhizoma is not only in antidote group but also in neutralizer group and showed 28.5% fall of serum glucose level. In neutralizer group, Paeoniae Radix (30 mg/kg) showed 31.1% fall of serum glucose level. Crude drugs in cathartic group and diuretic group did not affect the high level of serum glucose in STZ-diabetic mice.

3.2. Effect of Composed Crude Drugs in 6 Groups of BOF, Which Lowered the High Serum Glucose Level, on Serum Insulin Level in STZ-Diabetic Mice

BOF (300 mg/kg) significantly elevated the serum insulin level in STZ-diabetic mice. Effects of composed crude drugs in 6 groups of BOF, which lowered the high

serum glucose level, were examined on the serum insulin level (**Figure 2**). Ephedrae Herba (10 mg/kg) in diaphoretic group, Saposhnikoviae Radix (10 mg/kg) and Schizonepetae Spica (10 mg/kg) in diaphoretic and antidote groups and Forsythiae Fructus (30 mg/kg) in antidote group significantly increased serum insulin level. Scutellariae Radix (100 mg/kg) and Gypsum Fibrosum (3 mg/kg) in antipyretic group and Paeoniae Radix (30 mg/kg) in neutralizer group also increased serum insulin level. However, Cnidii Rhizoma (100 mg/kg) in antidote group and Gardeniae Fructus (100 mg/kg) in antipyretic group did not affect serum insulin level, although reduced the high serum glucose level in STZ-diabetic mice.

3.3. Effects of Composed Crude Drugs in 6 Groups of BOF on Serum Triglyceride Level in STZ-Diabetic Mice

BOF (300 mg/kg) significantly lowered the high serum triglyceride level in STZ-diabetic mice. Effects of composed crude drugs in 6 groups of BOF, diaphoretic, cathartic, antidote, antipyretic, neutralizer and diuretic groups, were examined on serum triglyceride level (**Figure 3**). Platycodi Radix (100 mg/kg) in antidote group and diuretic group and Gardeniae Fructus (100 mg/kg) in antipyretic group significantly reduced the high serum triglyceride level. However, other 16 crude drugs did not affect the high level of serum triglyceride level in STZ-diabetic mice.

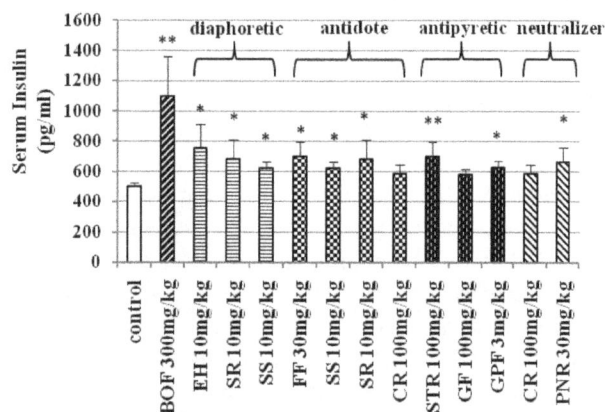

Figure 2. Effects of composed crude drugs in 6 groups of BOF, which lowered the high serum glucose level, on serum insulin level in STZ-diabetic mice. Serum insulin levels were measured at 6 hours after *i.p.* administration of BOF and each composed crude drugs which lowered the high serum glucose level into 3 hours fasting STZ-diabetic mice. The values were expressed as means ± S.E.M. of 5 - 13 data. $^*p < 0.05$, $^{**}p < 0.01$: Significantly different from control water group. EH (Ephedrae Herba), SR (Saposhnikoviae Radix), SS (Schizonepetae Spica), FF (Forsythiae Fructus), CR (Cnidii Rhizoma), STR (Scutellariae Radix), GF (Gardeniae Fructus), GPF (Gypsum Fibrosum), PNR (Paeoniae Radix).

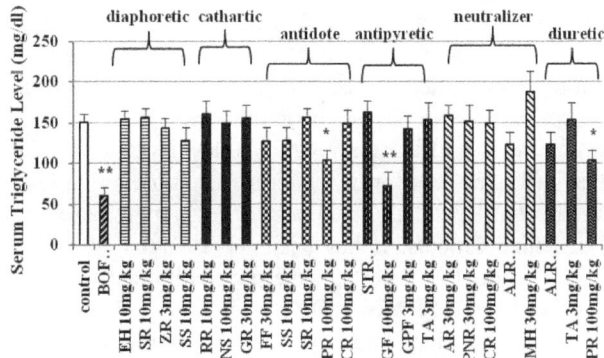

Figure 3. Effects of composed crude drugs in 6 groups of BOF on serum triglyceride level in STZ-diabetic mice. Serum triglyceride levels were measured at 6 hours after *i.p.* administration of BOF and each composed crude drugs into 3 hours fasting STZ-diabetic mice. The values were expressed as means ± S.E.M. of 5 - 15 data. $^*p < 0.05$, $^{**}p < 0.01$: Significantly different from the control water group. EH (Ephedrae Herba), SR (Saposhnikoviae Radix), ZR (Zingiberis Rhizoma), SS (Schizonepetae Spica), RR (Rhei Rhizoma), NS (Natrium Sulfricum), GR (Glycyrrhizae Radix), FF (Forsythiae Fructus), PR (Platycodi Radix), CR (Cnidii Rhizoma), STR (Scutellariae Radix), GF (Gardeniae Fructus), GPF (Gypsum Fibrosum), TA (Talcum), AR (Angelicae Radix), PNR (Paeoniae Radix), ALR (Atractyloidis Lanceae Rhizoma) and MH (Menthae Herba).

3.4. Effects of Composed Crude Drugs in 6 Groups of BOF on Serum Cholesterol Level in STZ-Diabetic Mice

BOF (300 mg/kg) significantly lowered the high serum cholesterol level in STZ-diabetic mice. Effects of composed crude drugs in 6 groups of BOF, diaphoretic, cathartic, antidote, antipyretic, neutralizer and diuretic groups, were examined on the high serum cholesterol level (**Figure 4**). Ephedrae Herba (10 mg/kg) and Zingiberis Rhizoma (3 mg/kg) in diaphoretic group, Schizonepetae Spica (10 mg/kg) in diaphoretic group and antidote group significantly lowered serum cholesterol level. Paeoniae Radix (30 mg/kg) in neutralizer group also lowered the high level of serum cholesterol in STZ-diabetic mice.

4. Discussion

STZ-induced diabetic model has been often used to the research about the diabetes mellitus according to the dosages used and experimental conditions [19]. Our STZ-diabetic mice showed high serum glucose level, low serum insulin level and high serum triglyceride and cholesterol levels. BOF lowered high serum glucose level and elevated low serum insulin level [11], indicating that our STZ-diabetic mice had the ability to release insulin from pancreatic β cell.

The effects of orally administered BOF on obesity [4-6], hypertension, hyperglycemia [6] and liver lipids [7,8]

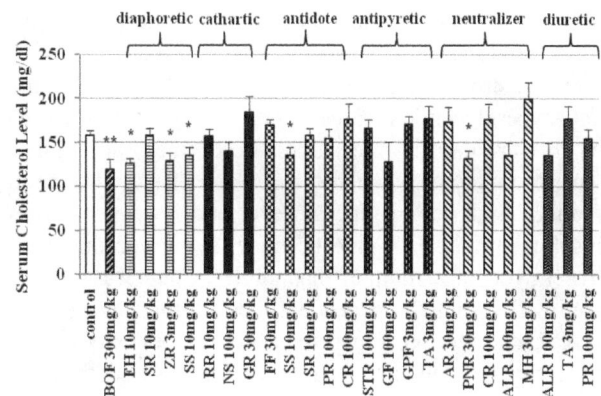

Figure 4. Effects of composed crude drugs in 6 groups of BOF on serum cholesterol level in STZ-diabetic mice. Serum cholesterol levels were measured at 6 hours after *i.p.* administration of BOF and each composed crude drugs into 3 hours fasting STZ-diabetic mice. The values were expressed as means ± S.E.M. of 5 - 15 data. $^*p < 0.05$, $^{**}p < 0.01$: Significantly different from the control water group. EH (Ephedrae Herba), SR (Saposhnikoviae Radix), ZR (Zingiberis Rhizoma), SS (Schizonepetae Spica), RR (Rhei Rhizoma), NS (Natrium Sulfricum), GR (Glycyrrhizae Radix), FF (Forsythiae Fructus), PR (Platycodi Radix), CR (Cnidii Rhizoma), STR (Scutellariae Radix), GF (Gardeniae Fructus), GPF (Gypsum Fibrosum), TA (Talcum), AR (Angelicae Radix), PNR (Paeoniae Radix), ALR (Atractyloidis Lanceae Rhizoma) and MH (Menthae Herba).

were certificated. Generally, oral administration method is often used when Chinese medicine is administered. However, in order to evaluate the drug evaluation with accurate amount and avoid the influence of digestion, we chose single intraperitoneal administration method. The effects of single intraperitoneal administration of BOF were the same as oral administered effects on diabetic parameters such as glucose, insulin, triglyceride and cholesterol levels in serum. High serum glucose level was improved by BOF. BOF also decreased high serum triglyceride and cholesterol levels in a dose-dependent manner in STZ-diabetic mice [11].

From the view of traditional Chinese medicine, diabetes is induced by toxin turned from extra nutrition. There are series of symptoms in diabetes, such as more thirty, more drink, more urine, high blood glucose level, hot feeling, etc. BOF is a typical Chinese medicine, which can discharge the extra toxins in the body. In this study we deeply investigated the respective efficacy of composed crude drugs in 6 groups of BOF, diaphoretic, cathartic, antidote, antipyretic, neutralizer and diuretic groups, on the parameters of diabetes.

It has been reported that BOF has the function on promoting the insulin secretion to improve high blood glucose level [6]. It is necessary to analyze which composed crude drugs were participated in the anti-hyperglycemic effect of BOF. Thus we studied to compare the actions of

BOF for the diabetic parameters with the actions of composed crude drugs in 6 groups of BOF. Both of recovery rate and drug dosages of crude drugs in BOF and the anti-hyperglycemic actions of crude drugs were measured in STZ-diabetic mice. Ephedrae Herba, Saposhnikoviae Radix and Schizonepetae Spica in diaphoretic group reduced high serum glucose level and improved serum insulin level in STZ-diabetic mice. It implied that anti-hyperglycemic action of diaphoretic group was associated with an insulin-dependent mechanism. Saposhnikoviae Radix and Schizonepetae Spica are not only in diaphoretic group but also in antidote group. Antidote group can dispose the toxins in the body to remove the source of diseases. In antidote group, Forsythiae Fructus and Cnidii Rhizoma also lowered the high serum glucose level. Forsythiae Fructus increased serum insulin level. However, Cnidii Rhizoma did not increase serum insulin level although lowered the high serum glucose level. The reducing effect of Cnidii Rhizoma might be associated with an insulin-independent manner. Antipyretic group was used to solve the symptoms in diabetes such as thirsty and hot feeling [20]. In antipyretic group, excepting Talcum, Scutellariae Radix, Gardeniae Fructus and Gypsum Fibrosum all reduced high serum glucose level in STZ-diabetic mice. At the same time, Scutellariae Radix and Gypsum Fibrosum significantly increased serum insulin level, but Gardeniae Fructus did not affect serum insulin level. It implied that there were insulin-dependent and insulin-independent manners on the action of lowering high serum glucose level in the antipyretic group. Paeoniae Radix in neutralizer group also lowered high serum glucose level and improved serum insulin level. However the other crude drugs in neutralizer did not show the effect of lowering high serum glucose level in STZ-diabetic mice. From the results of anti-hyperglycemic actions and insulin-increasing actions of composed crude drugs in 6 groups of BOF, the anti-hyperglycemic action of BOF had two mechanisms such as in insulin-dependent and insulin-independent manners. Actions of Ephedrae Herba, Saposhnikoviae Radix, Schizonepetae Spica, Forsythiae Fructus, Scutellariae Radix, Gypsum Fibrosum and Paeoniae Radix were associated with an insulin-dependent mechanism. On the other hand, actions of Cnidii Rhizoma and Gardeniae Fructus were associated with an insulin-independent mechanism. We must explore the mechanism of Cnidii Rhizoma and Gardeniae Fructus on lowering high serum glucose level in STZ-induced diabetic mice.

BOF lowered high serum triglyceride level in STZ-diabetic mice in a dose-dependent manner [11]. As the same with our single administration of BOF, Saito et al. [21] reported that BOF inhibited pancreatic lipase in vitro and suppressed the elevation of plasma triglyceride after oral administration of lipid emulsion. Morimoto et

al. [5] also proved that BOF inhibited triglyceride synthesis in the liver. From our results, Platycodi Radix in antidote and diuretic groups reduced the high serum triglyceride level in STZ-diabetic mice, but other 16 crude drugs did not affect serum triglyceride level. It implied that effect of BOF on the high serum triglyceride level should be dependent on effects of Platycodi Radix and Gardeniae Fructus. It has been reported that Platycodi Radix worked as a peroxisome proliferator-activated receptor gamma (PPAR-γ) activator in liver, and decreased serum triglyceride storage [22,23]. The inhibitory effect of Platycodi Radix on serum triglyceride level might be a direct reducing effect on triglyceride, being non-dependent on its anti-hyperglycemic action. Gardeniae Fructus also significantly lowered serum triglyceride level in STZ-diabetic mice. This reducing effect might depend on geniposide, the main compound of Gardeniae Fructus. Geniposide had the effect on lowering the quantity of visceral fat and showed an alleviating effect on abnormal glucose/lipid metabolism [24]. The lowering effect of Gardeniae Fructus on serum triglyceride was parallel with its anti-hyperglycemic action. It suggested that the reducing effect of Gardeniae Fructus might be an indirect reducing effect on serum triglyceride, being related to its anti-hyperglycemic action. These results indicated that the lowering effect of single administered BOF on high serum triglyceride level in STZ-diabetic mice had direct reducing effect such as the action of Platycodi Radix and indirect reducing effect such as the action of Gardeniae Fructus.

BOF also significantly lowered serum cholesterol level in STZ-diabetic mice [11]. This lowering effect may be useful for preventive therapy in lifestyle-related diseases since the Guidelines from the National Cholesterol Education Program recommended reduction of LDL cholesterol levels as the primary goal in cardiovascular risk-reduction therapy [25]. The study had been reported that orally administered BOF lowered total cholesterol and LDL cholesterol levels. We threw more light on the reducing effect of BOF on high serum cholesterol level in STZ-diabetic mice. Ephedrae Herba and Zingiberis Rhizoma in diaphoretic group, Schizonepetae Spica in diaphoretic and antidote group and Paeoniae Radix in neutralizer group significantly lowered the serum cholesterol level of STZ-diabetic mice. It has been reported that Zingiberis Rhizoma was able to lower the serum cholesterol level in hypercholesterolemia rabbit [26]. The reducing effect of Zingiberis Rhizoma on serum cholesterol level was not depended on its anti-hyperglycemic action. On the other hand, reducing effects of Ephedrae Herba, Schizonepetae Spica and Paeoniae Radix on serum cholesterol level were parallel with their reducing effects on high serum glucose level and increasing effects on serum insulin level in STZ-diabetic mice. These results indicated that effects of Ephedrae Herba, Schizonepetae Spica and Paeoniae Radix on high serum cholesterol level were associated with their effects on reduction of high serum glucose level and increase of serum insulin level. Their improving actions on abnormal glucose and insulin metabolism might cause reducing of acetyl-CoA. Acetyl-CoA was biochemical precursor of cholesterol. The excess of acetyl-CoA in STZ-diabetic mice causes an excess of hydroxymethylglutaryl-CoA reductase (HMG-CoA). HMG-CoA reductase is a rate-limiting enzyme in the cholesterol biosynthetic pathway. Inhibition of HMG-CoA reductase decreases cholesterol synthesis. The inhibition of HMG-CoA reductase is very effective in lowering serum cholesterol and LDL in most of animal species, including humans [27]. All of these results suggest that BOF has two mechanisms for lowering effects on serum cholesterol level. One mechanism is the direct action of Zingiberis Rhizoma on cholesterol biosynthesis in the action of BOF. The other mechanism is associated with their anti-hyperglycemic actions, inducing by Ephedrae Herba, Schizonepetae Spica and Paeoniae Radix in the action of BOF.

5. Conclusion

The present study demonstrated that single administrated BOF and composed crude drugs were investigated on the levels of diabetic parameters (serum glucose, insulin, triglyceride and cholesterol) in STZ-diabetic mice. The anti-hyperglycemic action of BOF had two mechanisms: one was insulin-dependent mechanism such as actions of Ephedrae Herba, Saposhnikoviae Radix, Schizonepetae Spica Forsythiae Fructus, Scutellariae Radix, Gypsum Fibrosum and Paeoniae Radix. The other was insulin-independent mechanism such as actions of Cnidii Rhizoma and Gardeniae Fructus. Platycodi Radix in antidote and diuretic groups and Gardeniae Fructus in antipyretic group reduced the high serum triglyceride level in STZ-diabetic mice. The action of Platycodi Radix might be a direct reducing action on serum triglyceride but no anti-hyperglycemic action. Gardeniae Fructus might be related to its anti-hyperglycemic action, although Gardeniae Fructus did not release serum insulin level. Lowering effect of high serum triglyceride level in BOF also included both direct effect and indirect effect on decrease of serum triglyceride. Zingiberis Rhizoma in diaphoretic group might be direct reducing effect on serum cholesterol level but no serum glucose level. The Ephedrae Herba in diaphoretic group, Schizonepetae Spica in diaphoretic and antidote groups and Paeoniae Radix in neutralizer group might have reduced serum cholesterol level by reducing serum glucose level. From these results, composed crude drugs in 6 groups of BOF show various mechanisms in the actions of BOF.

REFERENCES

[1] S. Hasani-Ranjbar, B. Larijani and M. Abdollahi, "A Systematic Review of Iranian Medicinal Plants Useful in Diabetes Mellitus," *Archives of Medical Science*, Vol. 4, No. 3, 2008, pp. 285-292.

[2] J. Yin, H. Zhang and J. Ye, "Traditional Chinese Medicine in Treatment of Metabolic Syndrome," *Endocrine, Metabolic & Immune Disorders Drug Targets*, Vol. 8, No. 2, 2008, pp. 99-111. doi:10.2174/187153008784534330

[3] K. Ohno, H. W. Chung, I. Maruyama and T. Tani, "Bofutsushosan, a Traditional Chinese Formulation, Prevents Intimal Thickening and Vascular Smooth Muscle Cell Proliferation Induced by Balloon Endothelial Denudation in Rats," *Biological & Pharmaceutical Bulletin*, Vol. 28, No. 11, 2005, pp. 2162-2165. doi:10.1248/bpb.28.2162

[4] T. Yoshida, N. Sakane, Y. Wakabayashi, T. Umekawa and M. Kondo, "Thermogenic Antiobesity Effects of Bofutsushosan in MSG Obese Mice," *International Journal of Obesity and Related Metabolic Disorders*, Vol. 19, No. 10, 1995, pp. 717-722.

[5] Y. Morimoto, M. Sakata, A. Ono, T. Maegawa and S. Tajima, "Effects of Bofutsushosan, a Traditional Chinese Medicine, on Body Fat Accumulation in Fructose-Loaded Rats," *Nippon Yakurigaku Zasshi*, Vol. 117, No. 1, 2001, pp. 77-86. doi:10.1254/fpj.117.77

[6] Y. Morimoto, M. Sakata, A. Ohno, T. Maegawa and S. Tajima, "Effects of Byakkokaninjinto, Bofutsushosan and Goreisan on Blood Glucose Level, Water Intake and Urine Volume in KKAy Mice," *Nippon Yakugaku Zasshi*, Vol. 122, No. 2, 2002, pp. 163-168.

[7] S. Sakamoto, S. Takeshita, S. Sassa, S. Suzuki, Y. Ishikawa and H. Kudo, "Effects of Colestimide and/or Bofutsushosan on Plasma and Liver Lipids in Mice Fed a High-Fat Diet," *In Vivo*, Vol. 19, No. 6, 2005, pp. 1029-1033.

[8] T. Nakayama, S. Suzuki, H. Kudo, S. Sassa, M. Nomura and S. Sakamoto, "Effects of Three Chinese Herbal Medicines on Plasma and Liver Lipids in Mice Fed a High-Fat Diet," *Journal of Ethnopharmacology*, Vol. 109, No. 2, 2007, pp. 236-240. doi:10.1016/j.jep.2006.07.041

[9] C. Hioki, K. Yoshimoto and T. Yoshida, "Efficacy of Bofutsushosan, an Oriental Herbal Medicine, in Obese Japanese Women with Impaired Glucose Tolerance," *Clinical and Experimental Pharmacology and Physiology*, Vol. 31, No. 9, 2004, pp. 614-619. doi:10.1111/j.1440-1681.2004.04056.x

[10] J. Yamakawa, I. Yasuhito, T. Fumihide, T. Takahashi and J. Yoshida, "The Kampo Medicines Orengedokuto, Bofutsushosan and Boiogito Have Different Activities to Regulate Gene Expressions in Differentiated Rat White Adipocytes: Comprehensive Analysis of Genetic Profiles," *Biological & Pharmaceutical Bulletin*, Vol. 31, No. 11, 2008, pp. 2083-2089. doi:10.1248/bpb.31.2083

[11] Q. Yu, M. Yasuda, T. Takahashi, M. Nomura, N. Hagino and S. Kobayashi, "Effects of Bofutsushosan and Gardeniae Frutus on Diabetic Serum Parameters in Streptozotocin-Induced Diabetic Mice," *Chinese Medicine*, Vol. 2, No. 4, 2011, pp. 130-137. doi:10.4236/cm.2011.24022

[12] C. Rerup and F. Tarding, "Streptozotocin and Alloxan-

Induced Diabetes in Mice," *European Journal of Pharmacology*, Vol. 7, No. 1, 1969, pp. 89-96. doi:10.1016/0014-2999(69)90169-1

[13] J. Movassat and B. Portha, "Beta-Cell Growth in the Neonatal Goto-Kakisaki Rat and Regeneration after Treatment with Streptozotocin at Birth," *Diabetologia*, Vol. 42, No. 9, 1999, pp. 1098-1106. doi:10.1007/s001250051277

[14] M. S. Gokhale, D. H. Shah, Z. Hakim, D. D. Santani and R. K.Goyal, "Effect of Chronic Treatment with Amlodipine in Non-Insulin-Dependent Diabetic Rats," *Pharmacological Research*, Vol. 37, No. 6, 1998, pp. 455-459. doi:10.1006/phrs.1998.0319

[15] N. Nakashima, I. Kimura and M. Kimura, "Isolation of Pseudoproto-Timosaponin AIII from Rhizomes of Anemarrhena Asphodeloides and Its Hypoglycemic Activity in Streptozotocin-Induced Diabetic Mice," *Journal of Natural Products*, Vol. 56, No. 3, 1993, pp. 345-350. doi:10.1021/np50093a006

[16] T. Miura, H. Toyoda, M. Miyake, E. Ishihara, M. Usami and K. Tanigawa, "Hypoglycemic Action of Stigma of *Zea mays* L. in Normal and Diabetic Mice," *Natural Medicines*, Vol. 50, No. 5, 1996, pp. 363-365.

[17] Y. Y. Liu, S. Kobayashi, T. Tsutsumi and H. Kontani, "Combined Effects of Stephania Radix and Astragali Radix in Antihyperglycemic Action of Boiogito (Fang-ji-huang-qi-tang) in Streptozotocin-Induced Diabetic Mice," *Journal of Traditional Medicines*, Vol. 17, No. 6, 2000, pp. 253-260.

[18] T. Tsutsumi, S. Kobayashi, Y. Y. Liu and H. Kontani, "Anti-Hyperglycemic Effect of Fangchinoline Isolated from *Stephania tetrandra* Radix in Streptozotocin-Diabetic Mice," *Biological & Pharmaceutical Bulletin*, Vol. 26, No. 3, 2003, pp. 313-317. doi:10.1248/bpb.26.313

[19] A. Junod, A. E. Lambert, L. Orci, R. Pictet, A. E. Gonet and A. E. Renold, "Studies of the Diabetogenic Action of Streptozotocin," *Proceedings of the Society for Experimental Biology and Medicine*, Vol. 126, No. 1, 1967, pp. 201-205.

[20] Y. Z. Zhang, L. M. Kuang, J. Zhou, M. Wang, H. Li and Q. Yi, "30 Case of Type II Diabetic Treated with The Method of Dissipating Heat Detoxifying," *Guangming Journal of Chinese Medicine*, vol. 23 No. 5, 2008, pp 632-634.

[21] M. Saito, T. Hamazaki, T. Tani and S. Watanabe, "Bofutsushosan, a Traditional Chinese Formulation, Inhibits Pancreatic Lipase Activity *in Vitro* and Suppresses the Elevation of Plasma Triacylglycerols after Oral Administration of Lipid Emulsion," *Journal of Traditional Medicines*, Vol. 22, No. 3, 2005, pp. 308-313.

[22] L. K. Han, Y. N. Zheng, B. J. Xu, H. Okuda and Y. Kimura, "Saponins from Platycodi Radix Ameliorate High Fat Diet-Induced Obesity in Mice," *The Journal of Nutrition*, Vol. 132, No. 8, 2002, pp. 2241-2245.

[23] D. Y. Kwon, Y. S. Kim, S. Y. Ryu, Y. H. Choi, M. R. Cha, H. J. Yang and S. Park, "Platyconic Acid, a Saponin from Platycodi Radix, Improves Glucose Homeostasis by Enhancing Insulin Sensitivity *in Vitro* and *in Vivo*," *European Journal of Nutrition*, Vol. 51, No. 5, 2011, pp. 529-540.

[24] K. Kojima, T. Shimade, Y. Nagareda, M. Watanabe, J. Ishizaki, Y. Sai, K. Miyamoto and M. Aburada, "Preventive Effect of Geniposide on Metabollic Disease Status in Spontaneously Obese Type 2 Diabetic Mice and Free Fatty Acid-Treated HepG2 Cells," *Biological & Pharmaceutical Bulletin*, Vol. 34, No. 10, 2011, pp. 1613-1618. doi:10.1248/bpb.34.1613

[25] Expert Panel on Detection, Evaluation, and Treatment of High Blood Cholesterol in Adults, "Executive Summary of the 3rd Report of the National Cholesterol Education Program (NCEP) Expert Panel on Detection, Evaluation, and Treatment of High Blood Cholesterol in Adults (Adult Treatment Panel III)," *The Journal of the American Medical Association*, Vol. 285, No. 19, 2001, pp. 2486-2497. doi:10.1001/jama.285.19.2486

[26] U. Bhandari, J. N. Sharma and R. Zafar, "The Protective Action of Ethanolic Ginger (Zingber Officinale) Extract in Cholesterol Fed Rabbits," *Journal of Ethnopharmacology*, Vol. 61, No. 2, 1998, pp. 167-171. doi:10.1016/S0378-8741(98)00026-9

[27] D. Amin, S. K. Gustafson, J. M. Weinacht, S. A. Cornell, K. Neuenschwander, B. Kosmider, A. C. Scotese, J. R. Regan and M. H. Perrone, "RG 12561 (Dalvastatin): A Novel Synthetic Inhibitor of HMG-CoA Reductase and Cholesterol-Lowering Agent," *Pharmacology*, Vol. 46, No. 1, 1993, pp. 13-22. doi:10.1159/000139024

28

Acupuncture and Moxibustion Theories of Zhang Ji[*]

Yong Chen[1,2#], Yinmin Le[1], Jia Wei[1]
[1]Jiangxi University of Traditional Chinese Medicine, Nanchang, China
[2]Fuda Cancer Hospital, Guangzhou, China
Email: [#]shanggongchenyong@163.com

ABSTRACT

This paper introduces the clinical experiences on acupuncture and moxibustion of Zhang Zhongjing, who was regarded as "medical Saint" of Traditional Chinese Medicine. He gave indications for acupuncture and moxibustion, developed robbing fire or inversing fire acupuncture principles to treat febrile diseases. His theories on acupuncture and moxibustion are precious and could be reference in clinical practice.

Keywords: Zhang Zhongjing; Treaties on Febrile and Miscellaneous Diseases; Golden Chamber Synopsis; Indication; Theory; Acupuncture Methods

Zhang Ji (about AD 150-219), also known as Zhang Zhongjing, was born in the Nieyang, Nangyang (known as Denxian, Henan province today) in the late age of East Han dynasty. The world honors him as Medical Saint. His works include 伤寒杂病论 (*Treaties on Febrile and Miscellaneous Diseases*), 金匮要略 (*Synopsis of Golden Chamber*). Even today, the two books are the compulsory classical courses in Traditional Chinese Medical Universities. His advocation on treatments according to syndromes differentiation by six channels and eight principles has great influences to the development of Chinese medicine afterwards.

On clinical, Zhang Zhongjing mainly treated diseases with formular medicine, however, there are dozens of terms related with acupuncture and moxibustion theropy. The acupoints mentioned in his books includ Fengfu (GV 16), Fengchi (GB 20), Qimen (LR 14), Dazhui (GV 14), Feishu (BL 13), Ganshu(BL 18), Laogong (PC 8), Guanyuan(RN 4) etc. The equipments and methods for acupuncture and moxibustion include needle (needling), moxa (moxibustion), fumigation, burning and warming acupuncture ect. are mentioned. Various diseases or symptoms were treated by not a few therapeutic methods of acupuncture and moxibustion, which have practicle influences to guidance of bedside acupuncture and moxibustion.

1. Theory of "当刺" (Need Acupuncture), "可灸" (Can Moxibustion)

The theory of "need acupuncture" often appeared in

Zhongjing's books. Such as, the 148th term from *Treaties on Febrile and Miscellanous Diseases* and the 22nd term from *Synopsis of Golden Chamber* (For each cited in the following passage, if not specifically indicated (the ××[th] term), the quotation is from *Treaties on Febrile and Miscellanous Diseases*, if the quotation is from *Golden Chamber Synopsis*, it will be specified in the text) reads: A woman was attacked by wind, fever, aversion to cold. Her menstruation was due and lasted for 7 to 8 days. After the fever was gone, her pulse was slow, cold body, chest fullness and stagnation sensation, delirious speech. These are the manifestations of heat entering blood chamber, acupuncture on Qimen is needed. The 221st term reads: When Yangming of a patient is attacked, the hematochezia and delirious speech suggested the heat entering blood chamber, if the patient had sweating head, need acupuncture on Qimen. The 147th term reads: If Taiyang and Shaoyang meridians of a patient is attacked at the same time, manifestations are headache and neck stiffness, or vertigo, sometimes feel stagnation of chest, stiffness associated with local rigidity in epigastric region, needs to acupuncture on Dazhui, Feishu, Ganshu. Be cautious that diaphoresis is not proper for the patient. If diaphoresis was applied to the patient, he or she would have delirious speech for 5 days, wiry pulse. It needs acupuncture on Qimen to slove the problem.

Sometimes, Zhongjing used the terminologies of "可刺"(can acupuncture), or "宜针"(acupuncture is appropriate). Such as, the 308th term reads: If Shaoyin is attacked, the patient has dysentery, bloody and purulent stool, can be treated by acupuncture. The 6th term from *Golden Chamber Synopsis* reads: For blood bi syndrome

[*]This paper is translated from *Acupuncture and Moxibustion Schools of Ancient Famous Practitioners*, which is edited by Wei Jia, Gao Xiyan. The work is sponsored by People's Healthy Publish House, China.
[#]Corresponding author.

(blood-arthragia)… using acupuncture to guide the Yang qi is appropriate. Sometimes, only "needling" is the word. Such as, the 112nd term describes the fever with aversion to wind, thirsty, abdominal distension, spontaneous perspiration… needle the Qimen. The 111st term reads: Fever with abdominal distension, delirious speech, floating and tight cun pulse… needle the Qimen. The 19th term from *Golden Chamber Synopsis* reads: Fujue (means the rigidity of foot, especially the flex function) [1], the patient can move forwards but hardly stop (by her/himself), needling 2 cun into the calf.

Generally, as to apply needles for treatment, "当刺" (need acupuncture),"可刺" (can acupuncture), "宜针" (acupuncture is appropriate), "刺" (needling) have the same meaning. The terms from the two books discussed 6 syndromes indicated by acupuncture, which are: Firstly, heat symptom of Sanyang (Triyang: Taiyang, Shaoyang, Yangming). Secondly, heat entering blood chamber, which means during the menstruation, before or after menstruation, the woman affected by external evils, heat evil lands in blood chamber (uterus). The manifestations include fever and aversion to cold, distension of chest and abdomen, delirious speech. Thirdly, stiffness and pain of neck, vertigo, and acupuncture should be the first choice with satisfied outcome. Fourthly, bloody and purulent stool, include the so called dysentery afterwards. Acupuncture proved to be very efficient for dysentery patients. Fifthly, blood-bi (blood-arthragia) [2], which mainly manifested as numbness of limbs. Acupuncture therapy is indicated for this type of diseases obviously. Sixthly, Fujue symptoms manifested as rigidity of acrotarsium, hard to walk. The clinical observation proved acupuncture has significant effectiveness for this type of diseases also.

Speaking of moxibustion, Zhongjing has the theories like "可灸" (can moxibustion),"当灸" (need moxibustion),"灸之" (apply moxibustion),"熏之" (fumigate). The 349th term reads: Fever with rapid pulse, cold extremities, can use moxibustion (to treat). The 304th term reads: Shaoyin disease, if lasts for 1-2 days, normal sense of mouth, chilly sensation in the back, the patient needs moxibustion treatment. The 17th term from *Golden Chamber Synopsis* and the 361st term reads: For diarrhoea, cold extremities, pulselessness patients, apply moxibustion… The 325th term reads: Shaoyin disease, diarrhoea, micro-astringent pulse, vomiting, sweating, the patient must change clothes frequently. Otherwise, apply moxibustion to warm Shaoyin.

Therefore, the indication range of moxibustion including: Cold extremities, aversion to cold, diarrhoea, weak pulse ect manifested in Sanyin (Triyin, which is Taiyin, Shaoyin, Queyin) diseases. It suggests that moxibustion treatment has function of restoring Yang saving inverse, which has differences compared using acupuncture to treat Sanyang diseases mentioned above. How-

ever, it is not absolutely impossible to treat Yang syndrome with moxibustion whilst acupuncture to Yin syndrome. Such as, in the 487th term applying fumigation to bi-yang disease; in the 308th term using acupuncture to treat diarrhoea of Shaoyin disease. We may infer that at bed side of patients, Zhongjing stressed the treatments according to syndromes differentiation.

2. Theory of "火逆" (Inversing Fire), "火劫" (Robbing Fire)

Zhang zhongjing, who was famous for his treatment of febrile diseases with decoctions, also persisting to the principles of treating cold diseases with heat medicine, while treating heat diseases with cold medicine (warm the cold, cool the heat). He thought the heat from the moxa fire same as the heat from herbals, and has vigilance on moxibustion treatment. He mentioned "火逆" (inversing fire),"火劫" (robbing fire), "火邪" (fire evil), "火动" (fire stirring), "火攻" (fire attack), "火盛" (surpassing fire), "被火" (burning/being on fire) ect. repeatedly, to raise attentions of following practitioners. The 119th term reads: Caused by fire evil, the patient manifested as irratation, reflex sensation. The 120th term describes, if the disease is located in external and treated mistakenly by moxibustion, fire would cause the disease severer, leads to inversing fire syndrome which is severe bi (arthralgia) of lower back. The 115th term describes if the fever with floating pulse was treated by moxibustion, may leads to the side effects of Yang depletion or mania. The 284th term describes the diarrhea, cough, and delirious speech of shaoyin disease is caused by robbing fire. The 117th term reads: Taiyang disease, treated by fumigation, no sweating, would cause the restlessness of the patient…, which is named fire evil. The 2nd term from Golden Chamber Synopsis reads: The patient with irritation and pain caused by dampness, needs diaphoresis, while attacking fire (moxibustion) is not appropriate. The 118th term reads: If pulse is floating, and the patient has extremely heat, this is excess. The excess needs to be treated by xu (difficiency). But if treated by moxibustion, the stirring fire can leads to dryness of throat, and hemoptysis. The 205th term reads: If Yangming is been burning by fire… leads to yellowish complexion. The 6th term describes: Taiyang disease, manifests as fever, thirsty, no aversion to cold is belong to warm disease. If treated by fire, could leads to epilepsy, clonic convulsion. One time of inversing fire may cause the delay of recovery, repeatedly inversing fire may shorten patient's survival time. The 205th term reads: If pulse is faint and rapid, no moxibustion. The fire seems mini, but have strength of inside attack, can burning bones and tendons, losing of blood. The 2nd term of Golden Chamber Synopsis reads: convulsion and skin ulcer caused by moxibustion are hard to cure. The 25nd term of Golden Chamber Synopsis reads: Drunk patients should not applied moxibustion in abdomina nor back. Otherwise the stagnation of intestine happens.

Above all, Zhongjing suggested the diseases and symptoms that need avoid of moxibustion include: Faint and rapid pulse, floating pulse, Taiyang syndrome, Yangmin syndrome, dampness causing the irritation and pain of the patient, heat syndrome (over excess of Yang or Yin differency), thirsty, excess, warm diseases ect., all of these regarded as Yang symptoms. He think the mismoxibustion may cause the side effects of irritation, reflex sensation, heavy bi in lower back, epilepsy, clonic convulsion, delirious speech, dry throat and hemoptysis, yellowish complexion... even leads to the disastrous effect like shortening life expectancy.

3. Theory of Warming or Burning Acupuncture

The theory of warming acupuncture and burning acupuncture is originated from Neijing (Internal Canon of Medicine). The 128th term describes that if fever of Taiyang disease treated by warming acupuncture would cause convulsion in the patient. The 226th term describes: If Yangming disease manifest as floating and tight pulse, dry throat, no aversion to cold but heat, then treated by warming acupuncture would cause apprehensiveness, irratation, and insomnia. The 267th term describes: Taiyang disease transfers to Shaoyang, and manifests as hypochondrium fullness and rigidity, retching and cannot eating, alternating of chills and fever, methods of diaphoresis, emetic therapy and purgation are done, if add warming acupuncture would lead to delirious speech. The 2nd term of *Golden Chamber Synopsis* describes: Taiyang attacked by summer heat could manifests as fever and aversion to cold, heavy body and general pain... diaphoresis may worsen the aversion to cold, warming acupuncture may worsen the fever. The 29th term describes: If fever with floating pulse... treated by diaphoresis and burning acupuncture can cause Yang depletion to the patient. The 121st term describes: Burning acupuncture may cause sweating of the location, if the acupuncture region attacked by cold may grow a red nut-like mass. One moxacone of moxibustion may be applied to handle the problem. The 122nd term describes: Burning acupuncture may cause irritation of the patient. The 158th term describes: After treat Taiyang disease with diaphoresis, both Yin and Yang qi are exhausted, if add burning acupuncture, which may cause irritation of the patient.

Due to the burning acupuncture and worming acupuncture needs fire during the process, Zhongjing regarded them as similar to the inversing fire or robbing fire in moxibustion. Burning and warming acupuncture are special treatment methods, which combine acupuncture and moxibustion together, and still in widely using

by far. The terminologies in Zhongjing's books are among the earliest recordations with relatively high historic value. Pitifully, Zhongjing didn't record the detail manipulation of the technicals.

4. Combination of Acupuncture and Drugs

At bed side, when give treatments, Zhongjing can combine acupuncture and drugs, fully use them advantages, which is estimable deeds. *Chapter 22nd pulse symptoms and treatments of woman miscellaneous diseases* in *Golden Chamber Synopsis* reads: ... of thirty-six diseases, with thousands of changes, practitioners need to feel the Yin and Yang of the pulses... combine acupuncture and drugs can cure severe diseases... Nowadays clinical dates show combination of acupuncture and drugs can bring better effectiveness for obstetrical and gynecological diseases like menstruation disorder, pelvic infection, mastitis, infertility, abnormal fetal position, dystocia ect. The 24th term reads: A Taiyang disease patient, treated by Guizhi decoction at first, more irritable without relieve. Add acupuncture on Fengchi, Fengfu, the patient recoered soon. The effectiveness of treating influenza (external syndrome of Taiyang) has been widely accepted today. The 4th term from *Golden Chamber Synopsis* reads: malaria... could be treated with diaphoresis, acupuncture and moxibustion. There are amounts of researches on acupuncture for malaria. For some diseases, acupuncture may have less effect, add drugs to make up the defect. For example, the 234th term discusses the wind attacks the Yangming, needling has less effect, the Xiaochaihu decoction can be helpful [3].

Besides the theories discussed above, Zhongjing also advocates the principles of prevention is better than cure, and treating diseases in early stage. The first part of *Golden Chamber Synopsis* states: "the pathogenic evils can enter the zang-fu organs by Jingluo (meridians and channels)", "if one pays attention to health, he/she won't let the evil wind interfere the Jingluo. If the evil attacks a Jingluo, he/she will seek therapies before it enter into zang-fu organs". Can apply "daoyin (physical and breathing exercise)... acupuncture and moxibustion..." to restrain the development of the disease. The 8th term states: When a disease is transferring from Taiyang to Yangming, "acupuncture on Yangming, can stop the transferring, and cure the disease", which indicates acupuncture can prevent the deterioration of diseases, and accelerates the healing process. These viewpoints are of great significances.

REFERENCES

[1] Q. X. Zeng, "Analysis of 'Fujue' Term of Golden Chamber Synopsis," *Chinese Journal of Basic Medicine*, Vol. 7, No. 8, 2001, pp. 568-569.

[2]   J. Z. Zhou and X. H. Liu, "Blood-Bi and Cardiovascular
      Diseases," *Chinese Journal of Integrative Medicine on Cardio/
      Cerebrovascular Disease*, Vol. 7, No. 7, 2007, pp. 612-613.

[3]   Z. J. Zhang, "Synopsis of Golden Chamber," Shanghai
      Press of Classics, Shanghai, 2010, pp. 152-154.

Permissions

List of Contributors

Aref Abu-Rabia
Ben-Gurion University of the Negev, Beer-Sheva, Israel

Anshul Shakya and Vikas Kumar
Neuropharmacology Research Laboratory, Department of Pharmaceutical Engineering, Indian Institute of Technology (Banaras Hindu University), Varanasi, India

Shyam Sunder Chatterjee
Stettiner Straße 1, Karlsruhe, Germany

Xiaojun Chen and Xuerui Tan
Department of Cardiovascular Diseases, The First Affiliated Hospital of Shantou University Medical College, Shantou, China

Liping Li and Xiaojun Chen
Injury Prevention Research Center, Shantou University Medical College, Shantou, China

Somya Dulani, Rajesh Dulani, Seema Lele, Sachin Diagavane, Sandeep Anjankar, Netra Jaiswal, Prem S. Subramaniam and Rakesh Juneja
Ophthalmology JNMC DattaMeghe, Institute of Medical Sciences, Wardha, India

Huanhua Lu, Yi'nan Wang, Yiying Song and Jia Liu
State Key Laboratory of Cognitive Neuroscience and Learning, Beijing Normal University, Beijing, China

John Wai-Man Yuen
School of Nursing, The Hong Kong Polytechnic University, Hong Kong, China

Mayur-Danny I. Gohel
Department of Medical Science, Tung Wah College, Hong Kong, China

Chi-Fai Ng
Department of Surgery, The Chinese University of Hong Kong, Hong Kong, China

Xixin Yan, Haibo Xu, Fangfang Qu, Yue Liu and Xiumin Zhang
Department of Respiratory Medicine, The Second Affiliated Hospital, Hebei Medical University, Shijiazhuang, China

Oluwagbemiga Sewanu Soyingbe, Albert Kortze Basson and Andy Rowland Opoku
Department of Biochemistry and Microbiology, University of Zululand, Empangeni, South Africa

Adebola Oyedeji
Department of Chemistry, Walter Sisulu University, Mthatha, South Africa

Xiaojun Chen and Xuerui Tan
Department of Cardiovascular Diseases, The First Affiliated Hospital of Shantou University Medical College, Shantou, China

David Racine
School of Physics, Trinity College, Dublin, Ireland

Anshu Rastogi
Department of Biophysics, Palack University, Olomouc, Czech Republic

Rajendra P. Bajpai
Division of Analytical BioSciences, Leiden University, The Netherlands

Jian-Rong Zhou, Kazumi Yokomizo and Takeshi Miyata
Department of Presymptomatic Medical Pharmacology, Faculty of Pharmaceutical Sciences, Sojo University, Kumamoto, Japan

Mohamed Aly M. Morsy
Department of Pharmacology, Faculty of Medicine, Minia University, Minya, Egypt

Kiyoshi Kunika
Division of Science and Medicine, Institute of International Kampo Co. Ltd., Nihonmatsu, Japan

Muhammad Shakil Ahmad Siddiqui
Rafah-e-Aam Dawakhana Ajmali (Clinics) and Rafah-e-Aam Herbal Laboratories, Karachi, Pakistan

Muhammad Shakil Ahmad Siddiqui, Khan Usmanghani, Ejaz Mohiuddin and Laeequr Rahman Malik
Faculty of Eastern Medicine, Hamdard University, Karachi, Pakistan

F. El Babili and C. Chatelain
Faculté des Sciences Pharmaceutiques, Laboratoire de BOTANIQUE, Toulouse, France

M. El Babili
Université Claude Bernard, Lyon I, Institut Michel Pacha, La Seyne sur Mer, France

I. Fouraste
Faculté des Sciences Pharmaceutiques, Laboratoire de Pharmacognosie, Toulouse, France

Qing Yu, Tatsuo Takahashi and Shinjiro Kobayashi
Department of Clinical Pharmacy, Faculty of Pharmaceutical Sciences, Hokuriku University, 3-Ho Kanagawa-Machi, Kanazawa, Japan

Masaaki Nomura
Department of Education Center of Clinical Pharmacy, Faculty of Pharmaceutical Sciences, Hokuriku University, 3-Ho Kanagawa-Machi, Kanazawa, Japan

Wen-Wan Chao
Department of Nutrition and Health Sciences, School of Healthcare Management, Kainan University, Taipei, Taiwan

Bi-Fong Lin
Department of Biochemical Science and Technology, College of Life Science, National Taiwan University, Taipei, Taiwan

Yau Lam, Cho Wing Sze, Yao Tong and Yanbo Zhang
School of Chinese Medicine, The University of Hong Kong, Hong Kong, China

Tzi Bun Ng
The School of Biomedical Sciences and School of Life Science, The University of Hong Kong, Hong Kong, China

Pang Chui Shaw
The School of Biochemistry and Faculty of Science, The Chinese University of Hong Kong, Hong Kong, China

Jia-Ming Tang, Jiong Liu and Wenbin Wu
Laboratory Animal Center, Shanghai University of Traditional Chinese Medicine, Shanghai, China

José M. Zubeldia, Aarón Hernández-Santana, Miguel Jiménez-del-Rio and Verónica Pérez-López
Polinat S. L. Taibique 4, Polígono Industrial Las Majoreras, Las Palmas, Spain

Rubén Pérez-Machín
Molecular Oncology Group (G-OncoMol) Research Unit, University Hospital of Gran Canaria, Canary Health and Research Foundation Barranco de la Ballena, Las Palmas, Spain

José Manuel García-Castellano
Department of Orthopaedic Surgery, Complejo Hospitalario Universitario Insular, Las Palmas, Spain

Lei Li and To Yau
School of Chinese Medicine, The University of Hong Kong, Hong Kong, China

Chuen-Heung Yau
School of Chinese Medicine, Hong Kong Baptist University, Hong Kong, China

Yan Zhang and Fenxia Gao
The Mental Health Center of Xi'an, Xi'an, China

Yanjun Cao and Hongying Wang
School of Medicine, Xi'an Jiaotong University, Xi'an, China

Haijie Duan
No. 5 Hospital of Xi'an, Xi'an, China

Shaodong Hua and Xiaoying Zhang
Department of Pediatrics, BaYi Children's Hospital of the General Military Hospital of Beijing PLA, Beijing, China
Shengli An
Department of Biostatistics, South Medical University, Guangzhou, China

Xiuxiang Liu
The Hospital Affilicated Binzhou Medicall University, Binzhou, China

Zhichun Feng
Department of Pediatrics, BaYi Children's Hospital of the General Military Hospital of Beijing PLA, Beijing, China

Jiangang Fu, Ling Dai, Zhang Lin and Hongmei Lu
College of Chemistry and Chemical Engineering, Central South University, Changsha, China

Shengyan Xi, Yanhui Wang, Linchao Qian, Xiaoyan Qian, Pengcheng Li and Dawei Lu
Department of Traditional Chinese Medicine of Medical College, Xiamen University, Xiamen, China

Yaochen Chuang
Center of General Education, Central Taiwan University of Science and Technology, Taichung, Taiwan

Hongmei Zhu
Department of Chinese Medicine, Medical School, Xiamen University, Xiamen, China

Minbo Lan, Dongying Lu, Hongli Zhao and Huihui Yuan
Research Center of Analysis & Test and Institute of Advanced Materials, East China University of Science & Technology, Shanghai, China

Zhengyou He
Sichuan Industrial Institute of Antibiotics, Chengdu University, Chengdu, China

Peishan Xie
Macau University of Science and Technology, Macau, China
Guangdong UNION Biochemical Development Co. Ltd., Guangzhou, China

Shuangcheng Ma
National Institute for Food and Drug Control, Beijing, China

Pengfei Tu
Peking University Modern Research Center for Traditional Chinese Medicine, Beijing, China

Zhengtao Wang
Shanghai University of Traditional Chinese Medicine,
Shanghai, China

Erich Stoeger
Plantasia GmbH, Oberndorf, Austria

Daniel Bensky
Independent Scholar, Seattle, USA

Qing Yu, Tatsuo Takahashi, Mai Yasuda and Shinjiro Kobayashi
Department of Clinical Pharmacy, Faculty of Pharmaceutical Sciences, Hokuriku University, Kanazawa, Japan

Masaaki Nomura
Department of Education Center of Clinical Pharmacy, Faculty of Pharmaceutical Sciences, Hokuriku University, Kanazawa, Japan

Kyoko Obatake-Ikeda
Department of Biochemistry, Faculty of Pharmaceutical Sciences, Hokuriku University, Kanazawa, Japan

Chen, Yinmin Le and Jia Wei
Jiangxi University of Traditional Chinese Medicine, Nanchang, China

Yong Chen
Fuda Cancer Hospital, Guangzhou, China

www.ingramcontent.com/pod-product-compliance
Lightning Source LLC
Chambersburg PA
CBHW080517200326
41458CB00012B/4238